TEXTBOOK OF MEDICAL-SURGICAL NURSING

VOLUME 2: ADVANCED SYSTEM-BASED AND SURGICAL NURSING CARE

Michele McCarthy

ALLIED
HEALTH
PRESS

Textbook of Medical-Surgical Nursing

Volume 2: Advanced System-Based and Surgical Nursing Care

Author: **Michele McCarthy**

Allied Health Press
4164 Lakeshore Road
Burlington ON L7L 1A4
Canada
www.alliedhealthpress.com
Email: orders@arclereducation.com

ISBN: 978-1-77956-820-5

ABOUT THE AUTHOR

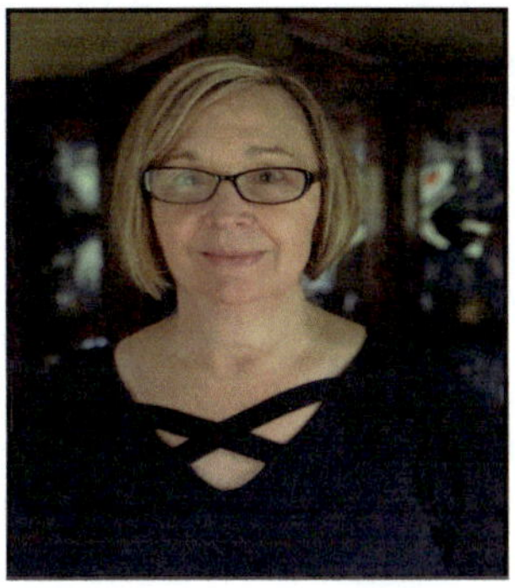

Michele is a registered nurse with over 25 years of clinical experience and a decade of service as a nurse educator. She holds national certifications as a Certified Nurse Educator (CNE) and Certified Healthcare Simulation Educator (CHSE), reflecting her commitment to excellence in teaching and experiential learning. Michele is passionate about advancing nursing education through learner-centered design, curriculum innovation, and the integration of simulation-based strategies.

Brief Table of Contents

Getting Started with This Book

Chapter Openers

A list of Chapter Outline is presented providing a brief Introduction to what will be covered in the chapter.

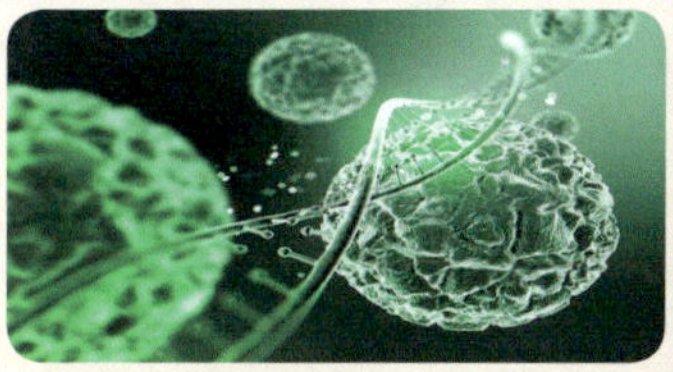

Introduction

Often referred to as the science of life, biology is a broad field of study aimed at comprehending the several kinds of life on Earth, from tiny creatures to sophisticated multicellular entities. Comprising several subfields, including molecular biology, ecology, and evolutionary biology, each of which advances our knowledge of living systems, this field clarifies the mechanisms controlling life events, including development, reproduction, and interaction with the surroundings, which is the central goal of biology. Moreover, biology fills in the void between the natural sciences and medicine by offering a necessary understanding of health, illness, and the interactions between organisms and their environments. Dealing with urgent global issues such as climate change, biodiversity loss, and new diseases depends on an awareness of these complex biological interactions, therefore highlighting the critical part biology plays in modern civilization. Fundamentally, biology explores and tests ideas about the living world using the scientific method. Through methodical observation and experimentation,

LEARNING OBJECTIVES

After studying this chapter, you will be able to:

1. Discuss the scientific method in biology;
2. Explain the cell theory;
3. Discuss the genetics and heredity;
4. Evolution and natural selection;
5. Focus on ecology and ecosystems;
6. Learn about human biology;
7. Evaluate the plant biology;
8. Explain the microbiology;
9. Focus on current trends in biology.

1.1. The Scientific Method in Biology

Learning Outcome

1. Describe the steps of the scientific method;
2. Focus on hypothesis formation;
3. Learn about experimental design.

Learning Outcomes

The beginning of each section of every chapter contains a set of Learning Outcomes that inform students of concepts they should understand. These outcomes help students understand what they should be able to do if they have mastered the material in that section.

Test Your Knowledge

Throughout each chapter, Test Your Knowledge cues you to note which topics have been covered and to self-test your understanding of the material presented.

Test Your Knowledge

1. Explain why correlation does not imply causation in scientific experiments.
2. How does the scientific method help reduce the influence of personal opinions in research?

Chapter Summary

The Summary Section appear at the end of each chapter and summarize main concepts covered throughout the chapter. These points provide key concepts in an engaging and meaningful way.

Summary

The investigation of biological principles highlights the importance of a comprehensive view of life by reflecting the intricate interactions that occur within living systems. The complexity of biology goes beyond individual species or systems, as this essay highlights; it also includes the interactions that mold ecosystems and affect biodiversity. Researchers can conduct in-depth analyses of metabolomic data using sophisticated technologies like MetaboAnalyst, which offer insights into the molecular mechanisms underlying these interactions. As demonstrated by the developments in MetaboAnalyst, for example, the integration of diverse omics data promotes a thorough understanding of metabolic pathways and helps identify important biological markers necessary for research on development and disease (Chong et al., 2018). Additionally, the phenomenon of ecological invasions is a key component of biological research and a vital field of study. The introduction of non-native species into unfamiliar habitats has significant ramifications and calls for multidisciplinary management strategies. Examining the origins and effects of these biological incursions, invasion science has become a crucial field that highlights the need to comprehend ecological dynamics and community interactions. As interest in biological invasions increases, new findings are emerging that put conventional ecological theories and practices to the test. The importance of incorporating various scientific viewpoints is shown by this developing discipline, which also highlights how invasive species shape ecosystems and advances our knowledge of ecological resilience (David et al., 2013). When taken as a whole, these discoveries from invasion science and metabolomics highlight the value of multidisciplinary biology research. Fostering cross-disciplinary collaboration and utilizing technological breakthroughs to improve our comprehension of intricate biological interactions are crucial as we look to the future of biological research. In addition to deepening our understanding of the complexities of life, this method lays the groundwork for tackling urgent environmental issues. Future studies can ensure the continued relevance of biology in a world that is constantly changing by acknowledging the interconnection of biological systems and opening the door to creative solutions that support sustainability and biodiversity conservation. We might imagine a thorough comprehension of life that serves both academia and society at large through ongoing investigation and integration of scientific knowledge.

Knowledge Assessment

The chapter includes material designed to review and reinforce each content. It includes Critical Thinking Questions to help test of your understanding of information presented in the chapter and Short answer Questions to review your understanding of the key concepts presented in the chapter.

Critical Thinking Questions

1. **Who is known as the "Father of Modern Biology"?**
   a. Aristotle
   b. Charles Darwin
   c. Gregor Mendel
   d. Louis Pasteur
2. **What is the basic unit of life?**
   a. Atom
   b. Molecule
   c. Cell
   d. Organism
3. **Which branch of biology studies the interaction of organisms with their environment?**
   a. Genetics
   b. Ecology
   c. Physiology
   d. Botany
4. **Which macromolecule is the main source of energy for living organisms?**
   a. Proteins
   b. Lipids
   c. Carbohydrates
   d. Nucleic acids
5. **DNA is primarily responsible for which function in living organisms?**
   a. Energy production
   b. Protein synthesis
   c. Storing genetic information
   d. Regulating body temperature

Short Answer Questions

1. What is biology, and why is it important to study biology?
2. What are the three main domains of life, and how are they different from one another?
3. Define homeostasis and give an example of how it works in living organisms.
4. What is the cell theory, and why is it fundamental to biology?
5. How do autotrophs and heterotrophs differ in the way they obtain energy?
6. What is the scientific method, and how is it applied in biological research?
7. Discuss how biology helps address global challenges such as climate change, disease, and food security.
8. Explain the levels of biological organization from the smallest unit to the largest. Provide examples at each level.
9. Describe the relationship between structure and function in biology, giving specific examples from cells or organs.
10. How has the discovery of genetics shaped our understanding of inheritance and variation among organisms?

Supplementary Materials

Key Terms: A list of key terms is given for quick reference

KEY TERMS FROM THIS CHAPTER

Annotation enrichment analysis	Biological structure	Cell
Cell theory	Cellular structure	Ecology
Ecosystems	Genetics	Human biology
Microbiology	Natural selection	Organism
Plant biology		

Further Resources: Recommendations for additional readings, websites, and multimedia resources.

References

1. Argelaguet, R., Velten, B., Arnol, D., Dietrich, S., Zenz, T., Marioni, J. C., Buettner, F., et al. (2018). Multi-omics factor analysis—A framework for unsupervised integration of multi-omics data sets. *Molecular Systems Biology, 14*. https://doi.org/10.15252/msb.20178124.
2. Bacher, S., Blackburn, T. M., Essl, F., & Genovesi, P. (2017). *Socio-Economic Impact Classification of Alien Taxa (SEICAT)*. https://core.ac.uk/download/286567949.pdf (accessed on 8th March 2025).
3. Barnett, R., Brace, S., Cucchi, T., & Dobney, K. (2013). *Divergent Evolutionary Processes Associated with Colonization of Offshore Islands*. https://core.ac.uk/download/20664364.pdf (accessed on 8th March 2025).

Detailed Table of Contents

CHAPTER 9

Endocrine Disorders and Diabetes Management for Nursing 269

CHAPTER 10

Renal and Urinary Tract Function: Assessment and Interventions 303

LIST OF FIGURES

PREFACE

Medical-surgical nursing is a vital discipline in clinical practice, where technical competence and theoretical expertise converge to promote patient recovery and enhance quality of life. Medical-surgical nursing spans a wide range of physiological systems and clinical conditions, and therefore, providers need to remain vigilant, critical, and reactive. From managing acute medical illnesses to leading patients through chronic illness and recovery post-operation, medical-surgical nursing is the foundation of hospital-based practice. It requires scientific expertise in human anatomy and physiology, as well as a humanitarian approach to personalized care. The dynamic nature of patients' needs, the evolution of treatment methods, and the nature of health issues in modern medicine have only increased the significance and relevance of this science.

As the population grows older and the burden of chronic disease escalates, new demands are being placed on medical-surgical nurses as never before. They often are the patient's first point of contact for serious health interventions—whether it is managing pain in palliative care, closely monitoring critical respiratory function, or guiding perioperative transitions. Their function extends beyond bed care to include patient education, case management with multidisciplinary teams, adherence to safety measures, and documentation. As technology improves and clinical guidelines evolve, continuous learning is no longer optional. High-quality educational resources are essential for equipping nurses with the necessary knowledge and skills to meet these needs and deliver evidence-based, ethical, and patient-centered care.

The *Textbook of Medical-Surgical Nursing – Volume 2* is specifically designed to support learners, educators, and practicing nurses with an overt, systematic, and comprehensive source of information on key subjects core to clinical nursing practice. Volume 2 further develops foundational skills from the past and diverges into system-based chapters that make unequivocal decisions about assessment, intervention, and condition-specific management. The textbook chapters are carefully designed to synthesize theoretical knowledge with clinical judgment and bedside practice. Case-based learning, diagrams, and practical models are incorporated throughout to ease understanding and assist recall. Language is rendered concise and straightforward to enable various types of learners, and clinical accuracy has been ensured by reference to up-to-date guidelines and peer-reviewed literature.

Chapter 1 presents the principles and concepts of palliative and end-of-life nursing care. In this chapter, the importance of symptom management, patient comfort, ethical decision-making, and psychosocial support for families and patients in the terminal phases of life is discussed.

Pain control, communication strategies, and interdisciplinary coordination are also presented in this chapter to guide humane care.

Chapter 2 describes perioperative nursing care, including the entire surgical procedure from preoperative preparation to intraoperative care and postoperative recovery. It addresses patient assessment, surgical asepsis, anesthetic issues, pain control measures, and prevention of complications. Chapter 2 aims to equip nurses with the skills to provide supportive and safe care during the surgical process.

Chapter 3 addresses respiratory function and care for pulmonary disorders. It includes physical and diagnostic assessment of lung function procedures, respiratory support technologies, and nursing interventions for pneumonia, COPD, asthma, and acute respiratory failure. There is a focus on early identification of respiratory distress and coordination of critical care.

Chapter 4 covers cardiovascular care, including management and assessment of arrhythmias, vascular disorders, and coronary disease. It covers electrocardiogram interpretation, hemodynamic monitoring, drug therapy, and nursing care of myocardial infarction, hypertension, and heart failure.

Chapter 5 covers the hematologic system, including regular blood function and the most common disorders. It is comprised of assessment of hematologic status, blood transfusion orders, and nursing care of conditions such as anemia, clotting disorders, and hematologic neoplasms.

Chapter 6 covers immune system disease and allergic reactions. It explains autoimmune diseases, hypersensitivity reactions, immunodeficiency disorders, and methods of regulating acute and chronic immune responses. Immunotherapy and nursing care of patients receiving immune-modulating therapy are also explained in the chapter.

Chapter 7 provides an in-depth examination of the musculoskeletal system, highlighting assessment techniques, trauma and injury detection, and the management of trauma. It discusses fractures, joint dislocations, soft tissue injuries, and posttraumatic rehabilitation theory. Patient mobility, pain control, and complication prevention are highlighted throughout.

Chapter 8 is GI system-oriented and covers information about upper and lower GI tract disorders. Information includes assessment tools, nutritional requirements, pharmacologic and surgical management, and the nurse's role in the treatment of conditions such as GERD, peptic ulcers, inflammatory bowel disease, and gastrointestinal bleeding.

Chapter 9 is dedicated to endocrine disorders, namely diabetes mellitus. It explains endocrine physiology, hormone regulation, diagnostic tests, and nursing implications of management of conditions such as hypothyroidism, hyperthyroidism, adrenal disorders, and type 1 and type 2 diabetes.

Chapter 10 addresses renal and urinary tract function, with a focus on current disorders, assessment strategies, and interventions by nurses. The discussion includes acute kidney injury, chronic kidney disease, urinary tract infection, dialysis, and fluid-electrolyte balance. The chapter is centered on early detection and comprehensive patient monitoring.

Chapter 11 addresses reproductive health, adopting a gender-sensitive approach to assessment and treatment. It deals with the normal status of the reproductive system, family planning care, reproductive system disorders, and practice care that considers patients' various identities and health needs on either side of the gender divide.

Chapter 12 ends with an overview of sensory and integumentary function. It includes assessment and management of wounds, prevention of pressure injuries, infections of the skin and burn, and sensory impairments like vision and hearing impairments. Nursing interventions that enhance sensory compensation and skin integrity are also discussed.

This book is designed for nursing students in diploma, undergraduate, or bridging programs, as well as nurse educators who design curricula and teach hospital-based or community-based clinical practice. Practicing nurses, particularly those working in general medical-surgical settings, perioperative areas, or critical care units, will find this book helpful as a resource for continuing professional development and at-the-bedside reference. It offers material for preparation for examinations, clinical decision-making, and patient safety programs. It encourages critical evaluation, reflection, and evidence-based practice to enhance the confidence and competence of healthcare professionals. Whether in a clinical setting, classroom, or simulation suite, this book is a trusted source of information and guidance for professionals dedicated to delivering high-quality patient care.

PALLIATIVE AND END-OF-LIFE NURSING CARE

1

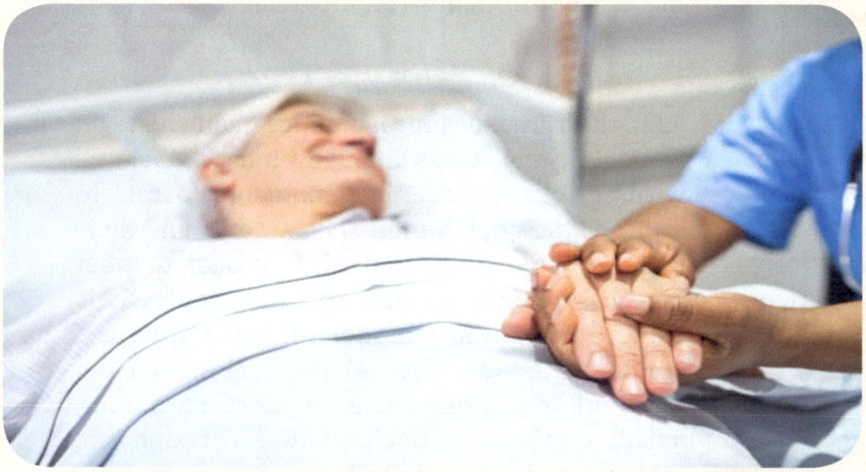

LEARNING OBJECTIVES

After studying this chapter, you will be able to:

1. Understand the historical context of palliative care
2. Explain the principles of palliative care
3. Discuss the pain management in palliative care
4. Focus on communication skills in end-of-life care
5. Learn about ethical considerations in palliative care
6. Evaluate the challenges faced by palliative care nurses

Introduction

The palliative and end-of-life nursing practice principle is an integrated approach to addressing the complex needs of patients nearing the end of life. As part of a fully operational healthcare system, effective palliative care aims to optimize the quality of life for patients and their families in critical situations. This refers not only to the control of physical symptoms but also to the provision of emotional, social, and spiritual care tailored to individual patient needs. It is of utmost importance to identify patients' wishes; most prefer dying at home, thus there is a need for special services that can honor their wishes and preserve dignity and comfort in the terminal stages of life. Therefore, research into innovative palliative care models, including hospice at home teams, is unavoidable in bridging patient preferences and accessible healthcare (Cartwright et al., 2008). Moreover, interdisciplinary collaboration plays an essential role in proper palliative and end-of-life care in enhancing the ability of healthcare workers dealing with patient care. Educational curricula, such as cross-faculty courses, enable health students to acquire essential competencies, providing them with firsthand exposure to palliative care settings. Through these educational processes, learners are empowered to engage with patients and families, leading to a more effective understanding and communication of sensitive issues. For instance, learning experiences from firsthand observation of patient contacts can have a lasting impact on future practice, shaping compassionate and empathetic health professionals. This emphasis on interdisciplinary teamwork not only encourages collaboration among different healthcare practitioners but also facilitates a more integrated approach to patient care during these life-defining moments (Breakwell et al., 2012). In total, palliative and end-of-life nursing care is an essential component of healthcare that requires a sensitive awareness of patient needs, interdisciplinary communication, and effective educational processes.

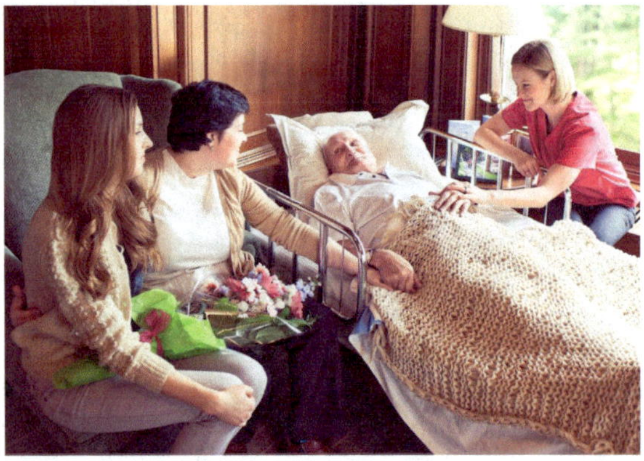

Figure 1.1. Palliative care.

Source: https://www.nursenextdoor.com.au/wp-content/uploads/2022/03/Palliative-Client-at-Home-with-Home-Care-Nurse-and-Family-1024x724.jpg.

As the medical environment continues to evolve, the imperative to equip healthcare workers with the expertise and skills they need to provide sensitive end-of-life care cannot be overstated. The implementation of innovative models and learning approaches provides opportunities to enrich the lives of both practitioners and patients. Through alignment with patient desires, interdisciplinary methods, and optimization of learning environments, palliative care practice can more effectively address the needs of patients with terminal disease, ultimately fulfilling the highest goal of maintaining dignity and quality of life within the context of death (Figure 1.1).

Definition of Palliative Care

Palliative care is a clinical practice that focuses on alleviating the stress and symptoms associated with serious diseases. Its main purpose is to improve the quality of life for patients and their families, employing a holistic approach to meet physical, emotional, and spiritual needs. It is a multidisciplinary model that demands the collaboration of medical professionals from different specialties, including doctors, nurses, social workers, and chaplains. Through the integration of services tailored to the particular patient, palliative care transcends routine curative care, prioritizing comfort and care amidst critical health challenges. Palliative care has been particularly dramatically developed in pediatric patients, where the wishes and needs of children with life-limiting conditions require compassionate and integrated care of both the patients and their families (Craft et al., 2013). One key element of palliative care is its flexibility in meeting the unique needs of patients with different life-limiting illnesses. This is manifested by the care strategy employed across various environments, ranging from in-hospital to outpatient environments, as well as in-home care environments. Palliative care can be initiated at any stage in the illness course, aligning with the patient's treatment goals and wishes. For instance, in the situation of care in dementia, the inclusion of spirituality care is vital in the overall well-being and health of patients approaching the end of life. A study found that spiritual care communication had a significant impact on the provision of comprehensive end-of-life care, highlighting the need to address spiritual needs alongside physical and emotional needs (Deliens et al., 2014). This multifaceted strategy is key to the delivery of well-rounded and individualized care for patients. Furthermore, in addition to alleviating current symptoms, palliative care encompasses long-term strategies for advance planning and anticipating future healthcare needs. Ongoing evaluations and honest communication among healthcare professionals and families facilitate decision-making between both groups, allowing patients to have an active role in their care planning. Family dynamics are particularly highlighted, as families often provide basic care and their services are crucial in ensuring patients' comfort and dignity. As the model of palliative care is continually developing, it further underscores the way spiritual and emotional care may be integrated into the care systems, which would ultimately provide an environment that is conducive to healing, acceptance, and peacefulness in life's darkest times (Craft et al., 2013; Deliens et al., 2014).

Importance of End-of-Life Care

The relevance of end-of-life care extends beyond symptom relief, encompassing a process that considers the social, emotional, and spiritual needs of the dying patient. As life nears its completion, the focus shifts from curative therapies to enhancing the quality of life. Palliative care bridges the gap by providing extensive support that is not merely medical in nature but also psychological and spiritual. By appreciating the complexity of the dying experience, it is possible for health professionals to better respond to patient-tailored preferences and cultural environments, thereby providing a more respectful and dignified end-of-life experience. This paradigm shift emphasizes the incorporation of such care as an integral part of everyday practice, as it indicates the substantial impact that effective end-of-life care has on patients' satisfaction and family well-being. The palliative care management of patients with illnesses such as dementia highlights specific challenges that must be addressed through the identification of effective end-of-life interventions. According to studies, almost 100,000 dementia sufferers die each year in the UK alone. Yet, many do not receive access to the services of palliative care that would directly assist their comfort and dignity of life during this critical period (Birch et al., 2008). Late-stage dementia patients usually possess specific needs that complicate the progression of their care; difficulties such as prognostication and communication deficits may hinder early availability to appropriate interventions. It has become increasingly apparent that enhancing end-of-life care in dementia involves overcoming these barriers, so a call has been made for quality to be urgently improved in palliative care and for more studies to be carried out to tailor resources for this vulnerable population better. Furthermore, spirituality emerges as an essential component of effective end-of-life care, transcending standard medical interventions to address deeper emotional and existential concerns of the patients and their families. More recent studies have demonstrated a growing recognition of the healthcare role of spirituality, highlighting the shift toward an understanding that incorporates historical and cultural context (Ascarya et al., 2016). By integrating spiritual care into models of palliative care, clinicians can provide a more comprehensive and respectful approach that honors individual beliefs and values. This addition to care not only supports the patient but also creates a soothing environment for families, ultimately improving overall end-of-life care. With the advancement of the discipline, integration of spiritual elements will be instrumental in evolving the optimum practice in end-of-life care so that it meets the diverse needs of patients undergoing this profound transition in life (Figure 1.2).

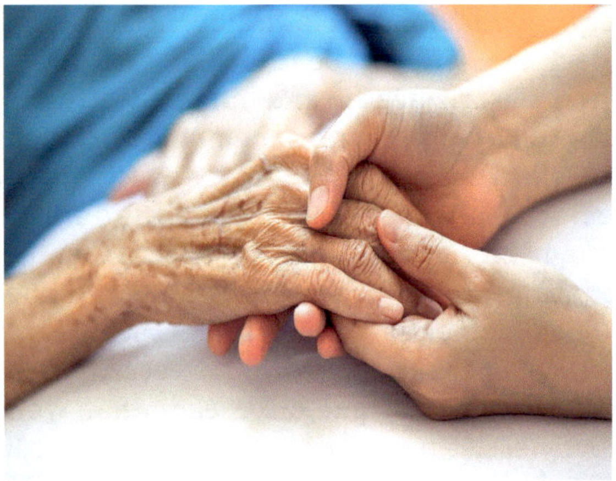

Figure 1.2. End-of-life nursing care.

Source: https://www.harwoodhouse.co.uk/wordpress/wp-content/uploads/End-of-Life-Care-2000x1200-1.jpg.

1.1. Historical Context of Palliative Care

Learning Outcome

1. Describe the evolution of palliative care practices
2. Focus on the development of palliative care
3. Learn about legislation and policies influencing palliative care

The background of palliative care reveals a gradual evolution that was primarily influenced by the societal attitudes towards dying and death. Death for societies in the past was often perceived as a normal process and not as a time to fear or postpone. Such societal consciousness of mortality provided the basis for communal practice with the same objective of comforting the dying. With the advent of modern medicine in the 19th century, the focus shifted towards a more technological and curative direction, generally relegating the emotional and spiritual needs of the patients to the background. This shift paved the way for the introduction of palliative care as a vital intervention, reflecting the importance of not only healing bodily pain but also psychological and spiritual dimensions of dying as well. As palliative care evolved, it incorporated more holistic practices, an increasing acknowledgment of the multidimensionality of end-of-life experiences. During the mid-20th century, innovators such as Cicely Saunders pioneered the development of hospice care, marking a turning point in palliative care. Saunders emphasized the need to emphasize quality of life, trying to provide a humane setting that preserved the dignity of patients during their final days. This movement resonated very much into broader societal changes, particularly as cultural perspectives regarding death transitioned from traditional conceptions to more individualized ideas about the process of dying. As a result, the principles of palliative care began to take form, creating systems that incorporated interdisciplinary symptom control and emotional support. The inclusion of spiritual care also became increasingly significant, recognizing the intangible spiritual realms that pervade terminal illness. This context sets the stage for contemporary palliative care, which is now attempting to address the integrative needs of patients and their families. As scholarship and debate within the field of palliative care expand, a growing interest in the historical and cultural contexts that shape spiritual beliefs and practices at the end of life emerges. Research indicates that spirituality can only be fully understood by analyzing its historical roots and cultural foundations, which reveal different perceptions of mortality and the afterlife. Critical reviews point out that much of the current literature, in fact, overlooks such contextual aspects, though, and focuses on individualistic spirituality strategies in healthcare. Considering how cultural frameworks may influence patients' and families' experiences can enhance the provision of care that is spiritually attuned. By recognizing the history of trajectories for spirituality as it relates to palliative care, practitioners can enhance approaches for patient care and facilitate their end-of-life experiences. Recognizing the growth in awareness of spirituality emphasizes the urgent need for integrating such an understanding into clinical practice, thereby providing holistic palliative care that is sensitive to the richness of human life (Inbadas et al., 2016, 2017) (Figure 1.3).

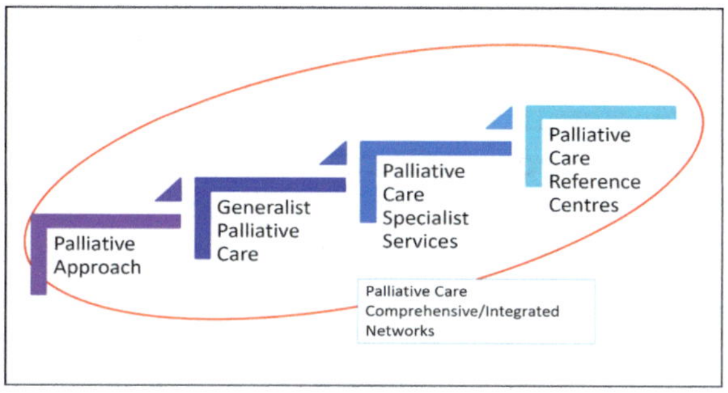

Figure 1.3. Development of palliative care.

Source: https://media.springernature.com/lw685/springer-static/image/chp%3A10.1007%2F978-3-319-77740-5_2/MediaObjects/333544_1_En_2_Fig1_HTML.png.

1.1.1. Evolution of Palliative Care Practices

The evolution of palliative care practice is a reaction to a growing recognition of the multidimensional needs of patients with life-threatening illnesses. In the past decades, palliative care has grown from being a specialty field primarily dealing with pain management into an integrated, holistic model of treating the multifaceted nature of suffering—physical, emotional, and spiritual. This movement has occurred alongside broader dispositions towards change in society, including heightened awareness of patient rights and quality of life in terminal care. New research attests to the value of incorporating spiritual care into palliative practice, but the majority of studies tend to overlook the historical and cultural forces that shape people's conceptions of spirituality in terminal contexts. The difference in contextual study reinforces the value of embedding cultural sensitivity into practice, thus revolutionizing the palliative care model into an open-ended discipline that resonates with varying patient needs (Inbadas et al., 2016). Moreover, the expansion of interdisciplinary teams has played a crucial role in advancing palliative care practice. The contemporary model increasingly emphasizes collaboration between health professionals, including physicians, nurses, social workers, and chaplains. This collaboration has enhanced the delivery of holistic care that addresses not only clinical symptoms but also psychosocial issues. Research funded by organizations like the Robert Wood Johnson Foundation has, to a considerable degree, influenced the development of end-of-life care strategies through the stressing of the need for goal-congruent care and policy change that is congruent with patient-centered care. With the integration of communication and evaluation practices, the art of palliative care continues to evolve, ensuring that it reflects the ethical obligations of healthcare providers to deliver humane and holistic care to patients and their families facing the challenges of severe illness (Spector et al., 2011). The future of palliative care practice is headed in the direction of mounting inclusion of personalized, culturally sensitive care that speaks to patients' individual experiences and values. As the field advances, the focus on understanding the historical and cultural contexts of spirituality becomes increasingly stronger. This strategy not only enhances the depth of knowledge about patient needs but also enhances the efficacy of spiritual care in the clinical environment. Through the identification of convergence between cultural beliefs and palliative care, the latter can better tailor their interventions to address patients' diverse values and beliefs. Ultimately, such a change indicates a shift in paradigm towards a patient-centric model that perceives the key role of contextual elements in ensuring comprehensive palliative care, so practices are as effective and inclusive as possible (Inbadas et al., 2016).

1.1.2. Key Figures in the Development of Palliative Care

Palliative care's emergence is primarily due to visionary thinkers who have worked tirelessly to ensure that the validation of holistic approaches to caring for dying patients has become a reality. Preeminently, Dame Cicely Saunders, the initiator of the modern hospice movement, was responsible for focusing attention not just on relieving the physical aspects of suffering but also addressing the emotional, spiritual, and psychosocial issues of patients. Her establishment of St. Christophers Hospice in London in 1967 was a radical shift towards how healthcare professionals attend to end-of-life care. Saunders' pioneering work set the path for subsequent innovation, based on the tenet that dying people have a right to dignity, respect, and integrated care. The model has remained influential for palliative care practice up to date, and as such it is vital to recognize her work in demystifying death and dying. Additionally, the contributions of Elizabeth Kubler-Ross to palliative care are invaluable. Her groundbreaking work, encapsulated in her book On Death and Dying, offered a model of the five stages of mourning, thereby presenting a psychological understanding of dying. Kubler-Ross not only drew focus to the affective processes of terminal patients but also summoned clinicians to discuss with patients and families regarding their fear of death and what they want. Her appeals for change ushered in a paradigm shift among healthcare professionals such that they now emphasize open communication and emotional support as integral aspects of palliative care. Palliative care has come a long way in integrating mental health considerations into palliative care, enhancing overall quality of life for people with serious illnesses. Additionally, the contemporary face of palliative care is characterized by academic advancements and an increased provision of education for healthcare professionals. Organizations such as the National Cancer Institute have been instrumental in educating practitioners in palliative care, as evidenced by programs like the two-day workshop specifically designed for Doctor of Nursing Practice (DNP) faculty and clinicians. The training focused on integrating the best palliative care practices into nursing curricula, the need for skilled practitioners in response to the growing number of aging populations, and the challenges posed by increasingly complex healthcare needs. By providing nursing professionals with critical knowledge and skills in palliative care, the quality of end-of-life nursing practice can be significantly enhanced, highlighting the crucial role played by education in the development of palliative care. More significant development is still needed, as highlighted by the challenges of incorporating adequate palliative care into nursing practice and education, issues that must be addressed systematically to meet the demands of an evolving healthcare landscape (Breakwell et al., 2018; Murray et al., 2013).

1.1.3. Legislation and Policies Influencing Palliative Care

Legislation and policy are at the forefront of developing the frameworks under which palliative care is delivered, ensuring that the ethical needs and functional demands of patients are met. Effective legislation requires that palliative care be an integral part of health systems, promoting quality and accessible care for individuals with serious illnesses. For instance, policies in integrated care models are crucial for addressing the fragmentation commonly observed in healthcare delivery. Integrated models (Veras et al., 2018) argues, that not only ensure proper communication among health providers but also ensure continuity of care, leading to improved patient outcomes. By establishing specific policy and funding pathways, legislation can help enhance the quality and accessibility of palliative care service provision among diverse population groups, particularly in vulnerable groups such as the elderly, who can have particular needs. Policies on advance care planning (ACP) further demonstrate how legislation can enhance the effectiveness of palliative care by encouraging patients and their families to have advance conversations about the patients' values and preferences for end-of-life care. Research has indicated that while attitudes are favorable towards ACP, translating them into practice remains challenging (Jiménez et al., 2018). Legislative support for ACP models has the potential to enhance communication between patients and clinical staff, fostering an environment where patients feel motivated to express their wishes. Incorporating elements such as decision aids and interactive dialogue into ACP programs enables policy to provide a more patient-centered approach to care. This not only improves care preference recording but also to treatment more consistent with patients' values and thus to overall palliative care quality. As healthcare continues to evolve, the constant reevaluation and fine-tuning of palliative care policies remain essential in addressing the needs of increasingly diverse populations. Policy-makers must consider cultural and contextual factors that influence the uptake and effectiveness of palliative care programs. For example, differences in societal views on dying and death have a significant impact on the adoption of ACP and palliative care services (Jiménez et al., 2018). With active collaboration with the communities and familiarity with their unique concerns, the legislators can formulate targeted interventions that appeal to those they are targeting. This adaptive approach ensures that legislative action is not only intellectually pleasing but also actually attainable, ultimately improving the efficacy and scope of palliative care initiatives in various settings (Figure 1.4).

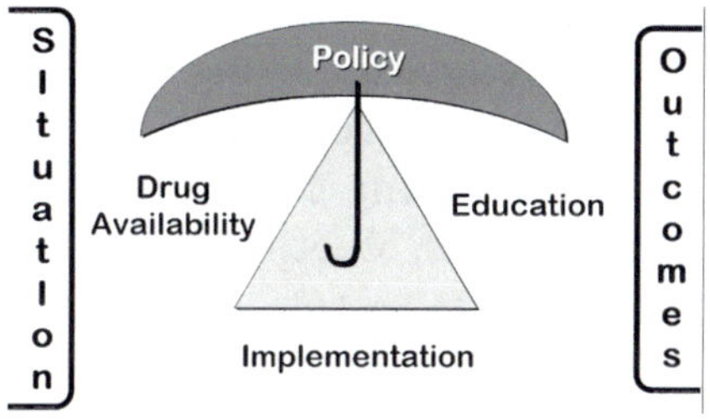

Figure 1.4. Palliative care in public policy.

Source: https://www.liebertpub.com/cms/10.1089/pmr.2020.0062/asset/images/pmr.2020.0062_figure1.jpg.

Test Your Knowledge

1. What is the primary goal of palliative care?
2. How does palliative care differ from curative treatment?

1.2. Principles of Palliative Care

Learning Outcome

1. Explain the holistic approach to patient care
2. Define the quality of life in patient care
3. Discuss the interdisciplinary team collaboration of palliative and end-of-life care

The palliative care guidelines are based on a philosophy of care centered on the quality of life for individuals with serious illnesses. The care model aims to reduce suffering by maximizing symptom control, providing psychosocial support, and facilitating communication about treatment intentions. Meeting the patient's and caregiver's physical, emotional, and spiritual needs will enable healthcare providers to establish an environment for healing that respects the dignity of both the patient and caregiver. The American Thoracic Society's push for the early integration of palliative care is indicative of the importance of early intervention in achieving improved overall patient outcomes. The policy statement by Theirs underscores the importance of developing delivery models that prioritize palliative interventions, which work to turn the use from solely curative interventions towards more balanced patient-centered care (Campbell et al., 2022). Advance care planning or talking about patients' preference for treatment and end-of-life care, is a central component of palliative care. Effective communication between healthcare providers, patients, and their families is crucial in ensuring that treatment and care align with the patient's values and expectations. Through this conversation, nurses help patients make sense of complex decisions so that they are more in control and less distressed. The inclusion of palliative care principles in nursing education also underscores the role of APRNs as key players in delivering this type of care. A study the growing recognition of education for palliative care for the next generation of healthcare leaders (Breakwell et al., 2018). Additionally, the principles of palliative care promote widespread caregiver support, recognizing the critical role family members play in the caregiving process. Caregivers experience significant stress and emotional toll during the care of a loved one with a terminal illness.

Through providing resources and respite care, medical staff can alleviate the burden, enhancing both the caregiver and patient experience. Reduction of health disparities is also an essential component of palliative care, as inequalities in access to treatment can significantly impact patient outcomes. Therefore, an integrative approach that includes community intervention and policy advocacy is crucial for making palliative care services accessible and equitable. By translating these principles into the care continuum, the healthcare system can better address the multifaceted needs of patients and their families throughout the trajectory of a serious illness (Campbell et al., 2022) (Figure 1.5).

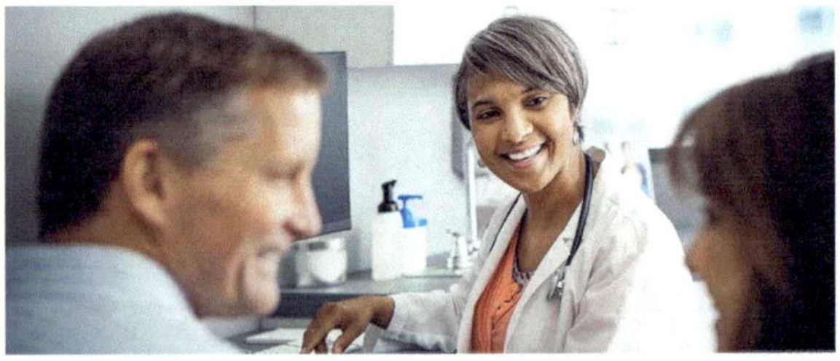

Figure 1.5. Advanced practice registered nurse (APRN).

Source: https://nursinglicensemap.com/wp-content/uploads/sites/62/2022/05/Advanced-Practice-Registered-Nurse.jpg.

1.2.1. Holistic Approach to Patient Care

Whole-person care is of utmost significance during end-of-life and palliative care, wherein patients' needs are not only physical but also social, emotional, and spiritual. The holistic technique encourages nurses to view the patient as a whole being, rather than a collection of symptoms or diagnoses. By engaging with patients and patient families, nurse personnel are able to build an empathic relationship founded on understanding, creating a partnership atmosphere where the patient is respected and valued. This approach fosters a culture of trust and honesty, enabling interventions to be tailored on a personal basis to the specific needs and desires of individual patients, particularly in long-term care settings where the complexity of health issues can make treatment plans and emotional status challenging (Chang et al., 2024). The incorporation of dietary dimensions in a holistic framework further enhances the quality of palliative care, addressing patients' nutritional needs during the complex phases of their condition. Since the majority of patients are seen with more than one life-limiting disease, control of diet becomes more complicated and essential. Nurses play a central role in identifying and addressing diet-related complexities that may arise, providing patients with optimal nutritional care tailored to their prognosis and stage of care. Assessment and screening instruments can facilitate well-educated and compassionate consultations about nutrition between families, patients, and healthcare providers. By categorizing dietary needs within the framework of the holistic model of care, nurses play a critical part in improving patients' comfort and quality of life while they are in palliative settings (Holdoway, 2022). Secondly, an integrated approach demands that nursing staff include interprofessional collaboration to formulate a more collaborative care plan that addresses all factors of a patient's journey. Collaboration with other healthcare practitioners, such as dietitians, social workers, and spiritual care workers, enables the development of an interdisciplinary plan of care that addresses the complex needs of patients and their relatives. By an embracing team-oriented approach, nurses can share relevant knowledge, experience, and skills that optimize patient care. In the long run, this comprehensive model not only enhances outcomes of better health but also maintains the dignity and autonomy of patients as they face terminal difficulties. This commitment to whole-person care embodies the palliative nursing spirit as a respected profession dedicated to enhancing the health and well-being of patients nearing the end of life and fostering meaningful relationships during their most vulnerable times.

1.2.2. Focus on Quality of Life

In palliative and end-of-life care nursing, it is essential to emphasize that the absolute priority must be maximizing quality of life. Palliative care is not only a technique for symptomatic relief from severe, life-limiting illnesses but also for enhancing general well-being, as exemplified by research indicating that formalized palliative interventions can lead to enhanced patient satisfaction and emotional support from loved ones. A systematic review showed that when nurses receive specialized training in palliative care, significant improvements can be observed in the nurses' skills and the quality of care provided, ultimately benefiting patients directly. In this sense, it is essential for nursing programs to incorporate palliative care education, enabling nurses to effectively address the holistic, multidimensional needs of patients nearing the end of their lives (Mohanty et al., 2025). End-of-life quality of care is particularly significant in chronic disease patients, such as those with chronic obstructive pulmonary disease (COPD). With the patients experiencing the debilitating effects of the diseases, there is a need to adopt an all-rounded care approach that addresses not only the physical but also psychosocial and spiritual aspects of patients and caregivers lives. Research examining patients' and families' perspectives has identified chief unmet needs, among which are the need for immediate and accurate communication about changing health status and end-of-life desires. Thus, an improvement in the quality of life for these patients involves not just cutting-edge medical interventions but also the implementation of supportive interventions, such as cognitive-behavioral therapy techniques and exercise protocols. That enhances physical functioning as well as emotional well-being (Johnston et al., 2017). The multifaceted approach of palliative care aims to maximize quality of life by facilitating dignified discussions, empowering patients, and fostering collaboration among healthcare providers, patients, and their families. Palliative care teams must be able to manage the complex emotions that arise from end-of-life discussions, where patients and their families are listened to and validated. The application of caregiving's technological advancements—such as telehealth care—can also enhance this care provision and interaction, improving the accessibility of information and support. Lastly, an unwavering focus on end-of-life quality in palliative care nursing not only relieves suffering, but also honors patients' dignity and desires at the end of life, because according to their own values and making their experience as a whole a better one (Johnston et al., 2017; Mohanty et al., 2025) (Figure 1.6).

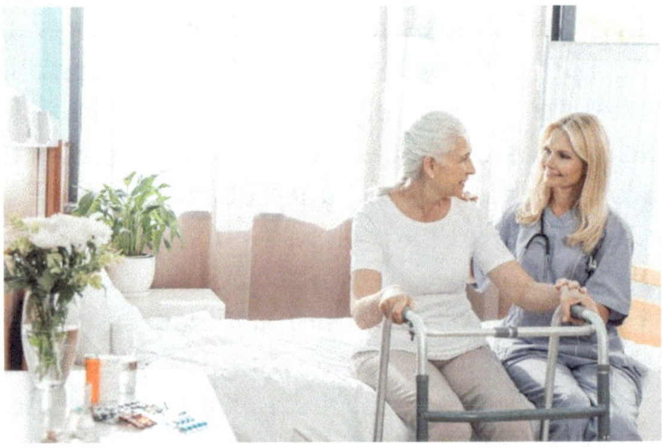

Figure 1.6. Nurses provide emotional support for patients.

Source: https://theresiliencysolution.com/wp-content/uploads/2021/02/care-givers-offer-support-to-patients-768x513.jpg.

1.2.3. Interdisciplinary Team Collaboration

Interdisciplinary teamwork is a crucial element in improving the quality of end-of-life and palliative care. The coordination of multiple healthcare professionals—such as nurses, doctors, social workers, and chaplains—permits a holistic approach to patient care that encompasses physical, emotional, spiritual, and social concerns. Successful collaboration ensures shared decision-making, resulting in patient-centered and family-valued integrated interventions. With an increasingly diverse patient mix presenting with high-complex needs, the roles of interdisciplinary teams are more important. As a combined effort, teams can also utilize their combined expertise by pooling different knowledge sets, which will ultimately result in improved outcomes and patient satisfaction. There is strong evidence testifying to the benefits of interdisciplinary collaboration in palliative care settings. Studies have shown that collaborative practice leads to improved patient outcomes and a more positive experience for the healthcare team. Studies, for instance, specify the functions of inter-team communication and formalized referral procedures in allowing timely care streams for patients with imminent end-of-life care requirements. Clinicians who participated in qualitative studies mentioned smooth collaboration through verbal handovers and a harmonious approach to managing patients and their families. However, indicators of a failure to prioritize and an inclination towards avoiding palliative care discussions at formal multidisciplinary team meetings point to potential areas for improvement. Addressing these issues will enable the health system to better manage patient care complexity and ensure that teams work in concert, thereby optimizing the palliative experience. The educational program on which interdisciplinary teamwork is based is also essential, particularly for medical students who are entering the field.

Participating in multidisciplinary studies not only introduces upcoming professionals to a general overview of palliative care principles, but it also imposes teamwork within practice in delivering effective care. For instance, students who participated in clinical observation exercises within interdisciplinary environments documented that they gained an appreciation of team member communication dynamics, as well as patient and family emotional cues. Acquiring the skill relationships best prepares students to be effective members of streamlined care teams. With the escalating demand for expert palliative care professionals, continuing emphasis on interprofessional collaboration in curricula for teaching will ensure that future healthcare professionals can engage synergistically in the multifaceted needs of dying patients (Breakwell et al., 2012; Borgstrom et al., 2024) (Figure 1.7).

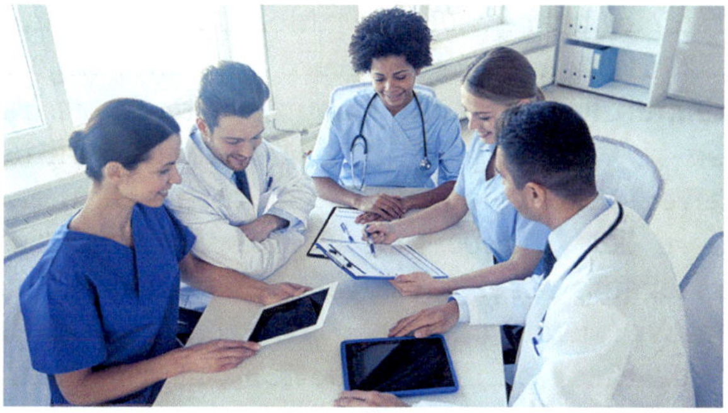

Figure 1.7. Interdisciplinary team collaboration for surgical nursing.

Source: https://external-content.duckduckgo.com/iu/?u=https%3A%2F%2Fwww.aarc.org%2Fwp- content% 2Fuploads% 2F2019%2F07%2F080119-interdisciplinary-teamwork-735x413 .jpg&f= 1&nofb= 1&ipt=80bd3d8e004ebe90b1dfc 5dfb7905abc4be91f929bb7450f7c6138556bda2b69.

Test Your Knowledge

1. What principle of palliative care focuses on relieving pain and other distressing symptoms?
2. Why is communication important in palliative care?

1.3. Pain Management in Palliative Care

Learning Outcome

1. Explain the assessment of pain in patients
2. Define the pharmacological interventions
3. Describe the non-pharmacological strategies

Pain management under palliative care is an elementary component with direct implications for the quality of life of patients suffering from life-limiting conditions. Effective control of pain can significantly contribute to comfort and mitigate the psychological distress usually resulting from agonizing pain. The guidelines of palliative care demand a holistic approach, which necessitates acclimatization to both pharmacological and non-pharmacological interventions. The combination of such therapies as opioids and adjuvant therapies is essential, yet patient preferences and individual response to treatment should also be considered by medical staff. Pain management education is also critical for nurses since training deficits may lead to ineffective pain control, which in turn will counteract the entire effectiveness of palliative therapy. These findings are supported by evidence that highlights the need for innovative methods of education in palliative nursing, where curricula must be adapted to equip nurses with core competencies in managing pain (Pfitzinger et al., 2016). The values of palliative care also align with the importance of individualized pain control strategies, acknowledging patients' clinical status, personal beliefs, and culture. The challenge is not merely in selecting appropriate drugs but also in engaging patients and their families actively in decisions regarding their treatment. There is evidence that open communication concerning assessment and treatment of pain is most crucial; patients with open discussions about their pain have better outcomes and greater satisfaction with care. The integration of practices that include psychological care and complementary therapies can also complement pharmacological treatment, establishing a comprehensive pain management model. The combined treatment approach is supported by previous research, which indicates the documented advantages of these interventions in enhancing patient experience in palliative care, ultimately leading to improved quality of life during the dying process (Bacon, 2008). Besides, with the advancement of the future of palliative care, increasingly, it is crucial to assess existing educational resources for nursing professionals. Aligning education curricula with the foundations of palliative care helps nursing students acquire the relevant competencies to manage pain effectively. Existing research indicates that while a significant step has been made in aligning nursing education with palliative care practices, gaps still exist, particularly in specialist areas such as pain control and symptom management. The necessity of allowing nurses to be competent and confident in the provision of best pain management is critical because their contribution plays a pivotal role in influencing patients' experiences. Continual assessment and revision of nursing education, with a focus on integrating effective pain control practices, are essential for fostering well-informed practitioners capable of meeting the complex needs of patients in palliative and end-of-life care settings (Pfitzinger et al., 2016) (Figure 1.8).

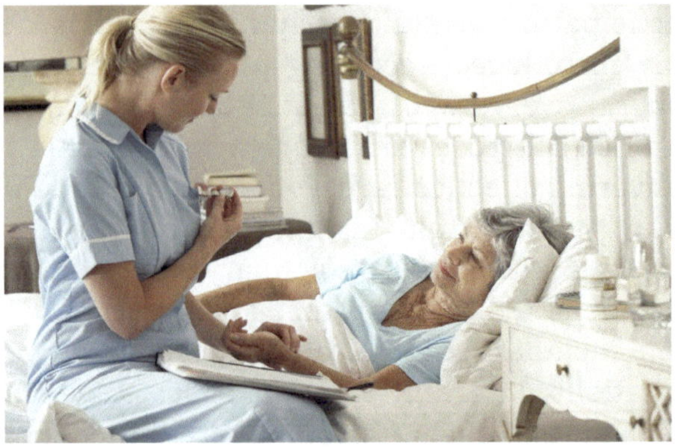

Figure 1.8. Pain management in palliative care.

Source: https://www.registerednursing.org/wp-content/uploads/2017/03/Palliative-care-nurse-image.jpg.

1.3.1. Assessment of Pain in Patients

Evaluation of pain among patients being under palliative and end-of-life care is a complex process that is based on both subjective and objective indicators. It has usually been described as a holistic experience, one that will vary with every individual, and therefore demands a clear understanding of its multiple dimensions. Accurate pain evaluation begins with a comprehensive evaluation of the patient's non-verbal and verbal signals and an in-depth clinical history that aids in identifying the etiology and character of pain. Since pain response and reporting may vary, clinicians must employ valid assessment methods, such as standardized questionnaires or behavioral rating scales, to measure the severity, quality, and impact of pain on the patient's global quality of life. Alongside this, an understanding of the subjective nature of pain and the potential for cultural differences in its experience serves to emphasize the need for a separate assessment process, ensuring that care plans are tailored to each patient's individual circumstances and needs. As life draws to a close, the need for accurate pain assessment becomes increasingly critical. It is at this point that sensitive communication takes effect, as patients may be in pain or uneasy and either do not verbalize it well because of fear or emotional distress. Health professionals must establish a trusting environment to make patients feel at ease expressing their pain and the problems associated. Pain assessment clinical education programs, designed to improve the skills of nurses and other healthcare providers, have been reported to show promising results in building knowledge and attitudes towards pain management.

Results have indicated that educational interventions improve the ability to assess pain accurately and disperse myths related to the use of opioids for pain relief (Alexander et al., 2016). By giving clinicians the correct information, clinicians can more effectively employ effective pain management techniques that are consonant with best practices in palliative care. Moreover, a key element in the assessment of pain is having knowledge of the psychological and social dimensions of the patient's experience. Pain is not only a physiological sensation; it also has emotional and social aspects, such as anxiety, depression, and support.

Pain assessment, which is a part of an integral approach, includes these elements to allow care managers to design holistic intervention plans addressing all aspects of pain in patients. Palliative care emphasizes the importance of education, where improvements in the knowledge base are strongly correlated with enhanced abilities for pain management (Divyalasya et al., 2017). It is not just about promoting physical comfort, but also about counseling patients on their emotional and social well-being during their final hours and thus aligning care strategies with the international objectives of palliative and end-of-life nursing (Figure 1.9).

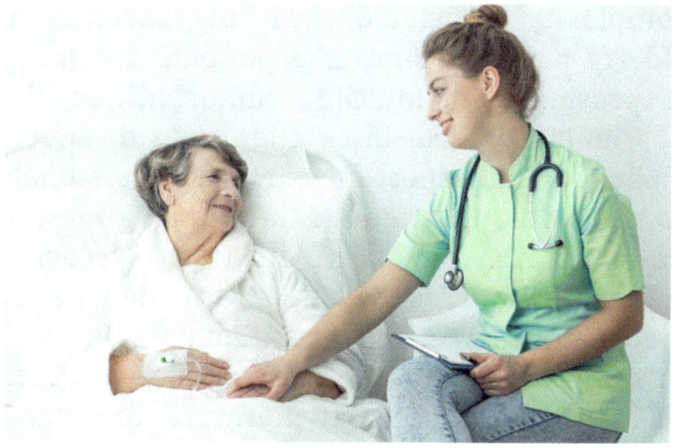

Figure 1.9. Assessment of pain in patients for end-of-life care.

Source: https://www.crossroadshospice.com/media/3478/why-is-palliative-care-important.png.

1.3.2. Pharmacological Interventions

Pharmacological interventions are the cornerstone of end-of-life and palliative nursing practice, with the predominant emphasis on symptom control and improving patients' quality of life who have advanced, chronic illness. Appropriate choice and administration of drugs can be a crucial factor in ensuring patients' comfort by reducing signs and symptoms like pain, dyspnea, nausea, and anxiety. Opioids, for example, are commonly employed in the management of advanced pain, especially where malignancies are concerned, providing much-needed relief when administered in the proper manner. Further, adjunctive therapies like anxiolytics or antidepressants can be used to treat psychological symptoms, and in doing so, promote a holistic care approach. Through incorporating these pharmacological interventions, nurses play an integral role in optimizing patient outcomes and providing for a dignified death experience, all of which reflects person-centered care in palliative settings. Additionally, the application of pharmacological treatment requires a profound understanding of the pharmacokinetics and pharmacodynamics in a specific patient, taking into account the complexity associated with polypharmacy in elderly patients. Since the patients are likely to present with multiple comorbidities, the possibilities of drug interaction and side effects make it a vital aspect for nursing professionals to consider. Continuous monitoring of the patient's reaction to medication is crucial; it enables nurses to adjust the dosage or medication as needed, maintaining symmetry in symptom control as needs evolve. Further, as mentioned in current literature, there is a recognized need for some information for both patients with severe dementia and caregivers regarding medication protocols at the end of life. Closing these gaps is key to enhancing standards of care for this vulnerable population (Ballard et al., 2006). Even the effectiveness of pharmacologic interventions for palliative care can be improved by interdisciplinary practice, wherein nurses, pharmacists, and physicians work together to produce balanced care plans. Interdisciplinary practice facilitates shared input on drug choices, informed by best practices and recent research. For instance, the production of annotated bibliographies, as done by researchers at the University of Sheffield, aids in synthesizing evidence on pain management among elderly individuals and in the terminal stages of palliative care (Aveyard et al., 2007). In addition to informing clinical practices, these resources also assist healthcare professionals in implementing evidence-based interventions with confidence, thereby facilitating an improved patient experience. Lastly, the reflective application of medication therapy in the palliative situation not just alleviates suffering but also honors the inherent human dignity of patients faced with the end of life.

1.3.3. Non-Pharmacological Strategies

In terminal and palliative nursing practice, the role of non-pharmacological interventions is a critical aspect of enhancing patient comfort and overall quality of life. Non-pharmacological interventions are beneficial in the management of complex symptoms such as pain, anxiety, and delirium, which occur frequently among terminally ill patients. Extensive literature reports several nursing interventions, including emotional support, active listening, and effective communication with the patients and their families. These practices are essential in laying out a therapeutic environment that promotes not only physical relief but also internal and spiritual ease. Primarily, the involvement of the kin family in treatment plans supports relational systems, offering emotional support to both patients and caregivers. Through the implementation of these non-pharmacologic measures holistically, nurses are in a position to provide holistic care that extends beyond symptom relief, embodying a more compassionate model of medicine. Further research identifies the essential contributions of multicomponent interventions as non-drug approaches in palliative environments, especially in delirium prevention among terminally ill patients. Studies confirm that routine practices, such as modifying the sleep environment, managing hydration, and engaging family, considerably contribute to improving patient well-being in end-of-life care. For instance, focus on fluids is an emerging practice among healthcare professionals because fluid intake is crucial in maintaining mental capacity. Despite the seeming appropriateness of such diverse interventions, there is a lag in their application, particularly on less common practices like bright light therapy. This dichotomy highlights the importance of ongoing training and development for nursing professionals, enabling them to employ the most effective non-pharmacological intervention strategies in clinically demanding contexts (Kanno et al., 2025). Moreover, effective non-pharmacological care interventions can significantly improve the quality of palliative care life, particularly through the provision of emotional and spiritual care. The implementation of humanization in nursing care serves as a bedrock for the delivery of dignified care. Evidence brought forth by research indicates that interventions such as control of pain, active listening, and spiritual care contribute greatly toward alleviating suffering during the process of dying. Even as limitations inherent in limited professional education and limited resources continue to confront the healthcare industry, the foundation laid by these interventions demonstrates them to be able to enhance patients lived experience. Through an emphasis on patient autonomy and the implementation of a person-centered system of care, nurses can facilitate not only physical comfort but also emotional healing. All these non-pharmacological interventions must be adopted and further researched to enhance nursing practice within palliative settings, ensuring that care for patients in the final stage of life is holistic in nature (Silveira et al., 2025) (Figure 1.10).

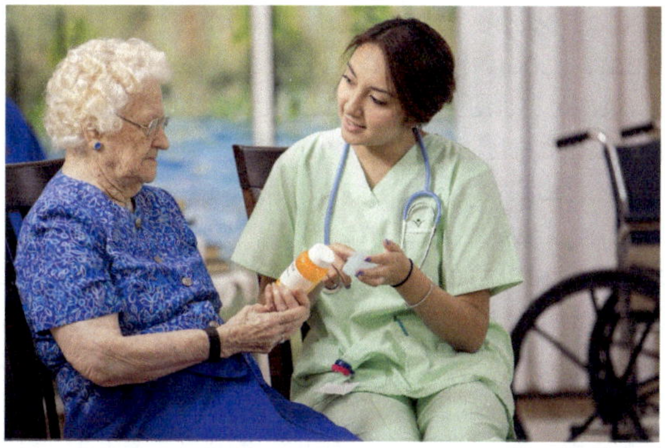

Figure 1.10. Non-pharmacological strategies.

Source: https://external-content.duckduckgo.com/iu/?u=https%3A%2F%2Fwww.crossroadshospice.com%2Fmedia%2F3189%2Fpalliative-patient-with-nurse.jpg&f=1&nofb=1&ipt=590edd97004e061e1463f1adc9c4dec36293b85385b88d08d2e89bd6ef1ef9cf.

Test Your Knowledge

1. What are the common methods used to assess pain in palliative care patients?
2. Why is individualized pain management important in palliative care?

1.4. Communication Skills in End-of-Life Care

Learning Outcome

1. Identify the importance of effective communication in palliative and end-of-life (EOL)
2. Define the techniques for discussing prognosis and options in palliative and end-of-life care
3. Describe the supporting families through difficult conversations in palliative and end-of-life care

Good communication is at the forefront in the field of end-of-life care, particularly in ensuring empathetic and multifaceted care for the patients and their families. It is most often the responsibility of palliative care nurses to be the initial point of contact in such communication, with the mandate of presenting a wealth of empirical medical information in a manner that is both reassuring and comprehensible. The psychosocial and psychological dimensions are no less critical in such cases. It is widely agreed that all professionals involved in the delivery of palliative care need to have a minimum understanding of the psychological dynamics of terminal illness and be able to communicate and assess psychological risk. The lack of clear guidelines for the role of psychologists in palliative care settings reflects a failure in the comprehensive training of health professionals, with a greater focus on communication skills as a core element of nursing training (Costantini et al., 2010). Nurse communication lies at the heart of responding to the concerns faced by patients receiving palliative care, especially near the end of their lives. Effective nurse-patient communication has been shown by research to significantly improve the quality of care and empower patients to accept reality. A study of pediatric oncology nurses highlighted that experienced nurses are committed advocates of their patients, and trust and open communication are built. Through embracing the essence of what they went through, such nurses are more likely to empathize and provide supportive talks regarding end-of-life issues. It also contributes to their ability to comprehend and appreciate individual reactions to loss, an aspect that is essential in guaranteeing that the care of patients is highly individualized and receptive to the emotional needs of patients and their families (Montgomery et al., 2013). Moreover, enhancing the communication skills of nursing professionals in end-of-life care facilities requires systematic training and education interventions.

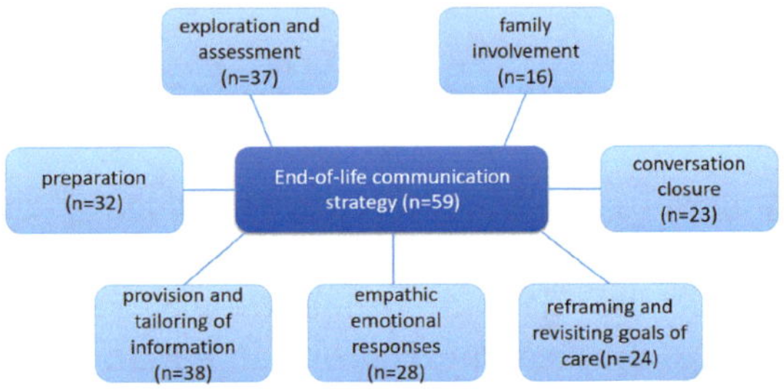

Figure 1.11. Communication skills in end-of-life care.

Source: https://external-content.duckduckgo.com/iu/?u=https%3A%2F%2Ftse2.mm.bing.net%2Fth%3Fid%3DOIP.kL28CDswu9Id_yykE84FXwHaDs%26r%3D0%26pid%3DApi&f=1&ipt=91e437bed867b119b7d702a7db6117dab5d34ca3dfa77c6a6aeaf736a3e669f0.

The introduction of formal curricula, simulation training, and mentorship can help bridge the gap between theory and practice. With exposure to diverse situations and support from peers, healthcare facilities can create a setting conducive to the development of effective communication models. Future research should evaluate the outcomes of such interventions, with a focus on whether improved communication not only enhances the caregiver experience but also has a profound impact on patient satisfaction and quality of life during the end stages of their illness (Montgomery et al., 2013). This is significant since the healthcare community is still seeking innovative ways to address the complexities of end-of-life conversations (Figure 1.11).

1.4.1. Importance of Effective Communication

Effective communication is central to the practice of palliative and end-of-life (EOL) nursing, providing the foundation to enhance understanding, empathy, and collaboration among the patient, family, and healthcare team. Since the essence of this communication revolves around the delivery of complex medical information, along with emotional and psychological requirements. Nurses, often the first and primary point of contact in such sensitive circumstances, must walk a fine line with conversations that involve not only the logistics of care but also the sheer emotional weight associated with discussions of dying. As is also the focus of newer research, enhancement of nurses' communication skills can lead to more patient and family-oriented environments, which in turn help them tackle the complexities of EOL care with dignity and respect (Montgomery et al., 2013). These skills are essential in establishing trust so that patients can share their choices and concerns freely. Furthermore, the quality of communication is particularly highlighted in nurse education and training. Curricula of nursing programs have recently come under criticism for giving EOL care communication short shrift, reinforcing the necessity of targeted educational interventions. By implementing focused training on evidence-based communication approaches, nursing students can become more comfortable and proficient in communicating with patients and their families to address end-of-life issues. As a demonstration, in one study, it was demonstrated that educational seminars significantly improved nursing students' confidence in defining EOL care concepts, with an improving trend in pretest and posttest comfort level scores (Boroughf et al., 2006). This supports the theory that robust educational programs with interactive sessions are necessary to better prepare future nurses for the unique challenges they will face in palliative settings. In addition to enhancing patient results and assisting nursing education, strong communication also empowers families during the EOL process. By ensuring families are clearly informed and actively involved in care decisions, nurses can eliminate confusion and helplessness related to terminal illness. Open communication facilitates the development of common goals and understanding between providers and families, resulting in the formulation of care plans that are congruent with the patient's values and preferences. The process is interactive and has been emphasized in research from a phenomenological study, which found that nurses should become advocates for their families and patients (Montgomery et al., 2013). In doing this, nurses not only fulfill their professional duty but also positively contribute to the experience of dying for patients, reaffirming the crucial role they play within palliative care.

1.4.2. Techniques for Discussing Prognosis and Options

Collaboration through discussions on prognosis and treatment planning within palliative and end-of-life care requires a sensitive, open communication, and patient and family dynamics-aware approach. Establishing meaningful discussions begins with active listening, which enables healthcare providers to determine the informational and emotional needs of patients and their families. When rendering a prognosis, it's also necessary to present information in a manner consistent with the patient's knowledge and preferences, so that it can be tailored to follow-up discussions on treatment. Interdisciplinary-related training activities are key, as they enable healthcare professionals to respond effectively to challenging conversations regarding prognosis and decision-making around care, backed by evidence that interdisciplinary monitoring enhances communication within palliative care settings (Breakwell et al., 2012). In addition, approaches such as the SPIKES protocol (Setting, Perception, Invitation, Knowledge, Emotions, and Summary) provide a step-by-step process for delivering difficult prognosis news. This framework supports an empathetic approach with ongoing sensitivity to the patient's and family's emotional signals throughout the conversation. Guiding conversations utilizing this framework, nurses can establish an environment that facilitates frank discussions of prognosis in a way that is sensitive to patients' emotional states. Furthermore, healthcare professionals should consider incorporating conversation about advanced care planning into the treatment process early on. It is recommended that well-educated oncology advanced practice nurses (APNs) improve patient understanding and readiness to participate in such significant discussions (Houldin et al., 2010). Secondly, ongoing education and training in communication skills will be a vital factor in optimizing discussions about prognosis and options. Evidence emphasizes that raising the knowledge and attitudes towards advanced care planning among healthcare professionals leads to improved patient outcomes. Identification of perceived barriers, including resistance from patients to disclose sensitive data, is vital in facilitating more effective conversations. Establishing rapport and trust enables practitioners to support patients and their families through the complexities of end-of-life decisions. In palliative care, the ultimate purpose is not only to provide extensive prognosis information, but also to facilitate patients and families in making value-based and preference-informed decisions. Enhancing practice behavior and knowledge in such communication guarantees a more compassionate, patient-centered approach to care (Houldin et al., 2010) (Figure 1.12).

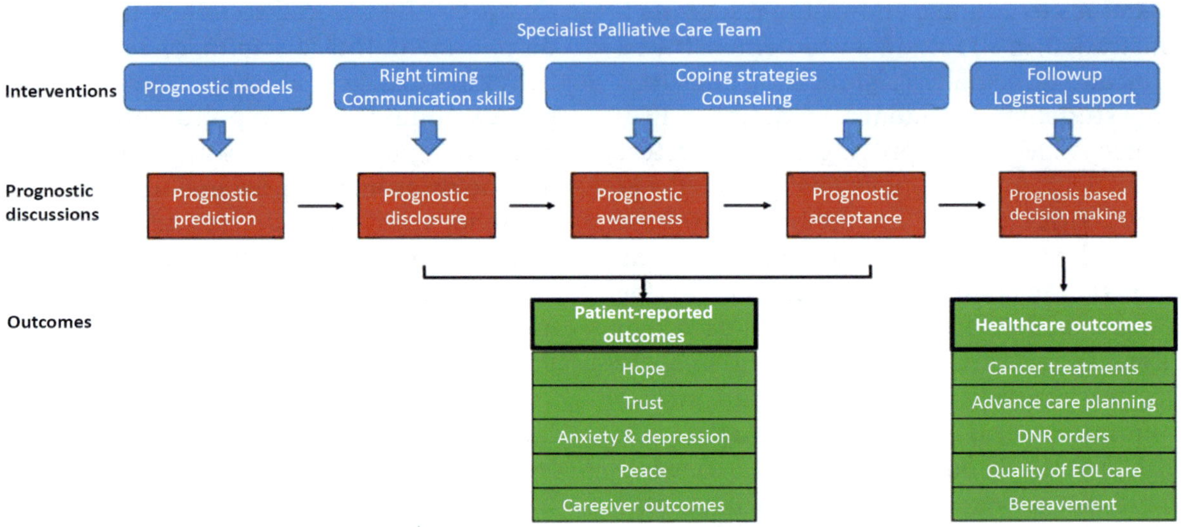

Figure 1.12. The continuum are prognostic prediction, prognostic disclosure, prognostic awareness, prognostic acceptance, and prognosis-based decision-making.

Source: https://www.researchgate.net/publication/348404599/figure/fig1/AS:11431281115414483@1674879327210/The-Prognostic-Continuum-The-5-key-steps-orange-along-the-continuum-are-prognostic.png.

1.4.3. Supporting Families Through Difficult Conversations

Involving families under challenging conversations throughout the end-of-life and palliative care process is a critical aspect of holistic nursing practice. Nurses are responsible for initiating open conversation about prognosis, treatment, and end-of-life planning while addressing the emotional and psychological needs of families, who are typically overwhelmed by the gravity of the circumstances. By providing a setting in which families can discuss their fears and concerns, nurses can offer relevant support at a time when open communication is most essential. Nevertheless, time constraints and even anxiety on the part of nurses in bringing up end-of-life topics can stand in the way of such discussions. Therefore, enhancing nurses' confidence through educational programs in disease progression and palliative care options can significantly improve their ability to engage in practical discussions with families (Battah et al., 2016). The value of interprofessional collaboration among healthcare team members cannot be overstated in family support. Research indicates that nurses are often not involved in significant discussions during prognosis disclosure, rendering them incapable of performing their roles optimally (Haglund et al., 2019). With the coordination of physicians and other medical caregivers, nurses can enhance the quality of information presented to families. Such a collaborative approach not only ensures wholeness in care but also supports the nurse's role as a key one in being a reassurance and support figure. The development of multidisciplinary teams with a robust emphasis on communication can yield better outcomes for families and patients, ultimately diminishing some of the emotional burden of end-of-life decision-making. By advocating for their involvement in such forums, nurses can play a crucial role in safeguarding the interests and needs of both families and patients. Furthermore, training programs that prepare nurses to have challenging conversations about end-of-life care are necessary to establish a supportive setting for families. These interventions enable nurses to acquire the skills necessary to assist patients and families in navigating challenging emotional terrain, alleviate family suffering, and ensure that families are properly educated about potential alternatives as patients approach the end of life. Assisting nurses in adopting an empathetic but firm communication style can make a big difference for family understanding and participation in care. By offering knowledge of the unease that nurses feel about talking about death and dying, organizations can establish a staff that is better placed to help families through the dialogue. Ultimately, adopting training and education in palliative care communication enables nurses to become active advocates for families in times of need, thereby enhancing the overall quality of end-of-life care (Battah et al., 2016).

Test Your Knowledge

1. Why is active listening important when communicating with a terminally ill patient?
2. How can healthcare providers show empathy during end-of-life conversations?

1.5. Ethical Considerations in Palliative Care

Learning Outcome

1. Describe the autonomy and patient rights
2. Define the decision-making in end-of-life scenario
3. Discuss the cultural sensitivity and ethical dilemmas

Palliative care ethics offer valuable guidance for nursing practice, since nurses often have to deal with complex ethical issues that arise in the face of end-of-life care. At the heart of such challenges lies the conflict between patient autonomy and adherence to ethical principles such as beneficence and non-maleficence. Nurses must navigate the clashing demands of patients, families, and the healthcare team in situations where there is medical aid in dying. The expanding use of euthanasia protocols, as seen in recent literature, requires careful reflection on the role of the nurse within such contexts, which abound with ethical issues. As Burgess et al. (2020) determine, nurses must reflect on their ethical ontology and the nature of the nurse-patient relationship when considering acting upon euthanasia, so that their actions align with individual ethics as well as professional requirements. Furthermore, the ethical climate becomes even more complex when cultural issues are introduced into palliative care. Providers must be sensitive to the fact that patient preferences regarding end-of-life interventions are often shaped by cultural beliefs and values. This involves understanding how these cultural factors can influence the dying experience and the types of interventions patients want. Employing intercultural mediators may be a solution to mitigating potential conflict due to cultural miscommunication, as families make tough choices. The data gathered through research on the effectiveness of intercultural mediators indicate a sensitivity to cultural diversity and the need to incorporate multiple perspectives into treatment planning (Campinha-Bacote et al., 2017). Through fostering intercultural communication, medical professionals can enhance patient care to the extent that it becomes ethical, inclusive, and respectful of patients' values. Further, ethical concerns in palliative care also involve considering the implications of resource allocation as well as the extent of interventions offered to dying patients.

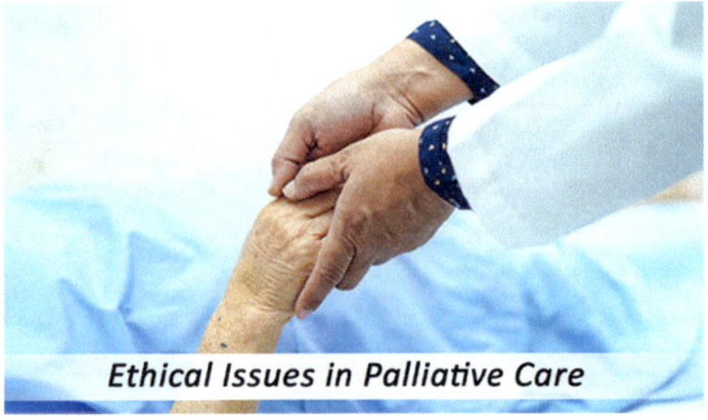

Figure 1.13. Ethical issues palliative care.

Source: https://www.rgcirc.org/wp-content/uploads/2024/07/ethical-issues-palliative-care.png.

During a time of healthcare shortages, decisions regarding the provision of palliative services typically depend on principles of justice and equity. Nurses must advocate for their patients against institutional policies that can limit the availability of specific types of care, such as effective pain management or palliative care. Ethical dilemmas arise when nurses discover a gap between what a patient requires and what is available or permissible under resource constraints. This emphasizes the need for ongoing debate regarding ethical and institutional responsibility in palliative care models, challenging the healthcare community to battle for greater accessibility and ethical care that honors patient requirements as well as healthcare necessities. In this scenario, continued advocacy remains a critical component of ethical nursing practice (Figure 1.13).

1.5.1. Autonomy and Patient Rights

The right to autonomy is one of the fundamental building blocks in healthcare, particularly in the context of palliative and end-of-life nursing care. Autonomy acknowledges the patient's right to make informed decisions about their own health care based on their values and preferences. It is especially significant in the context of palliative care, where not only emphasized, but also the optimization of the quality of life. Terminal patients have often struggled with choices regarding treatment options, symptom control, and end-of-life decisions. It is critically important that healthcare providers facilitate the exercise of autonomy by ensuring that patients are provided with information about their choices and the implications of their decisions. It allows patients in this manner to enhance their feeling of control as well as establish a therapeutic relationship with the caregivers, which indirectly promotes patient satisfaction and well-being. Identification of patient rights is intrinsic to the autonomy principle of nursing practice. Each patient carries inherent rights, including the right to informed consent, the right to refuse care, and the right to receive respectful care that honors their choices. These rights must be honored, particularly in the context of palliative and end-of-life care settings, where patients are vulnerable and care situations are often emotionally charged. The health care staff must collaborate to support these rights, combating any systemic factors that may restrict the practice of autonomy. Special attention must also be directed toward the special needs of marginalized groups, who may face compounded barriers through society's stigma or discrimination. By availing these rights, medical practitioners contribute to an inclusive and respectful model of care, acknowledging patients as dynamic participants in their health journey (Jeste, 2022). Furthermore, the integration of autonomy with ethical values cannot be overlooked. Healthcare professionals are often faced with complex ethical challenges that require balancing the patient's autonomy with other factors such as medical ethics and legal limitations. The evolving healthcare technological environment injects yet another level of complexity into the situation, with patient self-determination under attack from depersonalization. Ethically, promoting a fuller response that focuses on a person'spersonal dignity, quality of life, and informed choice is necessary. Reflective practice and continuous education in bioethics are necessary for healthcare professionals to manage such dilemmas successfully. Taking pride in compassionate communication and an ethical basis for patient rights upholds the autonomy principle, guaranteeing care that is patient-respectful and patient-centered, even during challenging situations (Mojzešová et al., 2018) (Figure 1.14).

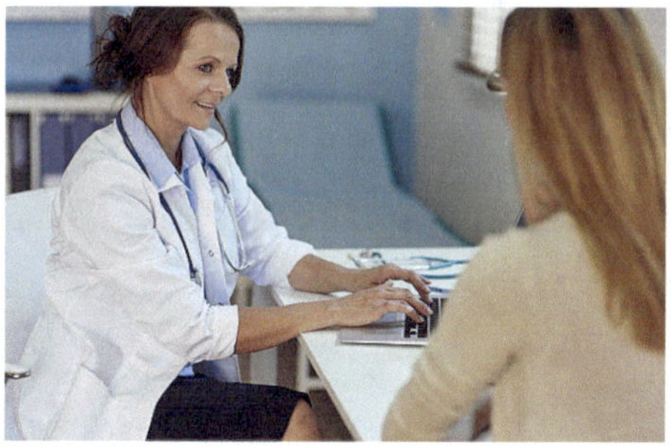

Figure 1.14. Autonomy and patient rights.

Source: https://domf5oio6qrcr.cloudfront.net/medialibrary/9451/conversions/iStock_78445461_MEDIUM-thumb.jpg.

1.5.2. Decision-Making in End-of-Life Scenarios

The complexity of decision-making in end-of-life care cannot be overstated, particularly when it involves palliative care. Effective decision-making models are imperative in guiding healthcare practitioners, patients, and families during these challenging moments. As patients are faced with terminal illnesses, including dementia, planning and making decisions on care preferences become pivotal. Palliative care aims at improving the quality of life for patients by maximizing their physical, emotional, and spiritual well-being. Although there are still hindrances, particularly regarding access to palliative care services among patients like individuals with dementia who might not be provided with suitable support. It has been found that improving the availability of these services can have a tremendous impact on overall comfort and dignity during end-of-life periods, which indicates the imperative necessity for efficient decision-making procedures (Birch et al., 2008). Pediatric palliative care decision-making is also a multi-faceted process that takes into consideration the unique needs of both the child and the family. Utilization of instruments like the My Choices booklets is promising in enabling families to voice their care and outcome preferences. The tools allow parents and children to be actively engaged in their care arrangements at the end of life, hence promoting a person-centered approach. It was observed that families tend to prefer care at home rather than in institutions, but this preference is not always acknowledged or accepted by medical professionals. The absence of professional confidence in prompting conversations about future care also makes the decision-making process more difficult. This discrepancy underscores the importance of teaching healthcare professionals communication and person-centered planning skills to bridge the gap between professional competence and family preferences (Bennett et al., 2013). Ultimately, patient autonomy, family involvement, and experienced guidance intersect to provide the basis for effective decision-making in palliative and end-of-life care. Freedom of choice is most critical, but it is typically defeated by ineffective communication among and between members of the healthcare team, as well as between teams and families. Providing an environment conducive to open discussion can facilitate a shared understanding and consent regarding care goals. Moreover, emphasizing active research and pilot studies aimed at increasing palliative care access can be a significant stimulus to the decision-making process in such instances. By eliminating the hurdles and strengthening the supportive infrastructure surrounding end-of-life care, health systems will be able to ensure that patients and families make these difficult choices with dignity and clarity, ultimately enhancing the overall palliative care experience (Birch et al., 2008) (Figure 1.15).

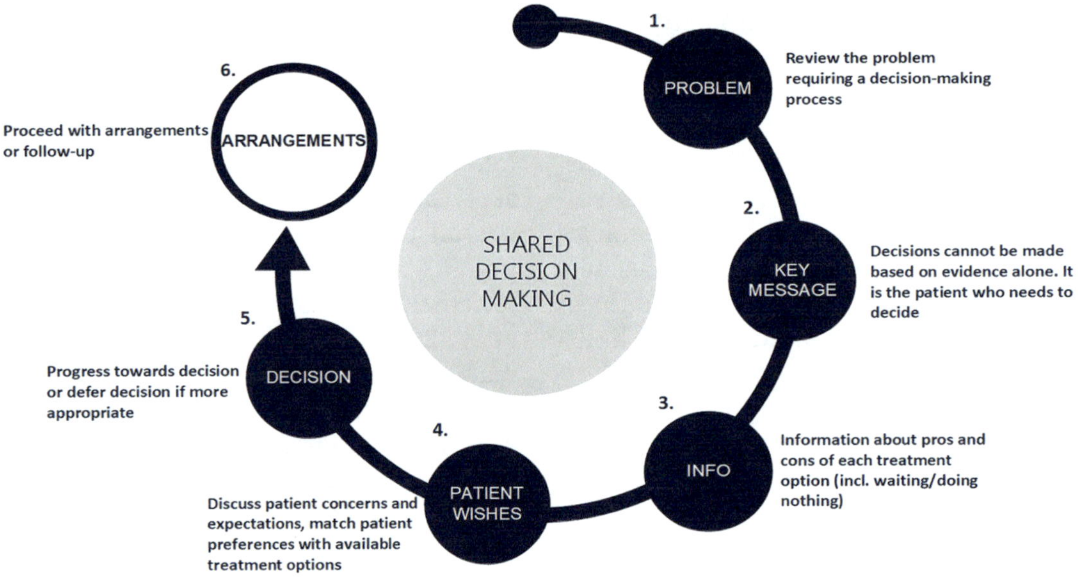

Figure 1.15. Shared decision making and advance care planning.

Source: https://media.springernature.com/lw1200/springer-static/image/art%3A10.1186%2Fs12910-023-00944-7/MediaObjects/12910_2023_944_Fig1_HTML.png.

1.5.3. Cultural Sensitivity and Ethical Dilemmas

Cultural sensitivity is vital in palliative and end-of-life care nursing, as it addresses the individual needs of patients and their families. Effective communication is the foundation, and nurses must actively listen and engage with patients to understand their culture and personal values. Sensitivity to cultural details enables nurses to create care plans tailored to patients' values and beliefs, thereby facilitating trust-building and comfort in challenging situations. Ethical issues usually arise where medical recommendation collides with cultural custom. In some communities, for example, the subject of death would be taboo, and therefore end-of-life care options would be hard to broach. Hence, healthcare professionals have to navigate these sensitive discussions skillfully while being respectful and empathetic to divergent cultures, such that treatment is not only medically recommended but also culturally compatible and ethically sound. Additionally, ethical dilemmas often intersect with the practice of bioethics, particularly in end-of-life care. The implementation of advance directives and shared decision-making illustrates how healthcare professionals can ethically engage patients in their care. Defined in the European Resuscitation Council Ethics guidelines, advance care planning prioritization allows for the integration of patients' personal and cultural values into their choice of care, thereby retaining autonomy and dignity even in the context of terminal illness (Mentzelopoulos et al., 2021). Nurses are often on the front line of such discussions, which require them to balance their ethical obligations against the very real pressure of family expectations that can vary dramatically across cultures. Creating a culture of cultural sensitivity, in short, not only enhances patient outcomes but also encourages ethical action in complex medical cases. In the care of patient management with end-stage disease, such as end-stage kidney disease (ESKD), nurses are faced with additional ethical issues. The International Society of Nephrology has cited ethics to have strong relevance to the overall picture of the integrated care of ESKD on the basis of discrepancies toward access and treatment availability among populations (Harris et al., 2019). For this purpose, clinicians need to be aware of the cultural determinants that influence health-seeking behavior and adherence to treatment. Such awareness can be translated into more effective and equitable care planning that is patient values-sensitive yet respects ethical principles. By linking cultural sensitivity with ethical issues, nurses can provide an integrated approach to palliative care that accommodates both the medical and ethical components of care in the delivery of end-of-life services (Figure 1.16).

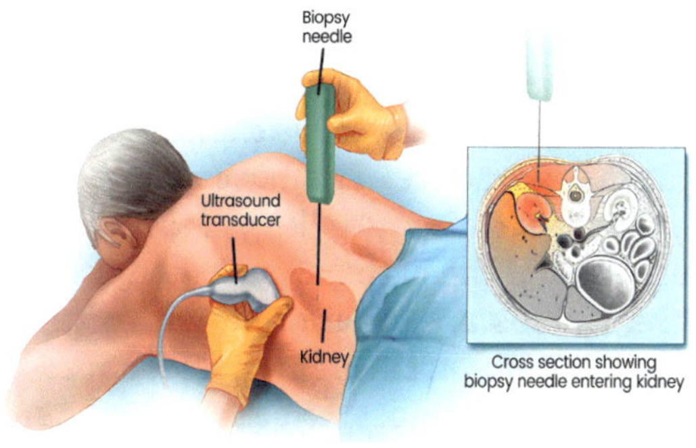

Figure 1.16. End-stage renal disease.

Source: https://www.mayoclinic.org/-/media/kcms/gbs/patient-consumer/images/2016/06/08/37/mcdc7_kidney_biopsy-8col.jpg.

Test Your Knowledge

1. Why is respecting patient autonomy significant in palliative care decisions?
2. What ethical dilemma might arise when a patient refuses life-sustaining treatment?

1.6. Challenges Faced by Palliative Care Nurses

Learning Outcome

1. Describe the emotional and psychological stress
2. Define the navigating healthcare systems
3. Identify the addressing patient and family needs

The role of palliative care nurses is central to managing the complexities of end-of-life care; however, they face numerous challenges that can impact their practice. The first of the primary dilemmas involves juggling ethical issues, namely in handling patients' autonomy and their welfare. Nurses are often faced with situations where patients' treatment preferences may conflict with the most effective management of symptoms, as evidenced by a systematic review of the ethical dilemmas that confront nurses on a day-to-day basis (Alanazi et al., 2024). These are challenges for which good communication skills are essential, but it can be difficult to learn them in stressful environments. In addition, the pressure to maintain respect for family relationships and dynamics, while simultaneously providing patient-centered care, heightens a level of complexity that can lead to emotional as well as moral distress for nurses. Finally, the COVID-19 pandemic has hastened any existing challenges within palliative care nursing practice. With the explosion of deaths in community settings, frontline healthcare workers, including nurses, have had to adjust rapidly to changing conditions and delivery systems, such as remote consultation (Mitchell et al., 2020). Lack of evidence-based guidelines in such an environment has left nurses ill-equipped and vulnerable, as they attempt to create meaningful end-of-life care amidst unprecedented challenges. This situation calls for the implementation of timely educational and organizational interventions to equip nurses with relevant competencies to handle both clinical and emotional challenges in the best manner. As palliative care settings evolve into newer paradigms in response to ongoing health crises, these transformations will play a crucial role in enhancing the quality of care provided to patients. In addition to ethical dilemmas and disagreements arising from external forces, the palliative care nurses also bear a significant emotional load from their work. Ongoing exposure to death and bereavement may lead to burnout, compassion fatigue, and moral distress, thereby making it even more difficult for them to provide optimal care. Research indicates that when nurses lack adequate support systems—i.e., access to mental health treatment and training in coping mechanisms—the risk of high turnover rates increases, resulting in instability within healthcare teams (Alanazi et al., 2024).

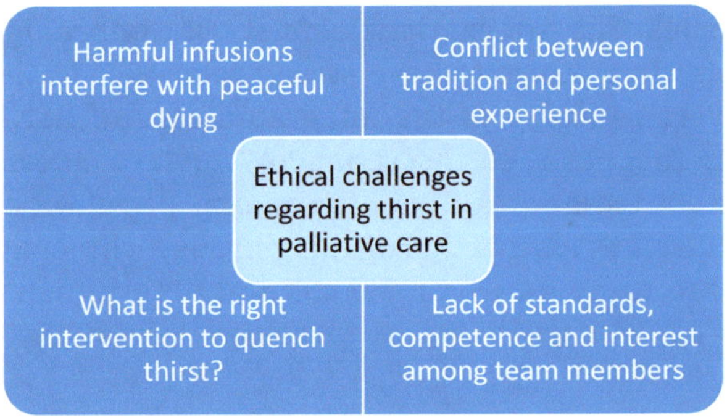

Figure 1.17. The four main themes in ethical challenges regarding thirst in palliative care.

Source: https://media.springernature.com/lw685/springer-static/image/art%3A10.1186%2Fs12904-024-01519-y/MediaObjects/12904_2024_1519_Fig1_HTML.png.

Substituting these problems necessitates organizations to build an environment centered on mental health and sustainability. Additionally, integrating empathetic communication skills into continuing professional development enables palliative care nurses, and thus healthcare institutions, to navigate the emotional subtleties of the nurse's role more effectively, thereby enhancing better outcomes for patients and nurses alike (Figure 1.17).

1.6.1. Emotional and Psychological Stress

Psychological and emotional distress is an actual phenomenon experienced by patients undergoing palliative and end-of-life care, which is compounded by the physical suffering of terminal illness. As the patients accept the scope of their prognosis, they are often faced with heightened anxiety, depression, and overall emotional disturbance. These psychological burdens can threateningly influence one's quality of life, leading to an escalated experience of pain, which necessitates the intervention of qualified nursing specialists. It is critical to recognize the intricate dynamic between emotional distress and physical pain in a bid to provide holistic care. Addressing both emotional pain and physical pain enables nurses to provide a comprehensive approach to care in respect of the patient's overall quality of life. Developing strong communication skills and emotional intelligence is crucial for nurses to effectively support patients through challenging moments, ultimately creating a healing environment that fosters emotional well-being. Additionally, emotional and psychological distress experienced by patients typically gets transferred to their caregivers, making a systemic shift necessary. Research has shown that caregivers tend to have their own emotional problems, including burnout and inadequacy, as they struggle with the complexities of their loved one's condition. This dynamic not only affects the caregivers' well-being but also the patient's quality of care. One must appreciate the interdependence of patient and caregiver experiences. According to a report presented by Henwood et al. (2017), information on the specific demands of caregivers enables health practitioners to develop targeted support systems that can withstand stress and promote resilience. By providing resources and emotional support, the well-being of patients and their caregivers can be enhanced simultaneously, while also facilitating relief from some of the emotional burden in palliative care situations. Finally, the integration of spiritual care in nursing practice is a possible means of reducing emotional and psychological suffering among dying patients. Spiritual care not only addresses the existential problems widely connected with terminal illness but also improves the emotional well-being of patients and families. Studies have demonstrated that spiritual support is associated with improved overall health outcomes, including reduced anxiety and enhanced emotional resilience, which are particularly vital in the palliative care context. Furthermore, Anisa et al. (2018) emphasize that spiritual care skills need to be taught to nurses to meet the total needs of the patients. Such training prepares nurses to engage in meaningful conversations with patients about their spiritual beliefs and emotional struggles, encouraging discussions that have the potential to bring solace and acceptance. As a result, prioritizing spiritual care as part of nursing procedures can enable healthcare professionals to address the various emotional and psychological issues of palliative care patients in an integrated way.

1.6.2. Navigating Healthcare Systems

Health system navigation is a challenging process, especially for professionals involved in end-of-life and palliative care nursing. Inherent complexity in health accessibility continually presents substantial barriers for patients and families. These barriers may include the misinterpretation of insurance coverage, varying levels of quality of care, and inadequate, unclear provider-patient communication. Healthcare providers, particularly nurses, are engaged in assisting patients through such systems and delivering them with holistic care that addresses their unique needs. This navigation is imperative even in palliative care settings, as early access to care can significantly affect the quality of life among patients who have life-limiting illnesses. Greater knowledge of healthcare resources, combined with effective communication, can empower patients and their families, making the process less daunting. Integration of technology in healthcare systems has added innovation and sophistication to palliative care. As suggested in recent discussions about the use of Artificial Intelligence (AI) and Machine Learning (ML), these technologies have the potential to improve patient outcomes. AI and ML can facilitate real-time monitoring and predictive analysis, which lead to tailored care plans and early detection of complications. Nurses, however, who work through such advancements, also have to address ethical issues and concerns related to data privacy. To harness the benefit of such technologies, ongoing education and interdisciplinary working are essential. By developing a context that is well-equipped to manage such technologies, healthcare systems can not only increase operational efficiency but also improve the quality of care overall for palliative patients (Ramoo, 2025). Furthermore, education on the economic effects of nursing care within a palliative setting is essential to ease navigation of the healthcare system. Research has documented excessive spending on preventable hospital admissions among palliative patients, highlighting the importance of optimizing resources and integrating effective care in health systems. For instance, a study identified that palliative care patients incurred heavy nursing costs due to avoidable emergency department visits (Afonso et al., 2025). Successful management of the health system demands knowledge of such economic determinants, which themselves influence decision-making and resource utilization. Minimization of process inefficiency and integration of palliative care into health systems better enables practitioners to reduce unnecessary financial burdens on patients and enhance care methods. Meeting not only the immediate needs of patients but also enhancing healthcare system sustainability in the face of increased demand, this combined effort is worthwhile (Figure 1.18).

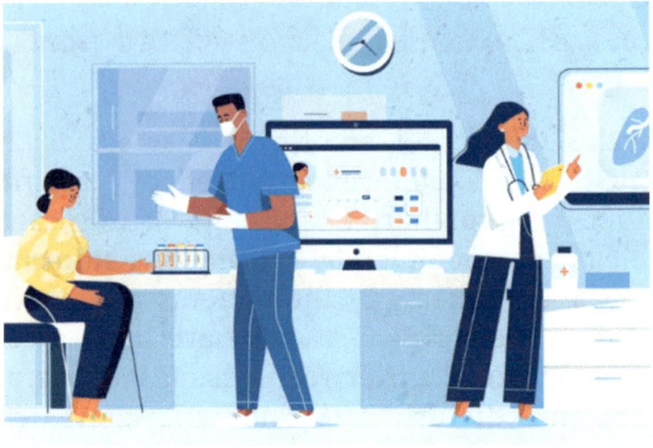

Figure 1.18. Navigation in healthcare.

Source: https://navigine.com//assets/web/news_files/2022/hospital-wayfinding-min.png.

1.6.3. Addressing Patient and Family Needs

In end-of-life and palliative nursing, it is crucial to manage the dual needs of patients and their families. Nurses play a significant role in facilitating communication, enhancing understanding, and guiding families through the intricacies of the healthcare system. This is especially significant for patients from culturally and linguistically diverse backgrounds who may have language limitations that complicate the process of palliative care. As highlighted in palliative care literature, cultural competency and trust can play a crucial role in enriching the caregiving interaction. Understanding migration history and culture educates nurses on how to deliver patient-centered care that respects individual choice while also accommodating family dynamics, thus creating a holistic approach to care that values the crucial role of the family within the process of palliation (Green et al., 2018). Shared decision-making is also a vital component for the management of the complex requirements of those patients who require palliative care, particularly those with dementia. The nursing staff not only have to manage the medical issues of these patients but also the ethical connotations of respecting their decisions and those of their families. The European Association for Palliative Care has presented detailed plans to incorporate shared decision-making models that involve empowering families and enabling them to participate in care decisions actively. Such inclusion is paramount in creating a collaborative setting whereby the voice of the patient is heard and ensuring that care plans honor their values and preferences. Using such strategies, nurses can create a supportive environment that addresses the psychological and emotional dimensions of end-of-life care, thus creating a respect and dignity-giving environment for the patient and family (Goodman et al., 2020). Besides, ethnic minority patients within the palliative care environment pose unique challenges that require an aggressive approach to delivering individualized care. The results reveal that patients are likely to experience treatment access gaps and varying survival rates; therefore, it is paramount that nursing practitioners acknowledge these disparities during the formulation of care plans. For palliative care experts to address disparities, they must be able to communicate effectively with families regarding clinical diagnoses and prognoses. This exchange not only soothes anxieties but also involves the families and makes them feel informed about the care process. By placing value on cultural competence and embracing the family's beliefs and values, nurses can significantly improve the quality of care they deliver to patients from diverse backgrounds, establishing an environment in which patients as well as their families can feel respected and nurtured (Green et al., 2018).

Test Your Knowledge

1. What emotional challenges might palliative care nurses experience while caring for terminally ill patients?
2. How can workload and staff shortages impact the quality of palliative nursing care?

SUMMARY

In drawing conclusions regarding palliative and end-of-life nursing care, it becomes clear that comprehensive attention is necessary to address the multifaceted issues involved in meeting the needs of patients and their families. Combining information from different perspectives provides a comprehensive understanding of the most effective ways to promote care during these critical life stages. Research exploring clinician experience with patient-reported measures different contexts, revealing the practice tensions associated with their use in various clinical settings. These practice tensions can impact the unencumbered implementation of patient-centered practices and, therefore, there is a need for ongoing discussion and professional education of healthcare practitioners to enhance their capacity to cope with such challenges (Cohen et al., 2018). Ultimately, the identification and addressing of these challenges will result in improvements in palliative care practice, with an emphasis on an integrated patient experience. Furthermore, cultural sensitivity is also a crucial dimension of palliative care, especially in multicultural societies. What has been learned from South Asian-based research highlights the significance of cultural beliefs about death and dying. Patients of such research indicate that their view of end-of-life care is not just about bodily issues, as it is enmeshed with their cultural and spiritual needs. This emphasizes the importance of healthcare professionals adopting culturally competent care practices that respect the values and traditions of diverse communities (Butt et al., 2014). Ultimately, incorporation of cultural dimensions into nursing care can also lead to improved patient satisfaction and harmony among family members throughout the end-of-life process. Finally, the development of palliative and end-of-life care nursing needs to be informed by empirical science as well as the lived experiences of patients from diverse backgrounds. As the healthcare climate evolves and continues to change, it is imperative that nursing practice and education incorporate an understanding of evolving demographics and patient needs, such as the requirement for cultural competency, to provide empathetic care. The merging of clinical science with an understanding of cultural knowledge will create a healthcare climate that not only alleviates physical pain but also honors the complex emotional and spiritual aspects of dying. By establishing improved communication, practicing tension recognition, and cultural adaptability, nursing professionals can actually enhance the quality of patients' and families' lives at this juncture.

In the context of palliative and terminal care nursing, the provision and coordination of services are crucial in ensuring patient comfort and dignity. Indicative abroad is a move towards expanding home care services for terminally ill patients. For instance, in the United Kingdom, there has been an attempt to enhance community care by establishing hospice-at-home teams. All these innovations are intended to be patient-initiated, specifically for patients who wish to spend their final days at home. Filling the gap between the desired end-of-life care and that which is actually provided, as discovered through the Bradford study, enables health practitioners to offer improved quality care to patients and their families during this fragile phase of life (Cartwright et al., 2008). Equally, however, caregivers' and health practitioners' perceptions are instrumental in shaping effective end-of-life care. The interplay between the caregivers' experience and the patients' needs is identified by the necessity of a multidisciplinary model with participation not only of nurses and doctors but also of mental health services and social work as well. Research has demonstrated that in the case of chronic diseases like COPD, there are far-reaching implications of unmet needs across varied care domains like physical, psychosocial, and spiritual care. Timely discussion of care options and advance directives enhances more patient-focused care, ultimately improving the quality of care towards the end of life. These innovative steps are significant in addressing the diverse aspects of care that patients and families experience at this stage in life (Johnston et al., 2017). Moreover, technological advancements and tailored therapeutic interventions are significant innovations in palliative care for patients with chronic, disabling diseases. New technology advancements, such as inhalation therapy and cognitive-behavioral therapy, demonstrate the changing nature of treatments available to foster patient outcomes. These developments underscore the importance of patient-centric care plans that respect individual choices in consideration of patients' physical and emotional needs. For medical professionals, the challenge is to integrate such breakthroughs into everyday practice while ensuring care is both holistic and humane. Through continual evolution in palliative and acceptance of multidisciplinary practice, the nursing practitioners can effectively respond to the complex needs of dying patients to provide them a peaceful and dignified death (Johnston et al., 2017).

KEY TERMS FROM THIS CHAPTER

- Advance directive
- Comfort measures
- Death anxiety
- Dying process
- Ethical dilemmas
- Grief counseling
- Interdisciplinary team
- Pain control
- Quality of life
- Symptom management
- Bereavement support
- Cultural sensitivity
- Do not resuscitate (DNR)
- End-of-life decision-making
- Family-centered care
- Hospice care
- Life-sustaining treatment
- Palliative sedation
- Spiritual care
- Terminal illness

CRITICAL THINKING QUESTIONS

1. **What is the primary goal of palliative care?**
   a. To cure terminal illness
   b. To prolong life at all costs
   c. To provide comfort and improve quality of life
   d. To perform advanced surgical procedures
2. **Which of the following best describes hospice care?**
   a. Focuses only on physical symptoms
   b. Is provided only in hospitals
   c. It is for patients who are seeking curative treatment
   d. It is for patients with a life expectancy of 6 months or less
3. **What is an important communication skill in end-of-life care?**
   a. Giving medical advice without discussion
   b. Using technical jargon to ensure accuracy
   c. Active listening and empathy
   d. Avoiding difficult conversations
4. **Which of the following symptoms is most commonly treated in palliative care?**
   a. Fever
   b. Pain
   c. Rash
   d. Infection
5. **Which ethical principle is most important in respecting a patient's end-of-life decisions?**
   a. Beneficence
   b. Justice
   c. Autonomy
   d. Non-maleficence

Short Answer Questions

1. What is the primary objective of palliative care?
2. List two common symptoms managed in end-of-life care.
3. Define hospice care.
4. Mention one difference between curative and palliative treatment.
5. What is the nurse's role in providing emotional support to terminally ill patients?
6. Explain the principles of palliative care and how they guide nursing practice.
7. Discuss the importance of communication skills in end-of-life nursing care.
8. Describe the ethical and legal issues commonly encountered in palliative care.
9. Explain the psychological and spiritual needs of dying patients and how nurses can address them.

Answers to Critical Thinking Questions

1. (c); 2. (d); 3. (c); 4. (b); 5. (c).

REFERENCES

1. Afonso, T. D. S., Capelas, M. L., & Martins, L. (2025). The economic cost of nursing care of palliative patients in the emergency department. *Healthcare, 13*(4), 421. https://doi.org/10.3390/healthcare13040421Alanazi, M. A., Shaban, M. M., Ramadan, O. M. E., Zaky, M. E., Mohammed, H. H., Amer, F. G. M., & Shaban, M. (2024). Navigating end-of-life decision-making in nursing: A systematic review of ethical challenges and palliative care practices. *BMC Nursing, 23.* https://doi.org/10.1186/s12912-024-02087-5 (accessed on 30th June 2025).
2. Alexander, S. (2016). A project to improve nurses' knowledge of, and attitudes towards, pain management at end of life. https://core.ac.uk/download/77511392.pdf (accessed on 30th June 2025).
3. Amador, S., Davies, S., Goodman, C., Handley, M., et al. (2014). Evaluation of the End-of-Life Care Train the Trainer (TTT) Education Model. https://core.ac.uk/download/29841285.pdf (accessed on 30th June 2025).
4. Anisa, N. R., Erika, K. A., & Rachmawaty, R. (2018). Nurse's spiritual care competencies to patient with end stage breast cancer. https://core.ac.uk/download/480549608.pdf (accessed on 30th June 2025).
5. Aveyard, B., Schofield, P., & Smith, P. (2007). Developing annotated bibliographies: A tool for education, collaboration and research development. https://core.ac.uk/download/177011.pdf (accessed on 30th June 2025).
6. Bacon, J. (2008). Hospice palliative home care in Canada: A progress report. https://core.ac.uk/download/71365021.pdf (accessed on 30th June 2025).
7. Ballard, C., Daley, S., Hughes, J., Keady, J., et al. (2006). End-of-life care and dementia. https://core.ac.uk/download/4145979.pdf (accessed on 30th June 2025).
8. Battah, C. (2016). End-of-life heart failure education with staff nurses; A quality improvement project. https://core.ac.uk/download/162578694.pdf (accessed on 30th June 2025).
9. Bennett, V., Hain, R., Hastings, R. P., Hobson, M., et al. (2013). Planning ahead with children with life-limiting conditions and their families: Development, implementation and evaluation of 'My Choices.' https://core.ac.uk/download/17205331.pdf (accessed on 30th June 2025).
10. Birch, D., & Draper, J. (2008). A critical literature review exploring the challenges of delivering effective palliative care to older people with dementia in the acute hospital setting. https://core.ac.uk/download/82906952.pdf (accessed on 30th June 2025).
11. Borgstrom, E., Gough, N., Hindley, E., Holti, R., et al. (2024). Practices, issues and possibilities at the interface between geriatrics and palliative care (InGaP): An exploratory study and knot working. https://core.ac.uk/download/603402902.pdf (accessed on 30th June 2025).
12. Boroughf, T. (2006). Addressing student nurses' concerns in end-of-life care. https://core.ac.uk/download/223074287.pdf (accessed on 30th June 2025).
13. Breakwell, S., Faut Callahan, M., Kim, M. J., Phillips, K., et al. (2012). Clinical observation reflections from students in an interdisciplinary palliative care course. https://core.ac.uk/download/213079311.pdf (accessed on 30th June 2025).
14. Burgess, M., Chambaere, K., Greig, M., Janke, R., et al. (2020). Nursing and euthanasia: A narrative review of the nursing ethics literature. https://core.ac.uk/download/200974626.pdf (accessed on 30th June 2025).

15. Butt, J., Charmaz, K., Department of Health (DH), HelpAge International, Office of National Statistics (ONS). (2014). Dying at home: A qualitative study of the perspectives of older South Asians living in East London. https://core.ac.uk/download/9991751.pdf (accessed on 30th June 2025).

16. Campbell, M. L., Courtright, K. R., Cox, C. E., Enguidanos, S., et al. (2022). Palliative care early in the care continuum among patients with serious respiratory illness: An official ATS/AAHPM/HPNA/SWHPN policy statement. https://core.ac.uk/download/543253969.pdf (accessed on 30th June 2025).

17. Campinha-Bacote, J., Crespo, E., García-Navarro, B., Martins Teixeira da Costa, E., Galao-Malo, M., González, M., et al. (2017). Intercultural mediation at the end of life: Different perceptions of the same process. https://core.ac.uk/download/186632139.pdf (accessed on 30th June 2025).

18. Cartwright, A., Daley, A., Grady, A., Strauss, A. L., Daley, A., Gomes, B., Lucas, B., et al. (2008). A reassuring presence: An evaluation of Bradford District Hospice at Home service. https://core.ac.uk/download/6251.pdf (accessed on 30th June 2025).

19. Chang, S., Choi, Y. R., Kim, D., & Lee, Y. (2024). Empowering palliative wound care in long-term care facilities: A comprehensive nursing competency for palliative wound care. *Journal of Korean Academy of Fundamentals of Nursing*. https://www.semanticscholar.org/paper/13a1c8c7699893804192223e21348e74e9eafc15 (accessed on 30th June 2025).

20. Clark, D., Inbadas, H., Whitelaw, S., Zaman, S., et al. (2016). Palliative care declarations: Mapping a new form of intervention. https://core.ac.uk/download/42371941.pdf (accessed on 30th June 2025).

21. Cohen, R., Krawczyk, M., Laforest, M., Reimer-Kirkham, S., et al. (2018). Micro-meso-macro practice tensions in using patient-reported outcome and experience measures in hospital palliative care. https://core.ac.uk/download/153444956.pdf (accessed on 30th June 2025).

22. Costantini, A., Jünger, S., Kalus, C., Payne, S., et al. (2010). EAPC task force on education for psychologists in palliative care. https://core.ac.uk/download/1547409.pdf (accessed on 30th June 2025).

23. Craft, A., Audit Scotland, Feudtner, C., Knapp, C., Humphreys, C., Bainbridge, D., Department of Health, et al. (2013). Evidence-based planning and costing palliative care services for children: Novel multi-method epidemiological and economic exemplar. https://core.ac.uk/download/17205342.pdf (accessed on 30th June 2025).

24. Deliens, L., Gijsberts, M. J. H., Hertogh, C. M. P. M., van der Steen, J. T., et al. (2014). Predictors of spiritual care provision for patients with dementia at the end of life as perceived by physicians: A prospective study. https://core.ac.uk/download/55762597.pdf (accessed on 30th June 2025).

25. Divyalasya, T. V. S., Pundarikaksha, H. P., & Vasundara, K. (2017). Impact of the educational session on knowledge and attitude toward palliative care among undergraduate medical, nursing, and physiotherapy students: A comparative study. https://core.ac.uk/download/539896832.pdf (accessed on 30th June 2025).

26. Goodman, C., Parker, D., Sampson, E. L., Bunn, F., Froggatt, K., Phillips, J. L., van der Steen, J. T., et al. (2020). Components of palliative care interventions addressing the needs of people with dementia living in long-term care: A systematic review. https://core.ac.uk/download/323056264.pdf (accessed on 30th June 2025).

27. Green, A., Green, M., Jerzmanowska, N., Lobb, E., et al. (2018). 'Death is difficult in any language': A qualitative study of palliative care professionals' experiences when providing end-of-life care to patients from culturally and linguistically diverse backgrounds. https://core.ac.uk/download/213607752.pdf (accessed on 30th June 2025).

28. Haglund, K., Newman, A. R., & Rodgers, C. C. (2019). Pediatric oncology nurses' perceptions of prognosis-related communication. https://core.ac.uk/download/228028413.pdf (accessed on 30th June 2025).

29. Harris, D. C. H., Davies, S., Finkelstein, F. O., Jha, V., Donner, J., Abraham, G., Bello, A. K., et al. (2019). Increasing access to integrated ESKD care as part of universal health coverage. *Kidney International, 95*, S1–S33. https://doi.org/10.1016/j.kint.2018.12.005 (accessed on 30th June 2025).

30. Henwood, M., Larkin, M., & Milne, A. (2017). Seeing the wood for the trees: Carer related research and knowledge—A scoping review. https://core.ac.uk/download/145186527.pdf (accessed on 30th June 2025).

31. Holdoway, A. (2022). Nutrition in palliative care: Issues, perceptions and opportunities to improve care for patients. *British Journal of Nursing, 31*(21), S20–S27. https://www.semanticscholar.org/paper/894fe60daf6132fa11e9026fc88ed58cd3a0dda1 (accessed on 30th June 2025).

32. Houldin, A. D., Parks, S. M., et al. (2010). Knowledge, attitudes, and practice behaviors of oncology advanced practice nurses regarding advanced care planning for patients with cancer. https://core.ac.uk/download/46969560.pdf (accessed on 30th June 2025).

33. Inbadas, H. (2016). History, culture and traditions: The silent spaces in the study of spirituality at the end of life. https://core.ac.uk/download/42371436.pdf (accessed on 30th June 2025).

34. Jeste, D. (2022). Caring for older adults with disabilities. *International Psychogeriatrics, 34*, 941–942. https://www.semanticscholar.org/paper/5fbaed29d248ef2aa3093df0cc1eb47e581b7292 (accessed on 30th June 2025).

35. Jiménez, G., Tan, W. S., Virk, A., Low, C. K., Car, J., & Ho, A. H. Y. (2018). Overview of systematic reviews of advance care planning: Summary of evidence and global lessons. *Journal of Pain and Symptom Management, 56*, 436–459.e25. https://doi.org/10.1016/j.jpainsymman.2018.05.016 (accessed on 30th June 2025).

36. Johnston, B., & Mathews, G. (2017). Palliative and end-of-life care for adults with advanced chronic obstructive pulmonary disease: A rapid review focusing on patient and family caregiver perspectives. https://core.ac.uk/download/96885466.pdf (accessed on 30th June 2025).

37. Kanno, Y., Nakano, K., Kajiwara, K., Kobayashi, M., Morikawa, M., Matsuda, Y., & Kako, J. (2025). Nursing practices for preventing delirium in patients with cancer with prognoses of months and weeks: A multi-site cross-sectional study in Japan. *The American Journal of Hospice & Palliative Care*. https://www.semanticscholar.org/paper/92abda2bc620adad3a4f9eeb02715a7c10330a2b (accessed on 30th June 2025).

38. Mentzelopoulos, S. D., Couper, K., Van de Voorde, P., Druwé, P., Blom, M. T., Perkins, G. D., Lulić, I., et al. (2021). European Resuscitation Council Guidelines 2021: Ethics of resuscitation and end of life decisions. *Resuscitation, 161*, 408–432. https://doi.org/10.1016/j.resuscitation.2021.02.017 (accessed on 30th June 2025).

39. Mitchell, S., Maynard, V., Lyons, V. S., Jones, N., & Gardiner, C. (2020). The role and response of primary healthcare services in the delivery of palliative care in epidemics and pandemics: A rapid review to inform practice and service delivery during the COVID-19 pandemic. *Palliative Medicine, 34*, 1182–1192. https://doi.org/10.1177/0269216320947623 (accessed on 30th June 2025).

40. Mojzešová, M., Capikova, C., & Trizuljakova, J. (2018). Bioethical challenges at the beginning of 21st century in education of healthcare professionals. *9*, 67–70. https://www.semanticscholar.org/paper/9d9826f19a3255842a3e5df1171106a6d9f4d7fd (accessed on 30th June 2025).

41. Montgomery, K. (2013). Communication during palliative care and end of life: Perceptions of experienced pediatric oncology nurses. https://core.ac.uk/download/217184783.pdf (accessed on 30th June 2025).

42. Murray, E., McLoughlin, K., & Foley, S. (2013). Access to specialist palliative care services and place of death in Ireland. https://core.ac.uk/download/71364943.pdf (accessed on 30th June 2025).

43. Pfitzinger, M. E. (2016). Evaluating baccalaureate curriculum end-of-life care content based upon End-of-Life Nursing Education Consortium (ELNEC) guidelines. https://core.ac.uk/download/322360300.pdf (accessed on 30th June 2025).

44. Ramoo, V. (2025). Advancing critical care nursing: Navigating artificial intelligence (AI) and machine learning (ML). *International Journal of Critical Care*. https://www.semanticscholar.org/paper/ab200d3e5ae551585a3834fba2326bd3ac8196d5 (accessed on 30th June 2025).

45. Sheldon, L., & Booker, R. (2023). Growth and development of oncology nursing in North America. *Annals of Palliative Medicine*. https://www.semanticscholar.org/paper/c1845720fd9f5b7a0bdd5aff8b9169aa62aae7a3 (accessed on 30th June 2025).

46. Silveira, A. D., Oliveira, L. F. de, Rodrigues, L. S., Pinheiro, P. L. L., & Martins, I. (2025). Enfermagem e cuidados paliativos: Conforto e qualidade de vida do paciente. *Revita ft*. https://www.semanticscholar.org/paper/74e817f78eea219a1e8b668e72800c404256c70c (accessed on 30th June 2025).

47. Spector, A., Thompson, E., & Patrizi, P. (2011). Improving care at the end of life. https://core.ac.uk/download/71358517.pdf (accessed on 30th June 2025).

48. Veras, R. P., & Oliveira, M. (2018). Envelhecer no Brasil: A construção de um modelo de cuidado. *Ciência & Saúde Coletiva, 23*, 1929–1936. https://doi.org/10.1590/1413-81232018236.04722018 (accessed on 30th June 2025).

49. Yoshioka, S., Murakami, S., & Oshita, R. (2025). Development of the Home Hospice Nursing Care Scale to support end-of-life patients with cancer and evaluation of its reliability and validity. *The American Journal of Hospice & Palliative Care*. https://www.semanticscholar.org/paper/f41ffafe9a682676ca4f8e7fbf47b26c1026a37a (accessed on 30th June 2025).

PERIOPERATIVE NURSING: PREOPERATIVE TO POSTOPERATIVE MANAGEMENT

2

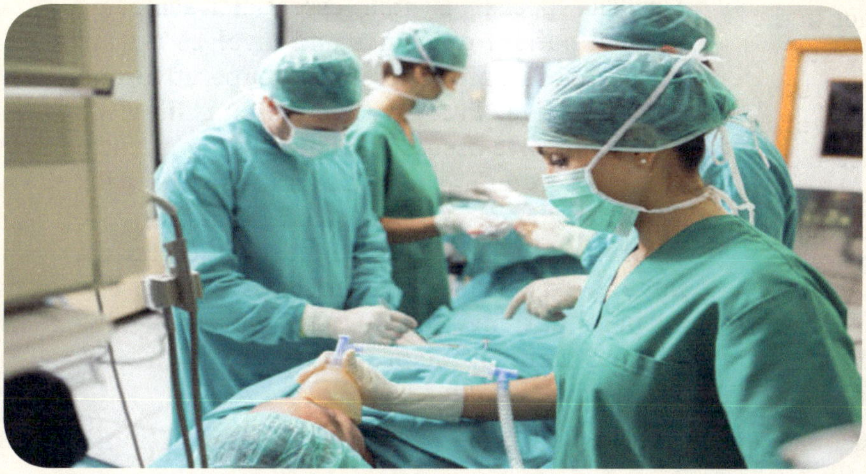

Introduction

The surgical process engages a care process ranging from preoperative to postoperative recovery all under the general rubric of perioperative nursing. Nurses take the central stage here in guaranteeing the safety, teaching, and psychological support of the patient throughout the various phases of surgical treatment. Each phase has its own challenges and requirements, hence the need for interdisciplinary care that harmoniously blends clinical expertise and patient-centered care. By emphasizing the significance of proper preoperative assessment, this essay aims to elucidate the foundational role that perioperative nursing plays in optimizing surgical results, patient satisfaction, and minimizing surgery-related problems. With increasing complexity of surgery, the role of preoperative education and preparation has gained prominence among healthcare professionals. This aspect of perioperative nursing is particularly critical for ostomy patients, as recent findings have shown that pre-surgical teaching can significantly

LEARNING OBJECTIVES

After studying this chapter, you will be able to:

1. Describe the role of perioperative nurses
2. Explain the preoperative assessment in nursing
3. Discuss the preoperative preparation in nursing
4. Identify the intraoperative nursing care
5. Learn about postoperative care
6. Evaluate the patient education and discharge planning

decrease levels of anxiety post-surgery and improve overall adaptability to body image alterations and self-care routines. Patients who are well-informed about their operations and the likelihood of outcomes are in a better position to manage both the psychological and logistical challenges of recovery. This shift towards a model of education fosters a healing and empowering environment, ultimately leading to improved long-term care for surgical patients (Harris et al., 2019). In addition, the importance of using appropriate warming techniques in the perioperative environment cannot be overstated, as they are essential in preventing perioperative hypothermia and its sequelae. Research indicates that implementation of evidence-based warming measures, accompanied by adequate staff training, can reduce patient outcomes by lowering rates of infection and other morbidities from hypothermia.

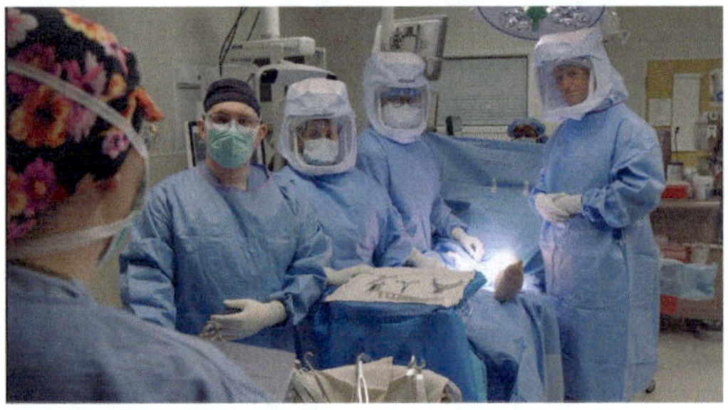

Figure 2.1. Perioperative nurse.

Source: https://jnj-connectivity.brightspotcdn.com/dims4/default/d12f139/2147483647/strip/true/crop/1400x787+0+1/resize/1000x562!/quality/90/?url=https%3A%2F%2Fjnj-brightspot.s3.amazonaws.com%2Fjnj-connectivity%2F57%2F77%2Ff704a5144834a500a908cca6acb7%2Fperioperative-care-promo3.jpeg.

Overcoming the barriers to the widespread application of these techniques, such as time constraints among perioperative staff, can allow healthcare organizations to create a culture of safety and efficacy in surgery. With nurses navigating the nuances of preoperative to postoperative care, their commitment to applying the highest practices is paramount for ensuring the best patient outcomes and advancing the science of perioperative nursing (Comans et al., 2021) (Figure 2.1).

Definition of Perioperative Nursing

Perioperative nursing is a subspecialty of nursing that encompasses the entire surgical process, from preoperative assessment to postoperative care. The specialty is vitally essential in achieving optimal patient outcomes and involves a triad of care phases: intraoperative, preoperative, and postoperative. Preoperative nursing involves comprehensive assessments, including medical history screening and identification of risk factors, to develop a personalized plan of care tailored to the surgical patient's unique needs. Not only do perioperative nurses psychologically prepare patients for surgery, but they also educate them on the procedure, complications, and recovery routes.

Preoperative preparation of this sort can significantly minimize patient anxiety and increase overall satisfaction with surgical care. Perioperative nurses play a crucial role in the intraoperative period, encompassing tasks such as maintaining the sterile field, monitoring vital signs, and assisting the surgeon and surgical team. This not only necessitates excellent technical competence but also demands the ability to communicate well under pressure. Effective intercommunication among surgical team members is essential to ensure patient safety, as communication breakdowns can lead to errors that pose risks to the patient's health. The perioperative nurse also maintains control of the patient's responses to surgery and anesthesia, continuously monitoring factors that may impact recovery after surgery. Their vigilance is crucial in anticipating problems and acting promptly, demonstrating why their contribution is essential throughout. In the postoperative period, the focus of perioperative nursing changes towards monitoring for recovery and pain. This is a valuable time as it involves monitoring the patient for complications like infection or delayed healing. According to existing literature, interventions at these stages significantly impact both short-term and long-term health outcomes, necessitating ongoing nursing care. As evidenced by reviews of non-surgical perioperative interventions, a combined holistic approach with psychology could enhance recovery experiences for surgical patients (Karl et al., 2018). Overall, the perioperative nurse plays a multifaceted role that combines clinical skills with compassion to provide a seamless experience throughout all stages of surgery, ultimately shaping the patient's journey to recovery.

Importance of Perioperative Care

The importance of perioperative care cannot be exaggerated because it falls under patient safety and general success of surgical outcome. The perioperative period encompasses various stages, including preoperative, intraoperative, and postoperative care, each of which requires careful coordination and management by healthcare professionals. Effective perioperative care ensures that patients are optimally prepared for the operation, which includes routine assessment and optimization of their underlying condition. For instance, diabetic patients, according to existing literature, can dramatically reduce their complication rates before surgery by evaluating and controlling HbA1c. Elevated glycosylated hemoglobin (HbA1c) is associated with an increased risk of postoperative complications and, consequently, requires specific perioperative measures to enhance patient safety and surgical outcomes (Breakwell et al., 2015). This proactive approach not only benefits enhanced surgical outcomes but also reduces the burden on healthcare systems by limiting the incidence of complications. Aside from medical assessment, the psychological aspect of perioperative care is also vital to patient recovery and satisfaction. Stress and fear of surgical procedures can harm a patient's ability to learn and successfully take care of themselves post-surgery. Preoperative education is a key component of this psychological support, through which patients can gain knowledge regarding their conditions, treatments, and processes of recovery, thus reducing anxiety. Studies have indicated that those patients who are provided with targeted education on their individual, specific surgical needs, such as ostomy patients, have significantly reduced postoperative anxiety compared to patients who receive general information (Harris et al., 2019). This reduction of anxiety not only enhances the learning environment but also enhances overall outcomes, as those patients who are better prepared are more likely to engage in self-care and adhere to postoperative protocols. Lastly, the integrated nature of perioperative care addresses both physical and psychological needs and, thus, is even more essential to contemporary surgical practice. Through the promotion of critical preoperative assessment, patient-specific education strategies, and effective postoperative management, healthcare professionals can significantly improve patient outcomes. Implementation of these practices not only minimizes complications but also motivates a compassionate environment, which facilitates patients throughout the surgical journey. Effective perioperative care is thus not merely a recitation of checks and steps; it is a system that integrates to ensure patients are equipped with the tools, information, and resources required to navigate their surgical ordeal with confidence and strength. By allocating equal emphasis to medical management and patient education, the nursing profession can elevate the quality of care and optimize the recovery options for surgical patients.

2.1. The Role of Perioperative Nurses

Learning Outcome

1. Describe the responsibilities in the surgical team
2. Focus on skills and qualifications required of perioperative nurses
3. Discuss how to impact patient outcomes

The perioperative nurse is not just confined to the operating room but also involves vital aspects of patient care in preoperative and postoperative care. The nurses, in the preoperative setting, have the responsibility to assess the needs of the patients, educate them, and instill confidence in them to erase anxiety. This is particularly vital for patients who are undergoing procedures involving significant lifestyle changes, such as ostomy creation. Evidence shows that preoperative stoma care education not only prepares patients for their new world but also minimizes levels of postoperative anxiety, enhancing their ability for self-management upon discharge from the hospital (Harris et al., 2019).

Through effective communication and empathetic support, perioperative nurses facilitate patients in becoming active participants in their healthcare process, ultimately leading to enhanced outcomes and a smoother transition through the surgical process. During the intraoperative phase, there is a significant variation in the roles of perioperative nurses. They closely cooperate with surgeons and anesthesiologists to ensure the operating room is sterile and safe. Their expertise in monitoring vital signs, assisting with surgical instrumentation, and anticipating the needs of the surgical team helps ensure procedural continuity. Effective planning reduces the likelihood of complications, resulting in higher surgical efficiency. Furthermore, the use of interventions such as the COUGH bundle is indicative of the proactive efforts perioperative nurses engage in to prevent postoperative complications, specifically respiratory complications, which are causally associated with rising morbidity and longer hospital stays (Hilton-Christie et al., 2020). Perioperative nurses lead the way in delivering high-quality surgical services through diligent adherence to best practice. In the postoperative phase, the perioperative nurses' function shifts to recovery and education, allowing the patient to be stabilized and discharged. Perioperative nurses assess patients for potential complications, aid in pain control, and educate patients on postoperative care. The teaching component is essential; patients given thorough instructions regarding self-care interventions will have improved recovery rates. For conditions such as ostomy care, successful teaching can yield long-term benefits, as knowledge-enabled patients are well-equipped to effectively manage their conditions (Harris et al., 2019). By also continuously raising awareness and promoting adherence to best practices, perioperative nurses help equip health systems with a safety and quality culture, with patient health at the forefront of the care received in surgery (Figure 2.2).

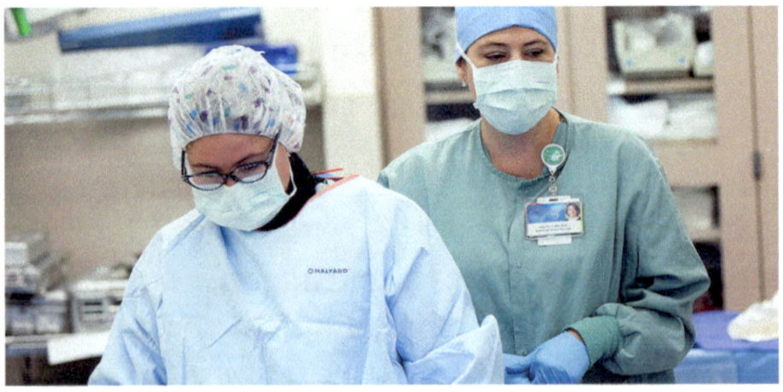

Figure 2.2. Role of perioperative nurses.

Source: https://college.mayo.edu/media/mccms/content-assets/academics/explore-health-care-careers/perioperative-nursing-career-3476002-0005-hero-tablet.jpg.

2.1.1. Responsibilities in the Surgical Team

The operating team comprises various professionals whose interdependent functions are crucial in achieving optimal patient outcomes during perioperative care. They all have different functions that make the successful conclusion of surgical procedures possible, from surgeons to anesthesiologists and nurses. The operating nurse, above all, has a vital role in ensuring a safe environment for operations through equipment preparation, care of surgical instruments, and implementation of patient safety measures. The introduction of a surgical safety checklist, as documented in recent literature, has demonstrated a significant reduction in complications and adverse events, emphasizing the importance of communication and teamwork among surgical team members (Bonner et al., 2011). Through the development of collaboration and the establishment of a shared understanding of each individual's role, operating teams can optimize the collective impact of perioperative practice. Outside technical tasks, emotional and psychological patient care is paramount within the operating room. Operating room staff must establish professional relationships with other staff members and patients, which can alleviate anxiety and increase patient satisfaction. Familiarity among staff and cooperation have been recognized as significantly influencing patients' perceptions and experiences of undergoing surgery (Bonner et al., 2011). The dynamics between members, the assignment of responsibility (such as initiating collaboration between surgeons, nurses, and support staff), can reduce conflicts in surgery and therefore enhance efficiency and safety. The role of the surgical teams must therefore not only be procedure-based but must also involve constructing a supportive environment for patients and colleagues. Moreover, the training and education of perioperative nursing students reveal the key position the practice holds in preparing future surgical teams. Observations by nursing students in Rwandan referral hospitals highlight how clinical placements enable students to apply theoretical knowledge in practice, thereby bridging the gap between classroom learning and practical application. These experiences enhance the students' understanding of surgical roles while promoting a teamwork culture that values cooperation and communication. On this note, the role of the surgical team is developed and established through collaborative experiences, understanding the need for effective partnerships among healthcare facilities and learning institutions. Lastly, professional development in the surgical team is paramount in promoting outstanding patient care along the perioperative journey (Figure 2.3).

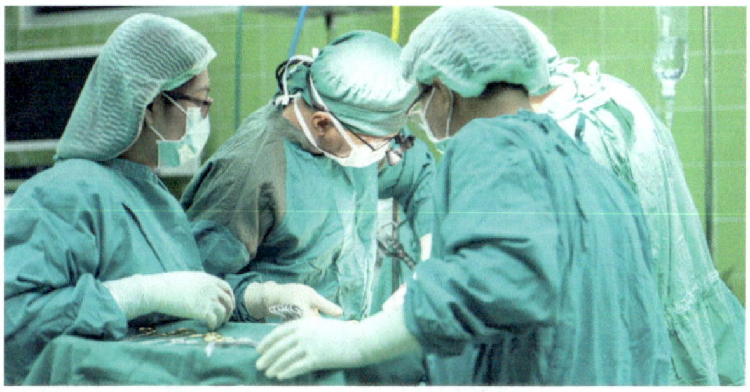

Figure 2.3. Responsibilities in the surgical team.

Source: https://www.betterteam.com/images/operating-room-nurse-job-description-4000x2669-2020122.jpeg?crop=40:21,smart&width=1200&dpr=2&format=pjpg&auto=webp&quality=85&format=jpg&quality=85.

2.1.2. Skills and Qualifications Required

In the dynamic perioperative world, qualification and skill are multifaceted and require both clinical competence and interpersonal skill. Practitioners must possess a thorough knowledge of anatomy, physiology, and surgery to support the adequate care of preoperative and postoperative patients. This is supplemented by further training in anesthesia and pain relief techniques, which are paramount in ensuring the patient's comfort and safety during their ordeal. Additionally, proficiency in the use of medical equipment and technology is crucial, as most modern surgical procedures require advanced tools. Competence in performing thorough assessments enables nurses to identify impending complications earlier, thereby prompting early interventions. Technical competencies plus elementary medical knowledge thus form the foundation of good perioperative care. Critical thinking and problem-solving competence are most essential when dealing with the unpredictable environment of operating rooms. Nurses must be able to analyze complex situations, make informed decisions quickly, and collaborate effectively within multidisciplinary teams to enhance patient outcomes. Communication is also essential, as nurses serve as intermediaries between patients, families, and surgical teams, educating and ensuring everyone's comfort with the procedure. Emotional intelligence is also essential in dispelling surgery fears in patients. Literature suggests that patients desire personalized communication and increased perioperative education, highlighting the need to discuss personal issues before and after surgery (Mooruth et al., 2016). Therefore, nurses must cultivate these soft skills to enable positive patient experiences through the challenging perioperative journey. Finally, ongoing education and professional development are essential components of a successful perioperative nursing career. With ongoing advancements in surgical techniques and technology, nurses must stay current with up-to-date evidence-based practice and emerging trends in the profession. Getting specialized in perioperative nursing via certifications such as those offered by the Association of Perioperative Registered Nurses (AORN) can significantly enhance the credibility and marketability of a nurse. Furthermore, participating in research and contributing to scholarly dialogue can advance the practice of nursing and foster a culture of continuous quality improvement. Likewise, the importance of understanding the complexities of diverse patient populations cannot be overstated, as customized treatment has the potential to significantly improve care outcomes. With the combination of formal education and a commitment to personal growth, perioperative nurses can meet the demands associated with this profession and provide better care to patients, including handling various forms of medications during operations (Bermano et al., 2014).

2.1.3. Impact on Patient Outcomes

For perioperative nursing, the impact on outcomes has been largely contingent upon complete preoperative education. Research has demonstrated that focused pre-surgery education enhances significantly patients' psychological readiness for procedures, particularly those undergoing ostomy surgery. Patients who receive initial education regarding their stoma management, as identified in research, exhibit less post-surgery anxiety. This decreased anxiety enables improved learning environments, allowing patients to acquire more effective self-care. Proper preparation of patients enables nursing practitioners to to influence their long-term adjustment of distorted body images and postoperative care in a significant way. Furthermore, the analgesic process performed during the perioperative period can significantly impact patient outcomes. For instance, the use of epidural analgesia (EDA) in patients undergoing pancreatoduodenectomy has been found to result in positive outcomes. Research has revealed that patients administered EDA not only experienced reduced pain scores but also fewer incidences of several serious complications like unplanned intubation and pulmonary embolism. These findings underscore the importance of vigilant pain management strategies within the perioperative framework, demonstrating how subtle nuances can lead to more effective recovery protocols and lower healthcare expenses, ultimately enhancing overall patient safety and satisfaction. Finally, the preoperative to postoperative continuum requires a focus on individualized patient care tailored to specific medical and psychological needs. As patient ostomy assessments indicate, education accompanied by anxiety control becomes the key to postoperative success. By such studies, lower anxiety via the best pre-operative education is found to result in greater adaptability and better control of home care. In addition, incorporation of newer analgesic regimens, e.g., EDA, further optimizes postoperative recovery. Together, these factors illustrate the profound influence that targeted perioperative nursing interventions have on outcomes in patients, ultimately to enhanced quality of life and effectiveness in healthcare as encapsulated within the perioperative model (Figure 2.4).

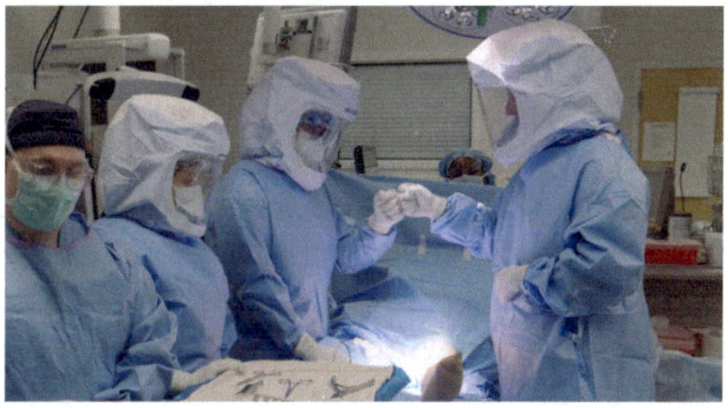

Figure 2.4. Impact on patient outcomes of perioperative nursing.

Source: https://jnj-connectivity.brightspotcdn.com/dims4/default/5a86d85/2147483647/strip/true/crop/800x450+0+0/resize/1200x675!/quality/90/?url=https%3A%2F%2Fjnj-brightspot.s3.amazonaws.com%2Fjnj-connectivity%2F35%2F35%2F2f8f242b4d509816fba9f8d951c3%2Fperioperative-care-promo2.jpeg.

Test Your Knowledge

1. What are the key responsibilities of a perioperative nurse during the intraoperative phase?
2. How do perioperative nurses help ensure patient safety before surgery?

2.2. Preoperative Assessment

Learning Outcome

1. Explain the patient history and physical examination
2. Define the risk assessment and management in perioperative nursing
3. Discuss the patient education and informed consent

In perioperative care, preoperative evaluation is a critical part of ensuring patient safety and optimal surgical outcomes. This stage aims to officially evaluate a patient's history, existing health, and potential risks associated with surgery. During the evaluation, healthcare practitioners have to consider various factors such as comorbidities, medication, and allergies, all key determinants in pre-surgery preparations. A comprehensive preoperative assessment not only identifies acute medical problems but also examines psychological and social issues that may influence a patient's readiness for surgery. By addressing these multidimensional factors, nurses can develop customized interventions that enhance patient well-being and overall perioperative satisfaction. This rigorous approach ultimately lays the groundwork for effective postoperative care, mirroring the inclusion of the preoperative phase within the overall continuum of care. Effective preoperative assessment incorporates educational aspects that have the potential to improve outcomes in patients greatly. An ongoing consideration is the need for pre-surgical education, which is highly effective in reducing patients' levels of anxiety for waiting for surgery. Research identifies that patients receiving extensive preoperative education, particularly those going through ostomy surgery, have considerably reduced anxiety scores compared to patients who are only provided standard education (Harris et al., 2019). This anxiety not only prepares patients psychologically for surgery but also increases their ability to learn needed information regarding postoperative care. In addition, transparent and timely education can lead to enhanced self-management and adaptation to postoperative alteration, thus enhancing a sense of autonomy and competence in patients. By integrating teaching strategies into the preoperative assessment, nurses can significantly influence the psychological readiness and long-term results of their patients. Furthermore, the impact that information technology contributes to the preoperative evaluation process cannot be discounted, as it is a significant contributing element in the improvement of patient assessment accuracy and productivity. The integration of digital technologies enables the cautious collection and analysis of patient data, ultimately leading to more informed decision-making and improved care coordination. With the implementation of combined hospital information systems, care professionals can simplify preoperative processes, reduce complexity, and identify areas for potential improvement more effectively(Daily et al., 2019). This technical advancement not only facilitates proper monitoring of patient status but also provides immediate access to critical information that informs treatment planning. As perioperative practice continues to advance, the integration of IT into preoperative assessment reaffirms the imperative to adopt innovative approaches to optimizing patient-centered care and improving outcomes across the entire spectrum of surgical interventions (Figure 2.5).

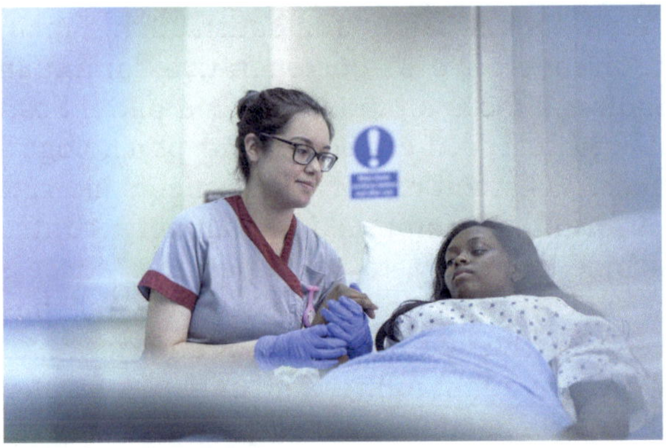

Figure 2.5. Critical importance of pre-operative assessment.

Source: https://www.pasadenauc.com/wp-content/uploads/2024/07/pre-operative-assessment.jpg.

2.2.1. Patient History and Physical Examination

One of the most essential elements of perioperative nursing is getting a thorough patient history and physical examination. Both are crucial beginning steps in establishing a baseline understanding of each patient's unique health status, allowing healthcare professionals to identify potential risks and comorbidities that can influence perioperative care. Thorough Patient histories must include surgeries in the past, current medical illnesses, drug use, and allergies, whereas physical exams provide hints about vital signs and overall health status. Such information is critical to the creation of a patient-centered perioperative care plan that addresses the individual needs and risk factors of the patient. Further assessment can also uncover issues such as opioid addiction or substance abuse, informing pain management and facilitating coordination with addiction specialists when necessary (Bifulco et al., 2017). After the initial evaluation has been performed, a comprehensive preoperative evaluation is crucial to ensure optimal patient safety and outcomes. The preoperative period is utilized to educate patients regarding the surgical process as well as to address any questions that they might have to minimize anxiety and facilitate a more effective perioperative course. Effective preoperative care involves providing written and verbal teaching tailored to the patients' understanding, enabling them to acquire knowledge about the surgical operation, postoperative recovery, and recovery techniques. Documentation of this learning process, as well as the patient's physical examination and medical history, must be completed, as it can serve as a guide for the entire healthcare team throughout the perioperative process (Ijäs et al., 2015).

Thorough scrutiny at this point can ultimately enhance the recovery time, reduce complications, and enable improved utilization of resources in the operating room. Ultimately, incorporation of patient history and physical exam into the model of perioperative nursing is contingent upon establishment of an in-depth understanding of the patient's overall health. Such an understanding sets the direction for effective communication among the interdisciplinary team, enabling collaborative decision-making that maximizes clinical outcomes. Conducting a proper evaluation also enhances the patient's autonomy in his or her care, as he or she becomes a more informed and involved actor in the process of surgery. Moreover, crossing cultural and linguistic barriers to communicate also optimizes the efficiency of patient interactions, removing obstructive obstacles that might be induced by misinterpretation or misunderstanding. Thus, the active process reflected in thorough preoperative assessment is vital for realizing patient safety, satisfaction, and success in the perioperative process (Ijäs et al., 2015; Bifulco et al., 2017) (Figure 2.6).

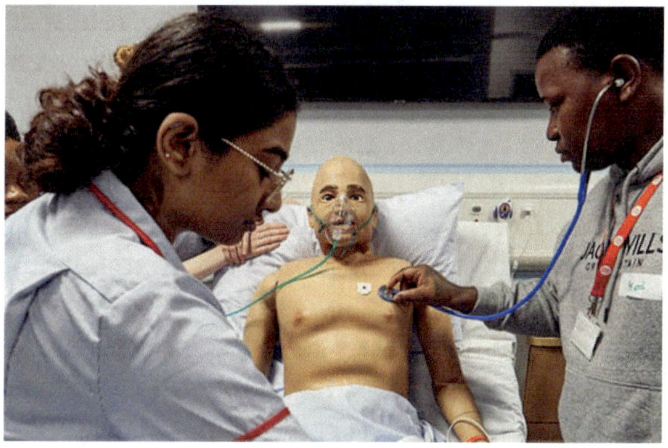

Figure 2.6. History taking and physical assessment.

Source: https://www.solent.ac.uk/media-library/images/courses/postgraduate/course-cards/history-taking-corse-card-min.xea8c2905.jpg.

2.2.2. Risk Assessment and Management

Practical risk assessment and management are part and parcel in perioperative nursing, particularly within the preoperative and postoperative stages of care. In the preoperative stage, individual patient-specific risk factors, including comorbidities, age, and psychological status, are determined and evaluated to facilitate appropriate preparation for the surgical procedure. Preoperative screening alerts the surgical team to potential complications associated with the procedure, facilitating tailored anesthetic and surgical plans. The importance of anesthetic techniques, i.e., epidural analgesia (EDA), has been highlighted in more recent research. EDA has demonstrated a reduction in postoperative complications, such as unplanned intubation and pulmonary embolism, thereby emphasizing the importance of selecting appropriate pain management methods and interventions to minimize risk factors during postoperative recovery (Ceppa et al., 2019). In addition to understanding physiological risks, perioperative nursing must also manage the psychological aspects of patient care. The majority of patients are more anxious than normal preoperatively and can be impaired in their capacity to learn from educational material and adapt to postoperative requirements. Preoperative teaching to address these problems is crucial for effective risk management. It has been shown that patients who have undergone extensive preoperative education demonstrate reduced postoperative anxiety, leading to increased involvement in their own care (Harris et al., 2019). This increased readiness can significantly enhance postoperative outcomes because the patient is better equipped to manage recuperation requirements, from adhering to medication regimens to fulfilling self-care obligations related to the new surgical changes. Following surgery, ongoing risk assessment remains vital as patients recover.

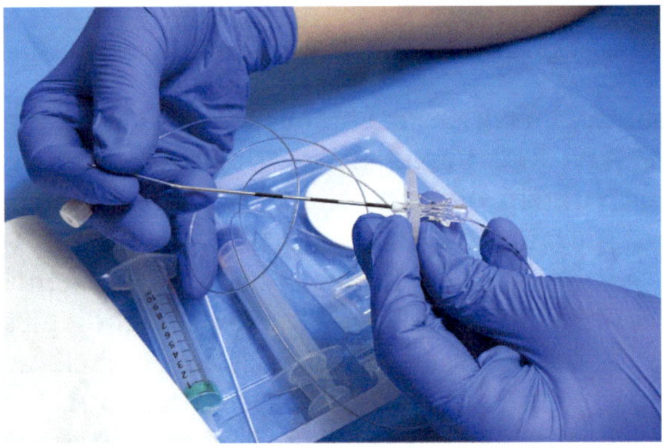

Figure 2.7. Epidural analgesia (EDA).

Source: https://external-content.duckduckgo.com/iu/?u=https%3A%2F%2Fanesthguide.com%2Fwp-content%2Fuploads%2F2023%2F05%2FEDA-set-kateter-genom-nal-demonstration.jpg&f=1&nofb=1&ipt=7ce70fe8348de3d341e490da35d48a92138029d9d9dcfc449e4061bfa7c5ba98.

Continual observation of clinical symptoms and signs enables nursing personnel to detect complications such as wound infections or respiratory disturbances promptly, which, if not immediately treated, can become significant issues. Having a standard policy for monitoring significant postoperative predictors facilitates easier management of potential risks for nurses as well as tailoring interventions based on each patient's needs. Moreover, incorporating multidisciplinary collaboration into the provision of postoperative care fosters co-responsibility for patient outcomes, creating an integrated care setting where risks can be mitigated through collaborative decision-making. Lastly, a combined approach in risk assessment and management throughout the perioperative continuum guarantees enhanced safety and quality of surgical care and provides substantial support towards improved patient outcomes (Figure 2.7).

2.2.3. Patient Education and Informed Consent

Informed consent and patient education in preoperative nursing are integral aspects that directly influence the success of surgery. They are not just ethical necessities but also elements that can enhance patient involvement and satisfaction. Effective patient education involves communicating concise and explicit information about the surgical procedure, associated risks, potential outcomes, and post-surgical treatment. By ensuring patients are well-informed about the entire process, anesthetic options, and recovery periods, nurses empower patients to make educated decisions about their own well-being, which leads to improved compliance and outcomes. The process must begin early enough before surgery to allow for good questions and dialogue, thus establishing a culture of partnership in which patients feel heard and committed to their care. The informed consent process reflects the ethical obligation to respect patient autonomy and to make certain ensure that patients give their consent based on a complete understanding of their treatment options. Perioperative nurses have an obligation to ensure that communication during this process is clear and specific; they must take the time to clarify the patient's understanding, ensuring that any jargon is translated into simple language. Additionally, it decisions free from coercion or misinformation. It is common in nursing practice, appropriate informed consent not only protects the rights of patients but also protects healthcare practitioners against legal action. According to (N/A, 2024), documenting the informed consent process in detail, including the information discussed and questions answered, is one of the most important steps in maintaining continuity and adherence to best practices in the healthcare field. Moreover, patient education and informed consent also extend beyond the preoperative setting; they are essential along the perioperative continuum. The implementation of Enhanced Recovery After Surgery (ERAS) principles, as described in Huang et al. (2025), emphasizes the importance of ongoing patient education after surgery. Patients must understand discharge instructions, recognize signs of potential complications, and be aware of the need for follow-up visits after surgery. By gaining confidence among patients via ongoing education, nurses can facilitate better postoperative compliance and self-management. Such an approach to care lays the foundation for a patient-centered care environment that ultimately leads to improved recovery patterns, reduced hospital stays, and overall patient satisfaction, eventually validating the central role of perioperative nursing in guaranteeing the best surgical outcomes.

Test Your Knowledge

1. Why is it important to evaluate a patient's medical history during the preoperative assessment?
2. What are typical components included in a standard preoperative assessment?

2.3. Preoperative Preparation

Learning Outcome

1. Explain the surgical site preparation
2. Define the medication management
3. Describe the psychological support for patients

Preoperative preparation is a key component of perioperative nursing, with the overall objective of having well-informed and ready patients for surgery. Preparation can range from the distribution of information materials to psychological interventions intended to cope with preoperative anxiety. Caregivers must ensure that they screen for patients' special needs because fear and anxiety have a significant impact on surgical outcomes. Evidence indicates that individually focused interventions, such as preoperative psychological preparation programs, are effective in reducing anxiety levels. By delivering matched information and directly involving patients and their families, healthcare professionals can maximize overall satisfaction with the surgical encounter, ultimately leading to better health outcomes (Ben-Amitay et al., 2018). Thus, systematic and individualized preoperative preparations are crucial in establishing a supportive climate that can alleviate preoperative distress. Effective Preoperative preparation is based on effective communication to inform and develop trust between clinicians and patients. Clinicians must provide clear and explicit information to patients during this stage about the surgical procedure, anesthesia, and recovery. This educational dialogue not only prepares patients for what is to come but also allows them to become active participants in their own treatment. Furthermore, for those patients with a background of chronic pain or opioid dependence, being informed of their own personal pharmacologic profiles is paramount. Identification of such comorbidities through preoperative screening can facilitate planning overall pain control strategies that mitigate the challenges of opioid tolerance and dependence (Bifulco et al., 2017). In the same vein, building an open communication culture can the quality of preoperative care and establishing the ground for effective postoperative recovery.

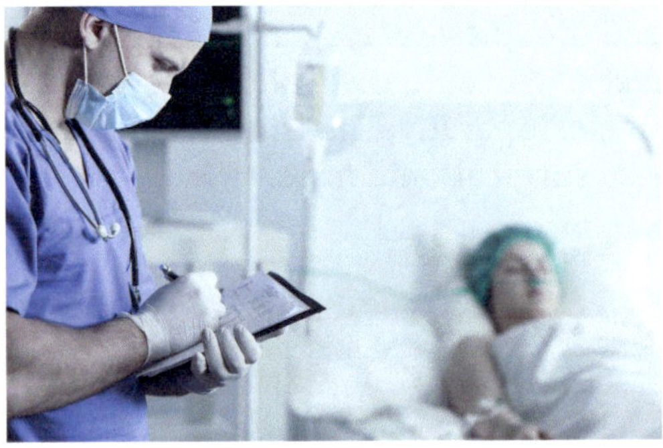

Figure 2.8. Preoperative preparation.

Source: https://www.verywellhealth.com/thmb/YbYKpd0JpktUmEycSd92qNhWjCQ=/1500x0/filters:no_upscale():max_bytes(150000):strip_icc()/iStock_72742951_XXLARGE-5764b8093df78ca6e42d0b8e.jpg.

In addition to its strengths and weaknesses, it is notable that the approach encompasses multidisciplinary perspectives in preoperative preparation, acknowledging that the outcome is predicated on a joint effort between multidisciplinary healthcare professionals. Multidisciplinary contributions by anesthesiologists, surgeons, nurses, and mental health professionals can be pivotal towards the accomplishment of customized care plans encompassing physical as well as psychological aspects of care. For instance, anesthesiologists would assess comorbidities and requirements of pain control, while mental health professionals would provide needed emotional support. There is evidence that preoperative preparation of both educational and therapeutic nature can reduce anxiety significantly and enhance patients' coping (Ben-Amitay et al., 2018). By adopting a multidisciplinary approach, healthcare teams are in a better position to optimize patient readiness, promote recovery, and deliver comprehensive care throughout the perioperative process (Figure 2.8).

2.3.1. Surgical Site Preparation

Adequate perioperative surgical site preparation is essential in minimizing the risk of surgical site infection (SSI), a frequent complication seen in 10-20% of procedures. The perioperative nurses' participation during surgical site preparation is necessary to ensure evidence-based practices deliver maximum patient safety. Recent advancements have highlighted the use of preoperative showering or bathing with antiseptic agents, yet their efficacy remains controversial. But application of 2% chlorhexidine in alcoholic skin preparations has also demonstrated a stunning reduction in SSI rates and is thus a mandatory component of surgeons' preparatory regimen (Astagneau et al., 2015). Strict adherence to these rules by nurses will enable them to ensure improved patient outcomes and establish a safety culture within the operating room. Moreover, a critical examination of patient-related factors is an essential ingredient of successful surgical site preparation. Preoperative evaluation should address risk factors such as diabetes, obesity, and current or history of infection that put patients at risk of SSIs. Care also needs to be taken concerning how opioid-tolerant patients are managed since inadequate pain control can complicate the surgical procedure. Their needs should be addressed through consultations with anesthesiologists and addiction medicine professionals to ensure their optimum perioperative care (Bifulco et al., 2017). This multi-disciplinary process guarantees not only that the operative site is well prepared, but also that the entire perioperative experience is optimized, and both are less anxious and recover faster. Finally, strict adherence to evidence-based care bundles is necessary to guarantee maintenance of consistent standards of operative site preparation. Examples of these bundles include preoperative regimes such as antibiotic prophylaxis, intraoperative normothermia, and glycemic control in a bid to further reduce the risk for SSIs. Application of negative pressure wound therapy post-operation has also gained popularity as a successful intervention to close surgical wounds (Astagneau et al., 2015). Perioperative nursing staff receiving ongoing education and training in best evidence-based practices will ensure a culture of excellence in surgical care and improve patient outcomes. By putting topmost priority on surgical site preparation, healthcare teams can collectively guard patients' health and enhance the efficacy of surgical procedures (Figure 2.9).

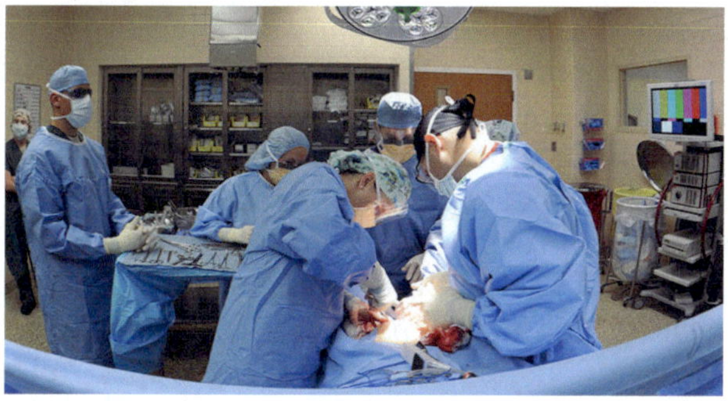

Figure 2.9. Perioperative nursing surgery center.

Source: https://www.myamericannurse.com/wp-content/uploads/2017/08/perioperative-nursing-surgery-center3.jpg.

2.3.2. Medication Management

Efficient medication management is a critical practice within perioperative nursing, with the effects extending to patient outcomes from preoperative to postoperative discharge. Precise identification of medication history, including all present conditions and treatments, allows practitioners to identify potential drug interactions and demand dosage changes. Pain management and minimizing complications are the primary goals at this stage. This involves a multidisciplinary crew in which anesthesiologists, surgeons, and nurses come together to create a tailored medicine approach that addresses individual patient needs. One example is the use of epidural analgesia (EDA), which is highly sought because it reduces postoperative discomfort and complications, as evidenced in studies showing lower rates of postoperative wound disruption and pulmonary complications among EDA patients compared to those who do not receive EDA (Ceppa et al., 2019). Postoperative medication management is also crucial, as effective pain management is related to patient satisfaction and rate of recovery. Intraoperative analgesia to postoperative pain management transition necessitates an extremely cautious reassessment of medications ordered. Medications need to be adjusted to prevent undertreatment or overtreatment, especially in patients with prior opioid exposure. Challenges arise due to the possibility of opioid tolerance and the associated phenomena of physical dependence and hyperalgesia, which necessitate that the entire surgical and nursing staff have an understanding of these phenomena (Bifulco et al., 2017). Preemptive strategies must include multimodal analgesia methods for pain reduction and lessening opioid consumption, hence enhancing recovery without enhancing the possibility of opioid-related complications. Ongoing monitoring of medication safety and effectiveness is also central to perioperative nursing care. The patient should receive education on their medications, dosing routine, and potential side effects, which enhances compliance and helps avoid complications. After surgery, the health care provider should be vigilant to monitor for evidence of opioid abuse or withdrawal in patients with a history of opioid use disorder. Coordination with mental health specialists and addiction experts can be achieved to offer comprehensive management to such high-risk patients (Bifulco et al., 2017).

During the patient's recovery process, the drug needs may have to be modified based on ongoing assessment of pain intensity and recovery function, ultimately resulting in a comprehensive and successful perioperative course (Figure 2.10).

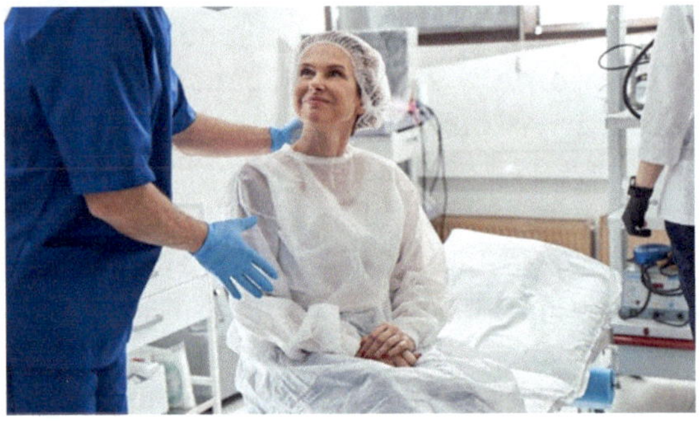

Figure 2.10. Perioperative medication management.

Source: https://www.pharmacist.com/Portals/0/EasyDNNNews/1218/images/0123_PT_42-525-350-p-L-97.jpg.

2.3.3. Psychological Support for Patients

Supporting the psychological well-being of patients through surgical procedures is a vital component of perioperative nursing, having an impact on both the short-term surgical process and long-term recovery. Anxiety before surgery can hinder the learning mechanisms involved in postoperative self-management since high levels of stress might impair attention and retention of essential information. For instance, ostomy surgery patients often encounter a cluster of emotions, including body image distortion, fear, and adjusting to a new illness. According to studies, preoperative education to minimize anxiety and equip the patient with an understanding of the reality of adapting to an ostomy helps significantly towards success following surgery and emotional well-being. With the delivery of holistic education coupled with directed psychological care, perioperative nurses can induce an ideal learning environment, which will further enhance patient outcomes and quality of life after surgery (Harris et al., 2019). Pain management patients, who may be opioid-tolerant, need a refined psychological care approach. As opioid dependents have several unique challenges common to them, including excessive anxiety regarding pain control and withdrawal anxiety, these patients must be adequately screened and managed by perioperative care providers with particular interventions. Psychological counseling is warranted in treating these conditions, resulting in greater knowledge regarding the comorbidities and psycho-social history of the patients. Effective perioperative care measures should, in turn, encompass a multidisciplinary cooperative approach by anesthesiologists, surgeons, and nurses to identify high-risk patients and provide holistic care, such as referral to addiction specialists on an as-needed basis. An integrated approach can lead to improved pain management strategies, thus improving patient satisfaction and recovery outcomes (Bifulco et al., 2017). Moreover, psychological care does not end with preoperative assessment and instruction; it also plays a crucial part in fostering resilience within the postoperative phase. Postsurgical patients can experience a variety of emotional responses, including depression, anxiety, and isolation. Continuous psychological care, through follow-up visits and support groups, helps patients deal with the psychological aftereffects of their surgical interventions. The development of targeted interventions, such as cognitive behavior therapy or mindfulness exercises, may also enhance emotional resilience. As patients learn to modify their lifestyle or adapt to chronic illness, consistent psychological assistance based on empathic nursing practice is necessary to make adaptation and healing recovery easier. The constant assistance materializes the significant role of integrated psychological care in enhancing overall patient-focused practice within perioperative nursing (Harris et al., 2019).

Test Your Knowledge

1. What instructions are typically given to patients regarding fasting before surgery?
2. Why is patient education important during preoperative preparation?

2.4. Intraoperative Nursing Care

Learning Outcome

1. Identify the monitoring of vital signs and anesthesia
2. Define maintaining a sterile environment
3. Describe the communication with the surgical team

Intraoperative nursing care is a crucial component of the broader field of perioperative nursing, encompassing patient care from the preoperative period through to postoperative recovery. Intraoperative nurses are responsible during surgery for multitasking and working alongside surgical teams to ensure that the operation runs smoothly and safely. Some of the most essential jobs involve providing a sterile environment, sterilizing and monitoring surgical devices, and ensuring the medical equipment is in good working order. The high-energy requirements of operating rooms demand rigorous attentiveness as well as responsiveness, as the nurses must address any adverse complications or changes in the patient's condition. Such attention is not only but also crucial for patient safety and for optimal surgical outcomes, as emphasized by clinical practice guidelines highlighting systematic intraoperative procedures for various surgical procedures (Irani et al., 2022). Additionally, utilizing ERPs in the intraoperative time reflects a progressive approach to surgical care focused on patient-oriented outcomes. ERPs are a set of evidence-based interventions designed to reduce postoperative complications and facilitate easier recovery. Intraoperative fluid management is one such area in which nurses are taught to observe fluid status and provide fluids cautiously to maintain hemodynamic stability, for example. Evidence indicates that optimal intraoperative fluid handling can lower postoperative complications such as acute kidney injury and myocardial injury, in line with guidelines suggested by senior surgical societies (Davis et al., 2022). In fulfilling the requisite enhanced recovery measures, intraoperative nurses play a crucial role in creating an environment that supports patients' quicker recovery and shorter hospital stays. Another significant aspect of intraoperative nursing practice is its effective communication and collaboration among surgical team members. Within high-risk operating theaters, effective communication enables all players to be on the same wavelength regarding the patient's care plan and any emerging complications during the procedure. Nursing practitioners facilitate the exchange of important information among anesthesiologists, surgeons, and other healthcare providers, ultimately creating a collaborative environment that enhances patient safety. Additionally, intraoperative nurses often serve as the patient's initial line of defense, as they monitor vital signs, levels of anesthesia, and overall well-being during surgery. This is indicative of the diverse nature of intraoperative nursing, which impacts not only the critical surgical moment but also long-term success in surgery by ensuring patients receive holistic care (Davis et al., 2022; Irani et al., 2022) (Figure 2.11).

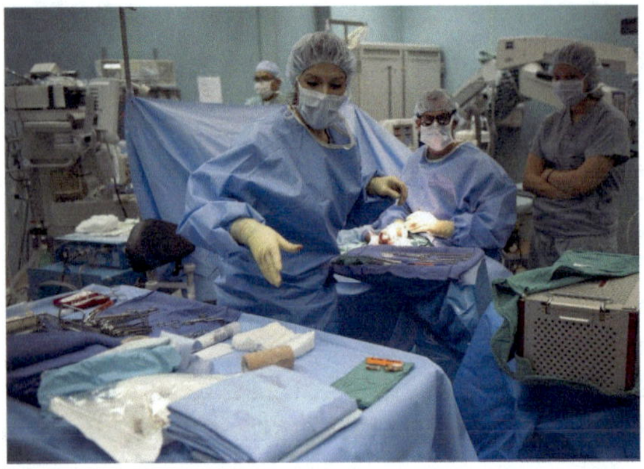

Figure 2.11. Intraoperative nursing care.

Source: https://wtcs.pressbooks.pub/app/uploads/sites/47/2023/12/medicine_medical_surgery_nurse_doctor_physician_operation_operating-1135815-1024x749.jpg.

2.4.1. Monitoring Vital Signs and Anesthesia

Accurate monitoring of vital signs is extremely critical during anesthesia, as it is directly linked to surgical success and patient safety. Monitoring typically involves continuous measurement of parameters such as heart rate, blood pressure, oxygen saturation, and respiratory rate. These vital signs are critical indicators of the patient's physiological state, allowing anesthesiologists and nurses to identify any adverse changes at an early stage. With better monitoring technology, data is captured in real time, and a response to any deviation from the normal can be taken instantly. Anesthesia management now includes sophisticated systems that integrate vital signs into comprehensive anesthesia information management systems (AIMS) to improve patient care and access to information. These advances are pivotal in coordinating the multidisciplinary responsibility in the operating room, where appropriate communication and the timely exchange of information are necessary to ensure the comfort of patients during the surgical period (Joseph et al., 2020). Anesthesiologists employ a balanced approach to general anesthesia, whereby several agents are administered simultaneously for synergistic action, maximizing effectiveness while limiting side effects. This method, multimodal general anesthesia, greatly reduces doses of single agents required and, thus, prevents likely side effects associated with opiates as well as other anesthetic agents. Continuous monitoring of vital signs during the procedure is essential, as it enables proper titration of anesthetic agents based on individual patient needs. Inclusion of advanced monitors provides invaluable information regarding postoperative pain and nociception, guiding clinicians in anesthesia-based interventions related to the operation. In addition, through their monitoring of patient response to inhaled agents, clinicians can dynamically adjust doses to maximize therapy while ensuring patient safety (Brown et al., 2018). Postoperatively, continuous monitoring of vital signs remains integral to successful recovery management. Patients may exhibit a variety of physiological responses on coming out of related to anesthesia with which require constant monitoring to keep vital signs stable before discharge from the recovery room. With the changes in blood pressure, heart rate, or respiratory status that occur during the recovery period, continuous assessment is needed to identify emerging complications and take action.. In addition, proper management of pain pathways used intraoperatively, such as the use of multimodal analgesia, can significantly influence postoperative recovery. Monitoring of the vital signs facilitates early intervention, whereby pain relief is optimized without enhancing opioid dependency, potentially exacerbating the current opioid overuse epidemic. Thus, through precise monitoring and assessment, perioperative nursing can facilitate a more secure postoperative state and best overall patient outcomes (Joseph et al., 2020) (Figure 2.12).

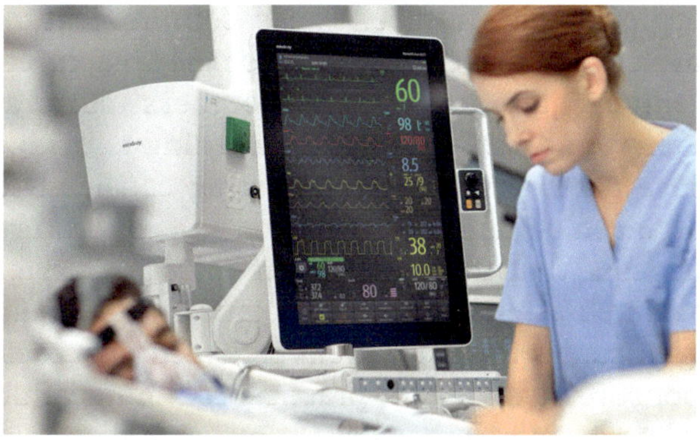

Figure 2.12. Intraoperative monitoring (IOM).

Source: https://www.mindray.com/content/dam/xpace/en_us/blog/patient-monitoring-pacu/6_Innov_Card_Component_894x566_PC.jpg.

2.4.2. Maintaining a Sterile Environment

Maintaining a sterile setup is crucial in perioperative nursing and forms the foundation for minimizing the potential for infection during surgery. Sterility cannot be overrated, for any slight compromise can lead to serious postoperative complications like wound infections and that could prolong a hospital stay. There are successful techniques of sterilization that encompass not only the surgical tools in isolation but also encapsulate the entire surgical site, including preparation of patients' skin and the environment as well. The protection of the patient's health is aided by the use of sterile protocols, such as surgical hand scrub, utilization of sterilized drapes, and personal protective equipment. Furthermore, education and training of nurses on a regular basis in the latest advancements in sterilization technology and optimal practices are essential to ensure effectiveness in always maintaining a sterile environment in the perioperative process. The application of Enhanced Recovery After Surgery (ERAS) principles significantly enhances the handling of a sterile environment. Incorporating these guidelines will enable perioperative nursing to optimize recovery while ensuring sterile conditions. In procedures such as total knee arthroplasty, the addition of ERAS protocols emphasizes preoperative education, fluid resuscitation, and ideal postoperative care protocols, which collectively contribute to a more controlled environment (*see* Huang et al., 2025). A major aspect of ERAS is also the preemptive action taken to decrease surgical stress, which not only lowers complications but also preserves the cleanliness of the operating field. Thus, a culture that emphasizes meticulous pre- and postoperative assessment enables the early detection and correction of any flaw that jeopardizes sterility, thereby optimizing patient outcomes overall and fostering a culture of increased safety among the surgical staff. In addition, emphasizing the importance of a meticulous preoperative assessment is crucial in maintaining a sterile environment throughout the entire perioperative period. A clear understanding of each patient's individual medical history and potential risk factors enables the implementation of individualized interventions to minimize exposure to harmful contaminants. In pediatric patients, for instance, as evidenced in neonatal care with complex conditions like biliary atresia, the nursing staff's role involves more than ordinary protocols but also includes special care to address complex concerns (*see* Zhang et al., 2025). Lastly, maintaining an atmosphere of sterility through close attention by nurses is a necessary safeguard, ensuring the delivery of the finest type of care from preoperative assessment to postoperative convalescence.

2.4.3. Communication with the Surgical Team

Effective communication with the surgical team is a core skill in perioperative nursing that significantly contributes to patient-level outcomes. Effective operation relies on seamless coordination between surgeons, anesthesiologists, nurses, and other team members. Correct communication of significant facts enhances not only care coordination but also fosters problem-solving in a team setting. Establishing open lines of communication encourages the sharing of vital patient information, ensuring that all team members are aware of the individual's special needs and potential complications. This collaborative atmosphere is particularly valuable in high-stress scenarios where rapid decision-making is necessary to impact the safety and success of the surgery, ultimately optimizing overall patient care and outcomes. Apart from that, education is also crucial in facilitating good communication within the surgical team. Preoperative education equips nurses with the knowledge necessary to communicate with the patients and the surgical team effectively. Through evidence-based educational interventions such as pre-surgical lectures or simulation training, nurses gain the knowledge they need to communicate patient concerns and relay pertinent information effectively. Not only do educational programs enhance the confidence of perioperative nursing staff members, but they also improve overall team skills in managing postoperative recovery and patient anxiety. Such a conceptual framework is reinforced by evidence that demonstrates better team member communication being correlated with reduced patient anxiety and high care satisfaction, and, therefore, highlights the importance of developing an educated nursing staff. In addition, communication barriers must be overcome in establishing an interdependent surgical team culture. These communication barriers may be due to hierarchical structures, technical jargon, or team members' cultural backgrounds. By continually working to bridge these gaps, perioperative nursing can lead to enhanced patient education and care. Literature suggests that adapting communication styles to match clinician-patient relationships could significantly impact patient satisfaction scores. Sponsored training in , practical communication skills not only empowers the surgical team but also enhances the patient experience, as they feel heard and are included in their care. Overall, a commitment to advancing communication in the surgical setting has significant implications for clinical effectiveness and patient-centered care, ultimately resulting in successful surgery (Figure 2.13).

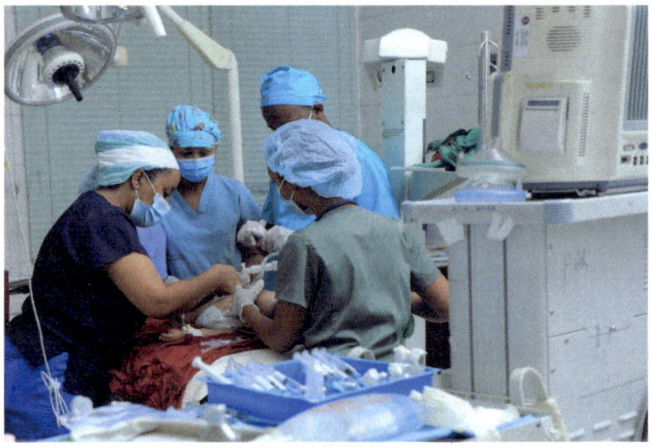

Figure 2.13. Strengthening surgical teamwork.

Source: https://www.lifebox.org/wp-content/uploads/2022/08/TikurAnbessaORTeamEthiopia.jpg.

Test Your Knowledge

1. What is the role of the scrub nurse during surgery?
2. How do circulating nurses help maintain a sterile environment in the operating room?

2.5. Postoperative Care

Learning Outcome

1. Describe the immediate recovery monitoring
2. Define the pain management strategies
3. Discuss the prevention of complications during the perioperative period

Ideal Postoperative care is a crucial component of perioperative nursing that is central to patient recovery and outcome. It begins immediately after the procedure and encompasses a comprehensive array of nursing interventions aimed at preventing complications and promoting healing. Some of the key problems in postoperative care include the risk of venous thromboembolism (VTE), which is most prevalent among those who have undergone primary operations. Studies have indicated that correct risk stratification and individualized prophylactic care are required to prevent this risk, as many of the patients are usually old geriatric or have prolonged postoperative immobilization (Kara, 2025). With the deployment of pharmacological and non-pharmacological measures, nurses play a vital role in the and protection of patients during this vulnerable period, thereby enabling better recovery and quality of life. The postoperative ward is a dynamic setting where interdisciplinary teamwork plays a key role in maximizing patient outcomes. Nurses continually monitor vital signs and assess for any evidence of complications such as infection, bleeding, or respiratory compromise. The implementation of formal rehabilitation programs in the postoperative period has also come into focus as a means of enhancing recovery times, particularly in patients undergoing thoracic surgery. Evidence suggests that incorporating pulmonary rehabilitation into postoperative care can considerably alleviate pulmonary complications and reduce hospital stays (Xu et al., 2024). It reflects the importance of adopting a holistic attitude, as nurses not only deal with physical recovery but also with emotional recovery, thereby serving the whole range of patient needs. Education of the patient is a crucial part of postoperative care, enabling patients to become actively involved in their recovery process. Providing clear information regarding medication adherence, pain control, wound care, and recognizing early complications is crucial in enabling informed patients. Furthermore, effective communication between the providers and patients facilitates a favorable environment, ensures compliance with postoperative instructions, and enhances patient satisfaction. As a result, this education reduces the likelihood of readmission and complications, thereby cementing the value of intensive postoperative care provided by nursing tailored to each patient's unique needs. Through attention to these details, nurses ensure that the transition between home and hospital goes more smoothly, which in turn promotes better long-term health (Figure 2.14).

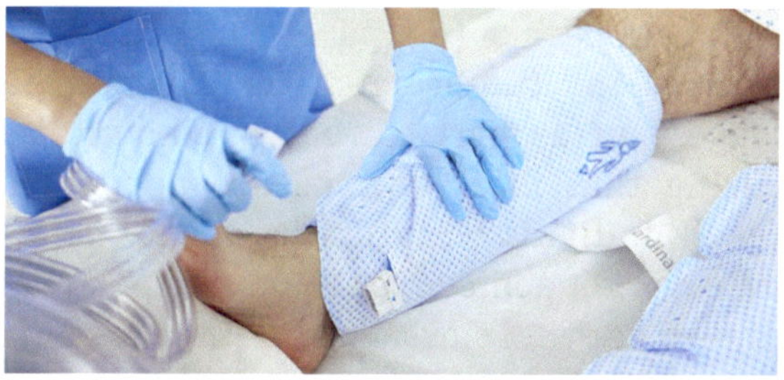

Figure 2.14. VTE prevention best practices.

Source: https://www.cardinalhealth.com/content/dam/corp/web/images/essential-insights/article-thumbnail/essential-insights-vte-best-practices-042424.jpg.

2.5.1. Immediate Recovery Monitoring

Routine recovery monitoring is an essential aspect of perioperative nursing after surgery. The monitoring during the immediate postoperative recovery phase directly affects the short-term and long-term recovery outcomes of the patient.

During this time, vital signs, pain, and reactions to anesthesia are closely monitored by healthcare professionals to ensure patient stability before they are transferred to a more permanent post-operative setting. Effective monitoring can significantly reduce the risk of complications, such as respiratory distress or hypotension, that could result from anesthetic agents or surgical intervention. Nurses can promptly detect abnormalities by using standardized protocols and implement effective interventions, thereby improving overall safety and patient satisfaction. In addition to monitoring vital signs, rapid recovery also requires an accurate assessment of the pain management plan. The use of modalities such as epidural analgesia (EDA) has been promising for decreasing postoperative pain as well as associated complications. Pancreatoduodenectomies data analysis showed that patients treated with EDA had lower incidences of adverse outcomes such as wound disruption and unplanned intubations compared to patients not treated with this form of analgesia (Ceppa et al., 2019). This addresses the requirement for tailored pain management as part of recovery monitoring, ensuring that interventions are appropriate to each individual patient's needs. This is necessary to achieve optimal recovery and minimize hospital stays. Furthermore, real-time recovery monitoring must include interventions to prevent perioperative hypothermia (PIH), which can cause serious complications following surgery. The implementation of a Thermal Care Bundle can potentially significantly improve prevention and early detection of PIH through risk assessment, temperature measurement, and the use of active warming techniques (Alexander et al., 2017). However, while the bundle supported better care practices, findings indicated that it was still not low enough in PIH incidence, demonstrating the complexity of this problem. Systematic continuous recovery observation, therefore, calls for a multifaceted intervention that spans prudent monitoring, successful analgesia, and judicious management of temperature regulation, underscoring the multilateral roles of perioperative nursing towards the creation of best patient outcomes.

2.5.2. Pain Management Strategies

Proper pain management methods rank at the forefront of the perioperative nursing cycle from preoperative assessment to postoperative recuperation. Perhaps the most utilized method is that of epidural analgesia (EDA), which has been noted as a successful approach for the reduction of postoperative pain. Studies reveal that EDA is associated with less wound disruption, fewer unplanned intubations, and improved overall pain scores following operations such as pancreatoduodenectomy. In fact, findings indicate that patients undergoing EDA treatment developed significantly less pain during the first three postoperative days compared to those receiving other pain treatment options, testifying to its worth in achieving maximum pain control in this crucial period of healing. The clinical relevance of these observations provides a rationale for the inclusion of EDA as a cornerstone of the management of surgical pain, particularly in high-risk patient populations where pain control can directly affect outcome (Ceppa et al., 2019). In addition to regional analgesia modalities like EDA, the complexity of pain management in patients with a history of opioid use or abuse poses unique challenges to healthcare providers. The growing incidence of opioid hyperalgesia and tolerance in chronic pain patients complicates postoperative pain management plans. Surgeons, anesthesiologists, and nurses must be sensitive to the signs of opioid dependence in preoperative assessment and modify their analgesic plans as a result. This includes stringent screenings for comorbidities, risk of withdrawal, and needs for altered medication regimens. By integrating multidisciplinary methods that involve surgical teams and addiction experts, clinicians can develop better-adapted pain management plans that suit the specific needs of opioid-tolerant patients. Thus, proper planning minimizes poor pain control and complications related to opioid abuse (Bifulco et al., 2017). In the postoperative period, application of multimodal analgesic plans can enhance pain management outcomes. This approach combines pharmacologic and non-pharmacologic treatments to provide comprehensive pain relief with lowered opioid dependence. Treatment may involve the application of non-steroidal anti-inflammatory medications (NSAIDs), acetaminophen, and adjuvants such as gabapentinoids, along with physical therapy measures aimed at maximizing mobility and alleviating pain and discomfort. This approach not only effectively relieves pain but can also lower opioid consumption, thereby minimizing opioid side effects and complications. With current research favoring the optimization of pain care to improve surgical outcomes, the synthesis of multimodal approaches in postoperative therapy underscores the evolving nature of perioperative nursing in providing comprehensive, patient-focused care during the recovery process (Ceppa et al., 2019) (Figure 2.15).

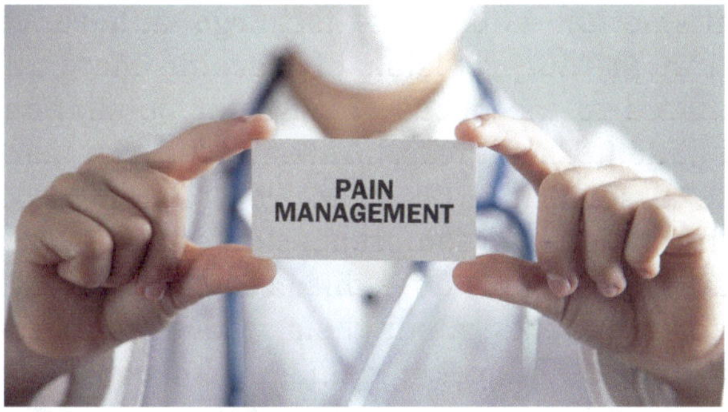

Figure 2.15. Interventional pain management treatment.

Source: https://images.squarespace-cdn.com/content/v1/5c828369d7819e1d4056a49f/1652084255467-00NGI4IKXB92BWXQSJA9/Doctor+holding+card.jpg.

2.5.3. Prevention of Complications

Prevention of perioperative complications is of utmost importance in ensuring patient safety and facilitating a smooth recovery. Various methods have been devised, and measures have been instituted to prevent postoperative complications, particularly respiratory complications, which are common and costly. Literature indicates the rate of postoperative respiratory complications ranges from 1% to 23% (Hilton-Christie et al., 2020). Adoption of protocols with an organized strategy, such as the COUGH bundle, has proven effective in preventing these complications from arising. The COUGH bundle promotes practices such as deep breathing, oral care, patient education, ambulation, and head-of-bed elevation, all of which contribute to improved lung function. Evidence suggests that, when used routinely, these interventions can significantly reduce incidence of conditions like pneumonia and unplanned intubation, hence reducing overall hospital stays and associated healthcare costs. Another essential element in complication prevention for perioperative nursing is the management of inadvertent hypothermia (PIH). Maintenance of normothermia during surgery is not only for patient comfort but to avoid major complications such as increased surgical bleeding, infection risk, and cardiac complications (Alexander et al., 2017). Implementation of the Thermal Care Bundle, such as risk assessment, temperature assessment, and active warming, is a preventive strategy to reduce the incidence of PIH. While one study found improved compliance with such practices, the overall incidence of PIH was unchanged after the implementation. The observation may indicate a need for quality improvement plan, including education and training of nurses, so that these guidelines are adhered to strictly and that the patients derive maximum benefit from enhanced thermal management. In the broader context of perioperative care, vigilance in avoiding complications extends beyond respiratory complications and hypothermia. A comprehensive approach towards patient care requires focus and coordination among surgical groups, anesthesiologists, and nurses. Coordination is crucial in identifying high-risk patients, as well as in the effective implementation of individualized care plans. Continuing education, regular audits, and quality improvement initiatives can enhance compliance with safety measures and significantly improve health outcomes. By creating a safety culture that focuses on standardizing best practices, health professionals can reduce the incidence of preventable conditions and intervention-related complications in surgery. This wide-ranging approach not only increases patient outcomes but also supports the quality of perioperative nursing care.

Test Your Knowledge

1. What are common complications that nurses monitor for after surgery?
2. Why is pain assessment important in the postoperative period?

2.6. Patient Education and Discharge Planning

Learning Outcome

1. Describe the instructions for home care
2. Define the follow-up appointments and resources in perioperative nursing
3. Identify the importance of patient engagement

Effective patient education and discharge planning are crucial components of perioperative nursing, having a significant impact on patient outcomes throughout the surgical continuum. Preoperative education prepares patients both mentally and physically for surgery, reducing anxiety and enhancing their potential to care for themselves postoperatively. Notably, studies indicate that educated patients adapt better to changes following surgical operations, for instance, those involving ostomy formation, in which specialized training is required for coping with long-term and emotional adaptation. Incorporating systematic education sessions with hands-on care practices and anticipated outcome information, nurses can develop knowledge that reduces post-operative complications and enhances overall health (Harris et al., 2019). Discharge planning is equally essential to continuity of care and patient satisfaction, pointing to the importance of effective communication among patients and healthcare providers. Research has established that modifiable factors, such as the quality of clinician-patient interaction and the information delivered, have a significant impact on patient satisfaction and post-discharge adherence. Through the provision of learning materials tailored to the needs of different populations of patients, healthcare professionals can make the association between complex medical information and comprehension on the part of patients. Not only does this proactive approach inform patients about their recovery process, but it also, induces a feeling of empowerment and ownership of their outcomes (Fortier et al., 2019). Additionally, a focus on the psychological aspects of patient education is essential for maximizing discharge planning. Anxiety levels can significantly impact the ability of a patient to learn and participate actively in their own care. Through the incorporation of psychological evaluations into preoperative assessment, nurses can determine those at greater risk for anxiety and take appropriate interventions. Having pre-operative education specifically for such cases as ostomies has been shown to alleviate post-op anxiety, thus equipping patients with information enabling them to create proper self-care. Therefore, an empowered and educated patient is more likely to adhere to directed postoperative care, resulting in a less complicated recovery and fewer opportunities for complications upon discharge from the hospital to return home (Harris et al., 2019) (Figure 2.16).

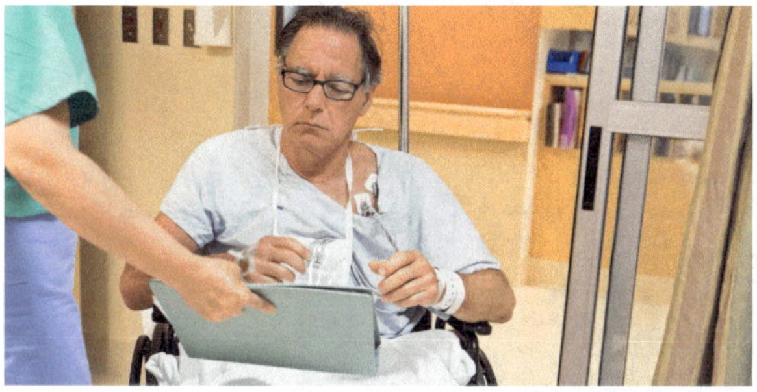

Figure 2.16. Nurses when performing patient discharge education.

Source: https://media.nurse.org/cache/b0/5d/b05d31c43a82f2fd098c6c79a7bdbce4.png.

2.6.1. Instructions for Home Care

Comprehensive and clear home care instructions are critical in perioperative nursing to facilitate a smooth transition from hospital to home recovery. After surgery, the patients might be susceptible due to anesthesia and surgical trauma itself. Accordingly, it is crucial to educate them comprehensively on wound care, adherence to medication, and signs of potential complications. This includes educating patients on how to dress and cleanse operating wounds, managing pain with medication, and staying active to prevent severe side effects such as deep vein thrombosis. By educating the patient with the skills and equipment needed to maximize their recovery, medical practitioners can significantly reduce the likelihood of acquiring postoperative complications. Evidence has shown that clear post-discharge instructions correlate with higher satisfaction rates and better health outcomes, indicating the necessity of structured home care education within the perioperative setting. Additionally, the use of evidence-based practices in postoperative home care instructions can provide maximum patient recovery. Adopting guidelines such as the Enhanced Recovery After Surgery (ERAS) principles helps instruct patients on early mobilization and proper hydration. These techniques not only alleviate pain but also facilitate overall healing, allowing patients to recover sooner. For instance, patients who are knowledgeable about early transfer are more likely to participate in rehabilitation exercises, which are vital for recovering strength and preventing complications. These methods are backed up by research, which indicates that ERAS methods lead to impressive decreases in postoperative complications and hospital length of stay (Huang et al., 2025). This provides evidence that proper implementation of formalized home care protocols that encompass these proven strategies is warranted. Moreover, the psychological aspects of postoperative care should not be overlooked when providing recommendations for home care instructions. Patients are also prone to may have fear about recovering alone, and this can detract from the recovery process. Providing direct instructions that include not only physical recovery, but also emotional support mechanisms can help instill confidence in patients to recover within prescribed guidelines. For instance, by encouraging the establishment of a support system—through family and friends, or community outreach—patients feel more supported and have a positive recovery outcome. Additionally, preoperative teaching about the expected postoperative course can help prepare patients psychologically for the transition, making the hospital-to-home transition smoother. Such a holistic strategy has proven effective in reducing postoperative complications and enhancing overall patient satisfaction (Xu et al., 2024). It reflects that accurate home care teaching is crucial for empowering patients as self-managers in their recovery (Figure 2.17).

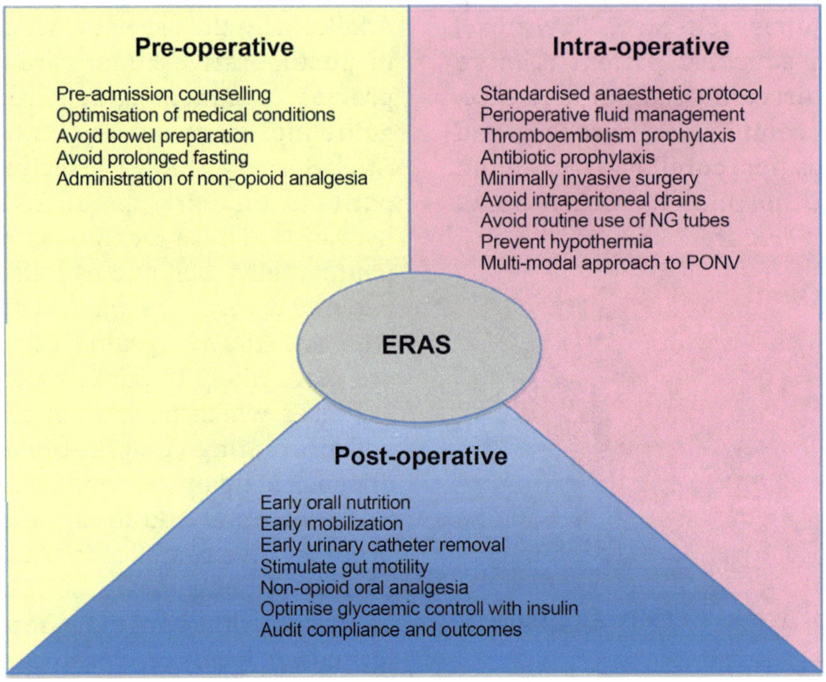

Figure 2.17. Enhanced recovery after surgery (ERAS).

Source: https://resources.wfsahq.org/wp-content/uploads/430-figure.png.

2.6.2. Follow-Up Appointments and Resources

Follow-up visits are critical for perioperative nursing as a transitional bridge between recovery and surgery. Follow-up visits provide an opportunity for healthcare professionals to assess the patient's healing, monitor for complications, and adjust treatment plans accordingly. Follow-up visits also provide the opportunity to determine the pain management interventions and the effectiveness of the interventions utilized in the postoperative setting. Participative patients who attend regular follow-ups tend to have higher rates of satisfaction and better outcomes. This indicates the importance of organized follow-up protocols in accordance with the individualized needs of each patient. Additionally, comprehensive educational materials that accompany follow-up visits enhance the efficacy of postoperative care. Patients must be provided with specific directions on how to recognize signs of complications, such as infection or increased pain, which can significantly impact their recovery. Sources may be written information or web pages with information on wound care, food, and levels of activity to be avoided. Through focused sources, the care team empowers patients to take responsibility for their recovery process, which enables them to become more independent and adhere to aftercare instructions more effectively. As the literature on immunosuppressive patients has indicated, tailored educational interventions can lead to better outcomes and reduced readmission following surgery, with an emphasis on educated interaction with follow-up treatment (Xiao, 2024). Moreover, recent advances in telehealth have provided increased access to follow-up visits and services, which enable patients to better communicate with their healthcare providers. Virtual consultations allow patients to discuss issues or symptoms without physical travel, a godsend particularly for mobility-impaired patients or those residing far from facilities. Telehealth may facilitate timely intervention and allow continued monitoring of the patient's status. Studies on minimally invasive procedures have underscored the value of protocolized follow-up strategies in outpatient settings, suggesting that telemedicine could be incorporated to provide support for ongoing patient care and care optimization (Mehmood et al., 2024). As technology advances further, perioperative nursing will likely incorporate these technologies to standardize and optimize follow-up processes, thereby enhancing the overall quality of care delivered to patients.

2.6.3. Importance of Patient Engagement

Practical perioperative nursing relies on successful patient engagement and has a significant impact on outcomes, from preoperative to postoperative recovery. Patient engagement in care enhances active involvement, instilling a sense of ownership in the health process. The process of interaction not only but also improves understanding regarding surgery, and facilitates better compliance with preoperative measures, leading to reduced complications. Evidence indicates that once patients are properly educated on the significance of preoperative education, e.g., expectation management and postoperative rehabilitation, they exhibit lower anxiety levels, ultimately resulting in improved clinical outcomes. Enhanced Recovery After Surgery (ERAS) guidelines, for example, emphasize patient involvement in the care process, resulting in a reduced length of stay and fewer postoperative complications, thereby highlighting the inherent link between engagement and quality of care (Huang et al., 2025). Finally, highlighting the importance of patient engagement is its contribution to perioperative interventions being tailored to each patient's specific needs, particularly in those with comorbidities. Collaborative decision-making facilitates effective risk stratification and preoperative optimization, enabling patients to receive individualized care plans that address their unique health concerns.

For example, bronchial asthmatic patients should be assessed preoperatively and educated on the planned strategy which will provide safety during the operative period. Employing the participatory approach enables physicians to utilize both pharmacologic and non-pharmacologic interventions effectively, promoting perioperative care safety and effectiveness. When patients are included in their treatment discussions, from adherence to medication to changes in lifestyle, they are more likely to adhere to the advice, resulting in improved health outcomes (Ilala et al., 2025). Patient involvement, beyond the immediate context of surgery, fosters a culture of continuous improvement in healthcare systems. The active of patients in their own care stimulates service delivery innovations, as patients can highlight areas of improvement that healthcare providers might not have identified. In perioperative nursing, ongoing conversation can improve processes, such as those in ERAS, for other patients to come. The integration of patient-reported outcomes (PROs) in the clinic setting enables care plans to be adjusted in real-time, ensuring they are both timely and effective. Finally, patient participation establishes an essential bridge across the preoperative, intraoperative, and postoperative care streams, resulting in an enlightened patient population that achieves enhanced levels of health and satisfaction throughout their surgical journey (Huang et al., 2025) (Figure 2.18).

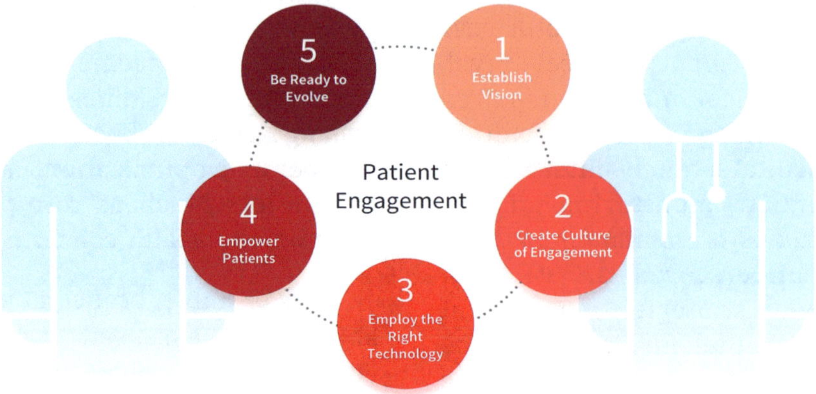

Figure 2.18. Patient engagement.

Source: https://www.tigahealth.com/wp-content/uploads/2021/05/patient-engagement-5.jpg.

Test Your Knowledge

1. What key information should be included in discharge instructions for a surgical patient?
2. Why is it essential to assess a patient's understanding during discharge education?

SUMMARY

The study of perioperative nursing study from preoperative to postoperative, it is evident that the complexity of patient care significantly influences the success of surgery. Preoperative patient health optimization is a crucial factor in minimizing complications. For instance, studies have established that preoperative optimization of diabetes control can tremendously reduce postoperative complication rates and enhance recovery (Breakwell et al., 2015). By sending diabetic patients to specialized clinics for better glycemic control, healthcare providers can be sure that patients present for surgery in the best possible state, thereby minimizing the risks usually associated with poor diabetes control. Lastly, this anticipatory preoperative care is an articulation of a key general principle of successful perioperative nursing: patient-specific strategies for successful surgical processes. Of equal importance is the mental dimension of perioperative nursing, particularly the education of patients. Providing sufficient preoperative education can help to reduce worry, a common but essential barrier to successful recuperation. Evidence suggests that condition-specific-educated patients have reduced rates of anxiety compared to those who are not provided with preparatory education (Harris et al., 2019). This anxiety reduction has hastened postoperative learning to support appropriate control of surgical aftercare and ultimately improve treatment compliance. These findings further underscore the importance of nurses adopting a holistic approach and addressing both physiological and psychological aspects of patient care throughout the perioperative continuum. The integration of holistic management practices into perioperative nursing not only enhances patient outcomes but also promotes the value of interprofessional practice. Smooth handovers of care throughout the surgical process depend greatly on effective communication among surgical teams, anesthesiologists, and nurses. Such interprofessional work can maximize preoperative preparations and follow-ups postoperatively, enabling every healthcare worker to have pertinent information that influences decisions about patient care. Additionally, continuing education and professional development within perioperative environments are essential to stay current with new technologies and innovations. The commitment to establishing such dynamic, interdisciplinary environments and advocating for patient interests characterizes optimal perioperative nursing practice and represents an unrelenting pursuit of excellence in healthcare delivery.

Perioperative nursing is a systems-based approach that spans preoperative, intraoperative, and postoperative care, all of which require a high level of attention to detail to achieve the best possible patient outcomes. One key element of preoperative care includes the taking and assessment of the patient's history, which provides the means to identify potential risk factors and guide diagnostic testing. Use of patient education, including informed consent, maintains keeps patients well-informed regarding their procedures and risks. Such preparations are crucial, as they form the foundation of a successful surgical experience, emphasizing the importance of individualized care tailored to meet patient-specific needs and medical histories. The emphasis on preparation is followed by recent trends in perioperative nursing, such as the integration of telemedicine, which provides interaction with patients before surgery (N/A, 2024). The perioperative nurse has a number of responsibilities aimed at ensuring safety for the patient and promoting successful surgery practice. This entails timely coordination with operating room staff to ensure open communication and adherence to evidence-based guidelines throughout the procedure. Some of the key interventions during this phase include rigorous infection control practices and effective anesthesia management. Vigilance in certain clinical risks that are associated with surgery, such as transurethral resection of the prostate (TURP),is also highlighted because they have a strong potential to influence the outcomes of surgery. The ability to respond promptly to any intraoperative issue is a key indicator of a well-prepared nursing team, which is essential for establishing a successful surgical setting (Le et al., 2024). Postoperative care is the final, yet most crucial, element of perioperative management, where recovery and complication prevention are emphasized. Perioperative nurses have a key role in assessing patients in the immediate post-recovery period, monitoring vital signs, and adhering to best practice in pain management that is individualized for the patient. All types of strategies, including urinary catheter management and early mobilization, are recognized as important in facilitating patient recovery. Education of the patient on home care and signs of potential complications is equally vital in ensuring continuity of care at discharge. As advances in surgical interventions and care integration techniques continue to evolve, ongoing education for perioperative nurses remains essential to meet staffing demands and deliver high-quality patient outcomes in this changing field (N/A, 2024).

KEY TERMS FROM THIS CHAPTER

- Anesthesia
- Deep breathing exercises
- Early ambulation
- Infection prevention
- Intraoperative monitoring
- Patient education
- Preoperative assessment
- Sterile technique
- Surgical site marking
- Wound care
- Circulating nurse
- Discharge planning
- Fluid and electrolyte balance
- Informed consent
- Pain management
- Post anesthesia care unit (PACU)
- Scrub nurse
- Surgical asepsis
- Vital signs monitoring

CRITICAL THINKING QUESTIONS

1. **What is the primary goal of preoperative nursing care?**
   a. To administer postoperative antibiotics
   b. To monitor anesthesia during surgery
   c. To prepare the patient physically and emotionally for surgery
   d. To discharge the patient early
2. **Which of the following is an essential preoperative nursing responsibility?**
   a. Start chemotherapy
   b. Obtain informed consent
   c. Perform the surgical procedure
   d. Discharge planning
3. **During the intraoperative phase, the circulating nurse is responsible for:**
   a. Suturing the incision
   b. Monitoring the sterile field and documentation
   c. Administering anesthesia
   d. Operating surgical instruments
4. **What is a priority assessment in the immediate postoperative period?**
   a. Bowel sounds
   b. Pain score
   c. Respiratory status
   d. Urine output
5. **Which intervention helps prevent postoperative complications like deep vein thrombosis (DVT)?**
   a. Encouraging prolonged bed rest
   b. Providing a high-calorie diet
   c. Administering stool softeners
   d. Early ambulation and leg exercises

Short Answer Questions

1. Define the three phases of perioperative nursing.
2. What are two key responsibilities of the preoperative nurse?
3. Mention one purpose of the surgical safety checklist.
4. Why is informed consent important before surgery?
5. Name two common postoperative complications nurses must monitor.
6. Describe the roles and responsibilities of the nurse in each phase of perioperative care.
7. Explain the nursing interventions to prevent postoperative respiratory complications.
8. Discuss the importance of patient education during the preoperative phase.
9. Explain the nursing management of pain in the immediate postoperative period.
10. Describe how nurses assess and manage infection risk in surgical patients.

Answers to Critical Thinking Questions

1. (c); 2. (b); 3. (b); 4. (c); 5. (d).

REFERENCES

1. Duff, J., Walker, K., Edward, K., Ralph, N., Giandinoto, J., Alexander, K., Gow, J., & Stephenson, J. (2017). Effect of a thermal care bundle on the prevention, detection and treatment of perioperative inadvertent hypothermia. *Journal of Clinical Nursing, 27*(5–6), 1239–1249. https://doi.org/10.1111/jocn.14171Alphonso, N., Beca, J., Blumenthal, A., et al. (2019). Study protocol: NITric oxide during cardiopulmonary bypass to improve recovery in infants with congenital heart defects (NITRIC trial): A randomized controlled trial. https://core.ac.uk/download/228026650.pdf (accessed on 30th June 2025).
2. Astagneau, P., Bayat, A., Blackham, J., Bonds, R., Bunn, F., Cabaluna, R., Daoud, F., et al. (2015). Evidence updates on prevention of surgical site infection. https://core.ac.uk/download/30731437.pdf (accessed on 30th June 2025).
3. Ben-Amitay, A., Bray, M., Brunton, C., Buckley, K., Capurso, M., Chieng, A., Chow, L., et al. (2018). A mixed-method systematic review of the effectiveness and acceptability of preoperative psychological preparation programmers to reduce pediatric preoperative anxiety in elective surgery. https://core.ac.uk/download/157856587.pdf (accessed on 30th June 2025).
4. Bermano, G., Bruce, A., Duff, C., Kirkpatrick, P., Stephen, J., et al. (2014). Competencies and skills to enable effective care of severely obese patients undergoing bariatric surgery across a multi-disciplinary healthcare perspective: A systematic review. https://core.ac.uk/download/222837400.pdf (accessed on 30th June 2025).
5. Bifulco, F., Coluzzi, F., Corcione, A., Cuomo, A., et al. (2017). The challenge of perioperative pain management in opioid-tolerant patients. https://core.ac.uk/download/127586677.pdf (accessed on 30th June 2025).
6. Bonner, J., Kearns, R. J., Robertson, J., Uppal, S., et al. (2011). The introduction of a surgical safety checklist in a tertiary referral obstetric center. https://core.ac.uk/download/110446.pdf (accessed on 30th June 2025).
7. Breakwell, S., Kallio, P. J., Nolan, J., Olsen, K., et al. (2015). Anesthesia preoperative clinic referral for elevated HbA1c reduces complication rate in diabetic patients undergoing total joint arthroplasty. https://core.ac.uk/download/213081699.pdf (accessed on 30th June 2025).
8. Brown, E. N., Pavone, K. J., & Naranjo, M. (2018). Multimodal general anesthesia: Theory and practice. *Anesthesia & Analgesia, 127*, 1246–1258. https://doi.org/10.1213/ane.0000000000003668 (accessed on 30th June 2025).
9. Ceppa, E. P., Colgate, C. L., Fennerty, M. L., House, M. G., et al. (2019). Post-pancreatoduodenectomy outcomes and epidural analgesia: A 5-year single institution experience. https://core.ac.uk/download/187423802.pdf (accessed on 30th June 2025).
10. Comans, T., Hays, Z., & Leach, C. (2021). Barriers to preoperative warming: Best practice guideline. https://core.ac.uk/download/483691872.pdf (accessed on 30th June 2025).
11. Daily, S., Doster, B., Lewis, C., Ryan, C., et al. (2019). Business process redesign in the perioperative process: A case perspective for digital transformation. https://core.ac.uk/download/289123784.pdf (accessed on 30th June 2025).
12. Davis, B. R., Valente, M. A., Goldberg, J. E., Lightner, A. L., Feingold, D. L., & Paquette, I. M. (2022). The American Society of Colon and Rectal Surgeons clinical practice guidelines for

ostomy surgery. *Diseases of the Colon & Rectum, 65*, 1173–1190. https://doi.org/10.1097/dcr.0000000000002498 (accessed on 30th June 2025).

13. Fortier, M. A., Kain, Z. N., & Trinh, L. N. (2019). Primer on adult patient satisfaction in perioperative settings. https://core.ac.uk/download/287622490.pdf (accessed on 30th June 2025).
14. Franson, H. (2020). A pain control optimization pathway to reduce acute postoperative pain and opioid consumption postoperatively: An approach to battling the opioid epidemic. https://core.ac.uk/download/389488233.pdf (accessed on 30th June 2025).
15. Harris, M. S. (2019). Does preoperative ostomy education decrease anxiety in the new ostomy patient? https://core.ac.uk/download/215413071.pdf (accessed on 30th June 2025).
16. Hilton-Christie, S., Livie, J., & Livie, V. (2020). Improving the use of the 'COUGH' bundle in Surgical High Dependency Unit, Ninewells Hospital, Dundee. https://core.ac.uk/download/323303779.pdf (accessed on 30th June 2025).
17. Huang, J., Wu, G., & Li, X. (2025). Application of perioperative nursing based on enhanced recovery after surgery (ERAS) principles in patients undergoing total knee arthroplasty. *Therapeutics and Clinical Risk Management, 21*, 829–839. https://www.semanticscholar.org/paper/2478f3bd5f4ca3d5b189ec10d5625488e13fdb5d (accessed on 30th June 2025).
18. Ijäs, E., & Suni, A. (2015). Preoperative assessment and patient teaching: Preoperative forms and guidelines for a LEIKO unit. https://core.ac.uk/download/38131033.pdf (accessed on 30th June 2025).
19. Irani, J., Hedrick, T. L., Miller, T. E., Lee, L., Steinhagen, E., Shogan, B. D., Goldberg, J. E., et al. (2022). Clinical practice guidelines for enhanced recovery after colon and rectal surgery from the American Society of Colon and Rectal Surgeons and the Society of American Gastrointestinal and Endoscopic Surgeons. *Diseases of the Colon & Rectum, 66*, 15–40. https://doi.org/10.1097/dcr.0000000000002650 (accessed on 30th June 2025).
20. Ismail, M. F. (2025). Opioid-sparing strategies in perioperative pain management: Current evidence, challenges, and future directions. *Asian Journal of Medicine and Health*. https://www.semanticscholar.org/paper/ecf4c4c0fff89b0424f618335d05594b11dcdaff (accessed on 30th June 2025).
21. Joseph, T. T., Wax, D. B., Goldstein, R., Huang, J., McCormick, P. J., & Levin, M. A. (2020). A web-based perioperative dashboard as a platform for anesthesia informatics innovation. *Anesthesia & Analgesia, 131*, 1640–1645. https://doi.org/10.1213/ane.0000000000005193 (accessed on 30th June 2025).
22. Kara, S. G. (2025). The role of prophylaxis for preventing venous thromboembolism in major urological surgery and nursing management. *The New Journal of Urology*. https://www.semanticscholar.org/paper/527579517de257cea4776bb05decb164d1e5d66b (accessed on 30th June 2025).
23. Karera, E., Karonkano, G. R., Mbonera, F., Mukamana, D., et al. (2018). Clinical experiences of perioperative nursing Masters students in selected Rwandan referral hospitals. https://core.ac.uk/download/478465964.pdf (accessed on 30th June 2025).
24. Karl, A., Porserud, A., Vidal Faune, A., Ghoneim, A. A., Jensen, B., Jensen, B., Jensen, B., et al. (2018). Supportive interventions to improve physiological and psychological health

outcomes among patients undergoing cystectomy: A systematic review. https://core.ac.uk/download/160606528.pdf (accessed on 30th June 2025).

25. Le, J., Ponto, J., Ying, Y., & Morlandt, A. (2024). Perioperative management for microvascular free tissue transfers for head and neck reconstruction–Commentary. *Journal of Diagnostics and Treatment of Oral and Maxillofacial Pathology*. https://www.semanticscholar.org/paper/30cec1260bbb6a549999adb7353f018559905094 (accessed on 30th June 2025).

26. Mehmood, A., Rupani, S., Teo, R. Y., & Redmond, H. (2024). Perioperative calcium monitoring in minimally invasive radio-guided parathyroidectomy: Early detection and management of hypocalcemia. *Annals of Quaid-e-Azam Medical College*. https://www.semanticscholar.org/paper/17fb8e14b7c63bf95a89ee7b6ba90cf07576a307 (accessed on 30th June 2025).

27. Mooruth, V. (2016). Knowledge and perceptions of patients regarding anesthetists and anesthesia. https://core.ac.uk/download/188768866.pdf (accessed on 30th June 2025).

28. Nash, R. (2013). Patient comfort and multimodal analgesia: Effects of preoperative ibuprofen. https://core.ac.uk/download/53025851.pdf (accessed on 30th June 2025).

29. Nelms, M. C. (2006). Patient satisfaction with the role of the nurse practitioner. https://core.ac.uk/download/480740997.pdf (accessed on 30th June 2025).

30. Slagle, J. A. (2015). Implementation of a warming protocol to prevent inadvertent perioperative hypothermia in the ambulatory surgical setting. https://core.ac.uk/download/216979786.pdf (accessed on 30th June 2025).

31. Xiao, B. (2024). Case report: A nursing challenge–Postoperative complications of pacemaker implantation in Behçet's disease. *Journal of Clinical Rheumatology and Immunology*. https://www.semanticscholar.org/paper/05c3c38b45a76b4a6d7933b274081691a529a119 (accessed on 30th June 2025).

32. Xu, M., Yang, X., & Guo, L. (2024). Effectiveness of preoperative and perioperative pulmonary rehabilitation nursing program for the management of patients undergoing thoracic surgery: A systematic review and meta-analysis. *Pakistan Journal of Medical Sciences, 40*, 1280–1286. https://www.semanticscholar.org/paper/8c1586ed319dea15d01f03a75333c69da4cbdc80 (accessed on 30th June 2025).

33. Zhang, H., & Zhang, M. (2025). Perioperative management of a neonate with congenital biliary atresia complicated by severe pneumonia undergoing hepatic hilar jejunostomy: A case report. *Nursing in Critical Care*. https://www.semanticscholar.org/paper/c8ec8f4e5ee7d1406bbc10fc57437dd7b34d7b2d (accessed on 30th June 2025).

34. Zhou, L., & Peng, L. (2025). Machine learning in perioperative management: Applications and progress. *Journal of Contemporary Medical Practice*. https://www.semanticscholar.org/paper/3aeaaf4c8604b8acd99e271d9fd5456538611b35 (accessed on 30th June 2025).

RESPIRATORY FUNCTION: ASSESSMENT AND MANAGEMENT OF PULMONARY DISORDERS FOR SURGICAL NURSING

3

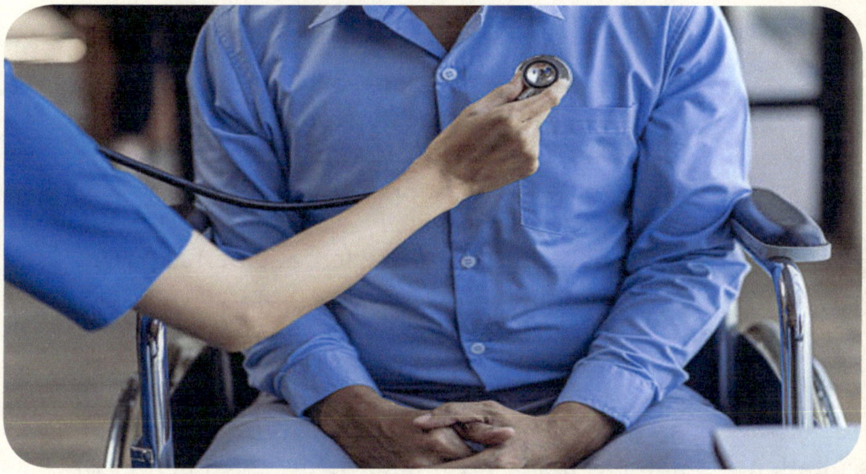

LEARNING OBJECTIVES

After studying this chapter, you will be able to:

1. Understand the anatomy and physiology of the respiratory system
2. Explain the common pulmonary disorders
3. Discuss the assessment techniques for respiratory function
4. Focus on management strategies for pulmonary disorder
5. Learn about the role of surgical nursing in respiratory care
6. Evaluate the challenges in managing pulmonary disorders

Introduction

Surgery nurses must understand the respiratory function as it is critical in patient care and post-operation. The respiratory system's function is to facilitate gas exchange by inhaling oxygen and exhaling carbon dioxide, a process required to ensure homeostasis. The lungs, airways, and respiratory muscles in the system facilitate intricate interactions that enable this exchange. Hence, a comprehensive understanding of respiratory function provides a foundation for nurses to detect abnormalities, monitor patients effectively, and respond to complications. Improved awareness of respiratory physiology enables nursing personnel to employ the correct interventions, resulting in better outcomes in surgical procedures. In the assessment of respiratory function, several significant parameters must be given attention, including lung volume and capacity, and the efficiency of gas exchange. Spirometric methods are one method that can provide insight into lung function by measuring the amount of air inhaled and exhaled over time. This is essential for diagnosing conditions such as COPD or restrictive lung disease, which can significantly affect the success of surgery. Furthermore, awareness of the effects of impaired respiratory function is crucial because it can lead to postoperative complications such as hypoxemia, atelectasis, and pneumonia. For operating room nurses, this reaffirms the value of thorough preoperative assessment and the establishment of postoperative monitoring regimens that are proportionate to the patient's respiratory status.

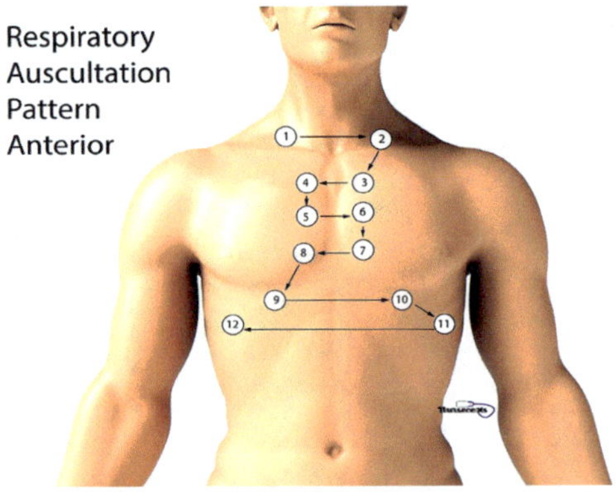

Figure 3.1. Respiratory assessment auscultation pattern.

Source: https://i.pinimg.com/originals/78/9c/3c/789c3c4311362367f9878c4cb8b1f9b8.jpg.

Management of pulmonary disease in the operating room nursing setting requires an anticipatory strategy that incorporates both preventive and interventional options. Comprehensive team interventions, with input from both respiratory therapists and physicians, are required for optimizing respiratory therapy. The development of evidence-based practice protocols enables nurses to effectively manage problems of compromised respiratory function. For instance, utilizing incentive spirometry and early mobilization can significantly minimize the risk of postoperative pulmonary complications resulting from compromised lung function. As the ESC Guidelines point out, doctors must remain updated with the latest guidelines to enhance their clinical skills and hence modify their strategies accordingly to the specific needs of the patient (Baumgartner H et al., 2020). Through this manner, nurses can directly influence the trajectory of patient recovery, and a full grasp of respiratory function in operating conditions is essential (Figure 3.1).

Definition and Importance of Respiratory Function

The Respiratory function is precisely described as the physiological process by which the body exchanges gases—oxygen and carbon dioxide—between the outside environment and the bloodstream. This fundamental process is executed through an elaborate system involving the muscles and lungs to enable efficient ventilation, diffusion, and perfusion. An understanding of respiratory function is crucial in surgical nursing since it directly affects a patient's ability to recuperate and respond to surgery. Normal respiratory function supports tissue oxygenation and carbon dioxide removal, helping maintain homeostasis. Dysfunction of this important process can lead to hazardous complications during and after surgery, making appropriate assessment and management important components of perioperative care. Respiratory function within the operating room cannot be overstressed. It plays a key role not only in patient stability but also in surgical outcomes. Effective respiratory management improves ventilation and ensures adequate oxygenation, which is required during several perioperative phases. Operations often involve general anesthesia, which can significantly compromise respiratory function due to the abolition of airway reflexes and potential airway obstruction. Therefore, operating nurses should carefully monitor the respiratory status of patients and identify any signs of hypoxemia or hypercapnia to launch associated interventions. Monitoring in this manner is crucial for minimizing respiratory complications, as per surgical care guidelines that aim to maximize respiratory function and enhance recovery outcomes (Baumgartner et al., 2020; Gustafsson et al., 2018). Furthermore, the assessment of respiratory function also involves the use of diagnostic tests, through which healthcare workers can measure lung capacity, airflow, and the efficiency of gas exchange. Pulmonary function tests, blood gas analysis, and imaging procedures all play a role in determining a patient's respiratory health. For surgical nursing, this assessment is not merely a matter of paperwork; it is essential to a preoperative risk assessment and to the formulation of future care plans. We also need to include any existing lung conditions of our patients that can complicate their surgical procedure. Effective management by careful assessment is paramount in optimizing patient recovery and averting postoperative pulmonary complications (Baumgartner et al., 2020; Gustafsson et al., 2018). Lastly, the significance of respiratory function in the operation further enhances the necessity of cautious and well-informed nursing practice in this realm.

Overview of Pulmonary Disorders

It is essential for the nursing personnel, especially in the operative scenario, to have a good understanding of pulmonary disorders, as adequate respiratory function is associated with surgical recovery. Certain conditions, such as COPD, asthma, and pulmonary fibrosis, are significant in the perioperative period. COPD, as a condition of airflow limitation, has significant implications for the postoperative course and length of hospital stay due to impairment of gas exchange and lung mechanics. Surgical nurses can learn to place the assessment of these conditions foremost and utilize focused care plans to reduce risks. Programs that specialize in maximizing pulmonary function preoperatively through preoperative teaching, smoking cessation, and bronchodilator therapy can significantly minimize patient complications. As a science, surgical nursing can value the complexity of these conditions to allow perioperative planning that considers individual respiratory needs for patients with compromised lung function. Recognition of pulmonary diseases and their pathophysiology is of the highest priority in surgical nursing. Asthma, for instance, is usually characterized by airway hyper-reactivity, resulting in intermittent airflow obstruction, wheezing, and dyspnea. Nurses must recognize symptoms and precipitating factors to give the best possible management pre-surgery. Additionally, perioperative care in asthmatic patients involves administering inhaled corticosteroids and bronchodilators, as needed, to achieve maximum bronchodilation prior to surgery. Moreover, the inclusion of guidelines such as those from the European Society of Cardiology enhances surgical clinical practice and confirms the importance of using evidence-based standards (Baumgartner et al., 2020). By keeping patients under close observation for respiratory status and implementing evidence-based practice interventions, surgical nursing can make an important contribution to the improvement of surgical outcomes in patients with pulmonary disease. Another important category of pulmonary disease is restrictive lung diseases, such as pulmonary fibrosis, which are responsible for a decreased lung volume and impaired gas exchange. These conditions pose unique challenges in the perioperative nursing setting, where it can be complicated to ensure patients are properly oxygenated. Due to its progressive nature, patients with pulmonary fibrosis require extensive preoperative testing to assess their respiratory function properly. The operating room nurses must work closely with the perioperative team to develop perioperative plans that include optimizing the intraoperative position of patients, as well as adjusting ventilation settings when indicated. As highlighted in the Enhanced Recovery After Surgery (ERAS) guidelines, the use of individualized interventions can potentially reduce complications and enhance recovery (Gustafsson et al., 2018). Therefore, an understanding of the full spectrum of pulmonary disorders and their implications on surgical patients is crucial to deliver effective and caring practice within surgical nursing (Figure 3.2).

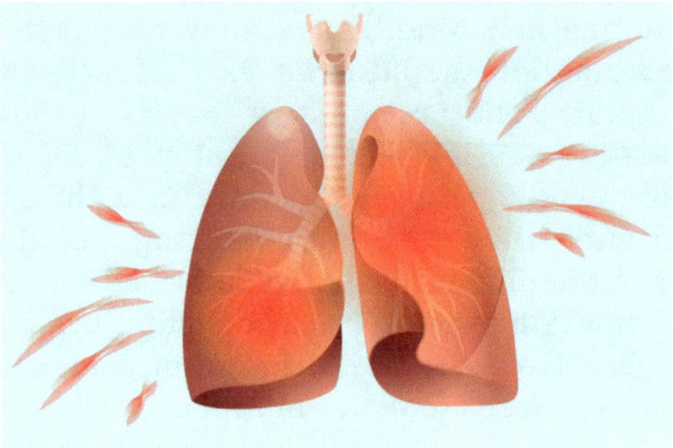

Figure 3.2. Lung disease can be deadly for rheumatoid arthritis patients.

Source: https://creakyjoints.org/wp-content/uploads/2018/12/1218_Arthritis-Lungs.jpg.

Relevance to Surgical Nursing Practice

In the practice of surgical nursing, respiratory function knowledge is essential not only for patient assessment but also in the care of possible pulmonary complications during the perioperative period. The dynamic interaction between surgery and respiratory health demands that the nurses are adept at assessing patients at risk for pulmonary disease, particularly in patients who have pre-existing respiratory illnesses such as COPD or asthma. Efficient assessment tools, such as auscultation and peak flow monitoring, are capable of facilitating early intervention and improving patient outcomes. Surgical nurses must also be vigilant, as compromised respiratory function can lead to complications such as postoperative atelectasis or pneumonia, which may increase hospitalization and healthcare costs. By integrating detailed respiratory assessments into their practice, surgical nurses can play a critical role in enhancing surgical care and patient safety. In addition, the implementation of evidence-based interventions in surgery nursing is important to improve the management of respiratory function in surgical patients. Systematic reviews provide valuable information on best practices and new methods that are relevant to clinical practice, providing maximum care. Adherence to the PRISMA 2020 guidelines enables the effective dissemination of high-quality evidence, informing nurses to make decisions that address specific patient needs and expectations individually. This evidence-based approach can lead to greater transparency about how various interventions work, ultimately resulting in improved patient care quality. Through the application of these outcomes in clinical care, surgical nurses can significantly reduce morbidity associated with pulmonary complications and improve recovery trajectories for surgical patients as they navigate the complexity of postoperative care (Page et al., 2021). Finally, the inclusion of suggestions from recognized organizations, such as the European Society of Cardiology (ESC), also underscores the importance of personalized nursing interventions for optimal respiratory function in surgical patients. The ESC Guidelines encourage the application of professional judgment supplemented with evidence-based guidelines for proper patient care. The surgical nurse must recognize the importance of considering individual patient factors during the assessment of respiratory functionality and when planning therapeutic interventions. Balancing individualized care with clinical guidelines is important because it fosters improved communication among healthcare team members and promotes shared decision-making with patients and their families. With the inclusion of both evidence-based guidelines and individualized care strategies, surgical nurses can enhance their practice to provide adequate care for respiratory complications arising within the chain of surgery (Baumgartner et al., 2020).

3.1. Anatomy and Physiology of the Respiratory System

Learning Outcome

1. Describe the structure of the respiratory system
2. Focus on mechanisms of gas exchange
3. Learn about the regulation of breathing

The anatomy of the respiratory system is human physiology. It begins with the upper respiratory system, which is made up of structures such as the nasal cavity, pharynx, and larynx. They essential function warm, and humidify air as it enters the lower respiratory system. The lower component consists of the trachea, bronchi, bronchioles, and alveoli, where oxygen and carbon dioxide are exchanged. The alveolar sacs, with dense capillary supply and enormous surface area, are key to the success of diffusion. Understanding of this anatomical structure is key to surgical nursing, particularly in the treatment of conditions interfering with normal respiratory function, since each part of the structure can be a target for disease processes altering overall respiratory efficiency. Physiology complements the anatomical structure of the respiratory system with its several processes that permit adequate oxygenation and carbon dioxide removal. The mechanics of ventilation, specifically inhalation and exhalation, depend on the contraction and relaxation of the diaphragm and intercostal muscles, which generate changes in pressure within the thoracic cavity. Moreover, the action of surfactant, a substance secreted by type II alveolar cells, is vital as it reduces surface tension within the alveoli so they do not collapse during exhalation. This biochemical feature is particularly significant in the neonate patient group, as its absence may lead to conditions such as respiratory distress syndrome (RDS). Since these surgical interventions typically involve an understanding of physiological principles, surgical nurses need to be proficient in recognizing abnormalities in function as they may manifest clinically, especially in individuals with underlying pulmonary disease. Physiological and anatomical integration provides a foundation for assessing and managing pulmonary disorders, which guides patient outcomes and nursing interventions. For instance, abnormal breath sounds during auscultation could indicate pulmonary complications that require immediate intervention.

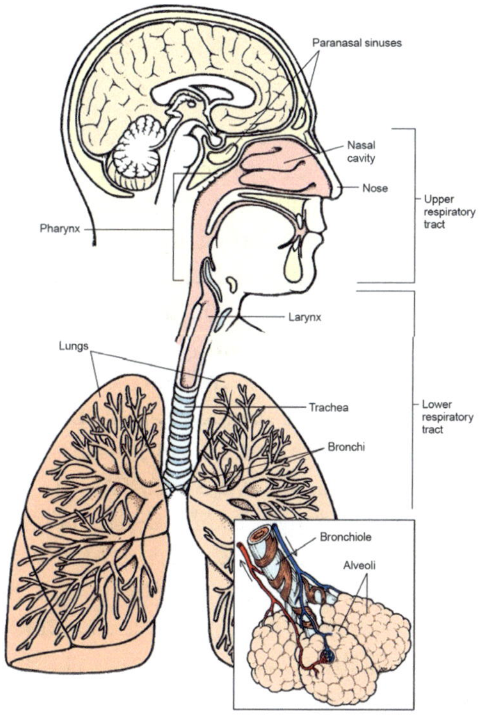

Figure 3.3. Anatomy of the respiratory tract human physiology.

Source: https://img.brainkart.com/article/article-Anatomy-of-the-Respi-Kth.jpg.

Recent advances in therapeutic modalities, such as exogenous surfactant administration, have revolutionized the management of conditions like RDS in neonates, demonstrating the applicability of respiratory physiology knowledge in informing clinical practice. Implementation of such treatments has drastically reduced morbidity and mortality rates caused by immaturity of lungs and other lung conditions, underlining the applicability of precise anatomical and physiological knowledge in surgical nursing. As pulmonary disorders present special challenges in operative settings, there should be proper knowledge of the structure and function of the respiratory system to provide good patient care and treatment (Figure 3.3).

3.1.1. Structure of the Respiratory System

The structure of the respiratory system is finely tuned to support the process of gas exchange, essential for the survival of human beings. It consists of various main components, including the upper respiratory system, which comprises the nose and pharynx. The function of the nasal cavity is very important because it warms, humidifies, and filters inhaled air, making it suitable for the more sensitive areas of the lungs. Having traversed the nasal cavity, air continues through the larynx, or voice box, into the trachea. The rigid tube is supported by C-shaped cartilage rings that direct air into the bronchi and, finally, into the lungs. An understanding of this system is crucial in surgical nursing because changes to any portion of the system have a direct impact on respiratory function and patient outcomes. Once they reach the lungs, the bronchial tree further divides into smaller bronchi and bronchioles, eventually terminating in the alveoli, where gas exchange occurs. Alveoli are very small air sacs lined with a thin epithelial cell wall, surrounded by capillaries through which oxygen and carbon dioxide pass. Their structure is designed for this purpose, with a huge surface area that accommodates millions of alveoli within a single lung. Moreover, the pulmonary surfactant, produced by alveolar cells, reduces surface tension, thereby preventing alveolar collapse induced by exhalation. This information highlights the importance of assessing the structure and functional integrity of the alveoli in the treatment of pulmonary diseases, as bronchiectasis is likely to severely impair gas exchange, with adverse health consequences (Chang et al., 2021). Apart from the anatomical structures, the respiratory system's supportive structures like the diaphragm and intercostal muscles also play a crucial role in ventilation. The diaphragm is a dome-shaped muscle located at the bottom of the lungs, which contracts and relaxes to create pressure differences that allow air to enter and exit the lungs. Intercostal muscles assist in opening and closing the rib cage to expand lung capacity. Proper functioning of these structures aids in proficient respiratory mechanics, which is important because surgery can affect thoracic capacity or mobility of the diaphragm in patients. Pulmonary disease in the operating theatre should be evaluated and treated with a deep understanding of these structural dynamics, as their influence largely dictates postoperative respiratory function and patient recovery (Ibrahim et al., 2023) (Figure 3.4).

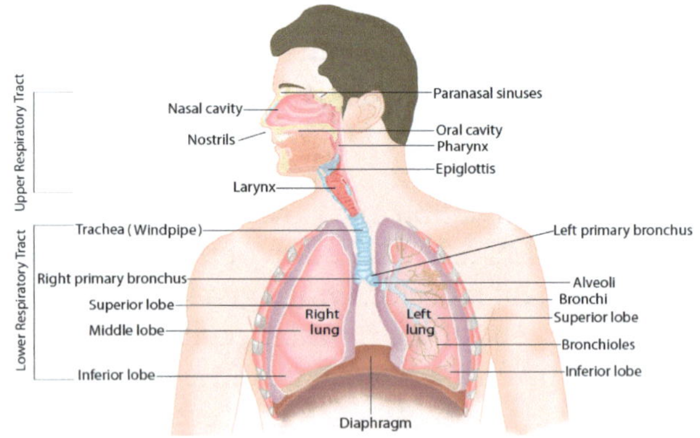

Figure 3.4. Structure of respiratory system.

Source: https://www.howtorelief.com/wp-content/uploads/2017/11/respiratory-system.jpg.

3.1.2. Mechanisms of Gas Exchange

The mechanisms of gas exchange in the lungs are essential to healthy respiratory function, particularly in handling pulmonary diseases that surgeons can expect to deal with in surgical nursing. Gas exchange occurs in the alveoli, where oxygen is moved from the incoming air into the blood and carbon dioxide is expelled from the blood into the lungs to be exhaled. Such exchange is facilitated by diffusion, which occurs due to partial pressure gradients of gases across the alveolar-capillary membrane. Efficiency in such exchange is primarily determined by surface area, membrane thickness, and partial pressure of gases. In acute lung injury (ALI) and acute respiratory distress syndrome (ARDS), all these mechanisms can be impaired, thereby leading to impaired ventilation and oxygenation. An understanding of these fundamental processes is essential for operating theatre nurses when assessing respiratory function and planning management for patients who have compromised pulmonary status (Chimbira et al., 2001).

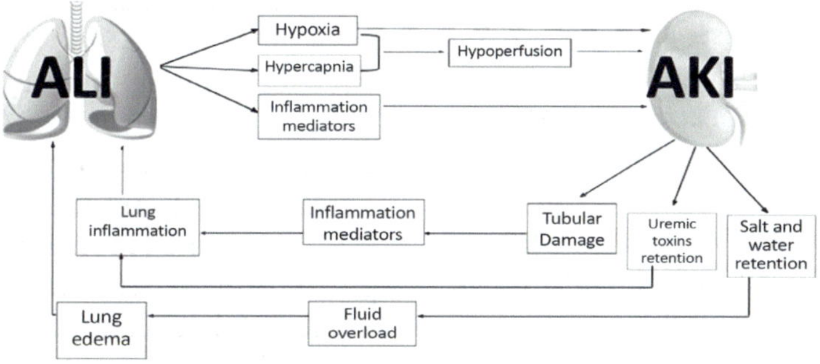

Figure 3.5. Acute lung injury (ALI).

Source: https://www.researchgate.net/publication/359389737/figure/fig3/AS:1142770764922882@1649469190612/Kidney-Lung-Crosstalk-ALI-acute-lung-injury-AKI-acute-kidney-injury.png

Furthermore, assessment of gas exchange efficiency can be quantified in terms of several clinical parameters, including the arterial-alveolar (A-a) gradient and the PaO2/FiO2 ratio. A significant A-a gradient can indicate shunting or ventilation-perfusion mismatches, which are stereotypical markers of widespread pulmonary impairment. For instance, in a clinical study involving pediatric patients with respiratory failure, a lower PaO2/FiO2 ratio was associated with greater mortality, indicating the prognostic value of gas exchange disturbances in patient outcomes (Chimbira et al., 2001). Detection of these relationships allows surgical nurses to determine the severity of pulmonary disease better and modify interventions accordingly. Close monitoring of these parameters during surgery is necessary to maximize benefit without causing complications secondary to compromised gas exchange. Therapeutic interventions for several conditions also aim to optimize gas exchange in patients with compromised respiratory function. High-frequency oscillatory ventilation (HFOV) and pharmacologic agent delivery, like nitric oxide, are among the methods used to counteract the challenges posed by diseases like ALI and ARDS. While HFOV can be used to improve oxygenation with minimal secondary lung injury, its use is associated with increased mortality due to the severity of the underlying illness (Chimbira et al., 2001). Thus, operating room nurses must be well-versed in such interventions and their roles in facilitating gas exchange. There must be a solid evaluation and management plan that prioritizes the optimization of respiratory function, particularly crucial for surgical patients, in whom the risk of respiratory complications can be serious (Figure 3.5).

3.1.3. Regulation of Breathing

Regulation of respiration is a complex process responsible for maintaining homeostasis and ensuring the adequacy of oxygenation and carbon dioxide removal. The respiratory centers in the brainstem mainly regulate the control of breathing, the medulla oblongata, and the pons, which react to different physiological stimuli. Central chemoreceptors sense changes in the concentration of carbon dioxide and blood pH, and peripheral chemoreceptors, which are found in carotid and aortic bodies, sense changes in oxygen concentration. They provide information to the respiratory centers, which in turn regulate the breathing rate and depth based on this information. For perioperative practice, understanding of this elaborate regulatory process is extremely crucial, as the patient undergoing surgery or under anesthesia has compromised respiratory function. Therefore, it is essential to monitor and intervene with caution to prevent respiratory complications. Under surgical conditions, the regulation of respiration gains greater significance with the risk of respiratory depression due to anesthetic agents. Anesthetics interfere with normal feedback mechanisms controlling respiration and lead to hypoventilation or apnea. It is crucial that surgical nurses assess a patient's baseline respiratory function to evaluate for any underlying pulmonary diseases that may complicate these conditions. Finally, the postoperative stage is also at high risk for developing complications such as atelectasis and pneumonia, especially in patients with poor mobility. Effective management practices like early mobilization and incentive spirometry can avoid such risks and promote the best recovery. The historical backdrop to the development of intensive care underscores the need for specialized nursing expertise in monitoring and supporting respiratory function, as attested by the developments catalyzed by the polio epidemic and subsequent elaboration of respiratory treatment procedures (Reynolds et al., 2011). Secondly, latest developments in pulmonary care and monitoring technology have enhanced surgery nursing procedures related to respiratory function. Technological advancements in non-invasive ventilation and sophisticated monitoring equipment enable the real-time measurement of respiratory parameters, allowing nurses to respond immediately to changes in a patient's respiratory status. For instance, the application of continuous capnography during operating room procedures enables the detection of complications, such as hypoventilation, at an earlier stage, allowing for prompt interventions. Additionally, nursing education has placed greater emphasis on the role of respiratory assessment and intervention, resulting in improved patient outcomes in the operating room. Based on various scholarly accounts, ongoing education and training in respiratory care remain focal points, reflecting the evolving landscape of surgical nursing and its role in addressing clinical concerns related to pulmonary disease (Copeland et al., 2018).

Test Your Knowledge

1. What is the primary function of the alveoli in the lungs?
2. How does the diaphragm contribute to the process of breathing?

3.2. Common Pulmonary Disorders

Learning Outcome

1. Explain the chronic obstructive pulmonary disease (COPD)
2. Define asthma and its implications
3. Discuss the pulmonary embolism and its risks

Gross acquaintance with Understanding the prevalent pulmonary ailments is necessary for surgical practice, particularly as these conditions can immediately influence respiratory function and surgical recovery. Chronic Obstructive Pulmonary Disease (COPD) involves adult patients having chronic respiratory symptoms and airflow limitation secondary to airway and alveolar defects. COPD patients typically develop exacerbations that may complicate the surgery; therefore, they need to be adequately assessed before the surgery to prevent complications. Surgical nurses are rehabilitation. Guidelines are available to use, which highlight the utilization of strict assessment measures like pulmonary function tests in determining interventions appropriately (Page et al., 2021). Moreover, understanding the nuances of COPD management can lead to improved patient communication regarding their disease, further enhancing the quality of care as a nurse. Asthma is another essential pulmonary disease that must not be forgotten in an operating theater and involves inflammation, hyper-responsiveness, and airway obstruction. Asthma can cause acute bronchospasm, particularly in or following a surgical procedure that involves general anesthesia or intubation. For perioperative nurses, identification of patients' asthma triggers and a management plan are essential in minimizing perioperative complications. Preoperative optimization may include pharmacological measures in the proper use of pharmacotherapy, such as corticosteroids or bronchodilators. Systemic implications of poor asthma control may lead to life-threatening conditions, including respiratory failure, and thus close monitoring of such patients is of utmost importance (Baumgartner et al., 2020). The addition of a multidisciplinary staff that includes anesthesiologists and respiratory therapists can further enhance the management policy, ultimately delivering patients holistic care that addresses their unique respiratory needs. Lastly, pneumonia is also a common pulmonary condition that can be contracted preoperatively or postoperatively and has a considerable influence on surgical nursing. This inflammatory respiratory disease of the lung tissue is capable of producing impaired exchange of gases, resulting in hypoxia and subsequent respiratory failure. Current patients with COPD or asthma are highly susceptible to pneumonia and, as such, surgical nurses need to be keen on its early signs.

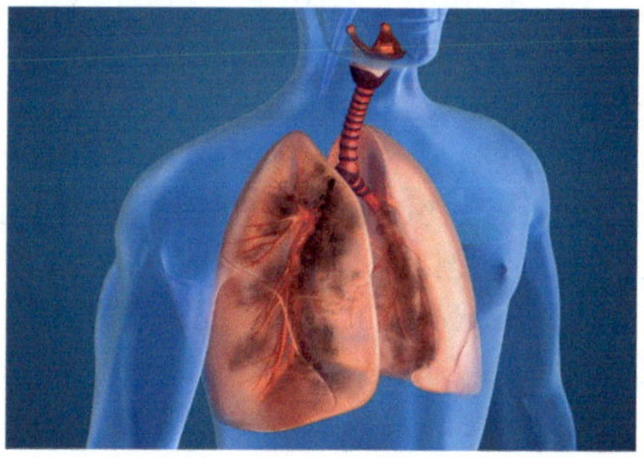

Figure 3.6. Common pulmonary disorders.

Source: https://external-content.duckduckgo.com/iu/?u=https%3A%2F%2Fpulmonarypracticeassociates.com%2Fwp-content%2Fuploads%2F2018%2F11%2FServices-LungDisease-img.jpg&f=1&nofb=1&ipt=ce0b60b2ba606b9dcad09d136cbddab83f14dca38309b1849a9116314cc88542.

Care strategies should incorporate thorough assessments of respiratory status, in addition to the use of prophylactic interventions through therapy, such as administering antibiotics when necessary and promoting early mobilization.

Additionally, preventive education on smoking cessation, pneumococcal disease, and influenza vaccination can play a key role in reducing the incidence of pneumonia among high-risk surgical patients. Similar to other pulmonary disorders, adherence to recommended guidelines can facilitate more effective patient management (Baumgartner et al., 2020; Page et al., 2021) (Figure 3.6).

3.2.1. Chronic Obstructive Pulmonary Disease (COPD)

Chronic Obstructive Pulmonary Disease (COPD) is a progressive respiratory lung disease that significantly reduces the quality of life of patients and represents a rapidly growing burden to healthcare systems globally. Characterized by irreversible airflow limitation due to chronic lung diseases such as emphysema and chronic bronchitis, COPD leads to chronic cough, sputum hypersecretion, and dyspnea. By the year 2020, COPD will rise as the third leading cause of death worldwide with major economic and societal costs. In addition, the incidence of severe to moderate airflow obstruction is very high, with about 10% of adults aged 40 years and above in various international studies (Zhou et al., 2015). This emphasizes the importance of surgical nurses being well-versed in COPD assessment and management to minimize patient outcomes and maximize overall quality of care. Optimal management techniques of COPD include both pharmacologic and non-pharmacologic therapy aimed at symptom relief and improvement in the quality of life of the patients. Standard pharmacological therapy typically includes predominantly inhaled bronchodilators, corticosteroids, and other supportive treatments, which are necessary for symptom control. Unfortunately, at later stages of the disease, a standard therapy can only produce minimal benefits, and patients accrue heavy symptom burdens and high comorbidities, including depression and anxiety (Zhou et al., 2015). Therapies like lung volume reduction surgery may be considered in highly selected patients with severe COPD, benefiting from improved lung function and enhanced survival. All these operative interventions, however, require careful patient selection and preoperative evaluation by surgical nursing teams themselves, who must be proficient in assessing lung function and health status of potential applicants. In addition to standard treatment approaches, new approaches, such as palliative care and integrated symptom management methods, are increasingly recognized as critical components of COPD management. Palliative care relieves the symptoms and stress of the illness, as well as helping patients and their families achieve a better quality of life. Research shows that advanced COPD patients tend to have poorly controlled distressing symptoms, with the inclusion of palliative care being essential (Zhou et al., 2015). Moreover, respiratory nursing should develop based in a broader perspective of symptom management with an emphasis on individualized therapies like opioid administration for refractory dyspnea. By integrating palliative care concepts, surgical nursing can become a key contributor to the development of improved care trajectories for COPD patients, leading to holistic and patient-centered treatment throughout the disease course.

3.2.2. Asthma and Its Implications

Asthma is a chronic respiratory condition consisting of airway inflammation and hyperreactivity, which results in wheezing, breathlessness, chest tightness, and cough. Asthma knowledge is essential in the clinical practice of surgical nursing, particularly in the perioperative period. Asthmatic patients have an increased risk for the intra- and postoperative occurrence of respiratory complications due to their reactive airways. This makes preoperative assessment significant; nurses must determine the severity of the patient's asthma, how effectively it is controlled, and whether or not there has been any recent deterioration. Ineffective management techniques must be tailored to each individual patient, typically through optimization of control medication in the lead-up to surgical intervention, thereby minimizing complications resulting from ineffective management, like bronchospasm or hypoxemia. Beyond immediate respiratory effects, asthma can travel a long way in complicating anesthesiology procedures. The presence of asthma also facilitates airway challenges during intubation and anesthesia management. It is recommended that anesthetists conduct extensive assessments of asthmatic patients in order to predict possible complications, especially among children, where obesity may complicate the clinical scenario (Jacob et al., 2015). Due to the systemic nature of asthma and the comorbidities that accompany it, surgical teams should embrace an interdisciplinary approach to provide integral management. This entails collaborative planning between anesthetic, surgical, and nursing staff to optimize patient outcomes and prevent hazards of the respiratory condition. Postoperative care also includes vigilant monitoring of patients with asthma. Scholars indicate that asthma patients undergoing surgery have higher rates of respiratory complications, such as pneumonia and slow recovery from anesthesia, which contribute to prolonged hospital stays (Jacob et al., 2015). Thus, postoperative care must be directed toward meticulous monitoring of respiratory function, with provisions available to administer proper bronchodilators and anti-inflammatory medications. Effective discharge planning is also necessary; patients and carers must be instructed on how to recognize asthmatic precipitants following surgery, thereby improving their ability to provide optimal respiratory function upon discharge back home. By implementing a comprehensive care plan that addresses the individual needs of asthmatic patients, surgical nursing can significantly improve patient safety and recovery (Figure 3.7).

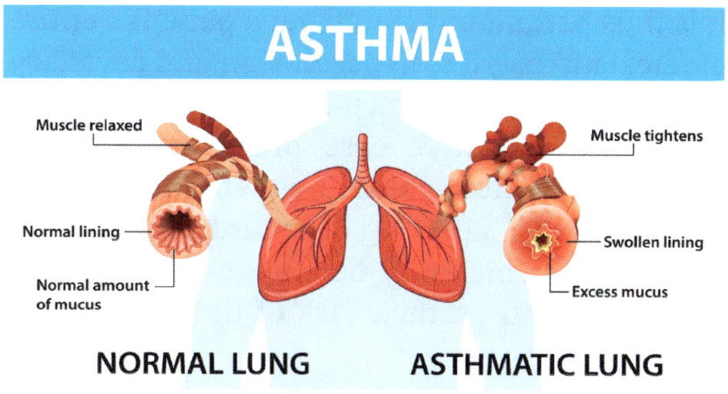

Figure 3.7. Asthma and its implications.

Source: https://static.vecteezy.com/system/resources/previews/003/244/384/original/asthma-diagram-with-normal-lung-and-asthmatic-lung-free-vector.jpg.

3.2.3. Pulmonary Embolism and Its Risks

The pulmonary embolism (PE) condition is a critical risk factor in the management of patients undergoing surgery, particularly thoracic cavity surgery. PE is defined as a form of venous thromboembolism whereby the blood clot travels to the pulmonary arteries, blocks the flow of blood, and results in severe respiratory dysfunction. This condition may manifest with a variety of symptoms, such as acute shortness of breath, chest pain, and hypoxia that complicate postoperative recovery in patients. The severity of PE not only lies in its sudden onset but also in the predisposing factors that increase the likelihood of its occurrence, such as prolonged bed rest, recent surgery, and underlying coagulopathies. Surgical nurses must remain vigilant and employ preventive measures, such as thromboprophylaxis, especially among high-risk groups, to prevent these potential adverse effects. When assessing the risk of pulmonary embolism, it is essential to consider patient-specific factors that may increase the likelihood of experiencing this complication during surgery. In research, pre-existing cardiovascular disease has been found to elevate operative mortality and serious complications, including PE significantly.

It is thus paramount to find out a patient's entire medical history, like hypertension and coronary artery disease, to determine surgical risk and tailor perioperative care plans accordingly. Clinical practice guidelines emphasize the importance of applying standardized tools to assess risk, which may be employed to stratify patients based on their risk of developing PE.

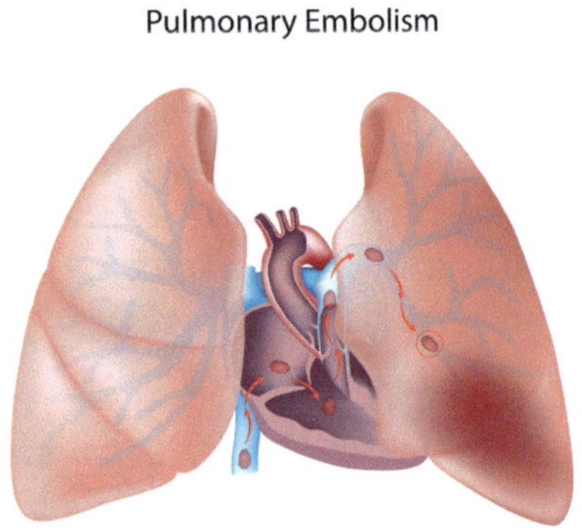

Figure 3.8. Pulmonary embolism.

Source: https://risks-of-surgery.com/wp-content/uploads/2022/05/pulmonary-embolism.jpeg.

Active management and identification of each patient's risk factors eventually lead to improved surgical outcomes and improved patient safety during the perioperative period. Besides respiratory consequences of pulmonary embolism, other fields of perioperative morbidity are also impacted. Notably, mortality from PE has been highlighted in recent evaluations with an operative mortality of 3.2%, and cardiovascular complications being the most frequent cause. Surveillance and assessment during surgeries facilitates early detection of PE, which may allow for more timely and effective treatment interventions. Adherence to evidence-based guidelines, encompassing both pharmacological and non-pharmacological interventions, forms the foundation of effective management in high-risk patients. Greater education and training of the surgical nursing staff regarding the pathophysiology and risk factors of PE are essential for establishing a proactive care culture, whereby patient safety is prioritized in every operating room (de Perrot et al., 2017) (Figure 3.8).

Test Your Knowledge

1. What is the main difference between asthma and COPD in terms of reversibility of airway obstruction?
2. How does pneumonia affect gas exchange in the lungs?

3.3. Assessment Techniques for Respiratory Function

Learning Outcome

1. Explain the patient history and physical examination
2. Define the diagnostic imaging and tests
3. Describe the pulmonary function tests and their significance

In surgical nursing care, evaluating respiratory function is crucial for detecting pulmonary disease and optimizing patient management. Various techniques are used to evaluate respiratory function, including spirometry, peak flow measurement, and pulse oximetry. Spirometry, for instance, allows for the quantification of volumes and rates of breathing, giving important information about obstructive and restrictive lung disease. The accuracy of this method is enhanced when tracked relative to normative standards, thus informing personalized patient care. Moreover, the application of peak flow meters allows tracking of individuals with diagnosed asthma or chronic obstructive pulmonary disease (COPD), offering a simple way to measure lung function in real time. Another key aspect of respiratory assessment involves the application of auscultation to detect abnormal lung sounds that may indicate underlying conditions. This is the foundation for diagnosing conditions such as pneumonia, pleural effusion, and bronchial obstruction. Differentiation of normal and abnormal breath sounds by the patient is essential for timely treatment. In addition, the utilization of sophisticated imaging techniques, such as chest X-rays and computed tomography scans, can complement auscultation findings, providing an overall picture of the patient's respiratory status. Most importantly, the practitioners' ability to integrate findings from diverse techniques and tailor them to specific care situations can significantly determine the reliability of respiratory assessment. In conclusion, the reliability of respiratory evaluation can only be ensured through meticulous reporting and documentation, as detailed in the PRISMA 2020 guidelines, where transparent reporting takes center stage in clinical practice (Page et al., 2021). Several recommendations and policies are implemented to inform healthcare workers through patient care, particularly in rapidly evolving medical environments. ESC guidelines focus on the fact that healthcare professionals must weigh evidence provided in clinical guidelines against individualized circumstances of their patients so that care is evidence-informed as well as personalized (Baumgartner et al., 2020). Thus, operating room nurses must continue to be skilled at evaluating respiratory function through a combination of assessment techniques and employing clinical judgments that adhere to established standards in responding to the specific needs of every patient. This multifaceted process ultimately results in enhanced care being delivered to patients with pulmonary disease (Figure 3.9).

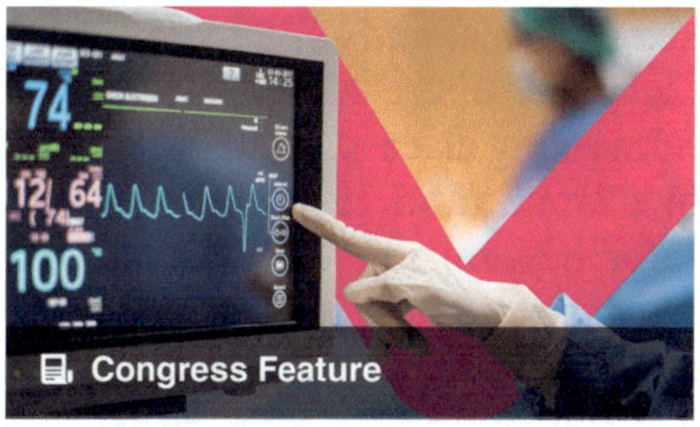

Figure 3.9. European society of cardiology.

Source: https://www.emjreviews.com/wp-content/uploads/2023/10/2023-European-Society-of-Cardiology-Guidelines-Feature-1-1.png.

3.3.1. Patient History and Physical Examination

A comprehensive patient history is critical in assessing respiratory function, particularly in the context of pulmonary disease, in surgical nursing. The process is the initial phase and most critical in gathering information on the medical history of the patients, including previous diagnoses, treatments, and comorbid conditions that may complicate the surgery. An example is a history of exposure to toxic chemicals, such as bleomycin in chemotherapy as a child, which can manifest with respiratory complications in adulthood. In one study, bleomycin patients are noted to exhibit pulmonary function abnormalities after therapy without exhibiting any respiratory symptoms, which underscores the significance of careful history-taking and ongoing follow-up under such circumstances (Özkan et al., 2025). Second, a thorough history of symptoms, such as dyspnea or cough, can reveal underlying pathologies that necessitate preoperative optimization. In addition to the patient's history, a complete physical examination is essential in determining respiratory function. With the physical examination, vital signs are taken, lung sounds are auscultated, and the total respiratory effort of the patients is monitored, which can detect significant dysfunctions or abnormalities that must be further evaluated. For instance, decreased breath sounds or adventitious sounds such as wheezes or crackles indicate obstructive or restrictive lung disease.In addition, the focused physical examination techniques can provide more information; for example, determining the diaphragmatic function can be particularly significant in neuromuscular disorders or after thoracic surgery (Mouratidou et al., 2025). As such, the physical examination must become systematic and detailed, encompassing both broad and targeted assessments to inform patient management. The integration of physical examination and patient history findings with diagnostic test findings results in a thorough approach to assessing respiratory function. Pulmonary function tests, chest X-rays, and other imaging modalities are helpful adjuncts that can support clinical evaluation and help detect specific impairments. In patients with prior exposure to bleomycin, for instance, PFT abnormalities revealed through careful assessment may not present as symptoms, thus requiring frequent follow-up and investigations to identify complications early (Özkan et al., 2025). In turn, where diaphragm dysfunction is suspected after immune checkpoint inhibitor administration, as in newly reported cases, early and targeted testing can lead to effective management measures, e.g., non-invasive ventilation (Mouratidou et al., 2025). Thus, application of an integrated model of history, examination, and diagnostics is crucial in safeguarding optimal respiratory function assessment in the operating room setting.

3.3.2. Diagnostic Imaging and Tests

The role of examination and diagnostic imaging in evaluating respiratory function plays a key role in surgical nursing, particularly in the treatment of pulmonary illnesses. They offer ways to observe the structure and process of the body within the thorax, hence enabling precise diagnosis of diseases such as pneumonia, emphysema, and lung cancers. Chest X-rays, CT scans, and magnetic resonance imaging (MRI) are typical imaging techniques. Each technique has distinct insights; for example, chest X-rays can show airspace opacities that suggest infection, whereas CT scans provide detailed cross-sectional images so that can detect subtle lesions. Furthermore, it is essential to understand the appropriateness and limitations of diagnostic tools, as they are directly related to decision-making and management strategies in patient care within the field of surgery (Baumgartner et al., 2020). In addition to imaging, pulmonary function tests (PFTs) constitute an important element of the comprehensive assessment of respiratory function. These track rates of lung capacity and airflow, enabling the diagnosis of obstructive or restrictive lung diseases. . Compulsive parameters that are quantified are forced expiratory volume in one second (FEV1) and forced vital capacity (FVC), both important in making a diagnosis and the severity of conditions like chronic obstructive pulmonary disease (COPD) or asthma. Interpretation of tests requires a highly sensitive understanding of normal values and how age, sex, and ethnicity affect results. Therefore, surgical nursing specialists ought to be proficient in the interpretation of PFTs, given that they have the propensity to influence preoperative risk assessment and guide postoperative care strategies (Stupp et al., 2017). The integration of diagnostic imaging and pulmonary function testing into the standard examination enables surgical nurses to provide holistic and effective care to individuals with respiratory disorders. Additionally, the ever-evolving advancements in imaging science and pulmonary evaluation methods necessitate nursing practitioners to remain constantly updated in their education. By staying current with developments, nurses can use the most proficient evaluation methods and serve as patient advocates in the operating room. Lastly, inter-professional collaboration with radiologists and respiratory therapists further establishes the nurse's function by encouraging a multi-disciplinary team approach to patient care. As the nursing profession evolves, nurses must adopt a role that combines technical competencies with logical thinking to enable them to make informed decisions regarding diagnostic methods for optimal respiratory health management (Baumgartner et al., 2020) (Figure 3.10).

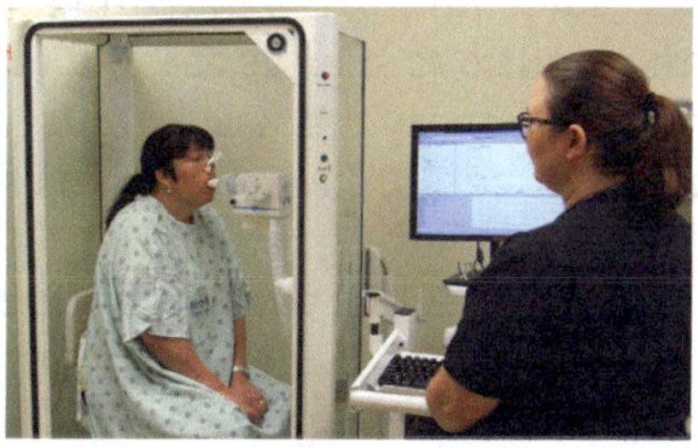

Figure 3.10. Pulmonary function tests.

Source: https://www.mercy.net/content/dam/mercy/en/images/mercy_carthage_plethysmograph.jpg.

3.3.3. Pulmonary Function Tests and Their Significance

Pulmonary function tests (PFTs) are a vital component of patient evaluation and care for patients with a pulmonary disorder, particularly within surgical nursing roles. PFTs quantify various determinants of lung function, including airflow, lung volume, and the efficiency of gas exchange. Understanding respiratory mechanics is essential in surgical nursing, as it enables one to more accurately assess the patient and tailor preoperative preparation. For instance, patients with COPD can present with reduced lung function and impaired diffusion, necessitating changes in surgical strategies to prevent perioperative complications. Thus, PFTs provide not only diagnostic data but also prognostic markers that guide operating rooms to maximize patient outcomes during the perioperative period. Incorporating PFT results into intraoperative decision-making can significantly impact preoperative evaluation. Specifically, the results are beneficial in identifying patients at high risk of postoperative complications, such as respiratory failure or prolonged hospitalization. For surgical nurses, awareness of the risks is crucial in making proper plans for interventions and postoperative care. In addition, quantification of the severity of pulmonary function impairment enables the surgical team to balance surgical urgency against the risks involved. According to professionals, systematic testing of pulmonary function can enhance the surgical care of patients suffering from pulmonary disease, underscoring the importance of interprofessional communication among healthcare experts (Halvorsen et al., 2022). The value of accurate and correct reporting of pulmonary function test results cannot be overstated, particularly in surgical nursing. A systematic approach to conducting and reporting PFTs, as advocated by the PRISMA guidelines, ensures consistency and accuracy across studies, thereby building confidence in clinical findings (Page et al., 2021). By adhering to such protocols, operating room nurses enhance their effectiveness in applying PFT results to clinical practice, optimizing patient-centered care. Furthermore, continued research and innovation in new PFT technologies have the potential to enhance diagnostic capabilities and therapeutic interventions. This evolving development requiring surgical teams to keep up to date with current advances in pulmonary function testing in order to achieve the best possible patient outcomes and to offer safe surgery (Figure 3.11).

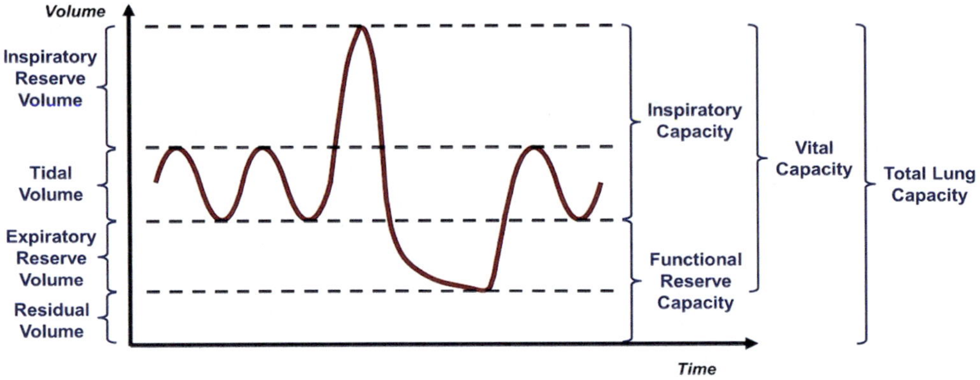

Figure 3.11. Pulmonary function tests (PFT).

Source: https://i.ytimg.com/vi/6TApeMJ-rkc/maxresdefault.jpg.

Test Your Knowledge

1. What are common signs a nurse looks for during inspection of a patient's respiratory status?
2. How is auscultation used to assess lung function?

3.4. Management Strategies for Pulmonary Disorders

Learning Outcome

1. Identify the pharmacological interventions of pulmonary disorders
2. Define the non-pharmacological therapies of pulmonary disorders
3. Describe the surgical options and considerations

Effective management of respiratory disease depends on a strategy that combines clinical assessment, education, and tailored treatment. A thorough assessment of respiratory function is essential in determining the individual needs of those with conditions such as asthma or chronic obstructive pulmonary disease. Surgical nursing encompasses a comprehensive understanding of such tests, including pulmonary function tests and imaging tests, to assess the severity of the disorder. Use of evidence-based practice as outlined in clinical guidelines is critical in enhancing the quality of care provided to such patients. Notably, the PRISMA guidelines promote transparent reporting and alignment with high-quality scientific standards, ensuring that management guidelines based on systematic reviews are valid and practical (Page et al., 2021). Of the many strategies used for managing pulmonary disease, pharmacologic therapies are a cornerstone. Treatment with bronchodilators, corticosteroids, and mucolytic agents can significantly improve lung function and overall quality of life in those with the condition. In children, treatment must be particularly sensitive to the developmental needs of young children and adolescents. It may require specially designed interventions addressing the physical and psychosocial aspects of their illness. Recent recommendations for disorders like bronchiectasis have highlighted the requirement for a multimodal strategy by pediatric specialists, nurses, and patient advocacy organizations (Chang et al., 2021).

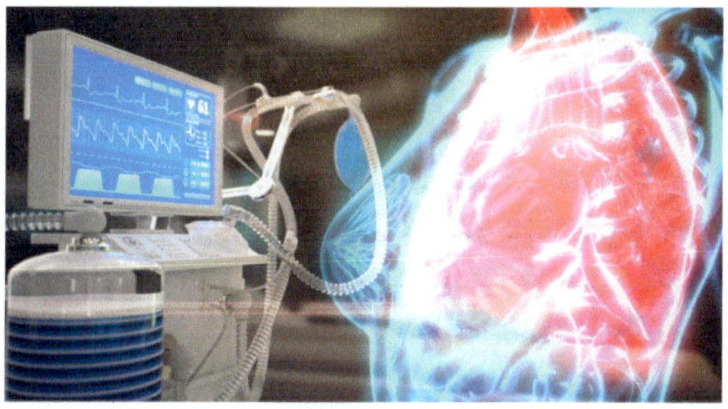

Figure 3.12. Protective lung strategy protocol in ARDS management.

Source: https://external-content.duckduckgo.com/iu/?u=https%3A%2F%2Fstatic.wixstatic.com%2Fmedia%2Fe4917c_ca0803fc45f342c7b7d09b1d5c72218a~mv2.jpg%2Fv1%2Ffill%2Fw_4200%2Ch_2363%2Cal_c%2Cq_90%2Cenc_auto%2FICU%252004.jpg&f=1&nofb=1&ipt=887604eac68022bdfe1bc0b6758d89f8bdb788b63b70be0f33cf5c3fdf5050e4.

Follow-up and monitoring are also essential components of effective management regimens for pulmonary disorders. Periodic assessment enables the re-prioritization of treatment modalities in response to evolving patient needs and their response to therapy. In operating room nursing, continuous assessment is of paramount significance, particularly for patients under consideration for surgery, as their pulmonary function must be closely monitored to minimize perioperative risks. In addition, teaching patients self-management techniques—i.e., recognizing symptoms of exacerbation and executing airway clearance maneuvers—enables individuals to take an active role in managing their own care. Developing quality care measures, as proposed by new recommendations for a number of pulmonary illnesses, enables clinicians to make regular practice improvements and also to direct additional research (Chang et al., 2021) (Figure 3.12).

3.4.1. Pharmacological Interventions

Pharmacological care in surgical nursing plays a crucial role in treating respiratory disorders, particularly in maximizing pre- and post-procedure respiratory function. Proper management typically involves the administration of bronchodilators, corticosteroids, and mucolytics, each of which serves a distinct function in alleviating symptoms and improving airflow. For example, bronchodilators are used to cause airway dilation, providing rapid relief from bronchospasm, which is particularly helpful for patients with diseases such as asthma or chronic obstructive pulmonary disease (COPD). Corticosteroids may be used to reduce inflammation, thereby addressing underlying issues that potentially endanger. Lastly, judicious utilization of these pharmacologic agents encourages not just relief of symptoms but also patient comfort and overall success of surgery. Pharmacological treatments within the context of Enhanced Recovery After Surgery (ERAS) protocols have demonstrated significant advantages in perioperative care for patients with respiratory issues. These clinical guidelines emphasize the importance of using pharmacological treatments to reduce complications, expedite recovery time, and improve clinical outcomes. For instance, preoperative bronchodilators have been proven to decrease pulmonary complications after surgery. Also, early postoperative use of corticosteroids is able to can reduce the frequency of inflammatory reactions and ensure quicker rehabilitation. As outlined in recent consensus guidelines, the combination of pharmacologic treatments aligns with a comprehensive approach to treating respiratory diseases, emphasizing the role of individualized patient care within surgery, thereby leading to improved outcomes (Engelman et al., 2019). Continuing pharmacotherapeutic improvements necessitate that operating room nurses stay informed about new therapies and their capabilities for patient care. Understanding current practice guidelines and engaging in ongoing education ensures that interprofessional teams are well-equipped to effectively implement pharmacological strategies tailored to each patient's unique health profile. As highlighted by the ESC Guidelines, healthcare practitioners are invited to evaluate critically the suitability of the current treatment options and adapt these to reflect best current evidence with regards to the individual patient's needs (Baumgartner et al., 2020). With the addition of pharmacologic interventions supported by robust research and evidence-based best practices, surgical nurses can enhance the assessment and management of pulmonary disease. This therapy not only benefits respiratory function but also significantly contributes to the overall success of operations and the postoperative recovery of patients.

3.4.2. Non-Pharmacological Therapies

In nursing, as applied to pulmonary disease, non-pharmacologic therapy is increasingly being discovered to be an essential adjunct to conventional treatments. It encompasses interventions of virtually all kinds, such as pulmonary rehabilitation, breathing exercises, and patient education, aimed at enhancing respiratory function and overall patient comfort. Through techniques that enhance lung function and promote patient participation in managing their own well-being, surgical nurses can be directly integrated into the comprehensive care of respiratory illnesses. These therapeutic techniques not only assist in symptom reduction of pulmonary disease but also help patients adopt healthier habits, allowing for healthier surgical outcomes and quicker recovery levels. Pulmonary rehabilitation is one of the most effective non-pharmacologic approaches to the treatment of respiratory illnesses. This is an integrated program that combines physical training, nutrition counseling, and educational training, tailored to the individual needs of patients with diseases such as chronic obstructive pulmonary disease (COPD) or bronchial asthma. Due to their involvement in the rehabilitation process, patients enhance exercise tolerance, reduce dyspnea, and improve the quality of life. In addition, breathing techniques learned through rehabilitation enable patients to manage their symptoms more effectively, leading to a sense of mastery over their health. Bringing these techniques into preoperative assessment may have the power to affect readiness for surgery and postoperative recovery alike, thereby contributing to the imperative of incorporating nonpharmacological treatment into the framework of surgical nursing. Instruction in lifestyle modification is a crucial aspect of non-pharmacological interventions for respiratory management. Nurses may encourage smoking cessation, a proper diet, and exercise, all of which are essential for maintaining proper respiratory function. Lifestyle modification has been shown to not only reinforce conventional treatments but also to prevent the progression of disease in patients with chronic respiratory illness. As shown in complementary and alternative medicine studies, patients actually view such therapies as supplementary to traditional medical treatments, implying greater awareness of the role of holistic approaches to healthcare (Mu'in et al., 2015). The incorporation of non-pharmacological therapies into surgical nursing can thus lead to a more comprehensive and improved method of managing pulmonary diseases, with an emphasis on patient-focused practice that considers both the clinical and holistic aspects of care (Figure 3.13).

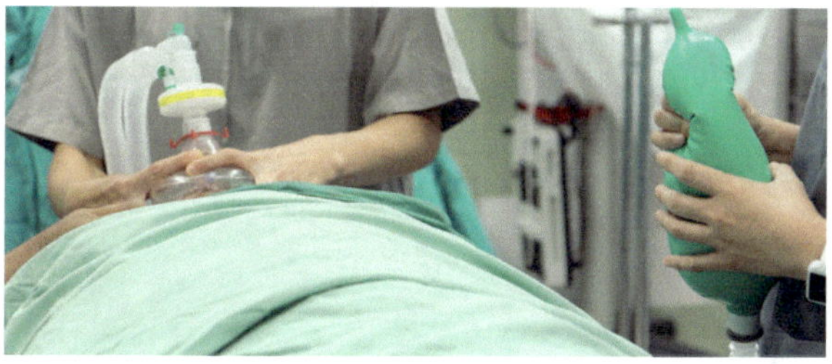

Figure 3.13. Non-pharmacological therapies.

Source: https://www.hgtc.edu/images/academics/programs/respitory-care-myrtle-beach-sc.jpg.

3.4.3. Surgical Options and Considerations

Surgical management of pulmonary diseases involves a complex interplay of decisions and variables crucial to achieving the most beneficial patient outcomes. Preoperative assessment must thus be elaborate to ascertain the patient's respiratory status and to establish the risk of various surgeries. It encompasses physiological measures such as spirometry, imaging examinations, and arterial blood gas analysis, which measure the functioning of the respiratory system. The surgeon's choices to undertake lobectomy, pneumonectomy, or video-assisted thoracoscopic surgery (VATS) is based on the nature and extent of the underlying pulmonary disease, as well as the patient's overall health status. Using clinical judgment combined with evidence-based guidelines, surgical teams can tailor interventions to the specific needs of individual patients without inciting perioperative complications. In the management of pulmonary conditions, surgical application should conform to the latest guidelines and standards. The ESC Guidelines are a benchmark that medical practitioners employ as a guide to practice, emphasizing that patient examination should not only encompass indications for surgery but also the patient's health status and preferences. The ESC also encourages practitioners to select the optimal option among various therapeutic practices and make well-informed choices through informed decision-making, informed by existing evidence-based research. The recommendations does not replace the clinician's responsibility to use judgment and make evidence-based decisions, but simply guide them towards the allocation of treatments to scientifically established practices to enhance the quality of care given to patients for surgery for respiratory diseases (Baumgartner et al., 2020). Additionally, postoperative issues in respiratory surgical nursing are of utmost importance, as they play a contributory role in the patient's recovery process.

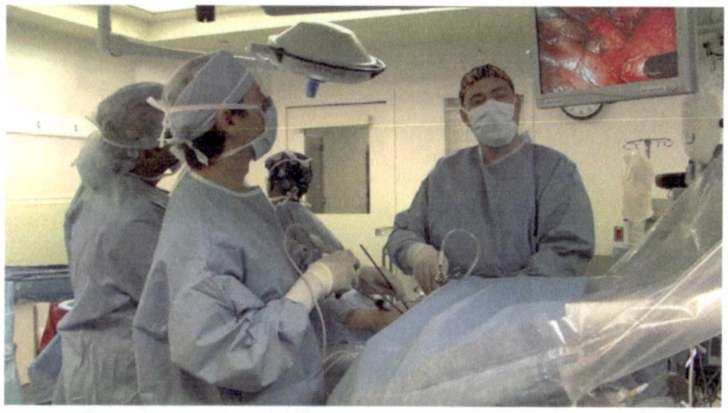

Figure 3.14. Video-assisted thoracic surgery.

Source: https://i.ytimg.com/vi/KoBw_-xj68E/maxresdefault.jpg.

Closely monitoring respiratory function after surgery is necessary to identify potential complications, such as atelectasis or pneumonia, which are more likely to occur due to compromised lung mechanics or secretions following surgery. Safe management practices, such as early mobilization and incentive spirometry, are well known to significantly enhance respiratory outcomes and reduce the hospital stay period. Furthermore, interdisciplinary surgical teams, respiratory therapists, and nursing staff must work in concert so that these measures can be implemented to the best possible extent. Such collaboration ensures that all the determinants of care are addressed, providing a comprehensive range approach to patient recovery from pulmonary surgery (Page et al., 2021) (Figure 3.14).

Test Your Knowledge

1. What is the role of bronchodilators in managing asthma and COPD?
2. Why is oxygen therapy used in patients with severe respiratory conditions?

3.5 Role of Surgical Nursing in Respiratory Care

Learning Outcome

1. Describe the preoperative assessment and preparation
2. Define the intraoperative management of respiratory function
3. Discuss the postoperative care and monitoring

Effective management of surgical respiratory care depends on various well-established assessment protocols, particularly to the evaluation of pulmonary function. Preoperative evaluations are of utmost significance, wherein surgical nurses conduct a thorough evaluation of patients' respiratory condition to identify any intrinsic pulmonary complications that may complicate surgery. This being a preventive measure ensures that respiratory complications can be prevented by early management before surgery, significantly enhancing recovery. Moreover, operating room nurses must be proficient at recognizing signs of respiratory distress, such as abnormal lung sounds or reduced oxygen saturation levels, in an attempt to make early interventions. Through adherence to rigorous assessment protocols, they greatly contribute to developing the cornerstone of safe surgical practices and ultimately improve patients' overall respiratory functioning (Page et al., 2021). Surgical nursing responsibilities in the postoperative phase include managing pulmonary complications that may arise after surgery. This is a critical area of care, given that patients are at risk for respiratory infection, atelectasis, and hypoxemia following surgery. Several techniques, such as incentive spirometry and deep breathing exercises, are utilized by surgical nurses to aid lung inflation effectively and ensure proper oxygenation. In addition, using evidence-based practice from guidelines established in Enhanced Recovery After Surgery (ERAS) protocols effective recovery without defensive complications of pulmonary disease. Continuous education and adherence to these protocols prepare surgical nurses to effectively manage respiratory complications, enabling patients to achieve optimal postoperative recovery (Gustafsson et al., 2018). Moreover, patient education and patient advocacy are responsibilities of the surgical nurse in respiratory care. Patient education on respiratory health, including adherence to postoperative orders and recognizing respiratory symptoms, is crucial. By equipping patients with education and strategies to help them maintain their respiratory disease, surgical nurses encourage autonomy in their own recovery process. This learning component also enhances nurses' ability to represent patients so that their ventilation needs are recorded and addressed in the sequence of surgery. Interprofessional collaboration between surgical teams and nursing practitioners is essential here since they collectively address the complex relationship between surgical procedures and respiratory care, significantly optimizing health outcomes and patient satisfaction (Page et al., 2021) (Figure 3.15).

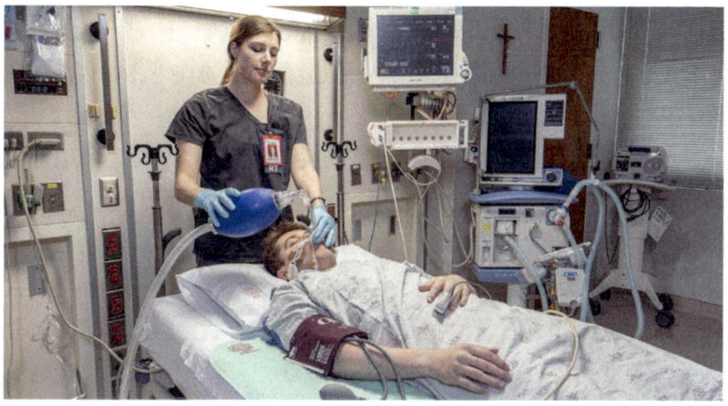

Figure 3.15. Role of surgical nursing in respiratory care.

Source: https://external-content.duckduckgo.com/iu/?u=https%3A%2F%2Fwww.umary.edu%2Fsites%2Fdefault%2Ffiles%2Fstyles%2Foptimized%2Fpublic%2F2021-09%2FAcademics-Undergraduate-Respiratory%2520Therapy-Respiratory%2520Therapist-%2520Intubating%2520patient.jpg%3Fitok%3DfRPscWDH&f=1&nofb=1&ipt=ce7543c9d562ffd52a1b48e21df9cab9096e0ca81457c8f021b6a0f1da1ff280.

3.5.1. Preoperative Assessment and Preparation

Effective preoperative evaluation and preparation are essential components of managing patients with respiratory disease who are undergoing surgery. It begins with a thorough review of the patient's medical history, particularly reviewing their respiratory function and the condition of any concomitant pulmonary disease. A comprehensive assessment can also include diagnostic testing, such as spirometry, arterial blood gas analysis, and imaging, to determine lung capacity and function. The identification of such risk factors as COPD, asthma, and other comorbidities is crucial since they have a pivotal role to play in postoperative results. Rigorous consideration of such risk factors enables surgical teams to devise personalized management strategies that may include maximum medical therapy, enhanced patient education, and anticipation of potential problems throughout the perioperative course, particularly regarding respiratory complications. The contribution of interdisciplinary coordination during the preoperative phase cannot be overemphasized. Team-oriented care among surgeons, anesthesiologists, respiratory therapists, and nursing staff ensures intensive care for the pulmonary patient. Interdisciplinary cooperation enables the development of an individualized care plan that addresses both the surgical and respiratory needs of the patient. Preoperative interventions may include pulmonary rehabilitation, smoking cessation therapy, and breathing exercise training. Moreover, psychosocial counseling is critical as the patients will likely have anxiety and fear about their surgery outcome. These emotional factors can be addressed through counseling and may make the recovery process less painful. Organized preoperative evaluation can diminish anesthetic risk and postoperative complications by enhancing the preparation of patients for surgery. The findings of practical preoperative evaluation are directly proportional to reduced morbidity and mortality among surgical patients, particularly those with compromised respiratory function. Research shows that preoperative care, if taken with caution, can lead to better overall outcomes of surgery, including lower operative mortality and lower incidence of potentially fatal complications like respiratory failure and myocardial infarction, especially in high-risk patients with such conditions as CAD and those who are ASA class 3 or 4 (de Perrot et al., 2017). Adherence to evidence-based guidelines also enhances the safety of surgical interventions. For example, preoperative management in children with neuromuscular conditions emphasizes the significance of such preparation while dealing with complex cases that may involve serious complications in the event of poor handling (Marsh et al., 2008). Therefore, the integration of proper preoperative evaluation practices is essential for ensuring positive surgical outcomes in patients with breathing difficulties (Figure 3.16).

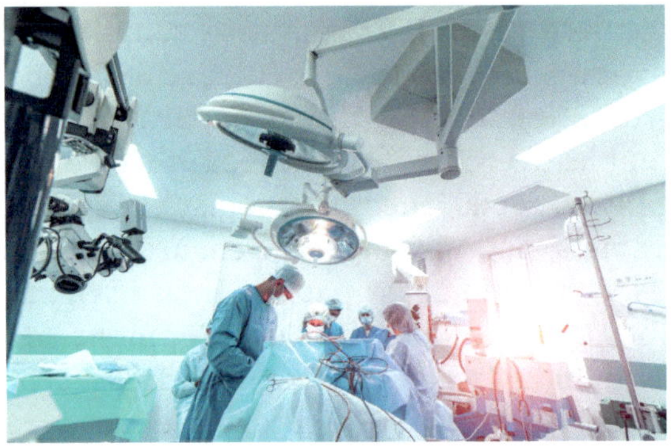

Figure 3.16. Preoperative assessment and preparation.

Source: https://lirp.cdn-website.com/627f2e53/dms3rep/multi/opt/AdobeStock_377279200-1920w.jpg.

3.5.2. Intraoperative Management of Respiratory Function

Intraoperative management of respiratory function is a crucial element in optimizing patient outcomes during anesthesia, particularly for patients with potential respiratory complications. Effective respiratory parameter monitoring, including oxygen saturation and airway function, enables surgical teams to recognize and address deterioration promptly. The application of guidelines and risk assessment methods plays a significant role in facilitating the monitoring process. For instance, the Modified Early Warning Score (MEWS) is a considerable instrument found to be beneficial in the detection of vulnerable patients for postoperative respiratory failure. According to research, the inclusion of MEWS in nursing documentation enables health practitioners to detect signs of patient deterioration early, thereby providing prompt interventions that can prevent significant complications, such as respiratory failure (Henley et al., 2011). Hence, watchful intraoperative monitoring during surgery remains at the heart of protecting respiratory function and ensuring patient safety. In addition to aggressive monitoring measures, care in anesthesia needs to be specifically tailored to meet the respiratory needs of high-risk patients, including those with pre-existing obstructive sleep apnea (OSA). OSA patients are particularly susceptible to perioperative disruption from respiratory and cardiovascular instability. Unfortunately, most OSA patients with moderate-to-severe disease remain undiagnosed and thereby increase the risk during surgery (Diamond et al., 2019). Thus, utilizing preoperative screening devices such as the STOP-BANG questionnaire can help detect OSA patients before anesthesia administration. Anesthesia protocols that are specific to combat potential threats of OSA can then be designed, for example, with careful selection of drugs to prevent respiratory depression. By resolving these problems, intraoperative respiratory care and, by extension, surgical outcomes in high-risk populations can be maximized by surgical nursing staff. Finally, the use of multimodal analgesia with prudent titration of narcotics is crucial in maintaining respiratory function during and after surgery. Postoperative respiratory failure, an emergent issue for surgical patients, has been linked to excessive narcotic administration. Research emphasizes minimizing opioid exposure in the perioperative setting, with higher doses of narcotics risking respiratory drive and having negative consequences (Henley et al., 2011). Utilization of adjunctive analgesic modalities, like regional anesthesia modes, will significantly minimize narcotic use administration and thus maximize respiratory stability. By prioritizing the management of respiratory function through integrative analgesic approaches, surgical teams can reduce the incidence of postoperative respiratory complications, thereby enhancing patient outcomes and surgical effectiveness. The integration of such interventions into surgical procedures is one form of commitment to evidence-based practice in nursing for patients who are at risk of pulmonary disease.

3.5.3. Postoperative Care and Monitoring

Adequate postoperative care and observation are crucial for preserving optimal respiratory function after surgery, particularly in individuals with chronic pulmonary disease. Initial observation involved a close assessment of vital signs, including respiratory rate, oxygen saturation, and heart rate. These are significant since they may indicate early signs of complications such as atelectasis or respiratory depression, which are known to be more frequent following thoracic and abdominal procedures. There should be proper oxygenation and ventilation; hence, the use of pulse oximetry and arterial blood gas analysis will provide timely feedback on the respiratory status of the patient. In addition, the use of incentive spirometry is essential in a bid to prevent postoperative complications by encouraging deep breaths and lung expansion to reduce pulmonary complication risk caused by immobility and anesthesia (Reynolds et al., 2011). In addition to observing vital signs and administering respiratory therapies, assessment for pain management is essential in postoperative care. Uncontrolled pain can significantly impair a patient's capacity to take deep breaths and execute other maneuvers necessary for optimal respiratory function. A multimodal approach to analgesia, including systemic as well as local anesthetic techniques, can therefore maximize comfort and allow for early mobilization. Early ambulation not only reduces pain but also improves pulmonary function and minimizes the incidence of complications such as deep vein thrombosis and pneumonia. The integration of patient education regarding pain management and respiratory maneuvers into the treatment schedule is necessary because it enables the patient to become an active participant in the healing process (Chimbira et al., 2001). Postoperative observation is also essential in the early detection of complications, which tend to have a profound impact on recovery. This entails frequent observation for signs of respiratory distress, including increased work of breathing and altered mental status. These symptoms could signify hypoxia or hypercapnia. Continuous monitoring equipment, such as capnometers, can also give helpful information regarding the carbon dioxide levels, making intervention on time possible if so needed. Additionally, having an organized protocol for respiratory monitoring after surgery in high-risk patients, such as those with obesity and chronic obstructive pulmonary disease, can improve outcomes. With the inclusion of stringent postoperative care and monitoring, healthcare providers can also offer a smoother recovery course, reducing the duration of hospital stay and enhancing overall patient satisfaction (Chimbira et al., 2001) (Figure 3.17).

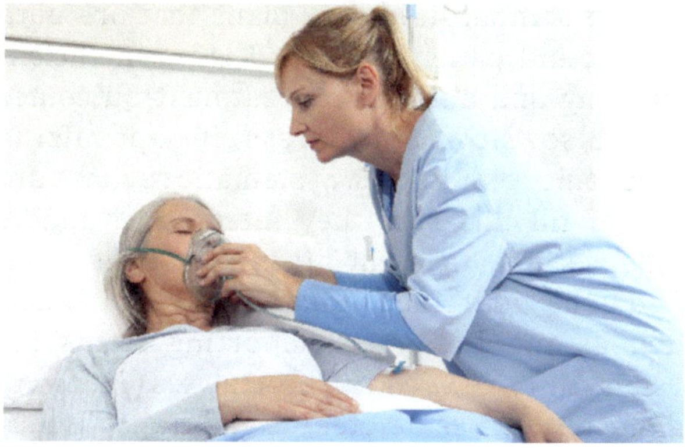

Figure 3.17. Postoperative care and monitoring.

Source: https://nursingeducation.org/wp-content/uploads/2023/09/Respiratory-Nurse.jpg.

Test Your Knowledge

1. What are key postoperative respiratory assessments a surgical nurse performs after thoracic surgery?
2. How does a surgical nurse help prevent respiratory complications such as atelectasis?

3.6. Challenges in Managing Pulmonary Disorders

Learning Outcome

1. Describe the patient compliance and education
2. Define the complications during surgical procedures
3. Identify the multidisciplinary approach to care

Management of pulmonary diseases creates multifaceted challenges that require profound understanding of respiratory physiology, particularly in the operating room nursing environment. The greatest challenge is patient variability in terms of reaction to treatment protocols, and this is based on comorbid conditions, age, as well as distinctive health histories. All these make it challenging to develop standardized care plans that are both effective and patient tailored. Besides, inefficient reporting and analysis of treatment outcomes have also slowed progress in optimizing management strategies. Systematic reviews are here to fill this gap; they integrate available evidence and highlight areas in practice that need to be addressed. Adherence to guidelines, such as the Preferred Reporting Items for Systematic reviews and Meta-Analyses (PRISMA), can foster data completeness and transparency in reporting the care of pulmonary disorders (Page et al., 2021). Preoperative assessment is another significant challenge, as it aims to identify potential pulmonary complications in patients undergoing surgery. Surgery can exacerbate underlying pulmonary conditions; therefore, accurate tests are necessary. Medical professionals may not have standardized assessment forms, and there will be inconsistent results and the possibility of under-inspection of crucial facts. An evidence-based process is crucial for improving preoperative evaluations and effectively managing the risks associated with pulmonary diseases. The ERAS Society emphasizes the importance of perioperative care guidelines in a well-structured format, with an integration of high-quality trials and consensus advice drawn up by rigorous research (Gustafsson et al., 2018). By enforcing such evidence-based guidelines, surgical nursing may enhance patients' outcomes and minimize the risk of postoperative pulmonary complications. Lastly, rehabilitation and postoperative recovery are fraught with challenges that require multidisciplinary approaches in pulmonary management. Postoperative patients recovering from a surgical procedure may have impaired pulmonary function secondary to extensive immobilization, pain, or inadequate control of comorbidities. This is particularly true in surgical nursing, where the primary role of the nurse is to monitor respiratory status and implement interventions aimed at improving respiratory function. This notwithstanding, inadequate resources or staff training in pulmonary rehabilitation may curtail successful recovery. Counter to these issues is following through with well-tested rehabilitation programs and incorporating respiratory therapists in the operating room team, which can significantly improve outcomes postoperatively. Thus, addressing multifaceted issues in managing pulmonary diseases calls for ongoing education, research, and interdisciplinarity among various healthcare professions (Figure 3.18).

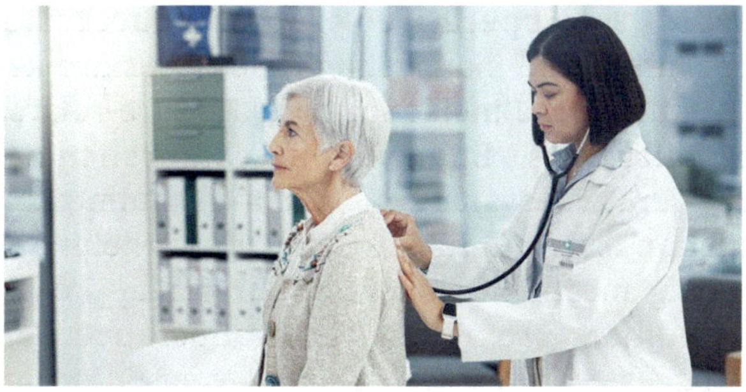

Figure 3.18. Evidence-based strategies for people living with chronic.

Source: https://www.mcmasteroptimalaging.org/images/default-source/blog-post-images/copd.tmb-blogpost.jpg?Culture=en&sfvrsn=4a5416d6_3.

3.6.1. Patient Compliance and Education

Effective compliance and education of the patient are crucial in the management of pulmonary disease, particularly in surgical care. Obtaining patients' information regarding their conditions, treatments, and the indication for particular interventions will enhance significantly enhance their adherence to prescribed therapy. Education is more than merely transferring information about medications and lifestyle modifications; it also encompasses symptom observation and awareness of complications. Through properly formatted educational programs and the dissemination of concise, comprehensible material, healthcare providers can empower patients, thereby creating an environment in which patients are actively involved in controlling their own health. Furthermore, active patients who are appropriately informed about their treatment procedures tend to make appropriate behavioral modifications, which can lead to improved surgical outcomes and overall respiratory function. In respiratory care, patient education includes demonstrating proper techniques for inhalation therapy, such as dispensing inhalers or nebulizers. Operating room nurses play a central role in the teaching process of educating patients to administer these therapies effectively. The emphasis on technique is critical because inadequate utilization can have unintended consequences, such as suboptimal symptom control and hospital readmission. Additionally, patient participation in education programs tailored to their own surgical procedure fosters a deeper appreciation of how their own respiratory status has a direct impact on recovery from surgery. Providing a personalized education plan helps to counteract specific obstacles to adherence, ultimately resulting in patient autonomy in treatment protocols.

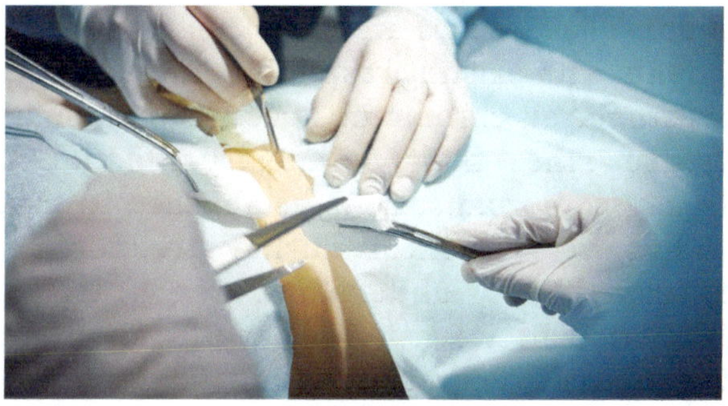

Figure 3.19. Post-surgical care.

Source: https://propelphysiotherapy.com/wp-content/uploads/2020/11/laminectomy-post-surgical-care-propel-physiotherapy.jpg.

Enhancing patient compliance is also made easier by regular follow-up and reinforcement of education messages. Postoperative care provides nurses with an excellent opportunity to assess the success of previous educational interventions and clarify any misunderstandings the patient may have concerning recovery and ongoing management of pulmonary disease. Follow-ups, in the form of in-person visits or telehealth systems, allow the healthcare provider to assess understanding and reinforce crucial information. Moreover, the identification and control of barriers such as health literacy, physical impairment, and emotional distress can significantly impact rates of compliance.

Through the use of a patient-centered approach with a focus on education and encouragement, hospital teams can optimize recovery procedures, leading to improved respiratory function and overall operative outcomes (Figure 3.19).

3.6.2. Complications During Surgical Procedures

The development of surgical complications can significantly impact patient outcomes, particularly regarding respiratory status. Surgery, especially thoracic surgery, can be related to a multitude of pulmonary complications like atelectasis, pneumonia, and respiratory failure. These issues are often compounded in patients with existing respiratory disease, such as asthma or chronic obstructive pulmonary disease, since their pulmonary function is already compromised. As established in case studies, it is critical during preoperative assessment to understand the intricate interaction between pulmonary function and surgical risk. The nursing staff must identify high-risk patients for pulmonary complications and apply the respective adequate measures to prevent such risks during the perioperative process (Cox et al., 2015). For lung resections, surgical nursing should consider specific post-operative complications. Specifically, evidence indicates that respiratory failure is one of the most common complications encountered in patients undergoing lung surgery, with associated morbidity potentially leading to long-term hospitalization and intensive care. Further, studies of patients undergoing surgery for lung cancer reveal that cardiovascular morbidity is one of the most significant causes of perioperative death and morbidity. Also noted in this area is the development of myocardial infarction and pulmonary embolism as significant determinants of surgical result (de Perrot et al., 2017). For perioperative nurses, understanding these multifactorial complications underlies the need for careful preoperative testing and vigilant monitoring across the operative process. Successful prevention and management measures are key to reducing the incidence of procedure-related complications. Engaging in comprehensive preoperative evaluations, such as pulmonary function tests and risk stratification, is helpful in guiding anesthetic choice and surgical approach. In addition, promotion of intraoperative best practices, such as avoidance of ventilation for as long as possible and optimization of pain control, can significantly influence respiratory outcomes. Mobilization and deep breathing exercises should also be emphasized during the postoperative phase to promote lung expansion and mitigate the risk of atelectasis. By adopting an active role in managing respiratory function, surgical nursing personnel can enhance patient recovery and minimize the adverse effects of surgical complications (Cox et al., 2015; de Perrot et al., 2017).

3.6.3. Multidisciplinary Approach to Care

Multidisciplinary care has gained increasing acceptance as part of the management of pulmonary diseases, and especially within surgical nursing practice. Such care brings together various healthcare professionals, including nurses, respiratory therapists, physicians, and pharmacists, to collaborate in addressing the complex needs of patients. Multidisciplinary care not only promotes facilitating inclusive assessment and management practices but also encourages care sharing across each patient's individual challenges. For instance, to manage respiratory function effectively, one needs not only a good understanding of pulmonary mechanics but also sensitivity towards the nutritional and psychological needs of surgical patients. Healthcare teams can develop more effective care routines within with their combined experience, achieving maximum recovery and minimizing respiratory- complications, resulting in improved patient outcomes. Its implementation is best observed under the umbrella of Enhanced Recovery After Surgery (ERAS) protocols, which emphasize evidence-based processes for the improvement of patient care. ERAS protocols advocate for a team approach where surgical teams collaborate with other experts to optimize perioperative care plans. Evidence suggests that the application of multiple disciplines yields significant enhancements in clinical outcomes and cost savings, affirming the value of a collaborative approach. Patient involvement in the recovery process through education and shared decision-making enhances adherence to prevention efforts and treatment measures for pulmonary complications too. Thus, these coordinated approaches not only aid in controlling present circumstances but also prevent postoperative respiratory complications, which are of prime significance in reducing the length of hospital stay and improving the quality of care. Furthermore, adherence to standard guidelines, such as those provided by the European Society of Cardiology (ESC), underscores the importance of a multidisciplinary approach in clinical practice. The ESC Guidelines recommend that medical practitioners consider the collective opinion of various specialties when managing complex patient situations, particularly those related to lung health. The guidelines reaffirm that it is within the scope of health professionals not only to adhere to clinical guideline principles but also to pursue personalized treatment modalities that are appropriate for the patient's specific health status and environment. Within the framework of surgical nursing, the application of these collaborative techniques ensures a thorough and multidimensional respiratory evaluation, ultimately leading to improved pulmonary disease management. Therefore, formulation of a multidisciplinary approach encourages a more patient-focused model of care consistent with professional and ethical standards in the healthcare setting.

Test Your Knowledge

1. What are common barriers to adequate medication adherence in patients with chronic respiratory diseases?
2. How do comorbid conditions complicate the management of pulmonary disorders?

SUMMARY

The intricate intertwinement of respiratory function and surgical outcome necessitates proper understanding and meticulous regulation of pulmonary conditions in the context of surgery in surgical nursing. Throughout the assessment and regulation process, clinical practitioners must apply evidence-based guidelines to inform their practices. As surgery tends to load the respiratory system, identification of underlying conditions and risk factors becomes necessary. This proactive approach not only enhances patient safety but also encourages enhanced clinical outcomes, which leads to increased patient satisfaction rates. Evidence-based assessments incorporated into nursing practice enable individualized interventions tailored to each patient's needs, reflecting the essential role of nursing in the healthcare continuum. Furthermore, the application of systematic review approaches in nursing practices provides a robust basis for clinical decision-making. According to the PRISMA 2020 guidelines, honest and complete reporting of systematic reviews is paramount in developing trustworthiness in outcomes. By adhering to these guidelines, surgical nurses can critically evaluate evidence on respiratory function management, enabling them to implement best practices effectively. Systematic synthesis of data from numerous studies will lead to improved care planning and standardization of protocols for managing respiratory complications among surgical patients. Hence, a strict review and use of evidence are necessary to promote nursing practice and patient care. Ultimately, the application of enhanced recovery protocols will significantly improve surgical outcomes among patients with pulmonary disease. There are findings to suggest that adherence to such guidelines might lead to better clinical outcomes as well as cost savings, particularly in the case of surgical care. Through the integration of findings from various meta-analyses and randomized clinical trials, nursing professionals can create an environment conducive to recovery and optimal perioperative management. Adherence to such evidence-based interventions not only reduces the incidence of postoperative complications but also enhances overall patient recovery pathways. As the field evolves, ongoing study and education in nursing will remain essential in refining these protocols to provide surgical patients with the best care related to respiratory function, ultimately upholding the vital role of nursing in the operating suite (Engelman et al., 2019).

A systematic understanding of respiratory function lies at the heart of assessing and managing pulmonary disease in surgical nursing. Most notably, extubation timing and technique after surgeries such as liver transplant have been emphasized in more recent guidelines, predominantly by the Enhanced Recovery After Surgery Society (ERAS) in 2022. The guidelines emphasize the importance of early extubation to minimize the adverse effects of prolonged mechanical ventilation, including ventilator-associated pneumonia and respiratory muscle deconditioning. But the issue remains in controlling early postoperative hypoxia, typically tied to such conditions as hepatopulmonary syndrome. The importance of understanding what causes hypoxia—such as through standard assessments or new modalities like electrical impedance tomography (EIT)—also highlights the essential role of operating room nurses in achieving optimal patient outcomes and facilitating early intervention to optimize respiratory function and recovery (Li et al., 2023). Management of bronchiectasis in children is no exception and represents a challenging task that requires a complex solution, which can only be met through a multimodal strategy. As the chronic nature of the illness is increasingly appreciated with associated impact on quality of life, clinical management has been codified by the European Respiratory Society (ERS) as guidelines to provide accurate algorithms for management. These guidelines provide a comprehensive review of evidence-based strategies, including diagnostics, treatment, and long-term care plans for children with bronchiectasis. Notably, a multidisciplinary team of healthcare professionals and patient representatives collaborated to address fundamental clinical problems so that the resulting recommendations are applied practically and from the patient perspective. Additionally, their integration into practice represents a step toward more individualized and informed care for patients who require surgical intervention for pulmonary conditions. The integration of new technologies, such as EIT, is beneficial for monitoring respiratory function during critical postoperative periods. With the use of new diagnostic methods, surgical nurses can more effectively assess and manage hypoxia and other respiratory disorders. In doing so, not only is the acute clinical state optimized, but also the long-term outcome of patients with respiratory dysfunction. These combined approaches, based on current literature and interprofessional models, are essential to the development of surgical nursing practice and ultimately patient outcomes in many pulmonary conditions (Chang et al., 2021; Li et al., 2023).

KEY TERMS FROM THIS CHAPTER

- Adventitious breath sounds
- Arterial blood gases (ABGs)
- Auscultation
- Chest physiotherapy
- Hypercapnia
- Incentive spirometry
- Nebulization therapy
- Oxygen therapy
- Pulmonary embolism
- Pulse oximetry
- Airway clearance techniques
- Atelectasis
- Bronchodilators
- Chest X-ray
- Hypoxemia
- Mechanical ventilation
- Oxygen saturation (SpO_2)
- Pneumonia
- Pulmonary function tests (PFTs)
- Respiratory Rate

CRITICAL THINKING QUESTIONS

1. **Which of the following is a primary nursing assessment for evaluating respiratory function?**
   a. Measuring blood glucose
   b. Assessing bowel sounds
   c. Auscultating lung sounds
   d. Checking capillary refill
2. **What is the purpose of incentive spirometry in postoperative patients?**
   a. To prevent constipation
   b. To reduce pain
   c. To promote lung expansion and prevent atelectasis
   d. To improve appetite
3. **Which arterial blood gas (ABG) value indicates respiratory acidosis?**
   a. pH 7.48, $PaCO_2$ 30 mmHg
   b. pH 7.35, $PaCO_2$ 40 mmHg
   c. pH 7.30, $PaCO_2$ 50 mmHg
   d. pH 7.45, $PaCO_2$ 35 mmHg
4. **A patient with a history of COPD is scheduled for surgery. What is a priority preoperative intervention?**
   a. Withhold bronchodilators
   b. Educate on chest physiotherapy and breathing exercises
   c. Encourage bed rest for 24 hours
   d. Increase fluid intake to 4L/day
5. **Which symptom is an early indicator of hypoxia in surgical patients?**
   a. Cyanosis
   b. Bradycardia
   c. Restlessness and confusion
   d. Decreased urine output

Short Answer Questions

1. What are two common postoperative respiratory complications?
2. Define atelectasis.
3. What is the purpose of performing a pulse oximetry test?
4. Name two nursing assessments used to evaluate respiratory status.
5. Why are breathing exercises important in surgical patients?
6. Describe the nursing interventions to prevent and manage postoperative pulmonary complications.
7. Explain the steps involved in a comprehensive respiratory assessment in a surgical patient.
8. Discuss the use and nursing responsibilities associated with oxygen therapy in postoperative care.
9. Explain how nurses identify and manage early signs of respiratory distress in the clinical setting.
10. Describe the pathophysiology, clinical manifestations, and nursing care for a surgical patient with pneumonia.

Answers to Critical Thinking Questions

1. (c); 2. (c); 3. (c); 4. (b); 5. (c).

REFERENCES

1. Baumgartner, H., De Backer, J., Babu-Narayan, S. V., Budts, W., Chessa, M., Diller, G., Lung, B., Kluin, J., Lang, I. M., Meijboom, F., Moons, P., Mulder, B. J. M., Oechslin, E., Roos-Hesselink, J. W., Schwerzmann, M., Sondergaard, L., Zeppenfeld, K., Ernst, S., Ladouceur, M., . . . Coats, L. (2020). 2020 ESC Guidelines for the management of adult congenital heart disease. *European Heart Journal, 42*(6), 563–645. https://doi.org/10.1093/eurheartj/ehaa554Chang, A., Fortescue, R., Grimwood, K., Alexopoulou, E., Bell, L., Boyd, J., Bush, A., et al. (2021). European Respiratory Society guidelines for the management of children and adolescents with bronchiectasis. *European Respiratory Journal, 58*. https://www.semanticscholar.org/paper/e49f20735adfd0d7e5ec16e9ebae8917353c2911 (accessed on 30th June 2025).

2. Chimbira, W., Crawford, H., Gupta, S., Legg, T. J., et al. (2001). Acute lung injury in pediatric intensive care: Course and outcome. https://core.ac.uk/download/pdf/8715345.pdf (accessed on 30th June 2025).

3. Copeland, L. I. B. T., James, Duinkerken, M. S. I., & Kelsey. (2018). Jefferson Digital Commons quarterly report: April–June 2019. https://core.ac.uk/download/220159103.pdf (accessed on 30th June 2025).

4. Cox, A. (2015). Thermal burns and smoke inhalation injuries. https://core.ac.uk/download/58826490.pdf (accessed on 30th June 2025).

5. de Perrot, M., Frey, J. G., Hühn, L., Licker, M., et al. (2017). Perioperative mortality and major cardio-pulmonary complications after lung surgery for non-small cell carcinoma. https://core.ac.uk/download/85212763.pdf (accessed on 30th June 2025).

6. Diamond, B., Guerrier, G., Holliman, C., Marrero, J., et al. (2019). A quality improvement project to determine the incidence and prevalence of obstructive sleep apnea, best practice anesthesia guidelines, and the incidence of perioperative cardiac and respiratory complications after the implementation of the STOP-BANG questionnaire. https://core.ac.uk/download/301296636.pdf (accessed on 30th June 2025).

7. Engelman, D. T., Ben Ali, W., Williams, J. B., Perrault, L. P., Reddy, V. S., Arora, R. C., Roselli, E. E., et al. (2019). Guidelines for perioperative care in cardiac surgery. *JAMA Surgery, 154*, 755–755. https://doi.org/10.1001/jamasurg.2019.1153 (accessed on 30th June 2025).

8. Fleming, F. J., Gaertner, W. B., Ternent, C. A., Finlayson, E., Herzig, D. O., Paquette, I. M., Feingold, D. L., et al. (2017). The American Society of Colon and Rectal Surgeons clinical practice guideline for the prevention of venous thromboembolic disease in colorectal surgery. *Diseases of the Colon & Rectum, 61*, 14–20. https://doi.org/10.1097/dcr.0000000000000982 (accessed on 30th June 2025).

9. Gustafsson, U., Scott, M. J., Hübner, M., Nygren, J., Demartines, N., Francis, N., Rockall, T., et al. (2018). Guidelines for perioperative care in elective colorectal surgery: Enhanced Recovery After Surgery (ERAS®) Society recommendations: 2018. *World Journal of Surgery, 43*, 659–695. https://doi.org/10.1007/s00268-018-4844-y (accessed on 30th June 2025).

10. Halvorsen, S., Mehilli, J., Cassese, S., Hall, T. S., Abdelhamid, M., Barbato, E., De Hert, S., et al. (2022). 2022 ESC guidelines on cardiovascular assessment and management of patients undergoing non-cardiac surgery. *European Heart Journal, 43*, 3826–3924. https://doi.org/10.1093/eurheartj/ehac270 (accessed on 30th June 2025).

11. Ibrahim, M. A., AbdElhafez, A. M. H., Hassan, E. A., & Alaswad, N. K. (2023). Impact of empowerment for pediatric nursing students on their knowledge about climate change and its impact on children health. *Egyptian Nursing Journal*. https://www.semanticscholar.org/paper/12fb84369ebd43486d44452644e3df73b9f2257f (accessed on 30th June 2025).

12. Jacob, J. (2015). Anesthesia implications of pediatric obesity. https://core.ac.uk/download/567882138.pdf (accessed on 30th June 2025).

13. Kitsiou, A., Caforio, A. L. P., Porta-Sanchez, A., Vahanian, A., Iung, B., Carrera, C., Szymanski, C., et al. (2013). ESC core curriculum for the general cardiologist (2013). https://core.ac.uk/download/55756305.pdf (accessed on 30th June 2025).

14. Konstantinides, S., Meyer, G., Becattini, C., Bueno, H., Geersing, G. J., Harjola, V. P., Huisman, M. V., et al. (2019). 2019 ESC guidelines for the diagnosis and management of acute pulmonary embolism developed in collaboration with the European Respiratory Society (ERS). *European Respiratory Journal, 54*, 1901647–1901647. https://doi.org/10.1183/13993003.01647-2019 (accessed on 30th June 2025).

15. Li, Z., Ding, C., Deng, Y., & Zhao, Z. (2023). Bedside electrical impedance tomography (EIT) for early assessment of lung function in liver transplantation. *QJM: Monthly Journal of the Association of Physicians*. https://www.semanticscholar.org/paper/d94e8509b100b030d368b1211190f38b6a711de0 (accessed on 30th June 2025).

16. Lu, L., Zhang, J., Xie, Y., Gao, F., Xu, S., Wu, X., & Ye, Z. (2020). Wearable health devices in health care: Narrative systematic review. *JMIR mHealth and uHealth, 8*, e18907–e18907. https://doi.org/10.2196/18907 (accessed on 30th June 2025).

17. Marsh, A., Smith, A. D., King, A. G., Van Vught, A. J., Padberg, A. M., Horemans, A. M. C., Manzur, A. Y., et al. (2008). A Dutch guideline for the treatment of scoliosis in neuromuscular disorders. https://core.ac.uk/download/pdf/15475783.pdf (accessed on 30th June 2025).

18. Mouratidou, N., Papadopoulos, D., Vrouvaki, I., Skouras, V., & Katsenos, S. (2025). Pembrolizumab-induced myasthenia gravis with isolated diaphragmatic involvement in a lung cancer patient: A case report. *Therapeutic Advances in Vaccines and Immunotherapy, 13*. https://www.semanticscholar.org/paper/3e578ebfd0a059a579fea8838e6b58c19e70bbb7 (accessed on 30th June 2025).

19. Mu'in, M. (2015). Pattern of complementary therapy used by patients in diabetes care regiment. https://core.ac.uk/download/76930622.pdf (accessed on 30th June 2025).

20. Özkan, E. M., Küpeli, S., Özcan, D., Özkan, A., Sezgin, G., & Bayram, I. (2025). Assessment of respiratory functions in pediatric oncology patients receiving bleomycin treatment. *Cukurova Medical Journal*. https://www.semanticscholar.org/paper/f643879ef670144a96288a7b2559b0233e4fa472 (accessed on 30th June 2025).

21. Page, M. J., Moher, D., Bossuyt, P. M., Boutron, I., Hoffmann, T., Mulrow, C. D., Shamseer, L., et al. (2021). PRISMA 2020 explanation and elaboration: Updated guidance and exemplars for reporting systematic reviews. *BMJ*. https://doi.org/10.1136/bmj.n160 (accessed on 30th June 2025).

22. Pisani, S. (2010). The nurse of the Mediterranean. https://core.ac.uk/download/46602269.pdf (accessed on 30th June 2025).

23. Reynolds, L. A., & Tansey, E. M. (2011). History of British intensive care, c. 1950–c. 2000. https://core.ac.uk/download/30696163.pdf (accessed on 30th June 2025).

24. Sheikhalishahi, S., Miotto, R., Dudley, J. T., Lavelli, A., Rinaldi, F., & Osmani, V. (2019). Natural language processing of clinical notes on chronic diseases: Systematic review. *JMIR Medical Informatics, 7*, e12239–e12239. https://doi.org/10.2196/12239 (accessed on 30th June 2025).

25. Stupp, R., Taillibert, S., Kanner, A. A., Read, W. L., Steinberg, D. M., Lhermitte, B., Toms, S. A., et al. (2017). Effect of tumor-treating fields plus maintenance temozolomide vs maintenance temozolomide alone on survival in patients with glioblastoma. *JAMA, 318*, 2306–2306. https://doi.org/10.1001/jama.2017.18718 (accessed on 30th June 2025).

26. Thorkildsen, K. (2016). The utilization of exogenous surfactant in the neonate. https://core.ac.uk/download/58827079.pdf (accessed on 30th June 2025).

27. Zhou, H., Ou, X., Tang, Y., Wang, L., & Feng, Y. (2015). Advanced chronic obstructive pulmonary disease. *Chinese Medical Journal, 128*, 2952–2959. https://doi.org/10.4103/0366-6999.168073 (accessed on 30th June 2025).

CARDIOVASCULAR CARE: ARRHYTHMIAS, VASCULAR, AND CORONARY DISORDERS FOR SURGICAL NURSING

4

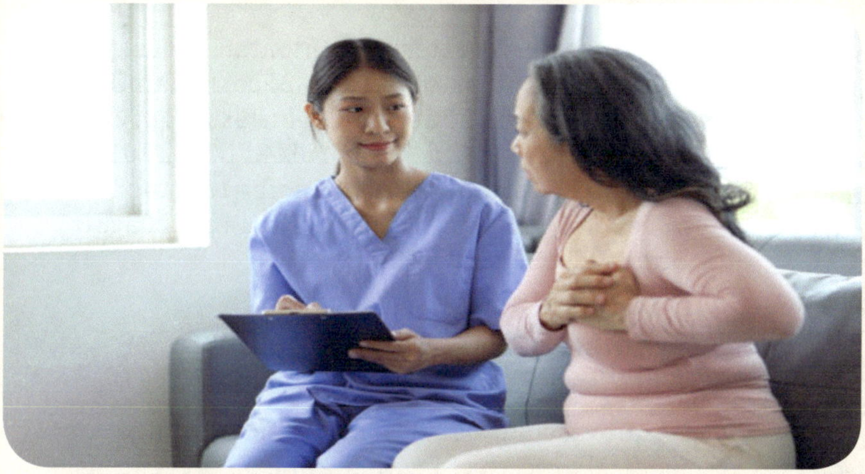

Introduction

The discipline of cardiovascular treatment is an integral part of contemporary medicine, particularly in the prevention and management of various heart conditions. The broad treatment strategy for the patient encompasses a wide range, from arrhythmias to more severe vascular and coronary diseases. Given the prevalence of cardiovascular disease, particularly among elderly individuals, as indicated by trends in research conducted in different settings, emphasis on early diagnosis and timely intervention cannot be exaggerated. For instance, hypertension and congestive heart failure are very prevalent among elderly individuals, and therefore it is crucial that medical professionals are equipped to diagnose and treat such conditions successfully (Kisenge et al., 2011). Technological advancements in diagnostic technology, as well as greater knowledge of the pathophysiology of such conditions, determine the model of cardiovascular care, ultimately determining the surgical nurse's role in advancing patient outcomes. In addition to an

LEARNING OBJECTIVES

After studying this chapter, you will be able to:

1. Understand the arrhythmias
2. Explain the vascular disorders
3. Discuss the coronary disorders: types and treatments
4. Focus on the role of surgical nursing in cardiovascular care
5. Learn about patient education and support
6. State the current trends and innovations in cardiovascular care

awareness of the physiological manifestations of cardiovascular disease, a major component of cardiovascular care is an awareness of the psychological effects on patients who are receiving treatment for surgical procedures. The preoperative phase is likely to cause significant anxiety among patients, particularly those suffering from advanced diseases that risk their cardiovascular health. Research on preoperative anxiety among cardiac surgery patients underscores the fact that the majority of patients experience mild or moderate levels of anxiety, which negatively affect postoperative recovery (Ali et al., 2023). Therefore, addressing these emotional issues is crucial, as they directly impact the patient's outcome. Surgical nurses must employ patient-centered communication skills and holistic nursing care practices to minimize anxiety and prepare patients for the reality of surgical treatment and rehabilitation. This emphasizes the intricate interdependence between physical and psychological health in the management of cardiovascular disease. As surgical nursing advances, interdisciplinary practice becomes increasingly critical to delivering integrated cardiovascular care. Healthcare professionals, including nurses, cardiologists, and mental health professionals, must collaborate to address the multifaceted nature of cardiovascular diseases. Working together, teams can provide comprehensive care that not only addresses the physiological and anatomical aspects of such conditions as arrhythmias, coronary heart disease, and vascular diseases but also incorporates patients' psychological and emotional health (Kisenge et al., 2011). This model of combined care yields improved outcomes by taking into account every aspect of a patient's health, ultimately resulting in a more efficient and empathetic treatment plan. The demand for an integrated approach to cardiovascular care that addresses both physical and psychological considerations is a sign of a commitment to delivering improved quality care for patients with such serious health conditions (Figure 4.1).

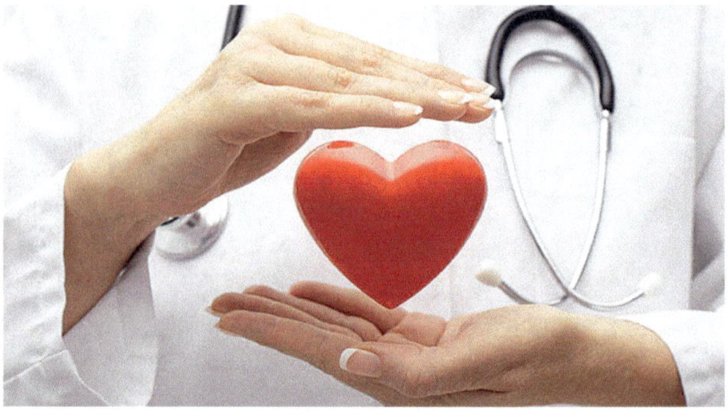

Figure 4.1. Cardiovascular care.

Source: https://external-content.duckduckgo.com/iu/?u=https%3A%2F%2Fcdn.dnaindia.com%2Fsites%2Fdefault%2Ffiles%2Fstyles%2Ffull%2Fpublic%2F2018%2F02%2F03%2F647631-cardiac.jpg&f=1&nofb=1&ipt=bbe9a3ee0cf6b113e2fcefba8e22217014bb8cbac386cacef08ee88ae0c7f908.

Definition and Importance of Cardiovascular Care

Cardiovascular treatment entails a range of medical procedures with the aim of preventing, diagnosing, and managing cardiac and blood vessel conditions. It is a sophisticated practice encompassing the management of arrhythmias, vascular illness, and coronary illness, all posing significant threats to health. With cardiovascular disease remaining a leading source of morbidity and mortality across the world, the importance of multidisciplinary cardiovascular treatment cannot be overstated. Such treatment not only addresses life-threatening illnesses but also emphasizes preventive interventions, such as lifestyle modifications and regular screenings, that are vital in reducing the risks associated with cardiovascular diseases. Increased awareness and accessibility of cardiovascular treatment enhance outcomes in health, making it an essential element of healthcare systems. Effective cardiovascular treatment is increasingly recognized for its ability to enhance the quality of life of those suffering from chronic disease, which in this context is atrial fibrillation (AF).

This indicates a shift toward value-based care, where patient-specific outcomes are the primary focus. A recent initiative by the International Consortium for Health Outcomes Measurement (ICHOM) aimed to establish a standardized set of outcomes relevant to treating AF, in response to the need to incorporate patient-reported outcomes alongside clinical outcomes. The incorporation of factors such as compliance with medications, lifestyle patterns, and demographics enables health care providers to tailor interventions according to patient-specific needs and ultimately optimize care delivery. The consensus on such standardized outcomes not only facilitates performance benchmarking but also identifies best practice, confirming that structured cardiovascular care significantly influences patient management. Furthermore, the use of multidisciplinary approaches in cardiovascular care is crucial for addressing the complexities associated with vascular and coronary diseases. Surgical nursing plays a key role in this cohesive care model.

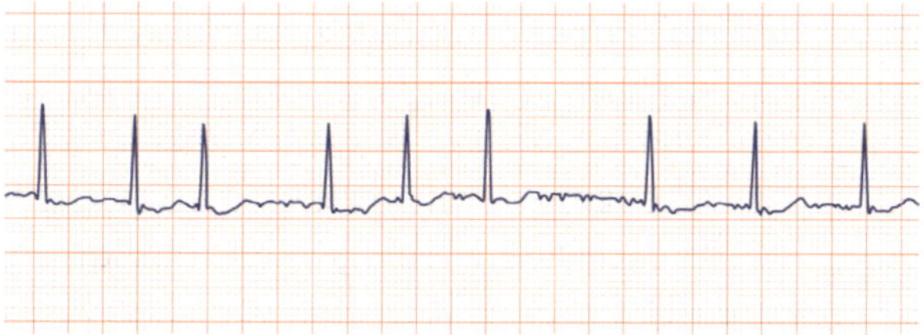

Figure 4.2. Atrial fibrillation (AF).

Source: https://www.aclsmedicaltraining.com/wp-content/uploads/2021/09/ACLS-Figure-30.jpg.

The patient is navigated to post-operative recovery. As increasingly sophisticated surgical procedures become feasible, so do the corresponding nursing techniques, which complement them. Placing great importance on education and mutual decision-making, the surgical nurse holds the authority to empower patients to actively engage in their own care. This collaborative practice has the potential to improve patient outcomes and treatment compliance. By creating an in-depth understanding of cardiovascular care, from surgery to prevention, healthcare providers can advance the science of cardiovascular management and ultimately result in healthier patients with these all-too-often disabling diseases (Figure 4.2).

Overview of Common Cardiovascular Disorders

Understanding the common cardiovascular diseases is vital in effective surgical nursing practice. Some of these common diseases include arrhythmias, which pose a significant challenge as they represent irregular heart rhythms that can lead to inadequate blood circulation. These irregularities could lead to palpitations, dizziness, or syncope in patients. Arrhythmias are usually treated using multiple techniques, including medications, lifestyle modifications, and invasive treatment by way of catheter ablation. Nurses have a critical role to play in monitoring symptoms in patients and educating patients regarding lifestyle factors leading to arrhythmias, such as diet and stress. Early recognition and treatment are also critical for better patient outcomes and highlight the importance of nurse vigilance in diagnosing and treating these disorders. Coronary disorders, including coronary artery disease (CAD), are a primary cause of morbidity and mortality globally. CAD occurs when the coronary arteries are narrowed or blocked by atherosclerotic plaque buildup, resulting in reduced blood flow to the heart muscle. This reduction of blood supply may lead to angina and, more dangerously, myocardial infarction. Angioplasty and CABG surgeries are usually needed for these patients. Surgical nurses must be empowered with preoperative and postoperative care for these procedures. They must understand not only the technical aspects of surgery but also the pathophysiology underlying the surgical procedure, as this optimizes patient education and leads to better recovery outcomes. Vascular disease, including peripheral artery disease (PAD) and aneurysms, are another category of cardiovascular diseases.. PAD is characterized by a decrease in blood flow to the extremities, often presenting as claudication pain in the leg or ulcers. It is most often associated with atherosclerosis, and such patients may require modifications in lifestyle, medication, or surgical interventions like angioplasty. Also, aneurysms, the pathologic dilatation of blood vessels, have the risk of rupture, for which early surgical intervention is essential. Nurses are also crucial in advising the patient about worsening risk factors like hypertension and smoking that aggravate these conditions. In addition, they coordinate critical circulatory monitoring of patients, which assists in the early detection of complications. Therefore, vascular disease highlights the complex and multidimensional aspects of cardiovascular well-being and the crucial role of nursing in addressing such diverse and complex conditions.

Role of Surgical Nursing in Cardiovascular Care

In the context of cardiovascular care, surgical nursing plays a critical role in managing arrhythmias, vascular diseases, and coronary artery disease. Surgical nurses play a key role in the multidisciplinary team of practitioners, fostering interprofessional collaboration among surgeons, cardiologists, and other healthcare professionals. Their function begins in the preoperative phase, where thorough assessments enable the identification of risk factors and development of patient outcome protocols. This is of utmost significance, considering the complexities involved in surgical procedures for cardiovascular diseases that require specialized knowledge and skills. Through comprehensive patient education, surgical nurses also prepare patients for what's to come, thus avoiding anxiety as well as improving compliance with postoperative regimens, which is instrumental for a successful recovery. In the operating room, surgical nurses play a pivotal role in administering interventions for various cardiovascular ailments. They are responsible for monitoring patients' vital signs, ordering medications, and ensuring asepsis throughout the procedure. Their keen observation and clinical acuity directly influence patient safety and surgical outcomes. Consistent with current guidelines, such as the 2023 AHA/ACC/ACCP/ASPC/NLA/PCNA Guideline for the Management of Patients with Chronic Coronary Disease, surgical nursing practice is informed by evidence-based practice, which promotes a patient-centered care approach. This guideline emphasizes shared decision-making and collaborative care, supporting the value of surgical nurses being competent at interpreting clinical information and participating in patient management decisions. This exchange not only supports improved recovery but also informs ongoing treatment plans. Surgical nurses are crucial after surgery in monitoring for complications of cardiovascular surgical interventions, such as infection, bleeding, or arrhythmias. Their ongoing assessment informs timely interventions to resolve any complications promptly. Operating room nurses also provide essential education on lifestyle modifications and medication compliance, addressing the social determinants of health that are at the core of managing chronic coronary disease. This combined approach is in line with the inclusive approaches advocated by Virani et al. (2023), such that care is not only reactive but also proactive. Furthermore, surgical nurses must remain aware of changing evidence and guidelines—such as emerging revascularization guidelines—so they can effectively advocate for their patients within a constantly evolving practice landscape. Their greater understanding positions surgical nurses to be in the best position to champion the implementation of best practices in cardiovascular care, ultimately leading to improved patient outcomes.

4.1. Understanding Arrhythmias

Learning Outcome

1. Describe the types of arrhythmias and their characteristics
2. Focus on diagnostic tools for arrhythmias
3. Learn about treatment options and nursing interventions

Arrhythmias, with disrupted rhythms of the heart's electrical conduction system, are formidable challenges in cardiovascular care. They can be harmless or even fatal and complicate the management of the patient in cases of underlying cardiovascular diseases. Preoperative and postoperative management of patients under the care of surgical nurses requires knowledge of the pathophysiology of arrhythmias to monitor and treat the patient appropriately. Various factors, including structural heart disease, electrolyte imbalance, and drug effects can typically explain the complexity of the arrhythmias. With the increasing incidence of arrhythmias, particularly in older adults, surgical nursing personnel must be equipped with the necessary knowledge and skills to assess and intervene accordingly in these cases, thereby leading to improved patient outcomes. An integral aspect of arrhythmia care is a holistic approach to patient care involving both short-term and long-term priorities. Surgical nurses must focus on the assessment of patients for risk factors of hypertension, smoking, and diabetes that contribute significantly to cardiovascular diseases, such as arrhythmias. Holistic care includes the "care, core, and cure" nursing approach, emphasizing that every patient has to be treated according to their unique requirements during the entire duration of treatment. The acute phase of treatment usually involves nurses feeling the "care" and "cure" more intensely, with prompt intervention being crucial to stabilizing the patient. While patients arrive at non-acute levels, however, education and rehabilitation come to the forefront, reminding us of the "core" aspect of the model, which aims to enhance self-management and promote healthier living (Umara et al., 2018). Education and collaboration are vital elements in the successful management of arrhythmias in the context of surgical nursing. Because arrhythmias can have severe effects on the outcomes of surgery, nurses must receive comprehensive professional development to be current with the latest research and guidelines for treatment. In addition, multidisciplinary care involving a cardiologist and other healthcare providers could improve patient detection and the timely management of arrhythmias, leading to earlier intervention, reduced complications during the operation, and ultimately, improved patient outcomes. This cross-professional collaboration enables comprehensive care that addresses not only the arrhythmia itself but also the overall impact of cardiovascular disease on the patient as a whole. By originating a culture of collaboration and intelligence sharing, surgical nurses will be better able to offer high-quality care, enhancing the standard of living for arrhythmia patients (Kitsiou et al., 2013) (Figure 4.3).

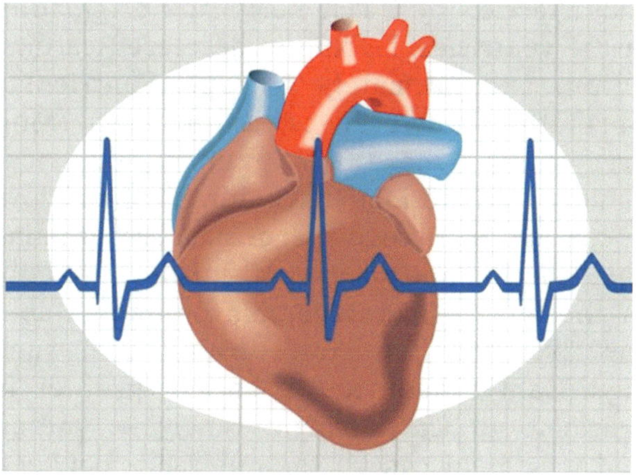

Figure 4.3. Heart arrhythmia.

Source: https://healthjade.com/wp-content/uploads/2017/08/heart-arrhythmia.jpg.

4.1.1. Types of Arrhythmias and Their Characteristics

The evaluation of arrhythmias is an integral part of understanding cardiovascular status, particularly in surgical nursing. Arrhythmias constitute a continuum of deviations from the normal heart rhythm that may compromise hemodynamic stability. Among the most frequent are atrial fibrillation (AF), ventricular tachycardia (VT), and bradycardia. Atrial fibrillation with rapid and irregular atrial contraction substantially elevates the risk of thromboembolic complications like stroke. This risk is compounded in older persons, and therefore careful screening and management of these conditions must be done in health facilities, especially as cardiovascular diseases are increasingly becoming more prevalent in older populations as noted in research where hypertension and heart failure are common indicators of arrhythmias (Kisenge et al., 2011). Successful surgical nursing care requires an awareness of these conditions to enhance patient care and minimize complications related to surgery. Another significant category of arrhythmias is ventricular arrhythmias, namely ventricular fibrillation and ventricular tachycardia. Ventricular tachycardia is characterized by a fast heart rate originating in the ventricles, leading to decreased cardiac output and ultimately syncope. Ventricular fibrillation, however, is—a life-threatening arrhythmia where disorganized electrical activity leads to ineffective quivering and loss of circulation. Recognition of such arrhythmias calls for instant treatment, most commonly in the form of cardioversion or implantable cardioverter-defibrillators. Understanding such significant differences in patient profiles is crucial to surgical nursing, as timely recognition and treatment can be the difference between life and death (Arbelo et al., 2020). Recognition of such comorbidities as heart failure or ischemic heart disease, often seen alongside these arrhythmias, can similarly inform treatment as well as improve patient outcomes. Bradycardia, abnormally slow heart rhythms, is another arrhythmia type worthy of attention in operating room nursing practice. Bradycardia may be due to intrinsic cardiac malfunction or extrinsic factors, such as the use of certain drugs or imbalanced electrolytes. Patients with bradycardia may experience symptoms ranging from dizziness and fatigue to syncope, making surgical care challenging. Monitoring of heart rhythms both pre- and postoperatively is vital to avoid bradycardia-related complications, especially among older patients who tend to have co-morbid cardiovascular disease. Given the prevalence of cardiovascular disease among various populations, a comprehensive understanding of arrhythmias—including their nature—enables surgical nurses to implement preventive strategies in assessing patient risk and improving care delivery (Kisenge et al., 2011). A successful whole approach to treating arrhythmia ultimately enhances surgical recovery and overall cardiovascular health (Figure 4.4).

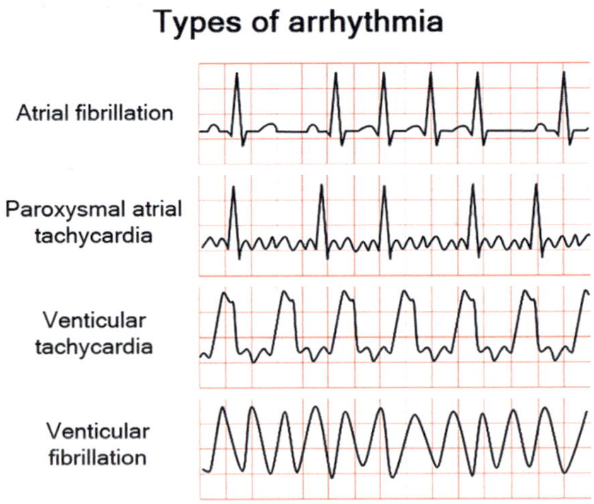

Figure 4.4. Heart arrhythmia treatment.

Source: https://newyorkcardiac.com/wp-content/uploads/2021/11/types-of-arrhythmia.jpg.

4.1.2. Diagnostic Tools for Arrhythmias

In cardiovascular practice, particularly in arrhythmia management, timely and accurate diagnosis is critical for suitable patient outcomes. Various diagnostic techniques aid in the detection of arrhythmic conditions, enabling management to be tailored appropriately. ECGs continue to be the backbone of arrhythmia diagnosis with real-time monitoring of electrical heart activity. With the advent of digital technology and remote monitoring, devices such as Holter monitors and implantable loop recorders have also contributed to the ability to capture infrequent arrhythmias that may not be present during a standard ECG. Not only do these technologies enhance diagnostic accuracy, but they also enable continuous patient monitoring, thereby improving the overall quality of cardiovascular medicine.

Hence, accurate diagnosis using these machines enables timely interventions and optimum treatment and management programs for the patient with arrhythmias. The roles of diagnostic machines extend beyond mere arrhythmia detection as they also yield information regarding the likely underlying pathology and associated risk. For instance, the application of echocardiography is helpful in assessing structural heart disease, which can make the patient susceptible to arrhythmias. Knowledge of atrial or ventricular morphology can be crucial in providing information regarding the treatment of the condition and prognosis. Additionally, techniques like electrophysiological studies can also be employed if non-invasive tests fail to clarify arrhythmic events. Such higher-level diagnostic testing enables the assessment of typical pathways that cause arrhythmias and provides insight into potential ablation therapies. Moreover, the application of emerging imaging technologies alongside traditional equipment facilitates a holistic evaluation of patients, ultimately enhancing surgical care and nursing treatment for arrhythmias. The interplay between psychological problems and arrhythmias underlines the requirement for an all-around treatment in cardiovascular care. Current evidence reveals that cardiac events such as arrhythmias are significantly aggravated by conditions such as anxiety and panic disorders. An understanding of this correlation is essential for surgical nursing, as it emphasizes the requirement of examining not only physiological factors but also those of psychological well-being among patients.

The imposition of strict screening for emotional illnesses can lead to better risk factor identification about arrhythmias. Especially, alleviation of anxiety by successful interventions will reduce the frequency of arrhythmic events and improve the overall quality of life in cardiac patients. Thus, a holistic approach that incorporates both physical and psychological evaluation is critical in determining treatment modalities and optimizing patient outcomes in the current challenging scenario of cardiovascular management (Abrignani et al., 2014) (Figure 4.5).

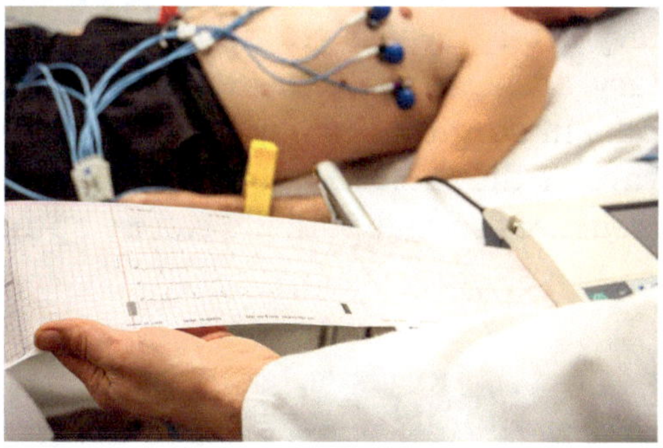

Figure 4.5. Electrocardiogram (ECG).

Source: https://external-content.duckduckgo.com/iu/?u=https%3A%2F%2Fdrarthurnasis.com.au%2Fwp-content%2Fuploads%2F2021%2F02%2Fshutterstock_1507886318-1.jpg&f=1&nofb=1&ipt=5000a28b104e5516b96c9ca2ca7533cc230347b13ac7782e60818fe86388bb0c.

4.1.3. Treatment Options and Nursing Interventions

In the management of cardiovascular disease, particularly arrhythmias and coronary disease, therapy must be individualized to meet the specific needs and clinical presentation of every patient. In the majority of situations, pharmacologic therapy is the initial treatment of choice, using antiarrhythmic drugs and anticoagulants to minimize risk for abnormal cardiac rhythms and thromboembolic events. ~~Besides, the nurses~~ play a pivotal role in monitoring side effects, medication adherence, and the interpretation of these medications on their conditions. The accurate assessment of the patient's response to pharmacotherapy enables timely intervention and adjustment, enhancing treatment outcome in general. Education is also crucial, as informed patients possessing information about their medications are more likely to use self-care measures that benefit their cardiovascular health, promoting collaboration among patients and healthcare providers to achieve improved health outcomes. Surgery may be indicated if conservative therapy is not able to stabilize life-threatening or highly severe cardiovascular disorders. Such procedures as catheter ablation for atrial fibrillation and coronary artery bypass grafting for obstructive coronary artery disease are examples of such methods. In surgical nursing, it is necessary to be aware of the indications, risks, and post-op care measures so that patients can ~~be~~ optimally recover and their safety is guaranteed. Nursing activities don't occur just within the operating room; they involve pre-operative education to prepare the patient psychologically and physically for the operation. Nurses play a crucial role postoperatively in monitoring vital signs, detecting complications, and providing supportive treatment, while also ensuring the patient's emotional and psychological well-being. The integration of all these whole-person nursing interventions has a critical impact on uneventful recovery and long-term success in the management of severe cardiovascular diseases. Emotional disease, particularly panic and anxiety disorders, is a significant factor in cardiovascular disease development, as outlined in recent studies. Anxious patients, for instance, can exhibit increased symptoms as well as poor control of their cardiovascular disease, leading to increased morbidity and mortality. Effective nursing interventions must therefore not only focus on the physical management of cardiovascular disease but also on the psychological issues of the patients. By incorporating anxiety management skills, coping strategy education, and appropriate referrals for psychological counseling, nurses significantly contribute to enhancing the overall quality of life for patients. Through the identification of the interconnectedness of mental and cardiovascular health, health providers can ensure the overall process of treatment, making patients lives and outcomes better (Abrignani et al., 2014; Kitsiou et al., 2013).

Test Your Knowledge

1. What is the difference between bradycardia and tachycardia?
2. Why is it essential to monitor patients with arrhythmias for signs of decreased cardiac output?

4.2. Vascular Disorders: An Overview

Learning Outcome

1. Explain the common vascular disorders and their implications
2. Define the risk factors associated with vascular disorders
3. Discuss the surgical nursing considerations for vascular patients

Vascular diseases comprise a range of illnesses that affect the blood vessels to a significant extent, so as to have a profound impact on quality of life and health. These include atherosclerosis, aneurysms, and peripheral artery disease, and if not attended to, they can result in very serious outcomes. Vascular diseases are also caused in part by lifestyle factors such as a bad diet, inactivity, and smoking.; Also, genetic susceptibility plays a prominent role in one's susceptibility to such diseases. Vascular disease pathophysiology is a concept that surgical nursing should have a thorough understanding of, and it often requires intervention at late stages of the disease. Effective management interventions, including lifestyle alterations and drug therapy, are crucial in preventing the spontaneous progression of these diseases and improving patient outcomes within the surgical setting. One of the most essential features of vascular disease management is the psychological and cardiovascular interaction. Findings from recent studies indicate that panic disorders and anxiety disorders are prevalent among vascular disease patients and that these contribute to treatment model difficulties. Anxiety patients could display excessive physiological responses, including increased blood pressure and heart rate, which could complicate existing vascular diseases. (Abrignani et al., 2014) reports that panic disorder is a significant risk factor for life-threatening arrhythmias and contends that mental health assessment should become an integral component of cardiovascular care. Such psychological components are specifically relevant to surgical nursing, where thorough evaluation can lead to individually tailored interventions that enhance both physiological and emotional well-being. Practice in surgical nursing is increasingly acknowledging the merits of an interdisciplinary approach to the care of vascular disease. Multidisciplinary treatment involving surgeons, nurses, psychologists, and nutritionists may lead to better patient health outcomes. With knowledge of all the factors in a patient's condition, such as the psychological implications uncovered by studies, healthcare providers can make more effective treatment strategies. An integrated approach not only addresses the physical signs of vascular illness but also prioritizes the importance of emotional care, care coordination, and patient education. Such comprehensive care can lead to an improved quality of life for patients, aligning with the principles of modern cardiovascular nursing practice. As healthcare evolves, the incorporation of psychological insight will have a pivotal role in enhancing surgical techniques and securing optimal recovery for vascular disease patients (Figure 4.6).

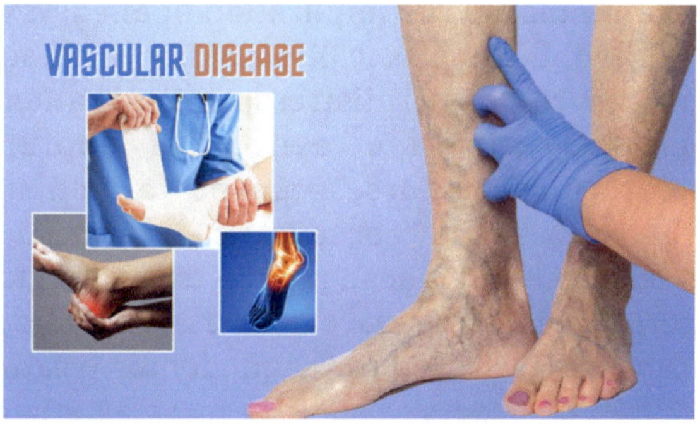

Figure 4.6. Vascular disease.

Source: https://www.professordigvijay.com/wp-content/uploads/2021/01/Vascular-Disease-750x450.png.

4.2.1. Common Vascular Disorders and Their Implications

Atherosclerosis leads to peripheral artery disease (PAD), one of the prevalent vascular disorders that presents enormous challenges in the field of cardiovascular care, particularly in surgical nursing. The condition leads to impaired blood flow to the limbs and clinically presents with symptoms of intermittent claudication. This will severely impair mobility and quality of life. The sequelae of PAD extend far beyond limb health because individuals afflicted with PAD are at increased risk for cardiac events, including heart attack and stroke. Early diagnosis and treatment are required, as lifestyle modification, medications, and surgical therapy can markedly reduce patient morbidity and reduce the sequelae of vascular injury. Understanding enhanced prognosis and quality of life. Another severe vascular illness is aneurysm disease, in which there is an abnormal enlargement of a blood vessel. Abdominal aortic aneurysms (AAA) are particularly of concern due to the risk of lethal rupture. Surgical intervention, typically in the mode of open repair surgery or endovascular aneurysm repair (EVAR), is required in the management of cases where the aneurysm is more than the threshold size or symptomatic. The implication of aneurysms goes beyond the physical morbidity; they also cause psychological distress among patients presented with the danger of rupture. Operating room nurses can be trained not only to assist with procedural care but also to provide, including those related to the surgical experience and potential outcomes. The addition of psychological care to the model for treating vascular disorders is crucial for maximizing both surgical efficacy and patient satisfaction. The relationship between vascular illness and psychiatric conditions should not be overlooked in combined cardiovascular treatment. Recent studies show that there is a solid connection between anxiety disorders and panic and cardiovascular illness development, such as arrhythmia. Specifically, studies demonstrate that panic disorders can provide a conduit for physiological changes that exacerbate vascular disease, thus impacting the overall health condition. Effective management of such mental illnesses is paramount since they affect the adherence of a patient to regimes of treatment and lifestyle modification required for vascular well-being. Also, treating anxiety has the added advantage of reducing the risk of life-threatening arrhythmias, thereby improving outcomes for patients. Operating room nurses must recognize the necessity for a comprehensive approach focusing on both the physical and psychological welfare to offer the optimal care and recovery for victims of widespread vascular diseases (Abrignani et al., 2014) (Figure 4.7).

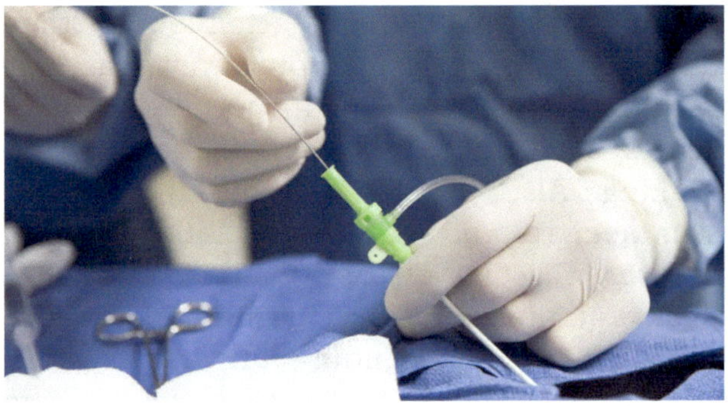

Figure 4.7. EVAR surgery (percutaneous endovascular aneurysm repair).

Source: https://res.cloudinary.com/broadcastmed/image/fetch/q_auto,c_fill,w_1300,h_731,g_faces:center,f_auto/http:%2F%2F55933-bcmed.s3.amazonaws.com%2Fbcp%2Fimages%2ForlVideoAssets%2FimgSource%2FAdobeStock_12968870.jpeg.

4.2.2. Risk Factors Associated with Vascular Disorders

The interplay of multiple risk factors is a significant contributor to the prevalence of vascular diseases, which encompass numerous disorders affecting the blood vessels. Among the most prevalent risk factors, hypertension stands out because it is an integral precursor to ailments such as stroke and aneurysms. Increased pressure not only strains the vascular system but also causes cumulative arterial damage over time. Other complications, including diabetes mellitus, contribute further to vascular impairment by inducing atherosclerosis—a condition where plaques accumulate within arterial walls. These diseases are frequently interrelated; for example, those with hypertension commonly develop diabetes, which repeats the process in a cycle of heightened danger. Treatment of these coinciding factors is highly crucial in the successful prevention process of surgical nursing because regulation of blood pressure and blood sugar levels can significantly reduce the risk of the occurrence of vascular complications and finally improve the results of patients in the long term. Lifestyle factors are also a pivotal element in the etiology of vascular diseases and are highly influenced by smoking and eating habits. Smoking, for instance, is an adjustable risk factor that hurts blood vessels, increases atherosclerosis, and raises the possibility of thrombus formation. Furthermore, eating habits high in saturated fats, sugars, and sodium cause obesity and dyslipidemia, which are both established risk factors for vascular disease. Cumulative effects of these habits make multifaceted patient education a mandatory component of surgical nursing. Nurses should include patients in individualized lifestyle alteration programs targeting smoking cessation and dietary improvement. By encouraging such alterations, healthcare workers can reverse the effects of these risk factors, ultimately leading to better control of vascular conditions and improved patient quality of life. Psychosocial determinants like stress and low socioeconomic status also contribute to the complexity of vascular disorder risk profiles. Chronic stress can lead to elevated cortisol, which in turn results in persistent hypertension and other cardiovascular dysfunction. Furthermore, individuals of low socioeconomic status have limited access to hospitals, hence their previous illnesses are not well treated and controlled, thereby facilitating the extension of vascular diseases. Identification of such psychosocial factors is essential in the nursing model, as it emphasizes a holistic approach to treating patients. By including social determinants and mental well-being in the assessment, the nurse is able to implement more effective interventions. This comprehensive knowledge not only addresses the physiological requirements for vascular health, but it also facilitates general care for patient experience, since being one of the fundamental principles of the nursing practice in the care, core, and cure model, all the more making surgical nursing reliant on the effective handling of risk factors more imperative (Kitsiou et al., 2013; Umara et al., 2018).

4.2.3. Surgical Nursing Considerations for Vascular Patients

In vascular surgical nursing, it is crucial to understand the following preoperative factors that can significantly affect patient outcomes. There is a need for a thorough history of the patient's medical history, comorbidities, and medications. They assist in identifying potential complications that may occur intraoperatively or postoperatively. Additionally, given that vascular surgery is a high-risk specialty, operating room nurses will need to adopt an interdisciplinary practice approach, with close physician interaction to develop personalized care plans. This integration enhances the general management of patients, particularly those with established cardiovascular backgrounds or significant lifestyle disorders, such as smoking and obesity. Lastly, the management of these preoperative concerns can lead to improved surgical results and reduced recuperation time for patients undergoing vascular interventions. During the perioperative period, intraoperative nursing considerations extend beyond the surgical procedure itself to the entire post-op monitoring and care of vascular patients.

Monitoring closely for complications such as bleeding, infection, or thrombosis is crucial. Operative room nurses should have the ability to assess and manage changes in vital signs, as patients can experience fluctuations due to anesthesia or changes in fluid status. Teaching the patient is equally crucial during this time, as thorough instruction on postoperative care can enable the patient to be actively engaged in the recovery process. Education should encompass medication adherence, wound care, and lifestyle modifications necessary for optimal vascular health. Therefore, postoperative care demands vigilance, education, and regular observation to facilitate effective and speedy recovery following vascular surgery. The psychological aspect of care cannot be overlooked when it comes to the surgical nursing of vascular patients. A vast majority of patients undergoing vascular surgery experience anxiety due to the perceived high risk associated with their surgery. The identification and management of such emotional responses are crucial for nurses, who must foster an open communication environment that provides support. By incorporating skills such as therapeutic listening and reassurance, patient anxiety may be minimized. Additionally, with the risk-high profile of vascular surgery uncovered in recent studies, defensive medicine has become a usual practice for this specialty. Thus, patient advocacy and nurse-physician communication in treatment planning can be enhanced by an increased understanding of how defensive medicine influences surgical practice. By addressing the psychological as well as physical health needs of vascular patients, the surgical nurses can enhance patient care and outcomes considerably (N/A, 1982; Busardo' et al., 2015) (Figure 4.8).

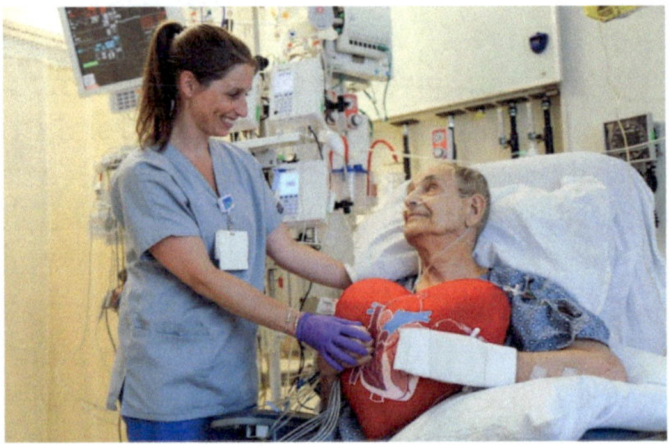

Figure 4.8. Cardiac surgery team improves care with pioneering ERAS protocol.

Source: https://external-content.duckduckgo.com/iu/?u=https%3A%2F%2Fwww.brighamhealthonamission.org%2Fwp-content%2Fuploads%2F2019%2F09%2F2-ERAS-1024x683.jpg&f=1&nofb=1&ipt=b7d7ed7a9b20e866cd3e0d12b885593acc1eb8faf835373c33ffb6ec88640cfa.

Test Your Knowledge

1. What are common symptoms of peripheral artery disease (PAD)?
2. How can hypertension contribute to the development of vascular disorders?

4.3. Coronary Disorders: Types and Treatments

Learning Outcome

1. Explain the coronary artery disease
2. Define the surgical interventions for coronary disorder
3. Describe the postoperative care and monitoring

Coronary disease, especially coronary artery disease (CAD), remains among the leading causes of illness and death globally. The disease is caused by the buildup of atherosclerotic plaques in coronary arteries, which will ultimately result in myocardial ischemia and infarction. The progression of CAD is based on various risk factors, including hypertension, hyperlipidemia, diabetes, and lifestyle choices such as smoking and physical inactivity. Early diagnosis by risk factor assessment and repeated screening is mandatory for effective prevention and management. Treatment strategies typically begin with lifestyle modification, followed by the addition of pharmacotherapy. Statins, antiplatelet agents, and beta-blockers are commonly used to manage symptoms and prevent cardiovascular events. ~~,~~the importance of a multidisciplinary treatment strategy for both ~~for~~ surgical and nursing management. Other patients may require more invasive treatments, such as PCI or CABG, to re-establish adequate blood flow to the myocardium. PCI is performed by deploying a stent to maintain the patency of the occluded coronary artery, whereas CABG necessitates grafting a different vessel to bypass the obstructed segment. Both procedures necessitate careful preoperative and postoperative care, with the nursing profession playing a key role in monitoring for complications and promotion of recovery. Coronary disorder treatment also involves comorbid condition management to minimize the risk of recurring events. Such treatment modalities pose clinical complexities that emphasize the importance of surgical nursing specialists having a comprehensive background in coronary pathophysiology, which has critical implications for patient outcomes and quality of care. Pharmacotherapy is also improving with the introduction of new agents that enhance therapeutic benefits in the treatment of coronary diseases. Calcium channel blockers (CCBs), for example, are a valuable drug class in the symptomatic treatment of diseases such as angina, hypertension, and some arrhythmias. The drugs exert their effect by inhibiting the entry of calcium, inducing relaxation of the vascular smooth muscle, and reducing myocardial oxygen demand with associated relief of symptoms. Yet, it is important to note possible complications, especially with an overdose, leading to dangerous hypotension and bradycardia, where interventions need to be specifically targeted (Rietjens et al., 2023). Additionally, coronary disorder management has to include an integrated approach that considers lifestyle factors and preventive care. The emphasis on early intervention and holistic risk assessment is a key factor that reduces disease progression and improves patient outcomes in surgical nursing practice, as illustrated by the attempts made towards personalized care (Hendriks et al., 2022) (Figure 4.9).

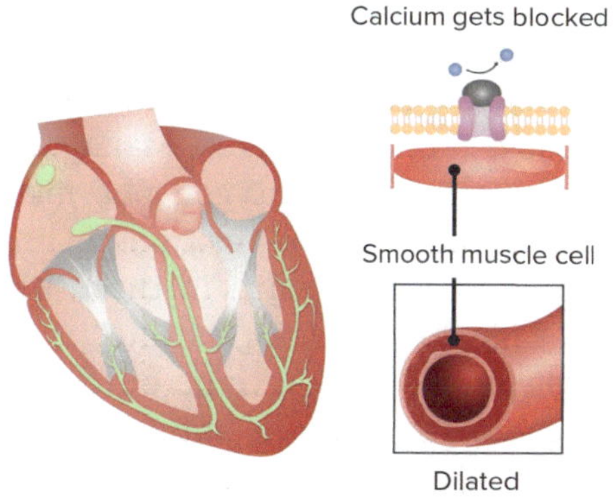

Figure 4.9. Cardiovascular effects of calcium channel-blockers.

Source: https://cdn.lecturio.com/assets/Cardiovascular-effects-of-calcium-channel-blockers-CCBs.jpg.

4.3.1. Overview of Coronary Artery Disease

Coronary Artery Disease (CAD) is a public health problem of immense scale since it is prevalent and of varied etiologies. It results from the gradual buildup of plaques composed of lipids, inflammatory cells, and fibrous tissue in the coronary arteries, leading to a reduction that restricts blood supply to the heart muscle. The clinical manifestation of CAD ranges from stable angina to myocardial infarction and acute coronary syndromes, for which an aggressive intervention is warranted in terms of diagnosis and management as it not only impairs the cardiovascular status but also compromises the quality of life of the patients. Cognitive knowledge of the risk factors, including hypertension, high cholesterol, diabetes, and lifestyle, is essential in the prevention of CAD and implies interprofessional patient care. CAD patients also present with disabling symptoms of dyspnea and angina pectoris, which impact their lives to a great degree. The interaction between CAD and comorbid disease, especially respiratory disease such as pneumonia, has been the target of recent studies. Dyspnea exacerbates cardiac symptoms and is a significant concern in the management of patients with concomitant CAD and respiratory illness. Acute intervention is excellent nursing practice that often identifies significant vital signs of cardiac distress, including increased blood pressure and tachypnea. Management of the symptoms, including oxygen, pharmacologic intervention, and ~~position~~ positioning, has been shown to decrease dyspnea in these patients. Incorporating these strategies into practice is crucial for improving patient outcomes and delivering holistic care to patients with CAD (Saraswati et al., 2024). The emerging paradigm in cardiovascular medicine also highlights the importance of biomarker monitoring for comorbidities that influence CAD progression. Albuminuria, a significant indicator of renal as well as vascular health, has come under growing identification for its implication in CAD risk. Albuminuria is a predictor of systemic vascular deterioration, heightened risk for adverse cardiovascular outcomes like heart failure and arrhythmias (Barzilay et al., 2024). As clinicians screen and manage CAD patients, screening for albuminuria must be standard, advancing their ability to identify those at greater risk for cardiovascular morbidity. This proactive approach can enable timely interventions that not only address the renal implications but also mitigate cardiovascular risk in a strategic manner. By incorporating existing evidence-based modalities, practice can contribute to the prevention of CAD progression and improvement of patient prognosis in surgical nursing (Figure 4.10).

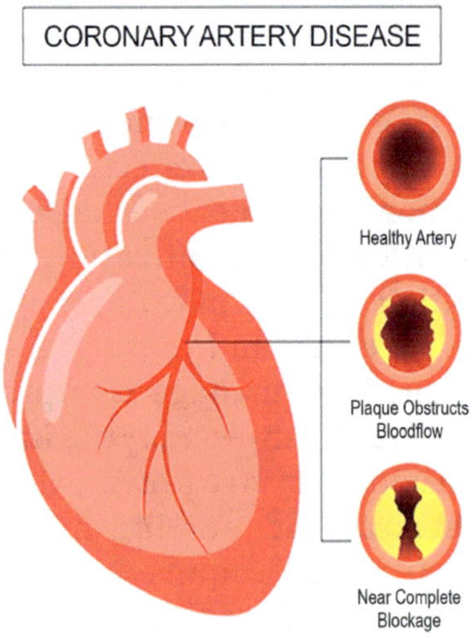

Figure 4.10. Coronary artery disease (CAD).

Source: https://modernheartandvascular.com/wp-content/uploads/2022/10/Coronary-Artery-Disease-CAD.png.

4.3.2. Surgical Interventions for Coronary Disorders

In the realm of cardiovascular therapy, coronary surgery for coronary disease is a critical focus of concern, namely addressing diseases that compromise myocardial perfusion. Coronary artery disease (CAD) is one of the most significant causes of morbidity and mortality worldwide and frequently necessitates surgical interventions to restore adequate circulation to the heart muscle. Two primary operations are widely used: coronary artery bypass grafting (CABG) and percutaneous coronary intervention (PCI). CABG is the surgical implantation of a graft for diversion of blood flow around occluded arteries, and PCI is the stenting for optimization of stenosis. Both are used to prevent ischemic occurrences and reduce adverse cardiac events. Successful surgery can significantly improve the health of CAD patients, leading to enhanced functionality and reduced cardiovascular risk (Wichmann, 2020). In addition to the procedures themselves, preoperative and postoperative care are equally crucial to optimize patient results. Preoperative evaluation should also include comprehensive assessments of cardiovascular status, and counseling of patients on the risks and benefits of surgery. Interventional planning also needs to consider patient comorbidities, lifestyle factors, and prognosis. Rehabilitation following surgery is typically a systematic approach with an emphasis on lifestyle modification, exercise, and monitoring for complications such as infection or thrombosis. Nursing input into this process is paramount; surgeons' nurses share in educating patients on adherence to medication, recognizing signs of complications, and speeding up recovery through rehabilitative mechanisms. This multi-dimensional approach places great importance on the role of nursing in the care cycle around surgical intervention for coronary disease (Wichmann, 2020). Implementation of evidence-based guidelines is also crucial for enhancing surgical outcomes in patients with coronary disease. The European Society of Cardiology (ESC) Guidelines are a guide for clinicians to make well-informed decisions for surgical management and postoperative care. These recommendations place top priority on the formulation of individualized treatment plans based on the latest scientific evidence and optimal practice. The strict adherence to these precise protocols by healthcare providers will enable them to navigate the complexities of coronary disease and optimize patient care. Priority on ~~the~~ following the patients' shared decision-making is needed to ensure that treatment approaches align with patients' values and preferences. This collaborative practice fosters trust and improves patient satisfaction, thereby significantly enhancing the overall patient experience of those undergoing surgical intervention for coronary disease (Baumgartner et al., 2020) (Figure 4.11).

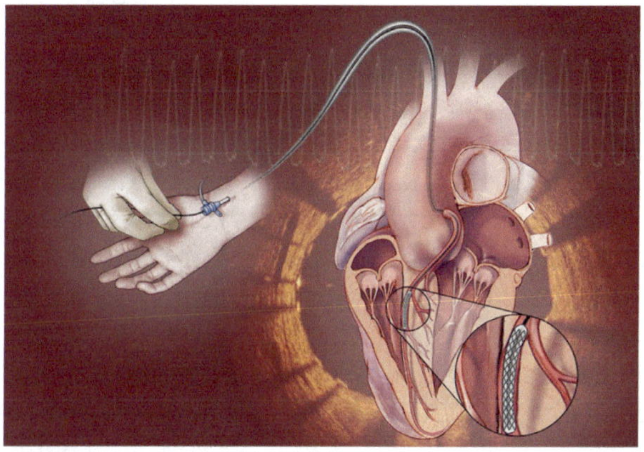

Figure 4.11. Cardiovascular diseases and cardiac surgery.

Source: https://www.mayoclinic.org/-/media/kcms/gbs/medical-professionals/images/2020/11/19/22/15/percutaneous_coronary_intervention_767x535.jpg.

4.3.3. Postoperative Care and Monitoring

Good postoperative monitoring and care are crucial for achieving optimal patient recovery, particularly in cardiovascular disease surgical interventions. Post-surgical patients are at an increased risk for thromboembolic complications, hemodynamic instability, and arrhythmias. A regimented monitoring protocol—vital signs, cardiac rhythm, and fluid status—lies at the foundation of postoperative care. Real-time monitoring of ECG is crucial for identifying arrhythmias early, which can occur due to surgical manipulation or the induction of anesthesia. Furthermore, vigilant monitoring enables the providers to identify any changes from the patient's baseline immediately, thus avoiding secondary complications. The value of an interdisciplinary process cannot be overstated, as it promises meticulous evaluation and intervention tailored to the postoperative needs of the cardiovascular patient (Halvorsen et al., 2022). In the case of cardiovascular surgery, postoperative treatment regimens should include frequent monitoring of not only vital signs but also neurological status and assessment of the surgical site. Patients are ~~usually~~ at risk for a wide range of postoperative complications that range from fluid overload, infection, or cardiac ischemia, which all require treatment appropriately. Interventions such as titration of medication doses, implementation of physical therapy, or application of therapeutic interventions ~~rely~~ are catered to ~~on~~ the specific needs of an individual patient. Healthcare providers must apply evidence-based guidelines to these interventions, which balance the most current research with clinical expertise. Regular postoperative follow-up and medication titration can significantly enhance recovery processes, allowing complications to be addressed proactively and enabling patients to progress smoothly towards recovery (Glikson et al., 2021). Patient education and activation are also crucial components of postoperative care in the cardiovascular setup. Discharge planning must include meticulous instructions tailored to the patient's status, psychosocial support systems, and follow-up requirements. Educating the patients on how to monitor for signs of potential complications—such as chest pain or trouble breathing—empowers them to be active players in the recovery process. Furthermore, incorporating family members into the educational process will create a support system that can monitor compliance with medical directives upon the patient's discharge to home. This collaborative strategy can reduce readmission rates significantly while enhancing overall well-being for patients undergoing cardiovascular surgery. Lastly, a holistic approach for postoperative care supplemented with zealous monitoring and patient participation results in improved patient outcomes (Halvorsen et al., 2022).

Test Your Knowledge

1. What is the primary difference between stable angina and myocardial infarction?
2. How do beta-blockers help in the treatment of coronary artery disease?

4.4. The Role of Surgical Nursing in Cardiovascular Care

Learning Outcome

1. Identify the preoperative assessment and patient education
2. Define the intraoperative responsibilities and techniques
3. Describe the postoperative care and complications management

Operating room nursing is essential to the intricate care of cardiovascular illnesses, particularly in the environment of arrhythmias, vascular disease, and coronary artery disease. Operating room nurses are essential in preparing patients for procedures such as catheterization, bypass grafting, and valve replacement, each of which requires careful assessment and monitoring. Their work commences preoperatively, where they educate patients on the procedure, assess their medical status, and identify personal risk factors such as hypertension and diabetes that can complicate surgical procedures. Their activity in creating this foundation during the preoperative period is essential because it that the patient is adequately informed and complications are reduced, leading to enhanced patient care and recovery procedures. Operating room surgical nurses are also critical team members, working in very close collaboration with surgeons and anesthesiologists to offer the unimpeded conduct of cardiovascular surgery. Their responsibilities include maintaining aseptic conditions, managing surgical tools and equipment, and monitoring patients' vital signs during surgery. Furthermore, surgical nurses must be competent in recognizing and managing intraoperative complications, such as arrhythmias or hemodynamic instabilities. Their skill and vigilance not only help the surgical team perform with greater efficiency but are crucial to ensuring the safety of patients through such high-risk procedures. With every interaction and every decision within the operating room, their contribution is brought to the forefront in delivering the best in cardiovascular care. Post-operatively, some of the responsibilities of surgical nurses include coordination of patient recovery, with an emphasis on the care and nursing intervention core.

Patients who have undergone cardiovascular surgery usually require monitoring for close observation of complications such as infection, bleeding, or arrhythmic episodes. Individualized care plans to manage these potential complications are created and implemented by surgical nurses as they strive to rehabilitate and educate patients for the lifestyle changes that follow. The focus on combined care, as highlighted within research into cardiovascular nursing practice, underscores the importance of responding to both the medical and psychosocial aspects of healing (Umara et al., 2018). The twofold emphasis on care and necessities underscores the importance of specialized nursing practice in enhancing health outcomes and quality of life for patients navigating the complexities of cardiovascular disease (Figure 4.12).

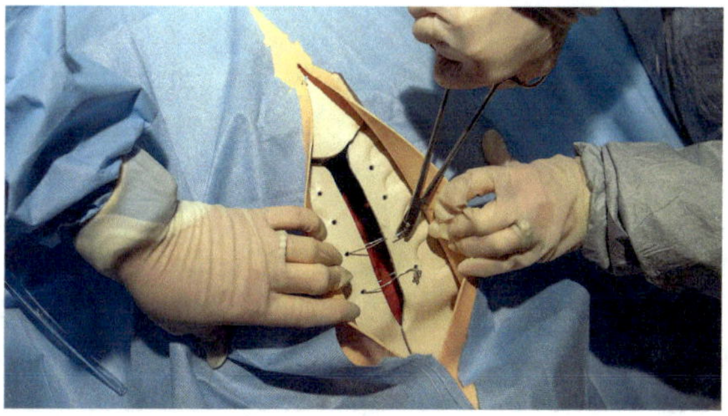

Figure 4.12. Role of surgical nursing in cardiovascular care.

Source: https://health.osu.edu/-/media/health/images/stories/2022/02/solving-complication-of-heart-surgery/training-closeup-sm.jpg.

4.4.1. Preoperative Assessment and Patient Education

Preoperative assessment is in cardiovascular surgery a critical component of ensuring the optimal patient outcome. It involves a detailed review of the patients' medical history, physical status, and psychosocial factors that affect their surgical management. Preoperative detection of conditions such as obstructive sleep apnea (OSA) is necessary, given its potential postoperative consequences. Studies have shown that patients with OSA have an enhanced risk for complications, including prolonged recovery times and respiratory distress during anesthesia (Jones et al., 2012). By systematically analyzing these factors, clinicians can tailor anesthetic and surgical plans to prevent or mitigate these risks, thereby improving the overall safety and efficacy of the procedure. This tiered approach to preoperative assessment aligns with the growing recognition of the multifaceted determinants of patient health status in the context of cardiovascular disease. No less central to the process of evaluation is the role of patient education, which significantly affects patient comprehension and compliance with preoperative instructions. Educational interventions designed to apprise patients of procedural expectations, potential complications, and postoperative protocols are essential in reducing preoperative anxiety. Research confirms that higher levels of preoperative anxiety can be detrimental to operative outcomes, as attested by the need for targeted educational interventions (Ali et al., 2023). By discussing patients' health, operative procedures, and care after the procedure, healthcare workers create an atmosphere of transparency and trust. This not only empowers patients but also encourages adherence to preoperative regimens, which is critical to reducing the risk of complications throughout the surgical process. Thus, the use of integrated educational techniques is essential to bolstering patient readiness and optimizing surgical outcomes. Moreover, the interplay between preoperative assessment and patient education underscores the need for a multidisciplinary approach to surgical nursing. Multidisciplinary collaboration among health professionals, including surgeons, nurses, and anesthesiologists, fosters an interdisciplinary understanding of every patient's unique health profile. This coordination is notably applicable among patients with serious cardiovascular ailments, who may suffer from additional complications during the perioperative period. For instance, an understanding of socio-demographic determinants of preoperative anxiety can guide particular educational interventions for reducing patient anxiety and enhancing their operating room experience (Ali et al., 2023). Such an integrated approach not only improves individual patient outcomes but also enhances general healthcare quality by creating a supportive environment in which patients are educated and involved in their care process. Essentially, the integration between thorough preoperative assessment and successful patient education is the most essential factor in effective surgical care in the cardiovascular specialty.

4.4.2. Intraoperative Responsibilities and Techniques

The intraoperative phase of surgical nursing is crucial, especially in dealing with patients with cardiovascular issues, given the complexities involved in arrhythmias, vascular, and coronary conditions. One of the key functions during surgery is the constant monitoring of patients to establish and maintain hemodynamic stability. The role of the anesthesia nurse is central, and it is the duty of the anesthesia nurse to closely monitor critical signs, such as heart rate, blood pressure, and oxygen saturation, and record them accurately. Because inherent danger is present in cardiovascular interventions, the possibility of myocardial ischemia indicates that intervention should be performed as soon as abnormalities are detected. Anesthetics, in particular, should be given with precision because agents such as propofol that have unfavorable impacts on hemodynamics can lead to severe postoperative complications if poorly monitored and controlled during the procedure (Brown et al., 2023). Hence, being aware of the physiological actions of anesthetic medications becomes crucial in optimizing the patient outcome and minimizing risks. Intraoperative responsibilities also involve adequate communication among the operating team. Coordination with surgeons, anesthesiologists, and surgical technologists ensures that all aspects of patient care are directed cohesively. Effective communication maximizes teamwork, which is essential in environments where operating protocols often deviate from planned to accommodate unforeseen complications. For instance, in situations where hemodynamic shifts occur rapidly, quick and coordinated responses by the intraoperative team are critical to maintaining the patient's stability before the procedure is initiated. In such instances, preoperative assessments are critical in guiding intraoperative strategies, since thorough assessments prepare the intraoperative team for potential complications during the process. By employing structured communication techniques, operating room nurses can help promote effective problem-solving and decision-making processes crucial to patient safety and quality of care. Additionally, the application of appropriate intraoperative techniques is at the heart of successful cardiovascular operations. Techniques such as proper positioning of the patient, meticulous prepping of the surgical site, and rigorous attention to sterile fields are critical in removing infection risk and obtaining the best possible surgical outcome. Moreover, employment of sophisticated technologies, such as intraoperative imaging and monitoring systems, can enhance the surgeon's ability to view and move through complex anatomical spaces. As indicated by recent literature on cerebrovascular diseases, refinement of procedures can have a substantial impact on surgery success and patient outcome (N/A, 2021). Therefore, continuous education and the adoption of new techniques in surgical practice are a priority in establishing an environment that prioritizes patient safety and optimal care in cardiovascular procedures (Figure 4.13).

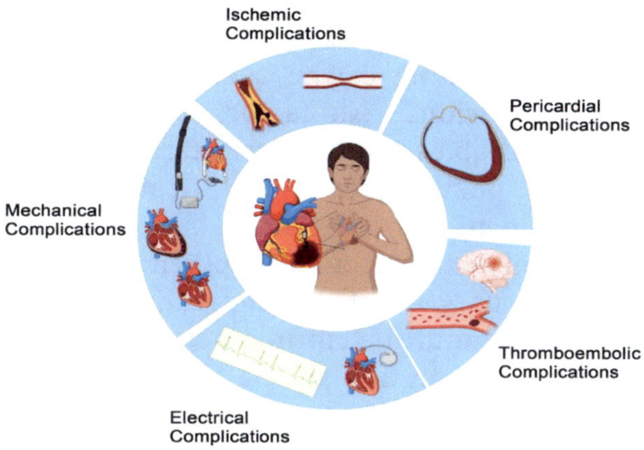

Figure 4.13. Complications in acute myocardial infarction.

Source: https://www.mdpi.com/hearts/hearts-05-00009/article_deploy/html/images/hearts-05-00009-g001.png.

4.4.3. Postoperative Care and Complications Management

Postoperative care is a significant part in the management of cardiovascular disease patients, namely those who have had surgery for arrhythmias, vascular, and coronary ailments. Through proper postoperative monitoring, recovery can be enhanced and complications prevented to a great extent. Throughout this period, healthcare providers exercise extra caution in monitoring vital signs, pain relief, and the detection of any complications that may be emerging. Special care needs to be taken for obstructive sleep apnea (OSA) patients, as they are at high risk of respiratory complications. Prolongation of anesthesia emergence and recovery times is more significant among these patients; therefore, specialty postoperative monitoring protocols are required that take into account the special challenges of OSA (Jones et al., 2012). Hence, such an understanding of risk factors ensures that nursing interventions are anticipatory rather than reactionary, facilitating improved patient outcomes and reduced healthcare costs. Beyond the observation of vital signs, skilled postoperative care requires an understanding of the complex interplay between various risk factors and patient-specific variables. For comorbid cardiovascular patients, postoperative complications can manifest in many forms, ranging from increased susceptibility to infection to potential for an acute coronary event. Intraoperative nursing involves a multidisciplinary process that ensures collaboration among the anesthetist, surgeon, and nursing team to create holistic care. Postoperative care measures must involve patient education, particularly on signs of complications and the importance of medication adherence. By combining these educational elements, nurses are in a position to promote active patient involvement in recovery, improving compliance with postoperative treatment regimens as well as overall health outcomes (Ohiienko et al., 2015). Effective management of postoperative complications requires that the nurses be observant and responsive to changes in the patient's condition. Since cardiovascular illnesses are very complex, there is a need for constant monitoring of the patient's respiratory function, cardiac output, and end-organ perfusion. As a case in point, OSA patients may require lengthy stays in the post-anesthesia care unit (PACU) to allow their respiratory status to return to balance. Studies have proven a correlation between OSA and hospital admissions of increased lengths and complications, placing greater importance on the timely and comprehensive postoperative evaluation (Jones et al., 2012). With the implementation of a systematic yet flexible patient management plan, operating room nursing staff enhance the quality of care rendered, ultimately decreasing risks involved in postoperative recovery while restoring patients to a level of stable health promptly.

Test Your Knowledge

1. What are the key responsibilities of a surgical nurse in the postoperative care of a patient after cardiac surgery?
2. How does a surgical nurse monitor for signs of cardiovascular complications?

4.5. Patient Education and Support

Learning Outcome

1. Describe the importance of patient education in cardiovascular health
2. Define the strategies for effective patient communication
3. Discuss the resources for patient support and rehabilitation

In cardiovascular medicine, specifically in the treatment of arrhythmias, vascular disease, and coronary disease, patient education is an essential aspect of treatment. The essence of these conditions necessitates effective and transparent communication by healthcare providers to patients. Educating patients on their individual diagnoses, treatment options, and the necessity of continuing medication enhances their ability to become active participants in their own care. This involvement is necessary because studies show that educationally well-prepared patients are more likely to adhere to prescribed therapy and lifestyle modifications that can halt further health decline. The nursing practice must thus play an active role in delivering education tailored to the patient's specific values, knowledge, and needs, empowering them to be responsible for their outcomes. The fundamental function of education cannot be overstated; it's a key doorway to increased patient engagement and improved clinical outcomes. Patient education in supportive interventions is essential for optimal cardiovascular disease management. For patients with complex diagnoses like heart failure or arrhythmias, support transcends information alone. Whole-person care elements, such as emotional and psychological support, play a crucial role in the patient experience. Nurses, being immediate care providers, are most qualified to deliver these intricate support systems, thereby facilitating a healing environment. Educational interventions aimed at enhancing patient knowledge can diminish anxiety surrounding such illnesses as well as the burden of caring for themselves. Additionally, patient support programs can reflect the theoretical underpinnings of "care, core, and cure," wherein nurses recognize individuals' emotional and practical needs, in addition to treating the disease. Such support steps strengthen patient resilience and adherence, facilitating better health outcomes and rehabilitation effectiveness as highlighted in research findings (Umara et al., 2018). Besides, the role of community support groups and resources in patient education cannot be overemphasized. Such organizations have the possibility of complementing health care professionals' individual health education efforts by promoting membership and mutual experience among patients who share similar health problems.

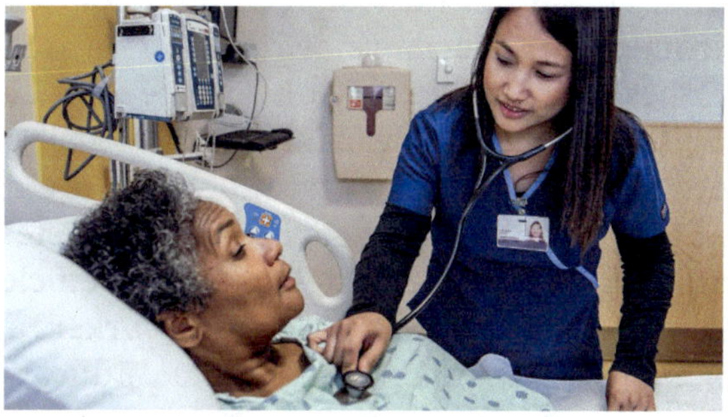

Figure 4.14. Patient education and support.

Source: https://www.nursingworld.org/globalassets/practiceandpolicy/workforce/what-is-nursing/largeimage-anais-42.jpg.

The peer support groups have also the possibility of significantly contributing to the educational process through practical advice, emotional support, and others' experiences that will remain with individuals longer than would professional contact alone. By integrating these community resources into the care process, a firmer base of support is established that can sustain patient education. Experience has shown that when professionals and their community facilitate patients, compliance with treatment plans and rehabilitation programs is maximized. Therefore, effective patient education, combined with a supportive community, creates a synergy of benefits that is imperative for ensuring the best cardiovascular care outcomes (Kitsiou et al., 2013) (Figure 4.14).

4.5.1. Importance of Patient Education in Cardiovascular Health

Effective patient education is the cornerstone of cardiovascular health, particularly in the care of arrhythmias, vascular disease, and coronary disease. The intricacy of these diseases demands that the patient not just understand their diagnosis but also its implications for overall well-being. An informed patient is in a better position to become an active participant in their own care, which significantly improves outcomes. Furthermore, education provides patients with information on recognizing early symptoms and warning signs, which can allow for timely medical treatment before any resulting complications. As healthcare systems increasingly prioritize value-based care, efficient communication between healthcare workers and patients becomes increasingly vital. Education interventions help fill knowledge gaps, thereby supporting treatment protocols and compliance with prognosis among cardiovascular patients (Kitsiou et al., 2013). Incorporation of patient-reported outcomes in cardiovascular care is essential to assess the actual impact of education on health care. Patient feedback has been shown to illuminate where education can make the most difference and where it is most required. For instance, once patients are aware of the long-term consequences of atrial fibrillation and associated complications, they are more consistently encouraged to adhere to recommended treatment regimens. The International Consortium for Health Outcomes Measurement (ICHOM) highlights the importance of patient opinion by developing a harmonized minimum structure of outcomes tailored to the needs of individuals with specific conditions (Arbelo et al., 2020). Involving patients in their own care choices instills a sense of responsibility that is essential for continuing required lifestyle adjustments and self-management, ultimately leading to improved cardiovascular health. Moreover, the role of healthcare professionals in facilitating effective patient education cannot be overemphasized. Surgical nursing, in particular, must integrate educational interventions that are individualized to meet patient-specific educational needs and learning styles. Nurses are likely to be the most involved in patient interaction and have a good sense of common misconceptions and barriers to patients' learning cardiovascular health.

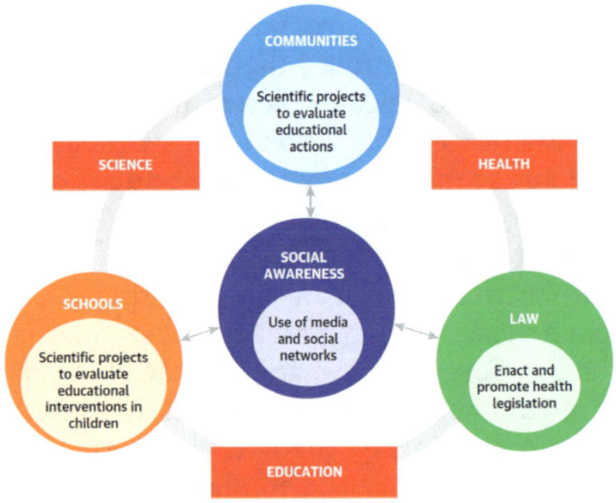

Figure 4.15. Patient education in cardiovascular health.

Source: https://www.researchgate.net/profile/Patricia-Bodega/publication/357893941/figure/fig3/AS:1146920575741953@1650458582845/Science-Health-and-Education-for-Promoting-Cardiovascular-Health.png.

Through teach-back strategies, visual display, and motivational interviewing, nurses can enhance learning and retention of significant information. This multi-factorial approach is critical in a population increasingly burdened by chronic cardiovascular conditions, where the efficacy of treatment interventions hinges on lifestyle decisions. Undeniably, an educated patient with the appropriate tools has a higher likelihood of achieving improved health outcomes, thereby emphasizing the critical importance of patient education within cardiovascular practice (Figure 4.15).

4.5.2. Strategies for Effective Patient Communication

Effective communication is paramount in cardiovascular practice, particularly with the management of complicated disorders such as arrhythmias and coronary disease. Open communication establishes a trusting relationship between health professionals and patients, which is the best for obtaining compliance and adherence to treatment regimens. Personalization of communications to fit the individual needs of each patient—either in language, information delivery rate, or treatment of specific concerns—ensures that patients feel heard and understood. Shared decision-making with patients not only empowers them but also enhances their ability to grasp the significance of their conditions and the need for interventions ordered. As defined by the American College of Cardiology, effective communication skills are crucial for all clinical cardiologists in their efforts to deliver quality care, which underscores the importance of strong patient relationships in achieving positive health outcomes (Book et al., 2017). No less important in facilitating effective communication is the understanding of health literacy. Multicultural patients will possess varying levels of awareness regarding medical treatments and terminology, and a flexible communication style will be required. Utilization of visual aids and materials with simplified explanations can prove helpful in bridging the understanding gap, thus ensuring that patients comprehend essential information concerning their cardiovascular diseases. Moreover, providing a platform where patients are not afraid to pose questions is a significant determinant in de-mystifying medical procedures and alleviating anxiety. The seriousness of cardiovascular diseases calls for healthcare providers to closely observe patients verbal and nonverbal cues to their level of comprehension and comfort. This is essential for facilitating adherence to the treatment plan and enhanced patient satisfaction (Aronow et al., 2007). Aside from direct communication strategies, the use of technological solutions also proves effective in enhancing patient engagement and information dissemination. Utilization of telehealth platforms provides convenient access to healthcare facilities, along with the power for patients to access consulting from their healthcare providers beyond geographical constraints. Educational platforms that provide tailored content regarding cardiovascular health can empower patients to be actively involved in their healthcare process. Thus, using technology alongside traditional methods of communication addresses the diverse needs of patients ultimately, allowing them to understand the various routes of treatment and changes in lifestyle. Through being attuned to the ever-changing phenomenon of patient communication, operating room nurses can potentially exert significant control over the quality of care provided to individuals with arrhythmias, vascular conditions, and coronary diseases (Book et al., 2017).

4.5.3. Resources for Patient Support and Rehabilitation

There has to be proper availability of resources for the patient's support and rehabilitation while treating individuals suffering from cardiovascular disorders. The rehabilitation programs, are adjusted to the specific needs of the patients, typically include aspects of physical therapy, diet counseling, and psychotherapy. These programs not only improve the physical recovery of the patients but also their mental and emotional health, which is crucial in coping with the issues related to chronic diseases such as coronary ailments and arrhythmias. Furthermore, incorporating educational material enables patients to make informed decisions about their treatment, as they are informed about their health and control measures, thereby providing them with a sense of control over their therapeutic process. One of the significant features of patient support is the use of evidence-based guidelines that inform practice. According to the 2023 AHA/ACC/ACCP/ASPC/NLA/PCNA Guideline for the Management of Patients with Chronic Coronary Disease, there is an emphasis on patient-centered care that integrates social determinants of health into the rehabilitation process. The guideline also emphasizes team-based treatment and shared decision-making that further improves the effectiveness of rehabilitation measures. It enables healthcare providers to recognize the diverse needs of patients, ultimately leading to improved outcomes. By regularizing care practices based on the available guidelines, nursing professionals can provide comprehensive care that addresses the clinical and psychosocial aspects of healing. Continuous resuscitation advanced cardiac care education and training are also crucial for healthcare professionals involved in patient rehabilitation. The 2021 European Resuscitation Council Guidelines are a rigorous overview of best practices in resuscitation, highlighting the importance of systems in saving lives and improving patient outcomes after cardiac arrest. This content is not only informative on emergency procedures but also directs post-resuscitation care for a return to normalcy. Surgical nursing specialists must integrate these discoveries into practice so that they can implement proper responses to various situations related to arrhythmias and other cardiovascular conditions. Continuous education of the professionals combined with efficient patient support systems has the ability to improve significantly rehabilitation processes, leading to higher quality of life for the patients post-surgery.

Test Your Knowledge

1. Why is it essential to assess a patient's understanding when providing health education?
2. How can nurses support patients in managing chronic illnesses at home?

4.6. Current Trends and Innovations in Cardiovascular Care

Learning Outcome

1. Describe the advances in surgical techniques and technologies
2. Define the role of telemedicine in cardiovascular care
3. Identify the future directions in cardiovascular nursing

Recent developments in cardiovascular medicine have been significantly impacted by the adoption of artificial intelligence (AI) technologies. The application of AI in cardiology has revolutionized every facet of healthcare, ranging from increasing diagnostic precision to optimizing treatment protocols. A systematic review supports the use of AI in enhancing innovation that enables accurate diagnostics and personalized medicine, which in turn redefine clinical practices in cardiovascular care. This shift is particularly significant for arrhythmia management, where AI-based devices can analyze cardiac rhythms in real-time and support enhanced monitoring and timely intervention. Not only do these integrations enhance patient outcomes but also enable optimized clinical workflows, thus making a strong case for continuous ouro development and deployment (Adertinto et al., 2024). In addition to AI, there has been a notable trend in cardiovascular care originating from new remote monitoring technologies. High-tech sensors embedded in wearable devices enable the real-time tracking of critical vital signs, such as heart rhythm and rate, allowing for early detection of any abnormalities. This feature is particularly beneficial for patients with chronic conditions, such as arrhythmias, as it enables them to take an active role in their own treatment decision-making. The use of remote telehealth services allows medical professionals to review patient data on a routine basis, making it simpler to adjust treatment plans accordingly. Remote monitoring also encourages a more patient-focused approach since patients are treated at home but remain well linked with their caregivers. The innovation of these technologies significantly influences the treatment of vascular and coronary diseases, enhancing both compliance and clinical outcomes (Touro College & University System, 2016). Moreover, the ongoing exploration of precision medicine for cardiovascular disease is a paradigm shift in therapy. With the precision of interventions based on individual genetic, environmental, and lifestyle factors, healthcare workers can optimize therapeutic effects while minimizing adverse effects. For instance, pharmacogenomics plays an important role in determining the optimal drug for patients with coronary artery disease, whereby therapeutic strategies are optimized for patients' specific biochemical profiles. This not only improves overall care quality but also enhances the efficacy of interventions, especially in managing complex cardiovascular conditions. With the evolving scenario of cardiovascular care, the integration of precision medicine, which hassped up with advances from the most recent studies, will surely be a unifying element in elevating the level of and enhancing patient outcomes in surgical nursing (Adertinto et al., 2024) (Figure 4.16).

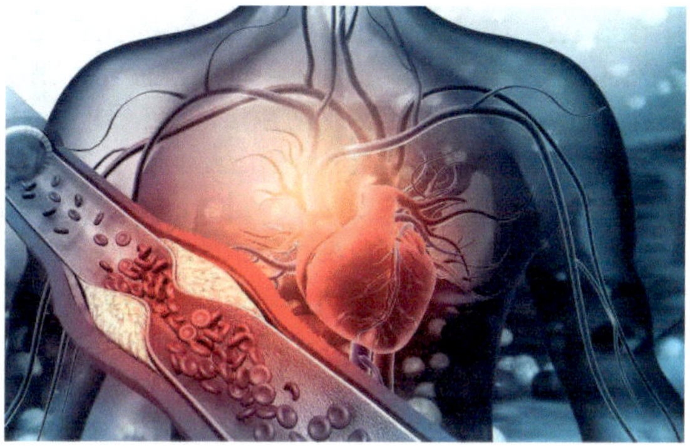

Figure 4.16. Current trends and innovations in cardiovascular care.

Source: https://etimg.etb2bimg.com/photo/104439885.cms.

4.6.1. Advances in Surgical Techniques and Technologies

The evolution of surgical techniques and technology remains central to cardiovascular treatment, particularly in the fields of arrhythmias, vascular disease, and coronary disease. These recent advancements have been toward less invasive surgeries, minimizing not only patient recovery time but also the likelihood of complications from open surgery. Techniques such as robotic-assisted surgery and sophisticated imaging modalities, i.e., intraoperative ultrasound and fluoroscopy, facilitate improved accuracy in cardiovascular procedures. Such innovations have transformed the way procedures such as coronary artery bypass grafting and valve repair are performed, enabling surgical teams to implement intricate techniques with greater precision and control. The combined effect of these technological innovations in the operating room yields improved patient outcomes, something that surgical nursing should adopt and adapt to the evolving realities of cardiovascular practice. In the field of arrhythmias, technological innovation in catheter-based ablation has revolutionized treatment conditions in patients with various cardiac rhythm disorders. The evolution of three-dimensional mapping technology has significantly improved arrhythmogenic focus localization, rendering interventions more effective and more straightforward. Not only does this precision-based approach minimize collateral damage to the local cardiac tissue, but it also decreases procedure times, thus lowering the cost factor for healthcare resources. Furthermore, newer energy sources, such as cryoablation and laser ablation, provide alternatives to traditional radiofrequency energy, meeting the specific needs of heterogeneous patient groups.

It is crucial to surgical nursing professionals to keep up with these new modalities to provide informed patient care, generate optimal results in surgery, and improve overall cardiovascular health. Furthermore, the integration of telemedicine and digital health technologies in surgery is a revolutionary step forward in managing cardiovascular care. Remote patient monitoring, facilitated by wearable sensors and mobile health applications, enables real-time assessment of vital signs and arrhythmia events, thereby facilitating pre- and post-operative care. This transition not only allows for timely interventions prior to cardiac complications becoming acute, but also enables patients to become more actively involved in their healthcare. Surgical nursing staff can gain significant advantages from this technology, enabling them to develop individualized care plans based on current data and patient feedback. With health care widely adopting these technologies, it will become crucial to have the ability to use digital technologies to maximize care efficiencies and maximize patient outcomes for the conditions of arrhythmias, vascular disease, and coronary disease, which are still at the core of cardiovascular surgical nursing (Kitsiou et al., 2013; Bouchlarhem et al., 2023).

4.6.2. Role of Telemedicine in Cardiovascular Care

Telemedicine has emerged as an essential resource in the treatment of cardiovascular illness, ~~particularly~~ including the treatment of arrhythmias, vascular disease, and coronary disease. Telemedicine enables physicians to treat patients remotely, and it gives patients regular monitoring and follow-up if managing appointments in person proved difficult . Telemedicine can mitigate risk potential in non-compliance due to missed appointments and delayed treatment for those with chronic cardiovascular illness. With the use of technology, practitioners can utilize real-time data from wearable devices to intervene promptly, assess symptoms, and fine-tune treatment regimens more effectively. These capabilities not only promote patient activation but also help enhance clinical outcomes by personalized care approaches, all in keeping with modern standards in cardiovascular nursing practices. The role of telemedicine is not only for consultation but also plays a vital role in holistic management programs among patients suffering from obstructive sleep apnea (OSA) and related cardiovascular comorbidities. OSA has a multifactorial relationship with a broad spectrum of adverse outcomes for overall health, including cardiovascular disease, making patient-specific treatment modalities imperative. Telemedicine facilitates individualized treatment, allowing for various treatment modalities to be executed in real-time. For example, patients may be advised on behavioral therapy or modifications to their continuous positive airway pressure (CPAP) treatment through virtual visits, augmented by ongoing data feedback from devices. As indicated by the recent research, novel phenotyping approaches are underway to personalize therapy better to suit the individual needs of the patient, in harmony with patient needs changing, and to promote compliance with treatment protocols, ultimately resulting in reduced cardiovascular risk of OSA (Chai-

Coetzer et al., 2017). Additionally, integrating telemedicine into cardiovascular care can significantly enhance the treatment of acute and chronic diseases by facilitating coordinated care among multidisciplinary teams. This interdisciplinary approach enables the rapid exchange of information among cardiologists, surgeons, and family doctors, ensuring coordinated and comprehensive patient care. Telemedicine systems can allow regular case conferences and consultations across different specialists, a necessity for patients with complex health histories. Through the use of technology to maintain solid lines of communication, health teams can effectively respond quickly to patient needs as they arise, leading to better control of arrhythmias, vascular, and coronary disorders. Working together is essential in conducting timely surgeries or interventions, thereby achieving overall patient success for cardiovascular health (Touro College & University System, 2018) (Figure 4.17).

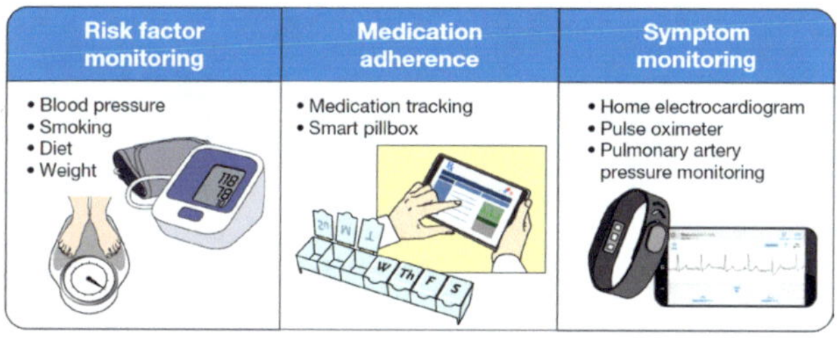

Figure 4.17. Role of telemedicine in cardiovascular care.

Source: https://www.ahajournals.org/cms/10.1161/CIR.0000000000001107/asset/ea6a0c74-351e-4c00-ad2f-6b7469542f9b/assets/graphic/cir.0000000000001107.fig02.jpg.

4.6.3. Future Directions in Cardiovascular Nursing

The future of cardiovascular nursing has a great ~~deal to transform~~ potential, primarily via technological innovation and improved patient-centered clinical practice. As the face of cardiovascular diseases continues to evolve, nurses will increasingly utilize digital health technologies, such as telehealth platforms and mobile health applications, to remotely monitor patients with vascular, coronary, and arrhythmia conditions and intervene early. These technologies not only facilitate patient activation but also allow for timely adjustment of treatment programs based on real-time data. Additionally, cardiovascular nurses will be at the forefront of educating patients about these devices, enabling them to take a proactive role in managing their health conditions. Through the inclusion of such digital solutions within their workflows, outcomes can be optimized, and a more independent approach to cardiovascular health management can be facilitated. At the same time, the emphasis on multidisciplinary care within cardiovascular care will shape the future of nursing practice. The Enhanced Recovery After Surgery (ERAS) protocols exemplify this, as they promote a team-based model of perioperative care, involving not only surgeons and anesthesiologists but also nurses, pharmacists, and dietitians (Grant et al., 2024). This partnership model will facilitate the sharing of knowledge and foster comprehensive patient management plans, thereby enhancing overall outcomes. As cardiovascular nurses occupy a position at the intersection of clinical practice and patient education, their role will be central in implementing ERAS guidelines effectively. Incorporating this culture of partnership will enable nurses to individualize their interventions more effectively according to the unique needs of patients, hence enhancing the standard of cardiovascular nursing care. Moreover, addressing the specific needs of the elderly in cardiovascular care is crucial to the future of nursing practice. As hinted by more recent studies, age is a substantial risk factor for conditions such as cardiogenic shock, but older individuals remain underrepresented in clinical trials and treatment protocols (Blumer et al., 2024). Therefore, cardiovascular nursing must adapt by prioritizing individualized assessments and interventions that are responsive to the unique needs of older patients. As a nod to the intricacies found with geriatric cardiovascular patients, nursing education would be compelled to focus on gerontology concepts in curriculum development. By cultivating a comprehensive understanding of the age-related factors affecting cardiovascular well-being, prospective nurses will become increasingly capable of providing supportive, evidence-based care that addresses the physiological and psychosocial needs of the elderly in clinical settings.

Test Your Knowledge

1. Why is it essential to assess a patient's understanding when providing health education?
2. How can nurses support patients in managing chronic illnesses at home?

SUMMARY

The significance of effective cardiovascular care cannot be overstressed, particularly in the scenario of arrhythmias, vascular disease, and coronary disease within surgical nursing. Based on the many studies that have been conducted, the swift progression of cardiovascular disease, especially with aging populations, emphasizes the incorporation of surgical nurses directly into the patient care process. The care, core, and cure model is an integrative care model that identifies not only the explicit medical intervention but also the importance of recurrent rehabilitation and patient education for health in patients of cardiovascular disease. Such a holistic approach allows nurses to provide care for patients' multifaceted needs and ensure patients receive treatment in the acute phase ~~but~~ and also sustained healthcare through long-term health management and behavior modification. This combined knowledge is essential in mitigating morbidity and improving overall patient outcomes across cardiovascular treatment (Umara et al., 2018). In addition, it is necessary to value the demographic trends that shape the landscape of cardiovascular disease since there is a significant burden of diseases such as hypertension and congestive heart failure, particularly among the elderly population. Current evidence has highlighted that the majority of geriatric admissions are a result of cardiovascular complications, hence the need for targeted interventions and screens on admission. Nurses play a central role in identifying such patients through vigilant assessment and preventive practices, as many will not initially present with cardiovascular issues. This proactive measure ensures the early identification and management of cardiovascular disorders, thereby reducing hospitalizations and improving the health of older patients. This commitment to understanding these trends and providing accurate care measures aligns with the overall goals of surgical nursing (Kisenge et al., 2011). Finally, advancements in the field of cardiovascular care require a joint effort on the part of all medical healthcare providers, and most notably surgical nurses, to foster a learning culture, rehabilitation culture, and interprofessional team environment. Continuous educational opportunities for nursing practitioners in light of emerging cardiovascular research and interventions are paramount. Additionally, improved communication among healthcare teams encourages a joint effort to care for patients, in which all aspects of a patient's condition are jointly addressed. Integration of evidence-based research into practice not only improves the delivery of care but also equips nurses with the tools necessary to advocate for patient demands and improve health outcomes. As the burden of cardiovascular disease continues to grow, maintaining a focus on overall cardiac care remains essential to creating patient population resilience (Umara et al., 2018).

In surgical nursing, it is crucial to have knowledge of guidelines for cardiovascular care, with a focus on arrhythmias and vascular disease. The recently released guidelines of the European Society of Cardiology provide valuable information for managing patients with cardiovascular risk factors who are undergoing non-cardiac surgery. The guidelines offer basic considerations, such as preoperative cardiac function evaluation and management of antithrombotic therapy. Surgical groups, particularly for lung cancer surgeries, must take into consideration the heightened risk of cardiovascular complications based on the patient-specific anatomical and physiological features of such surgeries. By adherence to these guidelines, surgical nurses can effectively work in advance to minimize risks and enhance patient outcomes, demonstrating the significance of evidence-based guidelines in clinical practice (Tacconi, 2022). Another critical aspect of the operating room nursing situation is the administration of red blood cell transfusions, especially in patients with varying hemoglobin levels. Recent research emphasizes the requirement to set optimal thresholds of transfusion so that the patient does not bear the risk of unnecessary exposure as well as ensuring safety. The findings indicate that restrictive transfusion strategies, operating at thresholds between 7.0 g/dL and 8.0 g/dL, can reduce the risk of receiving a transfusion without adverse effects on 30-day mortality rates or other notable clinical events. Notable is the model's suggestion of the need for tailored care strategies, particularly in patients with cardiovascular disease who may experience different physiological responses to anemia. Surgical nurses play a critical role in implementing these strategies, resulting in improved care and usage of resources in surgical departments (Carson et al., 2021). Finally, the implementation of these guidelines and continued research emphasize the dynamic nature of cardiovascular care in surgical nursing. With advancements in surgical techniques and patient management techniques still evolving, the need for continuous learning and adaptation is evident. With the integration of new cardiovascular guidelines and transfusion principles in clinical practice, surgical nursing can optimize recovery processes and enhance patient safety. Under a patient-focused policy, nurses can contribute to discussions about individual risks and benefits of specific interventions and make informed decisions, as guided by current best evidence. In bridging the gap between existing research and real application, surgical nurses play a pivotal role in influencing the successful outcomes of patients with arrhythmia, vascular, and coronary disorders (Carson et al., 2021; Tacconi, 2022).

KEY TERMS FROM THIS CHAPTER

- Angina pectoris
- Atrial fibrillation
- Cardiac monitoring
- Coronary artery disease (CAD)
- Electrocardiogram (ECG)
- Hemodynamic stability
- Myocardial infarction
- Postoperative arrhythmia
- Sinus tachycardia
- Vascular graft
- Anticoagulant therapy
- Bradycardia
- Cardiac rehabilitation
- Deep vein thrombosis (DVT)
- Heart failure
- Hypertension
- Peripheral arterial disease (PAD)
- Pulmonary embolism (PE)
- Thrombolytic therapy
- Ventricular fibrillation

CRITICAL THINKING QUESTIONS

1. **Which of the following arrhythmias is most life-threatening and requires immediate defibrillation?**
   a. Atrial fibrillation
   b. Ventricular fibrillation
   c. Sinus bradycardia
   d. Premature atrial contraction
2. **A key nursing intervention for a patient with deep vein thrombosis (DVT) is:**
   a. Massage the affected limb
   b. Apply cold compress
   c. Encourage ambulation without delay
   d. Administer anticoagulants as prescribed
3. **Which sign is most suggestive of myocardial infarction (MI)?**
   a. Sudden onset of sharp abdominal pain
   b. Burning chest pain relieved by food
   c. Chest pressure radiating to left arm and jaw
   d. Localized chest pain that worsens with deep breathing
4. **What is the purpose of telemetry monitoring in surgical patients with cardiac disorders?**
   a. To monitor temperature trends
   b. To assess gastrointestinal function
   c. To detect changes in cardiac rhythm continuously
   d. To improve sleep patterns
5. **In a postoperative patient with hypotension and tachycardia, what should the nurse assess first?**
   a. Blood glucose level
   b. Presence of surgical wound infection
   c. Signs of internal bleeding or hypovolemia
   d. Bowel sounds

Short Answer Questions

1. Define arrhythmia and give one example.
2. List two common signs of deep vein thrombosis (DVT).
3. What is the primary nursing action during a cardiac arrhythmia episode?
4. Name one risk factor and one complication of coronary artery disease (CAD).
5. Why is anticoagulant therapy important in patients with vascular disorders?
6. Describe the nursing management of a postoperative patient with atrial fibrillation.
7. Explain the signs, symptoms, and emergency nursing care for a patient with suspected myocardial infarction (MI).
8. Discuss preventive strategies and nursing interventions for deep vein thrombosis (DVT) in surgical patients.
9. Outline the pathophysiology, clinical presentation, and management of coronary artery disease.

Answers to Critical Thinking Questions

1. (b); 2. (d); 3. (c); 4. (c); 5. (c).

REFERENCES

1. Abrignani, M. G., Abrignani, V., Lo Baido, R., Novo, S., et al. (2014). Panic disorder, anxiety, and cardiovascular diseases. https://core.ac.uk/download/53296862.pdf (accessed on 30th June 2025).
2. Olawade, D. B., Aderinto, N., Olatunji, G., Kokori, E., David-Olawade, A. C., & Hadi, M. (2024). Advancements and applications of Artificial Intelligence in cardiology: Current trends and future prospects. *Journal of Medicine Surgery and Public Health, 3*, 100109. https://doi.org/10.1016/j.glmedi.2024.100109Ali, N. N. (2023). Assessment of preoperative anxiety, its contributing factors, and impact on immediate postoperative outcomes among cardiac surgery patients: A cross-sectional study. https://core.ac.uk/download/603659458.pdf (accessed on 30th June 2025).
3. Arbelo, E., Banerjee, A., Bollmann, A., Caffrey-Armstrong, M., et al. (2020). Development of an international standard set of outcome measures for patients with atrial fibrillation: A report of the International Consortium for Health Outcomes Measurement (ICHOM) atrial fibrillation working group. https://core.ac.uk/download/286716298.pdf (accessed on 30th June 2025).
4. Aronow, W. S., Fleg, J. J., Pepine, C. J., Artinian, N. T., et al. (2007). ACCF/AHA 2011 expert consensus document on hypertension in the elderly: A report of the American College of Cardiology Foundation Task Force on Clinical Expert Consensus Documents. https://core.ac.uk/download/56681322.pdf (accessed on 30th June 2025).
5. Barzilay, J. I., Farag, Y. M. K., & Durthaler, J. (2024). Albuminuria: An underappreciated risk factor for cardiovascular disease. *Journal of the American Heart Association: Cardiovascular and Cerebrovascular Disease, 13*. https://www.semanticscholar.org/paper/66c2ce93879da168389b7bedd4cf8dc0aa1a94cc (accessed on 30th June 2025).
6. Baumgartner, H., De Backer, J., Babu-Narayan, S. V., Budts, W., Chessa, M., Diller, G. P., Lung, B., et al. (2020). 2020 ESC guidelines for the management of adult congenital heart disease. *European Heart Journal, 42*, 563–645. https://doi.org/10.1093/eurheartj/ehaa554 (accessed on 30th June 2025).
7. Blumer, V., Kanwar, M., Barnett, C. F., Cowger, J., Damluji, A. A., Farr, M., Goodlin, S. J., et al. (2024). Cardiogenic shock in older adults: A focus on age-associated risks and approach to management: A scientific statement from the American Heart Association. *Circulation, 149*. https://doi.org/10.1161/cir.0000000000001214 (accessed on 30th June 2025).
8. Book, W., Cleveland, J. C., Dauber, I., Drazner, M. H., et al. (2017). 2017 ACC/AHA/HFSA/ISHLT/ACP advanced training statement on advanced heart failure and transplant cardiology (revision of the ACCF/AHA/ACP/HFSA/ISHLT 2010 clinical competence statement on management of patients with advanced heart failure and cardiac transplant). https://core.ac.uk/download/304664370.pdf (accessed on 30th June 2025).
9. Bouchlarhem, A., Bouchlarhem, A., Ismaili, N., Ismaili, N., Ismaili, N., El Ouafi, N., El Ouafi, N., et al. (2023). Cardiac intensive care unit: Where we are in 2023. https://core.ac.uk/download/595356241.pdf (accessed on 30th June 2025).
10. Brown, K., Campbell, Y., & Escobar, L. J. (2023). Remimazolam as an alternative induction agent in monitored anesthesia care: An educational module. https://core.ac.uk/download/622984208.pdf (accessed on 30th June 2025).

11. Busardo,' F. P., Fineschi, V., Frati, P., Gulino, M., et al. (2015). Does defensive medicine change the behaviors of vascular surgeons? A qualitative review. https://core.ac.uk/download/54534214.pdf (accessed on 30th June 2025).

12. Carson, J., Stanworth, S., Dennis, J., Trivella, M., Roubinian, N. H., Fergusson, D., Triulzi, D., et al. (2021). Transfusion thresholds for guiding red blood cell transfusion. *The Cochrane Database of Systematic Reviews, 12*, CD002042. https://www.semanticscholar.org/paper/99c12cd0b5820cae5a1e600b4078c4860bbd3ebd (accessed on 30th June 2025).

13. Chai-Coetzer, C. L., McEvoy, R. D., Vakulin, A., Yap, L., et al. (2017). Obstructive sleep apnoea: Therapeutic options and challenges. https://core.ac.uk/download/84868277.pdf (accessed on 30th June 2025).

14. Dantas, R. A. S., Dessotte, C. A. M., Furuya, R. K., Rodrigues, A. A., et al. (2019). Asociaciones de los síntomas de ansiedad y depresión preoperatorios con complicaciones postoperatorias de cirugías cardiacas. https://core.ac.uk/download/268299020.pdf (accessed on 30th June 2025).

15. Glikson, M., Nielsen, J. C., Kronborg, M. B., Michowitz, Y., Auricchio, A., Barbash, I. M., Barrabés, J. A., et al. (2021). 2021 ESC guidelines on cardiac pacing and cardiac resynchronization therapy. *European Heart Journal, 42*, 3427–3520. https://doi.org/10.1093/eurheartj/ehab364 (accessed on 30th June 2025).

16. Grant, M. C., Crisafi, C., Alvarez, A., Arora, R. C., Brindle, M. E., Chatterjee, S., Ender, J., et al. (2024). Perioperative care in cardiac surgery: A joint consensus statement by the Enhanced Recovery After Surgery (ERAS) Cardiac Society, ERAS International Society, and The Society of Thoracic Surgeons (STS). *The Annals of Thoracic Surgery, 117*, 669–689. https://doi.org/10.1016/j.athoracsur.2023.12.006 (accessed on 30th June 2025).

17. Halvorsen, S., Mehilli, J., Cassese, S., Hall, T. S., Abdelhamid, M., Barbato, E., De Hert, S., et al. (2022). 2022 ESC guidelines on cardiovascular assessment and management of patients undergoing non-cardiac surgery. *European Heart Journal, 43*, 3826–3924. https://doi.org/10.1093/eurheartj/ehac270 (accessed on 30th June 2025).

18. Hendriks, J., Elliott, A., Middeldorp, M., & Sanders, P. (2022). Contributing factors to personalized medicine in atrial fibrillation. *Heart, 109*, 164–165. https://www.semanticscholar.org/paper/c787650ddae744f0b603612e616fd68548a17c43 (accessed on 30th June 2025).

19. Jones, S. F. (2012). Obstructive sleep apnea and the effects of co-existing factors on PACU stay time. https://core.ac.uk/download/477679572.pdf (accessed on 30th June 2025).

20. Kisenge, P. R. (2011). Pattern of cardiovascular diseases among elderly patients admitted in medical wards at Muhimbili National Hospital Dar es Salaam Tanzania. https://core.ac.uk/download/pdf/16666639.pdf (accessed on 30th June 2025).

21. Kitsiou, A., Caforio, A. L. P., Porta-Sanchez, A., Vahanian, A., Iung, B., Carrera, C., Szymanski, C., et al. (2013). ESC core curriculum for the general cardiologist (2013). https://core.ac.uk/download/55756305.pdf (accessed on 30th June 2025).

22. Ohiienko, M. M., Redko, S. I., Shyshchuk, V. D., Огиенко, M. M., et al. (2015). General questions of anesthesiology. https://core.ac.uk/download/141448194.pdf (accessed on 30th June 2025).

23. Perkins, G. D., Gräsner, J. T., Semeraro, F., Olasveengen, T. M., Soar, J., Lott, C., Van de Voorde, P., et al. (2021). European Resuscitation Council Guidelines 2021: Executive summary.

Resuscitation, 161, 1–60. https://doi.org/10.1016/j.resuscitation.2021.02.003 (accessed on 30th June 2025).

24. Rietjens, S., van Riemsdijk, T. E., Sikma, M., & de Lange, D. D. (2023). High-dose insulin should NOT be used without vasopressors in calcium channel blocker toxicity. *British Journal of Clinical Pharmacology, 89*, 1275–1278. https://www.semanticscholar.org/paper/f038c852190b9a62f12eefa5c4a3d3ceb9a8684b (accessed on 30th June 2025).
25. Saraswati, N. P. S. D., Pratiwi, S. H., & Sari, E. (2024). Dyspnea management in patients with pneumonia and coronary artery disease: A case study. *Malahayati International Journal of Nursing and Health Science*. https://www.semanticscholar.org/paper/84bcdb3feeec15647b7c5b469457003eb2007d13 (accessed on 30th June 2025).
26. Tacconi, F. (2022). 2022 European Society of Cardiology guidelines on cardiovascular assessment and management of patients undergoing non-cardiac surgery: Which impact to lung cancer resection? *Heart, Vessels and Transplantation*. https://www.semanticscholar.org/paper/5b6ab3245db9a2392980c32417df4f311f5a1191 (accessed on 30th June 2025).
27. Touro College & University System. (2016). 2015 Touro College & University System faculty publications. https://core.ac.uk/download/217328920.pdf (accessed on 30th June 2025).
28. Umara, A. F. (2018). The model theory approach "Care, Core, Cure" for patients with cardiovascular disease. https://media.neliti.com/media/publications/277788-the-model-theory-approach-care-core-cure-62a50120.pdf (accessed on 30th June 2025).
29. Virani, S. S., Newby, L. K., Arnold, S. V., Bittner, V., Brewer, L. C., Demeter, S. H., Dixon, D. L., et al. (2023). 2023 AHA/ACC/ACCP/ASPC/NLA/PCNA guideline for the management of patients with chronic coronary disease: A report of the American Heart Association/American College of Cardiology Joint Committee on Clinical Practice Guidelines. *Circulation, 148*. https://doi.org/10.1161/cir.0000000000001168 (accessed on 30th June 2025).
30. Wichmann, D. (2020). Autopsy findings and venous thromboembolism in patients with COVID-19. *Annals of Internal Medicine, 173*, 1030–1030. https://doi.org/10.7326/l20-1206 (accessed on 30th June 2025).

HEMATOLOGIC FUNCTION: ASSESSMENT AND HEMATOLOGIC DISORDERS

5

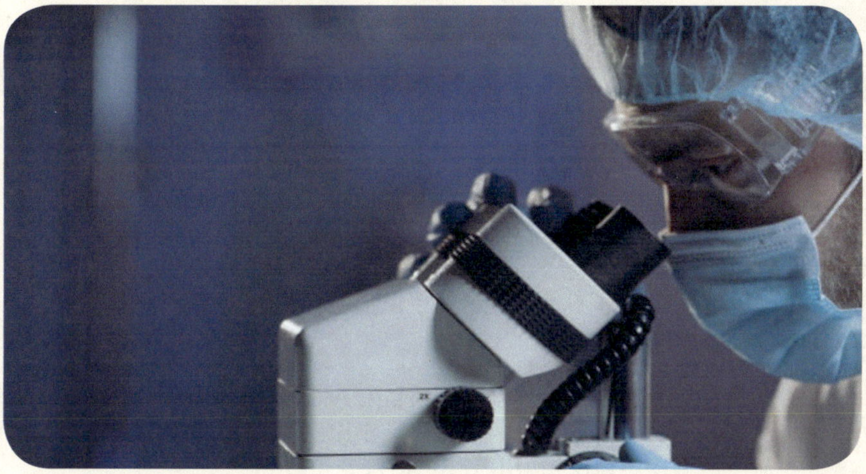

LEARNING OBJECTIVES

After studying this chapter, you will be able to:

1. Understand the anatomy and physiology of blood
2. Explain the assessment of hematologic function
3. Discuss the common hematologic disorders
4. Focus on hematologic disorders and surgical risk
5. Learn about nursing interventions for hematologic disorders
6. Evaluate the advances in hematologic care

Introduction

The hematologic system, which encompasses the blood and organs involved in its formation and maintenance, is crucial to health and homeostasis. The primary role of the hematologic system is to transport oxygen, nutrients, hormones, and waste products in the body. The most critical components of the hematologic system include red blood cells, white blood cells, platelets, and plasma. Red blood cells (RBCs) are most pertinent to oxygen transportation, while white blood cells (WBCs) act as one of the body's immune systems' defenses against infection. Platelets are tasked with providing adequate blood clotting and aids in regulating bleeding. Understanding these fundamental hematologic functions is significant to surgical nursing because patients undergoing surgery are capable of generating substantial alterations in their hematologic profiles due to trauma, anesthesia, or surgical interventions. Optimal evaluation and management of hematologic status ensure improved patient outcomes and can minimize potential complications.

In evaluating hematologic function, nurses must be able to interpret laboratory studies such as complete blood counts (CBC), coagulation tests, and blood smears. They provide information on various conditions such as anemia, leukopenia, thrombocytopenia, and other hematologic abnormalities. For instance, low hemoglobin levels may indicate anemia, and elevated platelet counts could signal an underlying inflammatory condition or malignancy. Coagulation tests also help evaluate a patient's hemostatic capability, which is critical in anticipating the risk of bleeding during and after surgery. Recognizing the significance of such tests enables surgical nurses to detect abnormalities from normal hematologic values, requiring early interventions. The use of this knowledge in the practice of medicine ultimately enhances the quality of care delivered to surgical patients and adheres to best practice standards. Hematologic diseases, represented by a wide range of disorders such as anemia, leukemia, and coagulopathies, present particular challenges to the operating room environment. These conditions hold high potential for complicating surgical decision-making, impacting not only the timing of the operation but also the care delivered by anesthesiology and postoperative recovery. For example, patients with untreated preoperative anemia are at increased risk for transfusion requirements and perioperative complications.

Similarly, individuals with clotting disorders will present with higher risks of intraoperative bleeding and require comprehensive preoperative evaluation and tailored perioperative plans of care. Operating room nurses must be adept at intervention planning, such as scheduling transfusions or administering clotting factor replacement, to ensure patient safety. Moreover, patient education about their hematologic conditions and associated risks is essential for obtaining informed consent and promoting increased compliance with treatment. By emphasizing hematologic studies and understanding their implications, surgical nurses are better equipped to advocate for patient safety and optimal surgical outcomes (Figure 5.1).

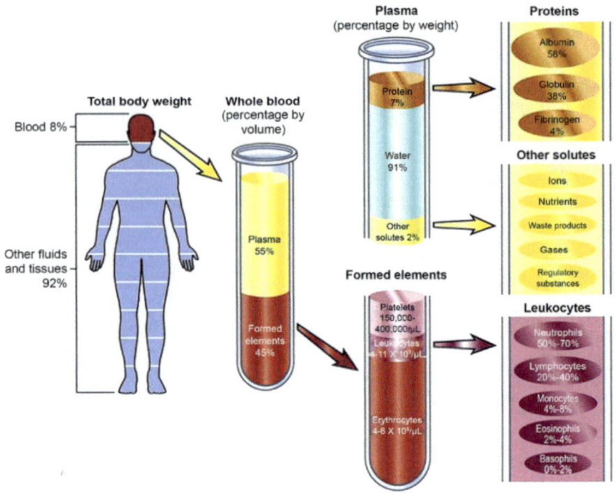

Figure 5.1. Nursing assessment: hematologic system.

Source: https://nursekey.com/wp-content/uploads/2016/11/B9780323086783000307_f030-002-9780323086783.jpg.

Definition of Hematologic Function

Hematologic function is mainly defined by the complex interaction between the blood elements engaged in various physiological processes, including oxygen transport, immune function, and hemostasis. Blood is composed of red blood cells, white blood cells, platelets, and plasma, with each playing a significant role in regulating homeostasis. Red blood cells play a critical role in delivering oxygen to tissues, while white blood cells play a crucial role in protecting against infection and orchestrating the immune response. Platelets play a crucial role in hemostasis by facilitating the clotting of blood and promoting wound healing. Awareness of these elements and their functions provide the fundamental ground for hematologic disorder evaluation, particularly when utilized in surgical nursing, where patients may be exposed to risk due to causes both preoperative and surgical. Hematologic function assessment is of utmost importance in surgical nursing for ensuring the best possible results for patients. Preoperative evaluation typically includes complete blood counts and coagulation tests to identify potential hematologic derangements that can affect surgical procedures. For instance, anemia can compromise oxygenation during surgery, while coagulopathies may cause a patient to bleed excessively. Finally, postoperative monitoring of hematologic function is essential because patients tend to develop complications like thrombosis or infection that affect blood cell counts and functions. The integration of this patient-specific data, such as comorbidities and treatment history, into hematologic studies enhances clinical decision-making and personalizes perioperative care. Evidence supports the use of prognostic models as a means of predicting hematologic complications in surgical patients. Although initially designed for use in overall intensive care populations, models such as the APACHE II, SAPS II, and SOFA have demonstrated varying degrees of predictive accuracy in cancer patients (Donnell et al., 2017). Models consider many different physiological measures, which allow caregivers to provide more informed risk estimation and optimize treatments. The findings of research assessing these tools can inform surgical nursing practice by demonstrating the value of vigilant monitoring and prompt intervention in accordance with hematologic status. Recognition of the value of hematologic function contributes not only to surgical patient care but also underscores the necessity for an integrative philosophy of care that treats both the physiological and psychological dimensions (Figure 5.2).

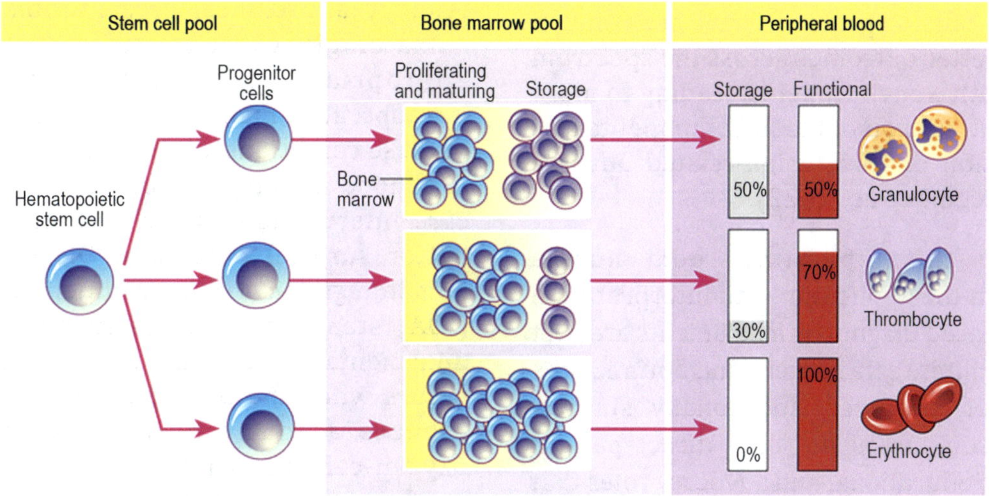

Figure 5.2. Structure and function of the hematologic system.

Source: https://basicmedicalkey.com/wp-content/uploads/2016/09/B9780323088541000278_f27-11-9780323088541.jpg.

Importance in Surgical Nursing

In surgical nursing, it is essential to have extensive knowledge of hematologic function to ensure patient safety and achieve the best possible outcomes of recovery. Surgical procedures tendency to disrupt normal hemostasis, and therefore, there is increased risk of hemorrhagic complications. Thus, surgical nurses must be competent in assessing the patient's hematologic status preoperatively as well as sustaining it intraoperatively. These skills not only assist in the identification of those patients who may require complementary interventions, such as blood transfusion, but also assist in the anticipation of potential future complications with hemostatic disorders. Knowledge of hematologic function enables surgical nurses to collaborate effectively with the surgical team, recognizing and promptly addressing any deviations from anticipated parameters, ultimately contributing to improved patient care (Copeland et al., 2019). Moreover, effective management of surgical bleeding relies on the interpretation and reaction of the surgical nurse to hematologic tests. Techniques such as thromboelastography (TEG) have come to the forefront in the operating room, as they provide dynamic insight into a patient's coagulation status. TEG, in particular, has advantages over traditional coagulation tests because it measures the dynamic clotting and lysis process. As has been emphasized, TEG-directed transfusion protocols have been shown to achieve better outcomes across the spectrum of perioperative environments, leading to more restrained utilization of blood components and the prevention of transfusion-related adverse effects (Buscemi et al., 2022).

Due to this, operating room nurses competent in the application and interpretation of such advanced diagnostic instruments are best placed to facilitate safe surgery and optimize the utilization of resources. Additionally, surgical nursing encompasses not only direct patient care but also educational and advocacy roles that promote patient safety in the surgical setting. Through fostering a culture of knowledge and expertise in hematologic testing among their peers and in their workplaces, surgical nurses can ~~plug~~ fill practice gaps in relation to newer technologies like TEG. This focus not only reiterates the critical need for the timely use of blood products but also emphasizes the necessity for an atmosphere of teamwork where multidisciplinary teams continually learn and improve. As surgical nursing continues to evolve, establishing an environment centered on learning about hematologic function will ultimately lead to improved clinical outcomes and patient satisfaction (Buscemi et al., 2022).

Overview of Hematologic Disorders

Hematologic disorders encompass a diverse range of diseases that affect various blood components, including red blood cells, white blood cells, platelets, and plasma proteins. They have the potential to significantly impact a patient's overall health, potentially leading to conditions such as anemia, a bleeding tendency, or increased susceptibility to infection. Anemia, for instance, is a prevalent disease characterized by a reduction in hemoglobin levels, which can result from nutritional deficiencies, chronic disease, or bone marrow disease. It is essential for operating room nurses to understand the etiology and clinical presentation of various hematologic diseases since it determines appropriate preoperative testing and intraoperative management. Proper knowledge of these conditions allows nurses to predict the likelihood of complications and adjust patient care interventions, which ultimately leads to better surgical outcomes. Of the numerous hematologic disorders, iron deficiency anemia (IDA) stands out due to its prevalence and detrimental effects on some populations. IDA occurs when the body lacks sufficient iron to produce adequate hemoglobin, resulting in oxygen-carrying capacity impairments. This condition occurs more frequently in pregnant women, who require increased iron intakes for fetal development and maternal health. The results of untreated IDA during pregnancy include compromised fetal growth and adverse neonatal outcomes, thereby necessitating targeted interventions to ensure iron sufficiency. Treatment of IDA is generally achieved through diet modification, incorporation of iron sources, and supplementation, especially in vulnerable groups. By understanding the specific issues of concern with IDA, surgical nurses are better equipped to promote prevention and health education, thereby contributing to improved patient care and perioperative safety (Cox et al., 2016). Hematologic disorders in the context of surgical nursing complicate surgical risk and operative and postoperative care. Diseases like thrombocytopenia, in which there are abnormally low platelet levels, increase the risk of bleeding during the procedure, can increase the risk of infection post-surgery. Furthermore, patients with pre-existing hematologic disease usually require careful monitoring and individually tailored anesthesia management as their physiologic response will tend to be quite different from that of a healthy patient. The utilization of prognostic models, such as APACHE II, SAPS II, and SOFA, aids in determining the risk profiles of surgical candidates with hematologic diseases. The utilization of these models aids in predicting outcomes and further enhances clinical decision-making, enabling surgical teams to optimize patient safety and treatment effectiveness (Donnell et al., 2017). Understanding the relationship between hematology status and surgical outcomes is key to enhancing the quality of surgical care (Figure 5.3).

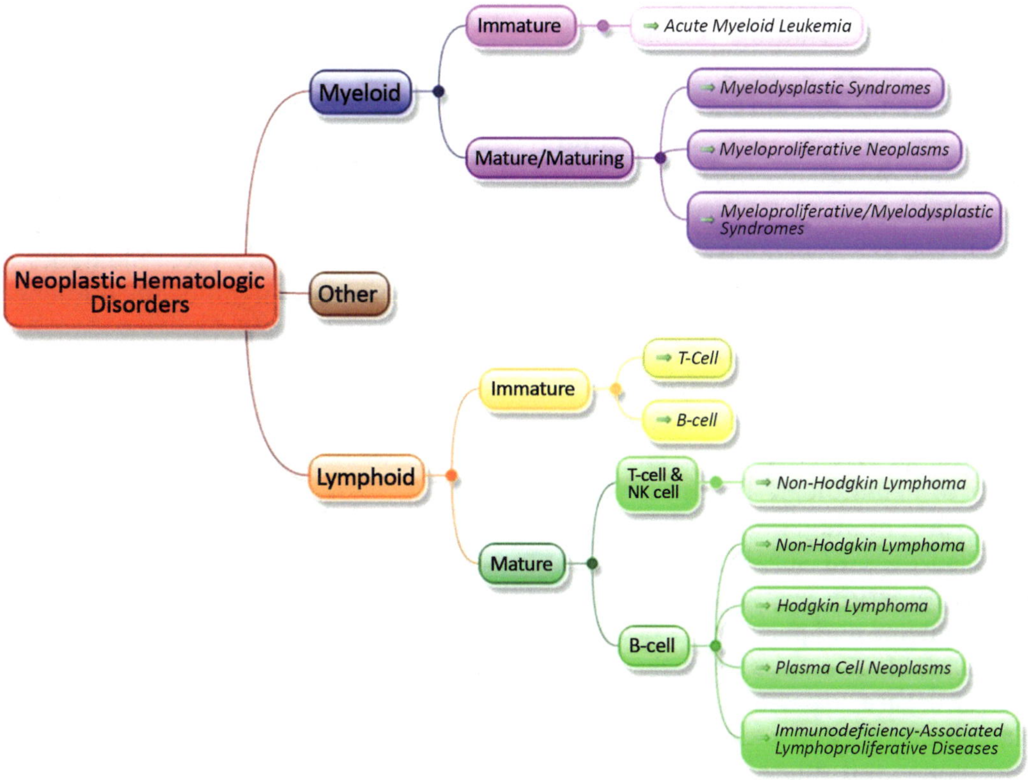

Figure 5.3. Neoplastic hematologic disorders.

Source: http://www.hematologyoutlines.com/images/neoplastic_hematologic_disorders_flowchart.jpg.

5.1. Anatomy and Physiology of Blood

Learning Outcome

1. Describe the components of blood
2. Focus on functions of blood cells
3. Learn how the role of plasma in hematologic function

The anatomy and physiology of blood form the foundation for comprehending its role in the human body. Blood is composed of various significant elements, including plasma, red blood cells, white blood cells, and platelets. Plasma, which accounts for approximately 55% of the blood's volume, serves as a medium for transporting waste products, hormones, and nutrients. Red blood cells, or erythrocytes, play a crucial role in oxygen transport due to their hemoglobin, which binds oxygen in the lungs and releases it in tissues. The white blood cells, or leukocytes, play a role in immune defense, and the platelets, or thrombocytes, are vital for hemostasis. This intricate composition facilitates homeostasis and provides a comprehensive understanding of hematologic function, which is crucial in the management of various hematologic disorders in surgical conditions. In hematologic function evaluation, several diagnostic instruments and parameters are used to effectively assess blood components. Complete blood counts (CBCs) are also widely used to track hemoglobin, hematocrit, and counts of different white blood cells and platelets, providing important information about a patient's overall health and indicating the presence of disorders. Deviation in the values of these parameters can reflect diseases such as anemia, infection, or clotting disorders. Surgical nurses should be competent in analyzing the results to facilitate appropriate clinical interventions. Furthermore, an understanding of the physiological reaction of blood under operating room conditions—i.e., the body's adaptive reactions to maintain perfusion and oxygenation during bleeding—is relevant to optimizing patient outcomes and enabling early intervention when hematologic irregularities are recognized. Understanding the physiology of blood is also pertinent to its role in coagulation and wound healing, particularly in operating room nursing. The coagulation cascade is a process that involves multiple factors leading to the formation of a stable fibrin clot. It is a critical process in hemostasis and the healing process. Being aware of diseases such as hemophilia or thrombocytopenia is crucial, as they can lead to several complications during surgery. Proper management of patients with such disorders relies on a thorough understanding of the underlying anatomy and physiology of blood, enabling healthcare providers to apply appropriate preoperative assessment and postoperative management measures. Prevention and management practices for such complications are critical elements of surgical nursing practice, significantly influencing patient outcomes (Figure 5.4).

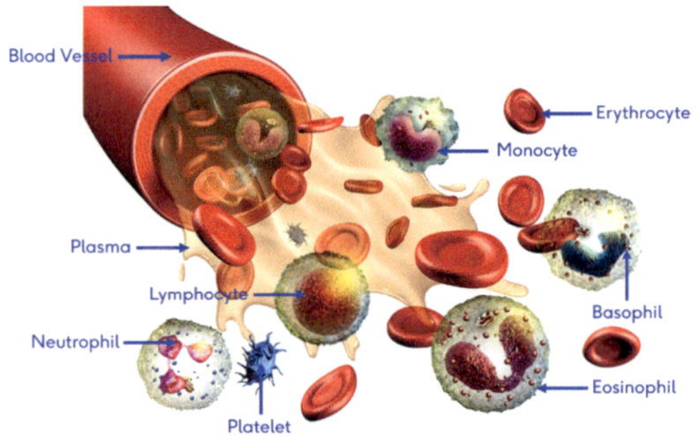

Figure 5.4. Blood vessels anatomy and physiology.

Source: https://www.physio-pedia.com/images/thumb/5/55/Blood_with_description.png/1000px-Blood_with_description.png.

5.1.1. Components of Blood

Blood is a connective tissue that plays a central function in the systemic and functional processes of the human body. Blood has four major components: plasma, red blood cells, white blood cells, and platelets. Plasma occupies about 55% of the total blood volume and is a yellowish liquid with high water content, electrolytes, nutrients, hormones, and waste products. It acts as a transport vehicle for carrying blood cells and other substances throughout the body. The cellular components play a significant role in maintaining hemostasis, oxygen transport, immunity, and overall homeostasis, and understanding these processes is crucial for surgical nursing professionals. Study of these components is capable of providing critical information regarding patients' hematologic status and help identify potential disorders before surgery. Red blood cells (RBCs), also known as erythrocytes, are the most abundant cellular component of blood and play a vital role in carrying oxygen. One molecule of hemoglobin is contained within each RBC, a protein that captures oxygen from the air spaces within the lungs and distributes it to tissues. Anemia, a deficiency of red blood cells or hemoglobin, can lead to tissue hypoxia in the body, complicating surgical procedures by increasing the risk of postoperative complications. Understanding the function and production of RBCs can help nursing practitioners assess the preoperative patient's health status and implement appropriate interventions. It is also worth noting that disorders of erythrocytes, such as polycythemia, can potentially affect blood viscosity and thereby hinder the outcomes of operative procedures, further emphasizing the need for correct monitoring and treatment in operating room nursing. The final blood components, platelets and white blood cells (WBCs), are responsible for the immune response and the coagulation cascade, respectively. White blood cells play a critical role in defense against infection and in response to inflammation. These values may indicate underlying infections or hematologic diseases necessitating surgical management. Leukocytosis, for instance, could represent an active infection, while leukopenia could cause difficulty due to immunocompromise. Conversely, the formation of a clot and the maintenance of hemostasis during and after surgery require platelets. Thrombocytopenia, or an insufficient number of platelets, may result in serious bleeding hazards, whereas thrombocytosis may develop into thromboembolic complications. Thus, the total quality analysis of blood components is crucial in surgical nursing, as it informs clinical decision-making and helps maintain patient safety throughout the surgical continuum, encompassing the preoperative, intraoperative, and postoperative periods (Figure 5.5).

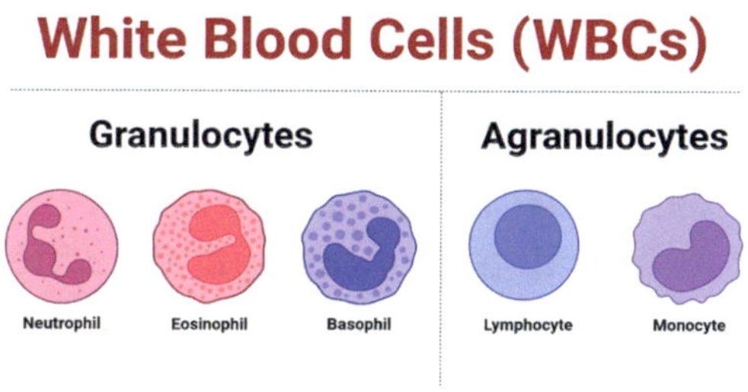

Figure 5.5. White blood cells (WBCs).

Source: https://microbenotes.com/wp-content/uploads/2024/04/White-Blood-Cells-WBCs.jpeg.

5.1.2. Functions of Blood Cells

In the intricate process of human physiology, blood cells perform a range of essential functions required for maintaining homeostasis. Red blood cells (RBCs) basically have the responsibility of delivering oxygen from the lungs to the tissues of the body and transporting back carbon dioxide for excretion. This capacity to transport oxygen can be mainly attributed to hemoglobin, a protein that can bind oxygen molecules, providing the tissues with the energy needed for metabolic processes. Red blood cells also play a role in maintaining acid-base balance by acting as blood pH buffers. Their lifespan of approximately 120 days requires constant production in the bone marrow to replace old and damaged cells, a process that, when disrupted, can lead to anemia —a condition commonly assessed during surgical consultation because it can have a significant impact on patient outcomes in the perioperative period. White blood cells (WBCs) or leukocytes are a vital part of the immune response to attacks by pathogens and foreign bodies. Composed of several different types, including neutrophils, lymphocytes, and monocytes, the cells work together to identify and destroy infectious pathogens. Neutrophils, the most abundant type, are typically the first to arrive at sites of infection, utilizing phagocytosis to engulf and destroy bacteria. Lymphocytes, such as T cells and B cells, provide adaptive immunity, providing specific responses to some pathogens and creating immunological memory.

Their roles are not only vital in defense against infection but also in detection of malignancies. Understanding how these cells function is critical to surgical nursing, as surgical operations temporarily impair immune function and therefore the vulnerability to post-surgical infection is increased, and recovery of the patient is adversely affected. Platelets, also known as thrombocytes, are the primary component in the process of hemostasis, which involves stopping bleeding. These tiny fragments of cells are present in the circulatory system and are mobilized to the site of vascular damage, where they adhere to the exposed collagen of blood vessel walls. Upon activation, platelets transform and release granules containing signaling molecules, which cause further platelet aggregation and recruit additional platelets to secure the clot. This is a rapid response, which is crucial to prevent excessive blood loss after surgery. Platelet function deficiency or dysfunction can result in major hemorrhagic complications, thus making preoperative platelet number and function monitoring essential. By contributing to clotting and maintaining vascular integrity, platelets demonstrate their key function not only in hemostatic mechanisms but also in optimizing surgical success, making examination of hematologic disorders unavoidable (Figure 5.6).

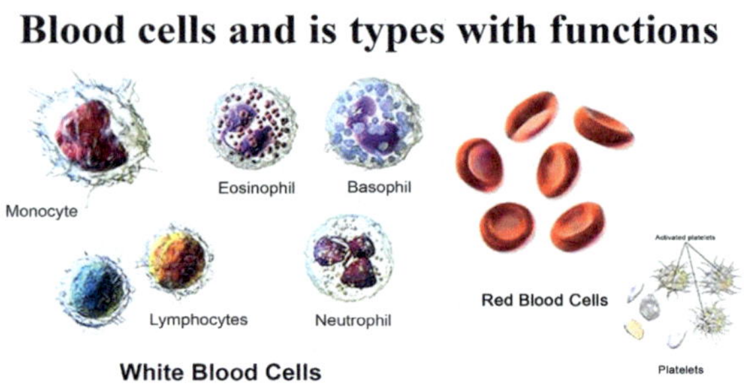

Figure 5.6. Blood cells and its types with functions.

Source: https://microbiologyinfo.com/wp-content/uploads/2017/04/Blood-cells-and-its-types-with-functions.jpg.

5.1.3. Role of Plasma in Hematologic Function

Plasma plays a central role in hematologic function, serving as the fluid portion of blood and as a vehicle for numerous significant processes. It comprises around 55% of blood volume and consists primarily of water, electrolytes, proteins, nutrients, hormones, and waste products. The plasma proteins, including albumin, globulins, and fibrinogen, play a significant role in functions such as maintaining osmotic pressure, regulating the immune response, and blood clotting. The availability of clotting factors in plasma is essential for hemostasis, which is the body's mechanism to forestall and arrest bleeding. When surgery is conducted, the need for a sufficient plasma volume to facilitate efficient blood clotting becomes intensely felt, underscoring its significance in surgical nursing and postoperative or operative management of patients. The make-up of plasma has a direct influence on hematologic function and patient outcomes in the surgical environment.

For instance, plasma protein composition disturbances, such as might follow liver disease or malnutrition, can lead to coagulopathy, which poses a risk for complications during surgery. Surgical patients are often under close monitoring of plasma components to offer sufficient amounts of clotting factors to minimize the risk of excessive blood loss, particularly in traumatic surgery or surgery with significant tissue dissection. Recent advances in the availability of thromboelastography (TEG) have highlighted the importance of employing plasma properties in real time to assess and control transfusion therapy, illustrating a trend toward more advanced, evidence-based practice in the treatment of surgical bleeding (Buscemi et al., 2022). Moreover, plasma's role in the transportation of gases and nutrients cannot be overstated. It permits the delivery of oxygen, carbon dioxide, glucose, and other required biochemical substances throughout the circulatory system, which is essential in surgery, where metabolic loads are placed on the body. For instance, pulmonary conditions such as acute lung injury and acute respiratory distress syndrome (ARDS) can arise after surgery, significantly raising mortality rates among surgical patients (Chimbira et al., 2001). Adequate plasma function offers efficient circulation and oxygen delivery to tissue sites with minimal risk of hypoxia and organ failure. Therefore, a correct concept ofplasma function not only facilitates efficient surgical nursing practice but also emphasizes the significance of ongoing assessment and management of hematologic function to enhance patient recovery in clinical settings.

Test Your Knowledge

1. What is the primary function of red blood cells in the circulatory system?
2. How do platelets contribute to the process of hemostasis?

5.2. Assessment of Hematologic Function

Learning Outcome

1. Explain the laboratory tests for hematologic assessment
2. Define the clinical signs and symptoms of disorders
3. Discuss the importance of patient history in assessment

To understand the assessment of hematologic function is critical to surgical nursing because it has a direct influence on patient outcomes and recovery. Hematologic tests comprise a range of laboratory examinations designed to assess various blood elements, including red blood cells, white blood cells, and platelets. All of these components are crucial for transporting oxygen, maintaining immune function, and facilitating clotting. Abnormalities in these values can be indicative of underlying disease states, such as anemia, leukemia, or thrombocytopenia, which require careful evaluation and monitoring. Laboratory investigations, such as complete blood counts (CBC), reticulocyte counts, and coagulation studies, provide critical information about a patient's hematologic status. Surgical nurses play a vital role in interpreting such findings and collaborating with the patient care team to instigate timely interventions and appropriate management regimens to rectify any identified dysfunction. In practice as surgical nurses, the interpretation of hematology function assessment in surgical practice is not merely based on values on lab reports.

Clinicians must contextualize these results within the patient's clinical setting, taking into account patient factors such as age, medical history, and current medications. For example, an abnormally low hemoglobin level may indicate anemia, but the nurse must identify the cause—chronic disease, nutritional deficiency, or acute blood loss—in order to decide on the treatment regimen properly. Finally, routine hematologic follow-up may be required in postoperative patients, especially those with underlying illnesses or those who underwent prolonged and complex surgeries. Impulsive conclusions based on isolated test findings can lead to improper therapy; therefore, a thorough approach to assessing hematologic function is essential in delivering optimal surgical care. Furthermore, surgical patients are commonly at risk for hematologic complications, given the surgery's physiological stresses.

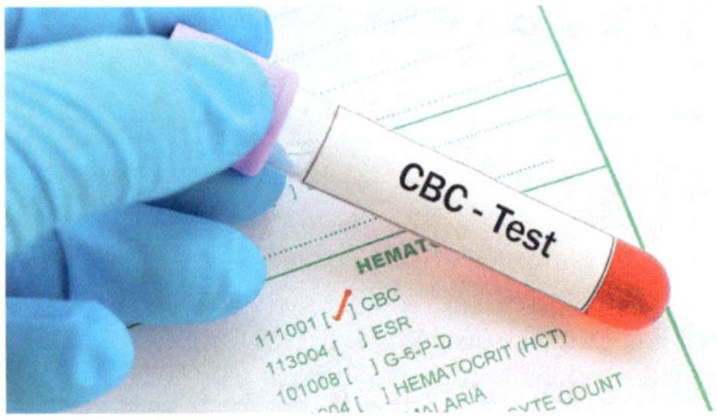

Figure 5.7. CBC test.

Source: https://arthdiagnostics.com/wp-content/uploads/2024/11/CBC-Test-in-Udaipur.jpg.

Preoperative investigation, therefore, must include tests of platelet function and coagulation function to screen out patients at risk of excessive bleeding or thromboembolic complications during surgery. Hematologic dysfunction can significantly impact the results of surgery and prolong recovery, so maintaining constant alertness is necessary. Postoperative monitoring must also be individualized by employing serial hematologic tests to detect any deviations that may predict infection or transfusion reaction complications. As medicine becomes more advanced, the integration of technologies such as point-of-care testing can enhance the speed and accuracy of hematologic testing, ultimately improving the quality of care administered to surgical patients (Figure 5.7).

5.2.1. Laboratory Tests for Hematologic Assessment

Labs play a significant role in hematologic assessment of patients, particularly in the surgical nursing environment, where total blood and coagulation management are at their best. A complete blood count (CBC) is one of the fundamental tests that provides information on red blood cells, white blood cells, and platelets. By measuring hemoglobin levels, hematocrit, and white blood cell differentials, clinicians can diagnose various hematologic disorders, including anemia, leukopenia, and thrombocytopenia. These diseases may have a significant impact on the outcome of surgery because they can expose patients to increased risks of bleeding or infection. Thus, the result of a CBC not only helps to direct diagnosis but also directs clinical decision-making for transfusion and administration of hematopoietic growth factors, which further determines perioperative patient management plans. Besides the CBC, other tests such as coagulation studies are necessary in establishing the hemostatic status of a patient before surgery. Prothrombin time (PT) and activated partial thromboplastin time (aPTT) are laboratory tests that help evaluate the extrinsic and intrinsic coagulation pathways, respectively. Both tests are of paramount significance in patient identification at risk of excessive bleeding intra-operatively. Furthermore, thromboelastography (TEG) has been a modern evaluation tool that provides real-time data on clotting and breakdown. As discussed in the literature, TEG-directed blood product transfusion has significant benefits in certain surgical categories, including cardiac and trauma surgery, by targeting the precise need for clotting factors and preventing the unwanted administration of blood products (Buscemi et al., 2022). It enhances the efficacy of surgical interventions, leading to improved outcomes for patients. Finally, a laboratory investigation to determine hematologic disorders not only determines the immediate need for surgery but also highlights the importance of continuous monitoring and follow-up. Thrombocytopathy or coagulopathy may be unapparent on routine tests but can have serious implications in the postoperative phase. Therefore, it is essential that surgical nursing practitioners remain well-informed of the laboratory findings and its clinical implications. Information regarding the complexities of these tests helps ensure that patients receive adequate preparation for surgery and receive assistance throughout their recovery phase. Detailed lab work interpretation provides nurses with the information needed to recognize potential complications before they occur, thereby enhancing overall care during surgery and improving patient safety (Deutsch et al., 2012) (Figure 5.8).

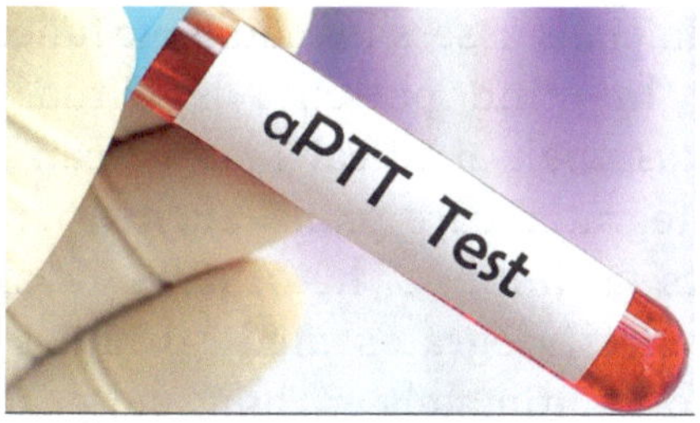

Figure 5.8. Activated partial thromboplastin time (aPTT).

Source: https://www.metropolisindia.com/upgrade/blog/upload/2023/01/Aptt-Test_-Procedure-Normal-Range-and-Result.jpg.

5.2.2. Clinical Signs and Symptoms of Disorders

The clinical presentation and signs of hematologic disease are significant indicators that aid in assessing surgical candidates. Signs such as pallor, dyspnea, and weakness can indicate anemia, a syndrome caused by a deficiency of red blood cells or hemoglobin. Anemia in the preoperative period is dangerous in surgical cases and poses various risks, such as an increased likelihood of transfusion and longer recovery times. Physicians must be adept at recognizing these symptoms early enough to request further diagnostic procedures. Hematologic disorders are made worse by chronic kidney disease and nutritional deficiencies. As such, it is crucial to understand the underlying etiology to carry out appropriate surgical planning and patient management. Prompt and effective intervention commonly rests on the clinician's ability to detect these clinical presentations; therefore, their identification is crucial in preoperative assessment for surgery in which hematologic function will be compromised. Another range of clinical presentation required for surgical nursing assessment is thrombocytopenia, or low platelet count. The patient may experience easy bruising, increased bleeding with lacerations, or, in a more severe scenario, spontaneous bleeding. The consequences of thrombocytopenia on surgical patients can be far-reaching, with the potential to lead to disastrous intraoperative and postoperative hemorrhagic complications. Surgical nurses need to exercise prudence in investigating platelet counts and observing any corresponding clinical signs to prevent surgical risks. Secondly, taking the history of a patient for previous bleeding or interventions such as anticoagulants increases the capability of surgical teams to prepare. Recognition of these clinical symptoms and signs not only influences short-term operative outcomes but also influences broader recovery trajectories and postoperative patient safety buffers, and because of this that accurate hematologic assessment within the operative setting is so important. In addition to anemia and thrombocytopenia, leukopenia, or loss of white blood cells, is also a significant clinical challenge in surgical nursing. Patients with leukopenia have a higher risk of infection, making recovery after surgery challenging and requiring sharp observation and preventive strategies. Clinical presentations typically include frequent fevers, unexplained malaise, and signs of local infection. Awareness of these signs alerts surgical teams to implement appropriate antibiotic prophylaxis and infection control. Effective leukopenia management depends not only on recognizing its presentation but also on being aware of its potential etiologies, which range from bone marrow dysfunction to chemotherapy. By critically monitoring such hematologic indices and presentations, surgical nurses can play a key role in optimizing patient outcomes and minimizing the risks associated with operations (Deutsch et al., 2012; Copeland et al., 2019) (Figure 5.9).

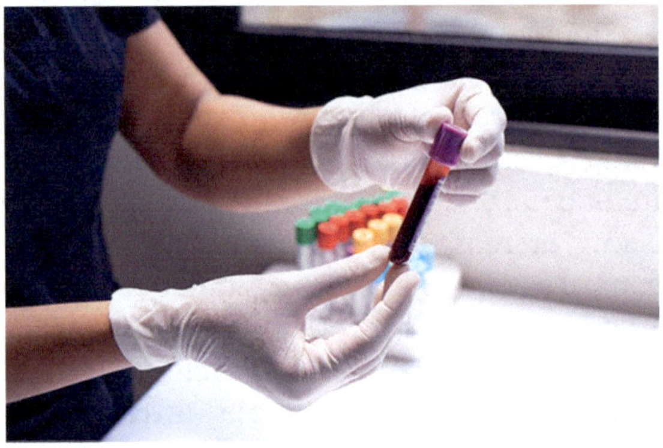

Figure 5.9. Rare blood disorders.

Source: https://health.ucdavis.edu/media-resources/contenthub/health-library/conditions/rare-blood-disorders-hero.jpg.

5.2.3. Importance of Patient History in Assessment

Compilation and analysis of a patient's medical history are necessary for determining hematologic function, particularly in surgical nursing. The knowledge of a patient's previous illnesses, current medication, and history of family who have hematologic disorders provides critical information to health practitioners. This overall picture enables nurses to identify potential risk indicators for surgical complications, as some hematologic disorders, such as anemia or coagulopathies, can significantly impact the outcome of surgery. Furthermore, a thoroughly documented patient history enables individualized interventions that consider the specific needs and reactions of each patient, ultimately leading to enhanced patient safety and quality of care. Complete history-taking not only informs clinical decision-making but also facilitates the establishment of trust and rapport with patients, which is imperative in the practice of surgical nursing through open communication and trust. Additionally, including spiritual well-being in assessment effectively offers an added dimension of comprehension to complex hematologic disorders. In populations like hemodialysis patients, who often have multiple health complications, spiritual well-being can influence adherence to treatment and quality of life.

For instance, spiritual well-being is connected to sleep quality, which may in turn affect physical health outcomes in these patients (Eslami et al., 2014). Consequently, when clinicians assess hematologic functioning, keeping in mind patients' spiritual health as well as their medical history can lead to more integrated care plans. Such a perception supports a holistic healthcare evaluation system that integrates medical and spiritual dimensions, ultimately enabling surgical nurses to provide care tailored to the diverse needs of their patients. Additionally, acquiring knowledge about the management of hematologic disorders may further enhance surgical nursing practices. The majority of congenitally genitourinary patients face unique challenges in transitioning from pediatric to adult care, where the severity of hematologic complications can increase (Bavendam et al., 2017). History assessment of a patient is critical in this regard since it can determine any lacuna in care that had manifested during the decades. Such patients may lack the ability to care for themselves, and hence rigorous assessments encompassing their medical, educational, and socioeconomic backgrounds are essential. By identifying a strong patient history as a priority, surgical nurses are best placed to educate and empower such patients to manage their health process. Thus, the addition of comprehensive patient history assessments is essential to optimize hematologic therapy during the life of a patient.

Test Your Knowledge

1. What common laboratory test is used to evaluate red blood cell levels in the body?
2. Why is a thorough patient history important in assessing hematologic disorders?

5.3. Common Hematologic Disorders

Learning Outcome

1. Explain the anemia: types and causes
2. Define the coagulation disorders: hemophilia and thrombocytopenia
3. Describe the leukemia: types and implications

Hematological disorders encompass a diverse group of conditions that affect blood cells, coagulation factors, and the bone marrow. The most common disorders are anemias, leukemias, lymphomas, and thrombocytopenias. Anemia, or the decrease in red blood cells or hemoglobin, causes symptoms that range from fatigue, pallor, and shortness of breath ~~to~~ that can significantly impact the quality of life and surgical recovery of a patient. Some types of anemia, such as iron deficiency anemia, for instance, are very prevalent and are caused by nutritional, chronic, or genetic disorders. Understanding their etiology and pathophysiology is an essential for surgical nurses because they must identify such complications prior to surgery and take proper control measures to prevent risks and ensure positive outcomes in the patient. Leukemias, more precisely acute lymphoblastic leukemia (ALL) and acute myeloid leukemia (AML), represent another important field of interest in the realm of common hematologic disorders. The leukemias disrupt normal hematopoiesis by excessive production of immature white cells that impair the immune mechanism. Leukemia patients typically present with a history of frequent infections, anemia, and bleeding as a consequence of thrombocytopenia. Surgical nursing is compounded when caring for such patients as treatment typically entails the coordination of chemotherapy regimens and potentially surgery. Effective communication between the treatment team, such as oncologists and nurses, is essential in achieving maximum patient care and scheduling surgical procedures in a way that prevents disease-related and therapy-related complications. Thrombocytopenia, characterized by a decreased platelet count, poses additional challenges in the surgical nursing scenario. It can be caused by some underlying diseases, including immune thrombocytopenic purpura (ITP), aplastic anemia, or bone marrow malignancy. Increased bruising, bleeding disorders, and wound healing signs are all delayed and add to surgical risk. In the operating room setting, monitoring and measurement of platelets, as well as preparedness for transfusions or intervention to alleviate coagulopathy, is crucial. Utilization of standardized assessment measures, like those highlighted under the Post-Acute Care Payment Reform Demonstration, ensures surgical nursing professionals are adequately equipped to handle these complexities and provide quality care (Copeland et al., 2019; Deutsch et al., 2012). Identification and control of recurring hematologic conditions are also aspects of enhancing surgical outcomes and patient safety (Figure 5.10).

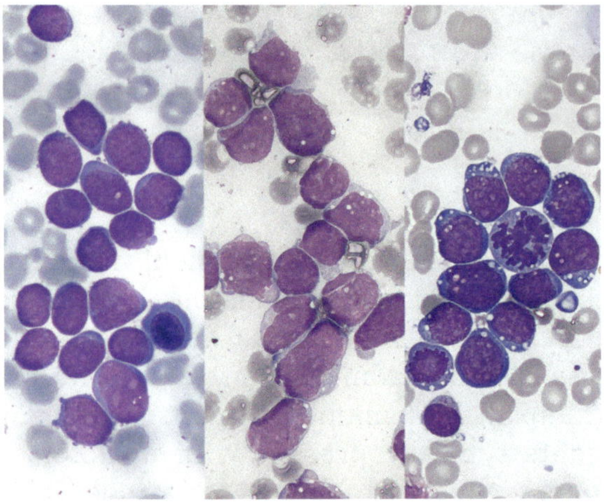

Figure 5.10. Acute lymphoblastic leukemia (ALL).

Source: https://upload.wikimedia.org/wikipedia/commons/f/f9/Morphological_types_of_acute_lymphoblastic_leukemia.jpg.

5.3.1. Anemia: Types and Causes

Anemia is a severe hematologic disease brought about by the deficiency of red blood cells (RBCs) or hemoglobin, thus a lack of adequate delivery of oxygen to tissues. Anemia may manifest in several forms, with the latter predominantly categorized into three: microcytic, macrocytic, and normocytic anemia. Microcytic anemia, also encountered with iron deficiency, possesses RBCs that are less than normal in size and produces weakness and pallor. Macrocytic anemia, on the other hand, is caused by a deficiency of vitamin B12 or folate and results in larger, but poorly functioning, RBCs. Normocytic anemia occurs when RBCs are of normal size but fewer in number and usually occur as a result of chronic illness or acute blood loss. Understanding the classification of anemia aids in adjusting treatment approaches to accommodate patients, especially in the instance of surgery, where the stability of the hematologic system is central to recovery and patient outcomes. Anemia etiology is multicausal and can be classified under three broad umbrella categories: decreased production of RBCs, increased destruction of RBCs, and blood loss. Reduced production may be due to dietary insufficiency, such as a lack of iron, vitamin B12, or folate, as in dietetic or malabsorptive deficiencies. RBC destruction is enhanced in the majority of instances owing to hemolytic anemias, with pathology such as autoimmune disorders or inherited diseases (e.g., sickle cell anemia) compromising the integrity of RBCs. Blood loss, acute secondary to trauma or chronic secondary to gastrointestinal hemorrhage, has a direct impact on the RBC pool and can have significant clinical ramifications. Careful assessment and understanding of each of these etiologies must be made so that surgical nurses and other healthcare professionals are able to make proper interventions and appropriately manage patient care during surgery. Identification of the effects of anemia is paramount in surgical nursing to enable optimal perioperative care. Anemia can also lead to an increased risk of surgery, longer recovery periods, and higher complication rates, such as infections or the need for blood transfusions. Anemia is typically treated before surgery with multimodal approaches that might include changing diet, supplementation, or even transfusion if necessary. Current practice stresses preoperative screening for anemia and encourages practitioners to implement extensive testing to help identify high-risk patients early in the surgical process. This fundamental aspect of care not only enhances patient safety but also improves surgical outcomes by improving patient preparation and the clinicians' ability to adjust their surgical technique or postoperative management plan based on the patient's hemoglobin status. Surgical nurses must remain attuned to the nuances of anemia management during the surgical process, facilitating improved patient outcomes and reduced risk of postoperative complications (Figure 5.11).

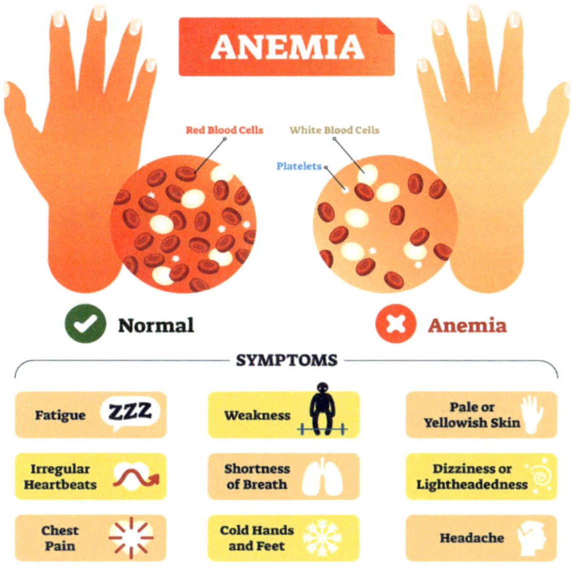

Figure 5.11. Anemia: cause, symptoms, diagnosis, treatment.

Source: https://samarpanphysioclinic.com/wp-content/uploads/2023/02/Anemia-1200x1271.webp.

5.3.2. Coagulation Disorders: Hemophilia and Thrombocytopenia

Coagulation disorders are a significant issue in surgical nursing, particularly illnesses such as hemophilia and thrombocytopenia. Hemophilia is a genetic disorder that incapacitates the body's ability to clot blood, required to stop bleeding. Hemophiliacs may experience spontaneous bleeding, even caused by minor traumas. The gene-related etiology of the disorder is attributed to the mutations of clotting factors, particularly factor VIII or IX. Understanding the complexity of this condition is paramount for operating room nurses, who must expect the risk of surgical bleeding complications. Prophylactic factor replacement therapy is often employed to manage hemophilia, a reason detailed coagulation parameter evaluation and monitoring in surgical patients are important as suggested in current hematology research initiatives aimed at improving clinical outcomes (Allard et al., 2016). Thrombocytopenia, or a decreased platelet count, further skews the coagulopathy profile. It results from a host of etiologies, including bone marrow disease, increased platelet destruction, or sequestration within the spleen. Clinical manifestations of thrombocytopenia can be theatrical, with patients being predisposed to hypoprothrombinemia bleeding that is secondary to ineffective platelet aggregation. For surgical nursing, understanding the etiology and assessment of platelet function is essential since they directly influence surgical planning and patient safety. The treatment modalities may vary from platelet transfusions to management of the etiology of thrombocytopenia. Moreover, the discrimination between acute and chronic thrombocytopenia influences therapeutic management, highlighting the importance of an adequate preoperative examination and personalized therapy against surgical procedure-induced bleeding complications (Allard et al., 2016). Such interaction between hemophilia and thrombocytopenia within the domain of surgical nursing highlights the significance of profound insight and quantification of coagulation disorders. Research initiatives, such as the EHA Roadmap for European Hematology Research, focus on addressing unmet needs in hematology, including the pursuit of targeted therapies and innovative treatments. This environment enables the surgical nurse to utilize evidence-based practice and optimize patient care. Patient education on their coagulation disorders, potential surgical complications, and compliance with treatment plans is crucial. By marketing this information, surgical nurses can take the forefront in optimizing outcomes for patients with hemophilia and thrombocytopenia, ultimately to improve quality of life and post-operative recovery (Allard et al., 2016) (Figure 5.12).

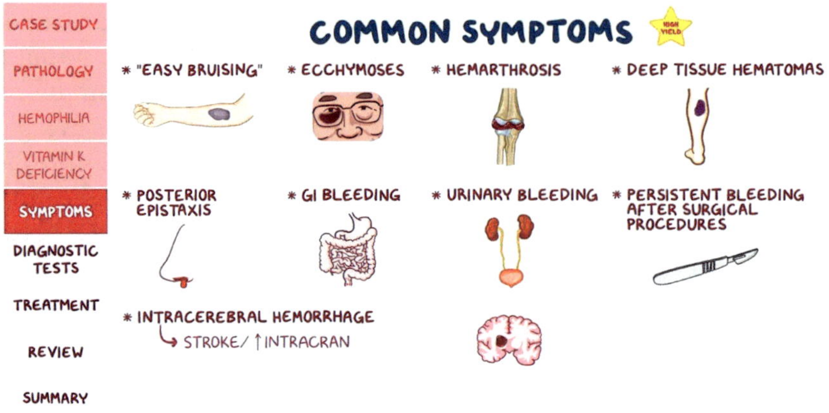

Figure 5.12. Coagulation disorders.

Source: https://www.osmosis.org/_next/image?url=https%3A%2F%2Fd16qt3wv6xm098.cloudfront.net%2F0PBSg_UfTGWSj8QK43Ht6ppgS9WqaBsN%2F_.jpg&w=3840&q=75.

5.3.3. Leukemia: Types and Implications

Leukemia, a cancer of the blood and bone marrow, is broadly categorized into two primary types: acute and chronic, each further differentiated into lymphocytic and myelogenous forms. Acute leukemias, characterized by the rapid formation of immature blood cells, require immediate treatment due to their virulent nature. On the other hand, chronic leukemias progress more gradually and will tend to have less severe presentations, offering an extended interval before intervention being necessary. Understanding the differences between these groups is ~~greatly~~ relevant to surgical nursing, given the varying therapeutic regimens and complications arising as a function of leukemia type. In addition, they establish the management of surgical patients based on their hematologic stability and supportive measures, such as blood transfusions or growth factor administration, to prevent complications from hypochromia. The impact of leukemia is broader than for the disease per se, having significant effects on the management of patients and surgical results. Leukemia patients often carry numerous comorbidities, like thrombocytopenia and anemia, that increase their predisposition to perioperative complications. Preoperative evaluation requires the surgical nursing staff to successfully recognize these hematologic insufficiencies and utilize the proper preoperative assessments in an effort to improve patient outcomes. As an illustration, open communication among the care team, ranging from oncologists and anesthesiologists to surgical staff nurses, is critically important in crafting tailored perioperative plans according to the unique hematologic status of each patient. Moreover, educating patients about the risk factors of surgery related to their leukemia will enhance their knowledge and adherence to postoperative practice as well as decrease the risk of complications. Care for the patient with leukemia undergoing surgery should be comprehensive and multidisciplinary, as well as combining oncology principles with surgical nursing protocols. For example, preoperative optimization may involve administering transfusions to correct low platelet counts or erythropoietin to treat anemia, thereby improving hematologic function. Use of technologies such as Vein Viewer has also been shown to improve vascular access and patient satisfaction in peripheral access procedures (Ramer et al., 2015). These advancements underscore the importance of surgical nursing in ensuring quality and safety for patients with complicated hematologic disorders. With the development of surgical nursing, an emphasis on understanding the implications of leukemia enables practitioners to provide specialized interventions, ultimately enhancing recovery and satisfaction for this at-risk population.

Test Your Knowledge

1. What are typical symptoms of anemia that nurses should assess for?
2. How does leukemia affect normal blood cell production?

5.4. Hematologic Disorders and Surgical Risk

Learning Outcome

1. Discuss the impact of anemia on surgical outcomes
2. Define the coagulation disorders and bleeding risks
3. Describe the management of hematologic disorders pre-surgery

It is imperative to comprehend the relationship between surgical risk and hematologic disorders to succeed in surgical nursing. Hematologic disorders, such as anemia, thrombocytopenia, and coagulopathies, can drastically complicate surgical outcomes. Anemia, a reduced red blood cell or hemoglobin concentration, can lead to inadequate oxygenation during surgery and postoperative complications such as myocardial infarction or impaired wound healing. Further, thrombocytopenia patients also show increased bleeding risks, preoperative transfusion, or the use of hemostatic agents. Operating teams must be adequately trained to assess these hematologic parameters to tailor perioperative care accordingly, enhancing patient safety and optimal surgical outcomes. Proper preoperative hematologic assessments should not be overemphasized. Through evaluation of the total blood count, coagulation parameters, and other pertinent hematologic measurements, health care providers can identify potential risks before they manifest during surgery. For instance, a detailed assessment can reveal underlying clotting abnormalities that can lead to excessive hemorrhage perioperatively. Understanding the patient's hematologic status enables individualized planning regarding the timing of elective procedures, the choice of anesthetic drugs, and postoperative monitoring protocols. As noted in several clinical trials, the inclusion of comprehensive hematologic screening in preoperative surgical planning leads to optimized patient care and a reduced incidence of perioperative adverse events (Copeland et al., 2019). Postoperative therapy must also address hematologic complications that may arise following surgery. Postoperative patients are susceptible to ~~a~~ hematologic complications, including deep vein thrombosis (DVT) and pulmonary embolism (PE), particularly following immobilizing or very manipulative surgeries. This risk highlights the importance of implementing preventive measures, such as pharmacological prophylaxis and early active mobilization. Moreover, continuous monitoring of postoperative hematologic indices reduces the latency in delayed identification and management of bleeding and thrombocytopenia complications. Information from several studies has established that effective postoperative care procedures significantly improve the outcome of patients and reduce risks for patients with active hematologic disorders (Deutsch et al., 2012). Through remaining holistic in the approach to the functionality of the hematologic system, surgical teams can significantly enhance short-term and long-term recovery for patients who have been impacted (Figure 5.13).

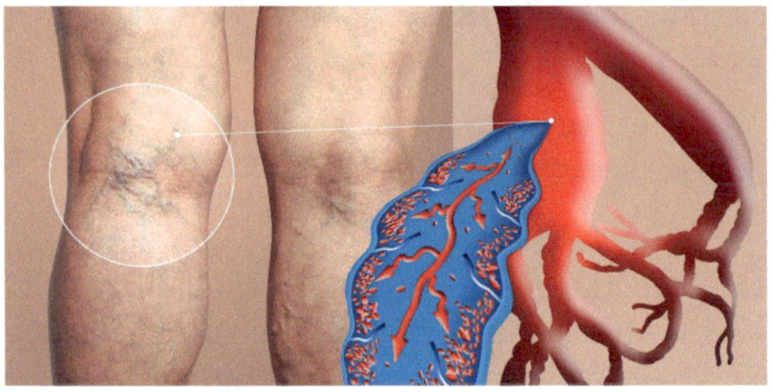

Figure 5.13. Deep vein thrombosis (DVT).

Source: https://knoxvascular.com/wp-content/uploads/2024/01/Deep-Vein-Thrombosis-min-scaled-2.jpeg.

5.4.1. Impact of Anemia on Surgical Outcomes

Anemia, typically characterized by lowered hemoglobin and red cell count, poses significant risk under surgical conditions. Tissues need to be adequately oxygenated for adequate recovery and healing are predisposed to tissue oxygen supply impairment, which has a chain of physiological complications in the form of increased cardiac load and impaired wound healing. Furthermore, anemia is associated with the postoperative risk of complications such as infection and higher mortality. The operating teams should therefore be proactively involved in the management and identification of anemia before surgery to neutralize these risks and enhance overall surgical outcomes. Patient preparation through transfusion or iron therapy also significantly enhances hemoglobin levels, thereby optimizing tissue oxygenation and potentially leading to a less eventful procedural course and recovery. Anemia's relationship to operative outcome is also further complicated by the patients' own physiological responses to surgery in and of itself. Anemia can magnify the systemic inflammatory reactions that are typically precipitated in response to surgical manipulation, potentially being related to postoperative delirium and other cognitive dysfunction. In cardiac surgical patients, for research has demonstrated that preoperative anemia is a predictor of postoperative delirium and that anemia could be a critical element to take into consideration in postoperative recovery pathways.

The intraoperative inflammatory response to surgery complicates recovery by interacting with underlying hematologic dysfunction, rendering it a risk for clinicians who manage postoperative care interventions. Comprehension of the importance of anemia in affecting surgical outcome is, hence, essential in organizing care and intervention to ensure more efficient patient management during surgery (John et al., 2017). Anemia management and its impact include a comprehensive pre-surgical assessment of hematologic function. Preoperative assessment must emphasize the identification of patients at risk by measuring hemoglobin levels and determining the etiology of the anemia, whether it is due to chronic disease, malnutrition, or acute blood loss. Such stratification enables health care providers to institute individually directed management commensurate with the individual patient's circumstances. Moreover, postoperative follow-up is also crucial in anemic patients since they are likely to be more at risk of experiencing complications such as extended hospital stays and prolonged recovery times. With the integration of focused interventions for managing anemia in both the preoperative and postoperative phases, surgical teams can play a significant role in impacting patient outcomes and, consequently, improving the quality of surgical nursing care (Taiju et al., 2017) (Figure 5.14).

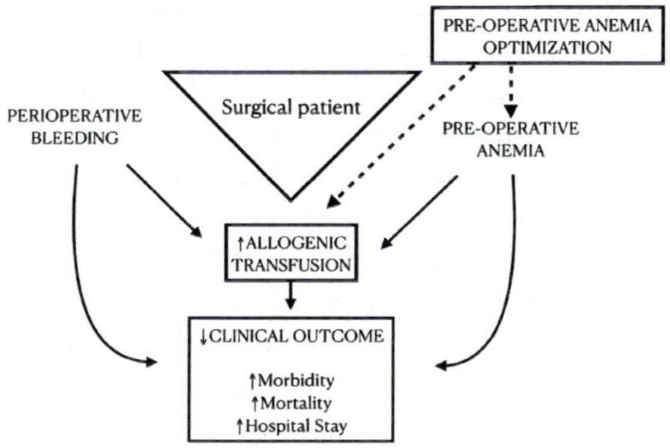

Figure 5.14. Clinical impact of preoperative anemia.

Source: https://www.mdpi.com/surgeries/surgeries-02-00027/article_deploy/html/images/surgeries-02-00027-g002.png.

5.4.2. Coagulation Disorders and Bleeding Risks

Coagulation disorders are a significant challenge in surgical nursing as they have the potential to enhance surgical and post-surgical bleeding risk. Hemophilia, von Willebrand disease, and thrombocytopenia all disrupt the hemostatic clotting cascade, which is essential for hemostasis. Such patients are thus predisposed to excessive bleeding, hematoma, and other complications that complicate the surgeries but can also prolong recovery times. Preoperative assessment should include a thorough review of coagulation studies, including prothrombin time and activated partial thromboplastin time, to identify potential bleeding dangers. Evidence-based practice is adequately applied to address these problems, thereby optimizing patient outcomes and the general safety of the operation (Hu et al., 2024). Patient care of surgical coagulation disorders involves individualized approaches to prevent the risk of bleeding while achieving optimal surgical outcomes. Surgical teams must coordinate closely to develop individualized care plans that incorporate both medical and nursing interventions. For instance, the application of prophylactic factor replacement therapy for hemophilia patients, along with rigorous monitoring and prompt management of excessive bleeding, can significantly reduce the risk. Moreover, evidence suggests that implementing enhanced recovery protocols will improve hemostatic function and overall patient satisfaction (Adeel et al., 2024). Such protocols may include judicious medication use, fluid resuscitation, and taking into account the timing of surgeries to reconcile the ,patient's coagulation profiles. Identification and management of risk for complications due to coagulation disorders are of utmost importance in postoperative management. Hemorrhage after surgery can necessitate transfusion and reoperation, adding further strain on healthcare resources and jeopardizing patient safety. Systematic surveillance for evidence of hemorrhage, including changes in vital signs and wound examination, should be incorporated into standard postoperative care in patients at risk. Evidence-based practices, such as the utilization of evidence-based nursing practice (ENP) interventions, have been shown to be effective in optimizing coagulation function and reducing complication rates in patients experiencing bleeding emergencies (Hu et al., 2024). The total approach to management eventually translates to better outcomes in recovery and enhanced quality of life in patients that are affected by coagulation disorders.

5.4.3. Management of Hematologic Disorders Pre-Surgery

Effective control of hematologic abnormalities before surgery is vital to the achievement of optimal surgical outcomes and minimizing complications. Preoperative evaluation refers to the process of careful examination of a patient's hematologic condition using blood cell count and the presence of coagulation disorders that can complicate surgery. Identification of anemia, thrombocytopenia, or clotting disorders enables the provision of individualized care measures, including possible transfusions, medication adjustments, or referral of the patient to specialists. All of these changes ensure that the patient is ready and safe for surgery, and eventually reduce morbidity due to surgical intervention. Furthermore, patient education on the need to treat such disorders increases compliance and cooperation, making combined changes by hematology experts and surgical teams a very effective approach. This, combined with changes made by hematology experts and surgical teams, is a crucial factor in this respect. In cases where hematologic disease has been diagnosed, treatment may include optimizing anticoagulation therapy or administering hematopoietic growth factors to stimulate red blood cell production. In patients with an underlying bleeding disorder, careful planning is necessary to provide successful hemostatic function through preoperative intervention. For example, patients with von Willebrand disease can be assisted with desmopressin treatment or platelet transfusion before surgery to increase von Willebrand factor levels and enhance the clotting function. The timing of these interventions is critical because it is directly related to the patient's hemostatic stability during surgery. Extensive communication between the hematology department and the surgical team can achieve significant risk minimization, thereby highlighting the interdisciplinarity required for managing hematologic disorders pre-surgery. Furthermore, ongoing research aimed at developing and enhancing hematologic examination techniques is crucial in strengthening the process of preoperative evaluation. Through the application of techniques such as point-of-care testing, the determination of coagulation profiles can be expedited, enabling effective decision-making within the surgical environment. In addition, integrating recommendations based on evidence, as presented in recent reports outlining post-acute care optimization, can inform practices focused on recovery and patient safety (Deutsch et al., 2012; Copeland et al., 2019). Through the integration of these guidelines into practice, healthcare providers are able to forecast more accurately the outcomes of hematologic disorders, allowing treatment policies to remain responsive and patient-centered. Thus, the deployment of advanced diagnostic tools and standard procedures is of paramount importance in influencing the care of hematologic disorders, with the ultimate goal of achieving optimal surgical outcomes (Figure 5.15).

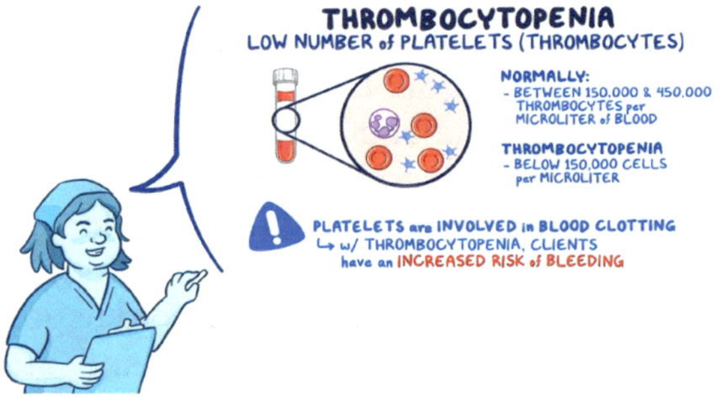

Figure 5.15. Thrombocytopenia in Surgical Nursing.

Source: https://www.osmosis.org/_next/image?url=https%3A%2F%2Fd16qt3wv6xm098.cloudfront.net%2F6ZJ53x_pTIaGwz0AOhxB78r2SfGhL1AY%2F_.jpg&w=3840&q=75.

Test Your Knowledge

1. Why is it important to assess clotting function before surgery in patients with hematologic disorders?
2. How can anemia increase the risk of surgical complications?

5.5. Nursing Interventions for Hematologic Disorders

Learning Outcome

1. Describe the monitoring and assessment techniques
2. Define the patient education and support
3. Discuss the collaboration with interdisciplinary teams for patients dealing with hematologic disorders

Effective nursing interventions in hematologic illnesses must depend on an understanding of the physiological impacts of these illnesses and the holistic needs of patients. Providing a complete assessment is crucial, particularly before surgery, as hematologic illness has significant effects on perioperative outcomes. Nursing evaluations should include testing blood to assess clotting factors, hemoglobin, and platelets, as these indicators can inform treatment plans. For example, patients with HMB must undergo a proper evaluation to identify potential underlying conditions that may complicate preoperative care (Hartanti et al., 2025). Nurses must also educate patients about the nature of their conditions and the benefits of management interventions, such as drug adherence in anticoagulation therapies, to prevent perioperative complications such as excessive blood loss. Another essential element of nursing interventions is the application of appropriate wound care techniques, particularly for patients with compromised hematologic function. Proper care of wound integrity not only enhances recovery but also minimizes pain and infection. The application of moist wound healing techniques has shown favorable outcomes in patients with tissue integrity disorders, particularly in cases related to diabetes mellitus (Hartanti et al., 2025). Nurses must assess mobile parameters such as patients' physical mobility and capacity to tend to these wounds on their own following surgery, identifying gaps in knowledge that hinder effective self-care. Through the provision of a formal learning process, nurses can empower patients to become active participants in their own care, which is essential in maximizing recovery and achieving positive health outcomes. Lastly, ongoing observation and evaluation are crucial to the success of nursing interventions for patients with hematologic disorders. Protocols for treatment should include frequent observation for signs of bleeding and frequent monitoring of vital signs to identify any deviation from baseline that may indicate complications. It is also crucial to be aware of the unique complexities involved in conditions such as disorders of platelet function, which may lead to an increased perioperative risk upon surgery (Delaney et al., 2025). Nursing intervention must also be responsive to changing patient needs, typically involving multimodal approaches, including hematologists and surgical teams, to deliver combined care. By establishing cooperative relationships between healthcare professionals, surgical nurses can ensure that hematologic disorders are effectively managed throughout the entire surgical process, thereby promoting patient safety and outcomes (Figure 5.16).

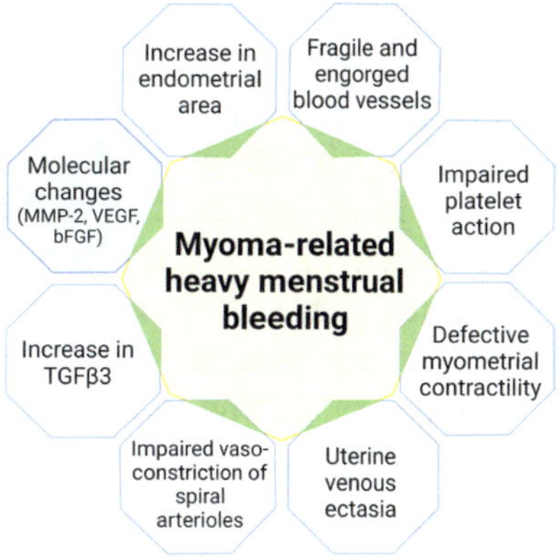

Figure 5.16. Conservative management of uterine fibroid-related heavy menstrual bleeding and infertility.

Source: https://www.mdpi.com/jcm/jcm-10-04389/article_deploy/html/images/jcm-10-04389-g002.png.

5.5.1. Monitoring and Assessment Techniques

The monitoring and assessment techniques in operating room nursing, particularly in relation to hematologic function, are of paramount significance in controlling patient outcomes. Effective monitoring begins with a thorough patient history and physical examination to identify risk for hematologic illness. Such an initial assessment should focus on the detection of preoperative states, such as anemia or coagulopathies, that complicate surgery (LeBoff et al., 2022). Following this, laboratory examinations such as complete blood counts (CBC) and coagulation profiles enable surgical nurses to assess the patient's hematologic status. Laboratory tests that measure the patient's hemoglobin level, platelet count, and coagulation factors are all critical for forecasting perioperative risks as well as guiding treatment modalities, thereby maximizing patient safety before, during, and following surgery. In addition to laboratory examinations, formal monitoring techniques are an excellent resource for providing a good postoperative recovery for patients with hematologic problems. Surgical nursing care should include continuous vital sign monitoring and specialized interventions for assessing bleeding or thromboembolic symptoms (Ajani et al., 2022). Patients with diagnosed hematologic disease might have specific postoperative complications, such as a higher tendency for bleeding or inadequate response to clotting. The use of advanced monitoring technologies, such as point-of-care testing, may enable rapid assessments of hematologic parameters and facilitate timely interventions. Anticipatory practice not only avoids complications but also helps to customize the treatment protocols based on real-time data, leading to better overall surgical outcomes. Finally, patient education forms part of monitoring to ensure that one is aware of his or her hematologic status and the importance of adhering to follow-up therapy. Effective communication channels should be employed to educate patients on monitoring for hematologic complications, such as unusual bruising or prolonged bleeding (LeBoff et al., 2022). Second, the importance of routine follow-up post-discharge blood work in monitoring for any abnormality that could indicate deterioration must be stressed to surgeons and nursing staff. It may maximize adherence and encourage active patients to seek timely medical counsel when needed. Therefore, a coordinated strategy involving observant monitoring, teaching slowly and deliberately, and interprofessional collaboration significantly enhances the management of hematologic functions under the umbrella of surgical nursing (Figure 5.17).

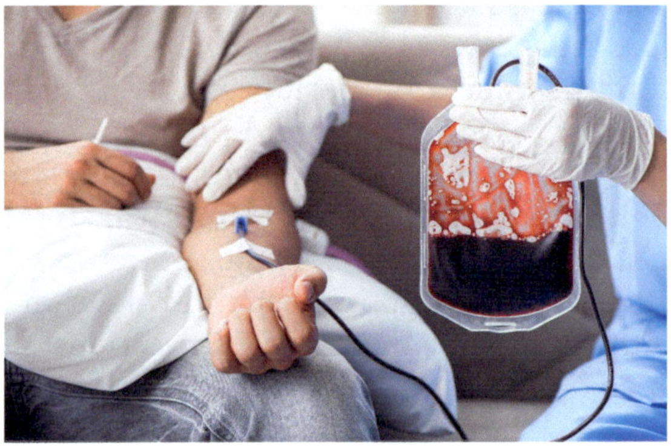

Figure 5.17. Monitoring and assessment techniques in hematologic functions.

Source: https://www.news-medical.net/images/Article_Images/ImageForArticle_745_16624283204238538.jpg.

5.5.2. Patient Education and Support

Patient support and education are crucial aspects of hematologic disease control in surgical settings within the nursing context. Adequate patient education not only addresses clinical issues in hematologic function but also enables the patient to become an active participant in their healthcare. Understanding their disease, options for treatment, and the importance of lifestyle changes enables patients to be involved in their healthcare. For operating room nurses, providing complete educational resources relevant to the patient's needs with a hematologic disorder is essential. It involves explaining medical terminology, treatment procedures, and potential complications in simple terms to foster an open and trusting environment where patients and medical professionals can communicate freely. With patient comprehension, there are more opportunities for adherence to treatment regimens and, ultimately, improved overall health outcomes. There must be support mechanisms put in place alongside education to handle the emotional and psychological components that come with hematologic disorders. Patients tend to experience anxiety about their diagnosis and the subsequent treatment implications, especially in surgical cases where intervention might be required. By developing a comprehensive support mechanism, surgical nurses can help patients overcome these emotional obstacles. Peer support groups, workshops, and counseling on an individual basis can make the setting conducive where the patients feel encouraged to open up their fears and seek assistance in managing their illness. Furthermore, educating relatives makes the support network more robust and helps patients face their disease more effectively. This complementary process of education and supportive care is key to improving resilience and coping, which can make a huge difference in recovery and good health. Finally, the effective integration of patient education and support into surgical nursing for hematologic disorders depends on ongoing evaluation and continuous improvement. The constantly evolving homologic function requires the medical professionals to remain aware and sensitive to their clients' shifting needs. Equipment such as thromboelastography (TEG) has emerged as an important tool in guiding treatment decisions and enhancing the management of surgical bleeding (Buscemi et al., 2022). However, there still remains an essential gap in the implementation of these tools, which necessitates better clinician training and education to allow them to implement such practices effectively in patient care. It is thus essential to concentrate on designing specialized programs that enhance both clinician competence and patient awareness, thereby bridging this gap and ultimately leading to improved outcomes and patient satisfaction in the area of surgical nursing for hematologic diseases.

5.5.3. Collaboration with Interdisciplinary Teams

Effective interprofessional teamwork is paramount to enhancing the quality of patient care in hematologic patients. Surgical nursing, in particular, involves a multidisciplinary team of health professionals, including hematologists, oncologists, and nurse practitioners, that come together to treat patients holistically. The shared expertise of the professionals facilitates thorough patient evaluation, diagnosis, and treatment. By combining their skills, team members can develop evidence-based care plans that are more tailored to the complexity of hematologic disorders, thereby providing improved patient outcomes and enhancing overall quality of life. Through this cohesive system, the importance of frequent communication and mutual respect among team members is emphasized in an effort to foster a unifying therapeutic environment. Furthermore, the interprofessional working observed in programs such as the comprehensive cancer programs supports the call for interdisciplinary working. Comprehensive cancer programs demonstrate how ordered team operation can support surgical nursing, calling for systematic responses to prevention, early detection, and treatment. Working structures developed in these collaborations provide crucial recommendations on best clinical practice. By utilizing experts' specialized skills, intensive care centers enhance operations in clinical trials and significantly improve the delivery of novel treatments, thereby focusing on better patient care outcomes. It relies on the establishment of a culture of collaboration among various healthcare providers (N/A, 2021). Nurse practitioners (NPs) are also a critical component of multidisciplinary teams, particularly in the assessment and management of hematologic disorders. Their training equips them with the knowledge to identify the correlation between systemic diseases and hematologic conditions so that they can determine what needs investigation. While they have promise, research indicates that the majority of NPs may not be aware of their competence in assessing oral health in terms of systemic disease, a trend also observed among healthcare professionals. Active promotion of NPs' involvement in collaborative care teams may enhance their confidence and improve assessment skills, ultimately leading to improved patient care. This partnership can help facilitate knowledge and experience exchange, advance enhanced competency in total patient management strategy, and enhance improved patient health outcomes (Haynes et al., 2020).

Test Your Knowledge

1. What nursing interventions are essential for a patient experiencing neutropenia?
2. How can nurses help manage fatigue in patients with anemia?

5.6. Advances in Hematologic Care

Learning Outcome

1. Describe the new diagnostic technologies in hematologic care
2. Define the innovative treatment options of hematologic care
3. Identify the research trends in hematologic disorders

The landscape of hematologic care has experienced dramatic advancements that significantly influence patient outcomes, particularly for surgical patients. Advances in diagnostics, including the use of next-generation sequencing and whole-genome profiling, enable a more precise interpretation of hematologic conditions. The advances enable early diagnosis and tailored treatment approaches through the use of unique personal genetic markers. With medical practitioners becoming increasingly skilled at diagnosing specific blood conditions, interventions grow more effective, ultimately reducing perioperative complications. In addition, the implementation of telemedicine platforms in hematologic education and patient care is a sign of ongoing evolution in healthcare delivery. Through remote consultation, patients can now receive timely evaluations and follow-up, eliminating travel congestion and enhancing treatment adherence (Copeland et al., 2019). Another significant evolution is the shift in transfusion practice towards patient-focused strategies. Evidence-based recommendations currently dictate transfusion thresholds, enhancing safety protocols that are sensitive to the subtle needs of surgical patients. For instance, the use of the restrictive transfusion strategy not only saves valuable blood products but also reduces the risk of transfusion-associated complications such as immunomodulation and transfusion-associated acute lung injury. Moreover, advances in synthetic blood products and cryopreserved stem cell technology are likely to expand therapeutic options for hematologic disorders to enhance preoperative care further. Proactive care enables more advanced treatment tailored to each patient, ultimately improving surgical outcomes in the context of hematologic risk factor management (Atyea et al., 2018). Ongoing studies in the area of hematologic disorders continue to uncover new treatment options, including targeted therapies that leverage the potential of immunotherapy. These therapies have great potential in combating hematologic malignancies, offering hope where traditional chemotherapy would not be effective. For surgical nurses, information about these new therapies is essential in helping patients receive adequate care and determining the best course of treatment.

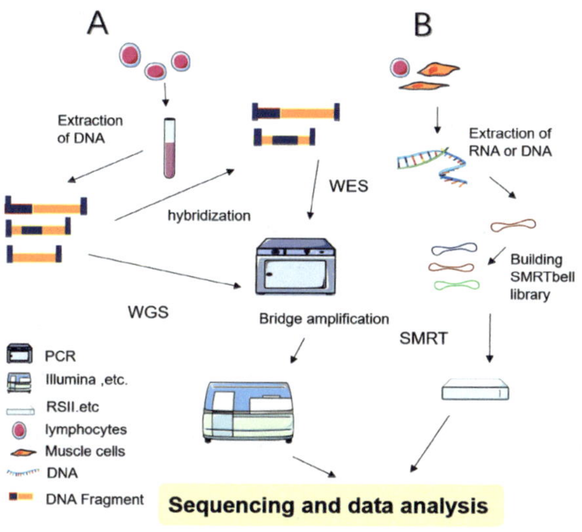

Figure 5.18. Next-generation sequencing technologies and neurogenetic diseases.

Source: https://www.mdpi.com/life/life-11-00361/article_deploy/html/images/life-11-00361-g001.png.

In addition, interprofessional models involving hematologists, surgeons, and nursing professionals provide an environment that fosters holistic patient care, ensuring the full consideration of the complexities of hematologic diseases. Such collaboration not only enhances the quality of care but also enables surgical nursing professionals to actively engage in minimizing the risks associated with hematologic diseases during surgery. The ever-changing nature of hematologic care continues to redefine the future of patient management and promote a holistic approach to surgical nursing (Copeland et al., 2019) (Figure 5.18).

5.6.1. New Diagnostic Technologies

The development of new diagnostic technologies is directly linked to the assessment of hematologic function and disease, particularly in surgical nursing practice. The more advanced blood diseases, such as anemias, coagulopathies, and leukemias, become, the more important the need for efficient and early detection methods is. The advancement of genomic profiling and chemical biology has facilitated the development of targeted therapeutics tailored to specific hematologic disorders. Not only do these technologies enhance diagnostic precision, but they also provide clues regarding the pathophysiology of blood diseases, thereby assisting in the formulation of effective treatment strategies. The integration of such diagnostic techniques into clinical practice aligns with the recommendations outlined in the European Hematology Association (EHA) Roadmap and focuses on the imperative for continuous innovation in diagnostic strategies to achieve improved patient outcomes in hematology (Allard et al., 2016). In addition, the application of advanced imaging modalities and laboratory diagnostics has transformed the surgical management of hematologic diseases. Technologies such as high-throughput sequencing and liquid biopsies have emerged as critical tools in the early detection of malignancy and monitoring of therapies. These technologies enable the identification of minimal residual disease, which typically hinders therapy regimens in surgery cases. Secondly, as highlighted in the EHA Roadmap, there is a constant need to optimize these technologies to enhance specificity and sensitivity, thereby improving accuracy in diagnosis. By focusing on research and development in these areas, healthcare practitioners can better understand patients' needs and apply treatments that are more effective and condition-specific (Allard et al., 2016). In addition to improving diagnostic accuracy, new technologies improve the cost-effectiveness of hematologic care. As evident from economic assessments associated with blood disorders, health system costs remain high. It is achievable to develop earlier interventions by applying sophisticated diagnostics, which can reduce the expense of long-term care for advanced complications and diseases. Hence, the EHA Roadmap emphasizes the importance of aligning research funding with such developments to ensure that innovations address real, unmet clinical needs in hematology. These strategic planning initiatives also help raise public awareness of the social consequences of blood disorders, leading to a more informed response to resource investment for research and treatment (Allard et al., 2016). With new technologies for diagnosis on the horizon, their potential to change the landscape of hematologic care is exceptionally bright and vital to patient outcomes for surgical nursing.

5.6.2. Innovative Treatment Options

The landscape of hematologic disorders has been changed by new treatment strategies that are enhancing patient outcomes in surgical nursing. Advances in precision medicine have enabled the development of targeted therapies specifically designed to address the root genetic mutation in various hematologic disorders. Such drugs can significantly enhance treatment efficacy with fewer side effects, which is essential for patients who typically have multiple comorbid conditions. The implementation of these targeted interventions into clinical care not only optimizes treatment regimens but also concords with the multidisciplinary models of care that are increasingly required in managing complicated health conditions. Hence, the development and implementation of new treatment strategies are critical for improving surgical nursing practice and patient outcomes in the management of hematologic disorders, both in terms of clinical presentation and patient quality of life. Another important advance in the management of hematologic disorders is the application of immunotherapies. These technologies utilize the body's immune system to recognize and kill cancer cells more effectively. For instance, CAR T-cell therapy has been highly effective in treating certain leukemias and lymphomas, indicating the potential of tailored immunological interventions. These treatments not only offer hope to formerly hard-to-treat patients but also represent challenges to coping with potential side effects, such as cytokine release syndrome. This syndrome highlights the importance of keeping operating nurses informed about the evolving treatment paradigm, enabling them to effectively monitor and treat complications as patients undergo these transformative treatments. The blending of these innovations in a harmonious way in treating the patients is the signature of the developments in the specialty. In addition to these therapy innovations, medication reconciliation is another significant practice that enhances safety during treatment. Application of formalized methods for effective medication management is important among patients with hematologic diseases who are often on complex regimens with anticoagulants and other critical drugs. The general overview of accidental medication order inconsistencies reveals shared potential clinical impacts that can be avoided by being vigilant during medication reconciliation. When implemented by a multidisciplinary team, these measures can substantially reduce adverse drug events, thereby improving patient outcomes (N/A, 2021). Incorporating pharmacists into the endeavor, for instance, has been beneficial in providing solutions to specific challenges, particularly with medications that can cause frailty or other issues associated with therapies such as androgen-deprivation therapy in prostate cancer (Buigues et al., 2020). This co-operative approach not only underscores the importance of novel treatment but also reaffirms an extensive viewpoint of patient care in surgical nursing (Figure 5.19).

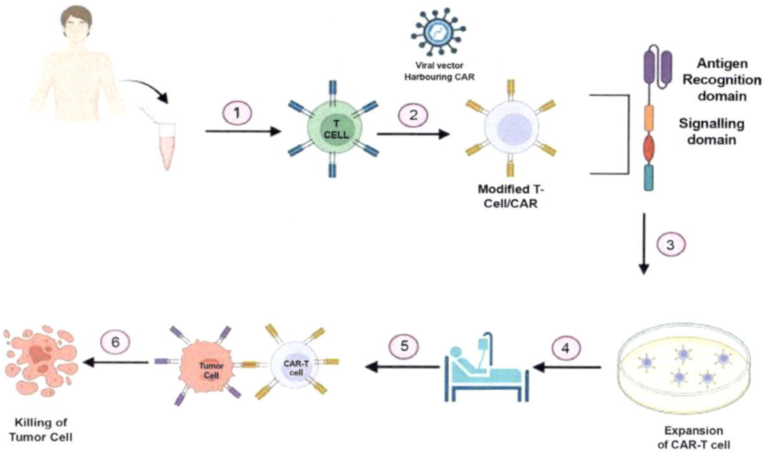

Figure 5.19. CAR T-cell therapy in cancer.

Source: https://ars.els-cdn.com/content/image/1-s2.0-S2347562524002014-gr1.jpg.

5.6.3. Research Trends in Hematologic Disorders

Recent research trends in hematologic disorders have increasingly focused on the genetic and molecular mechanisms underlying various conditions, including leukemia and hemophilia. Advances in genomics have enabled researchers to identify specific mutations and chromosomal abnormalities that contribute to disease onset and progression, thus paving the way for targeted therapies. The integration of precision medicine into clinical practice has provided a deeper understanding of patient-specific factors that affect treatment outcomes. This shift toward molecular characterization not only aids in the development of customized treatment protocols but also enhances prognostic accuracy. Understanding these genetic underpinnings is particularly crucial for surgical nursing, as it equips practitioners with knowledge about potential complications and the necessity for tailored perioperative care strategies (Copeland et al., 2019). Another significant trend is the use of novel therapeutic agents designed to improve outcomes for patients with hematologic disorders. For instance, the development of immunotherapy and CAR T-cell therapy has transformed the treatment landscape for certain hematologic malignancies, such as B-cell acute lymphoblastic leukemia. These innovative approaches aim to harness the body's immune response to combat cancer cells more effectively. Furthermore, advancements in hematopoietic stem cell transplantation techniques have led to improved survival rates and reduced complications, underscoring the importance of multidisciplinary care in achieving favorable patient outcomes. Surgical nursing plays a crucial role in this process, as practitioners must monitor and manage the complex side effects associated with these therapies while ensuring effective collaboration among medical teams (Callahan et al., 2019). As the field continues to evolve, research is increasingly directed toward improving patient management strategies and addressing disparities in care for various hematologic disorders.

For instance, researchers are investigating how socioeconomic factors and access to care influence treatment decisions and patient outcomes. There is also a growing emphasis on the use of telemedicine and digital health tools to enhance patient engagement and ensure continuity of care, particularly in underserved populations. These developments highlight the importance of incorporating a holistic, patient-centered approach in hematologic nursing practice. By leveraging research findings and technological advancements, surgical nurses can enhance their capability to provide comprehensive education and support throughout the treatment journey, ultimately optimizing care for patients with these complex disorders (Copeland et al., 2019).

Test Your Knowledge

1. How have targeted therapies improved treatment outcomes for patients with leukemia?
2. What is the role of stem cell transplantation in modern hematologic care?

SUMMARY

Hematologic function evaluation is essential in successful surgical nursing since understanding the interaction of blood components and surgical outcome may profoundly influence patient management. The subtlety of hematologic disorders, such as coagulopathies and anemia, necessitates meticulous evaluation and prompt intervention. With the integration of advanced hematological assessment methods and interpretation of findings based on evidence-based guidelines, nurses enhance patient safety and maximize surgical outcomes. The identification of potential complications resulting from hematologic abnormalities, both before and after surgery, plays a vital role in risk prevention, morbidity reduction, and recovery. Besides, the application of innovative diagnostic technologies, such as TEG, is revolutionizing blood management practices within operating rooms. TEG has the potential to provide valuable insights regarding coagulopathic conditions and may support individualized transfusion protocols, which can really improve patient outcomes. Such individualized approaches, under the direction of precise hematologic assessments, are critical in maintaining postoperative hemostatic balance and preventing excessive surgical bleeding. TEG-directed interventions have been shown to enhance transfusion efficiency and impact, aligning with overall standards of surgical competence and patient-centered care. To fully appreciate the significance of these advances in hematologic testing, an educational campaign targeting surgical nursing practitioners on these technologies is imperative. Closing the knowledge gap for the interpretation of TEG and its application in high-acuity surgical cases will enable informed clinical decision-making with confidence, leading to improved patient care. As the field of surgical nursing continues to evolve, integrating detailed hematologic screenings will not only address proximal surgical concerns but also foster a culture of continuous improvement in patient outcomes. Through education, cooperation, and innovative methods for managing hematologic function in surgical nursing, the discipline can effectively prevent complications from hematologic disorders, ultimately increasing the overall rate of surgical success (Chimbira et al., 2001; Buscemi et al., 2022).

Hematologic function evaluation is a critical area of preoperative analysis in surgical nursing that ensures the patients are optimized for the surgery. Understanding various constituents of blood, including red cells, white cells, and platelets, provides a basis for nurses to identify hematologic disorders. Anemia, for example, whether due to iron deficiency or a chronic disease, results in greater surgical risks and a prolonged convalescence. A further role of coagulation factors is crucial in hemostasis, with any alteration resulting in either a state of profuse bleeding or thromboembolic disease, both of which are high-risk states for surgical patients. Knowledge of certain hematology values enables surgical nurses to deliver the necessary interventions, such as blood transfusions or clotting factor administration, thereby improving patient safety and ensuring the best possible care. As essential as operating room nursing knowledge is, it is knowledge about common hematology disorders that complicate surgery. Leukopenia and thrombocytopenia, for instance, require careful observation and may require a change of the operation or perioperative treatment. The operating team must also be aware of the effects of underlying malignancies, as neoplastic hematologic cancers like lymphoma and leukemia will markedly alter the patient's body response to surgery and postoperative healing. Patients with chronic diseases also exhibit varying hematologic profiles, which can affect anesthesia management and surgical outcomes. Through up-to-date knowledge bases regarding such disorders and outcomes, OR nurses can provide patient-specific care that corresponds to each patient's unique hematologic disorder, closing the loop between intraoperative management and preoperative evaluation. Long-term continuous education and the integration of evidence-based interventions into surgical nursing structures will be required to enhance patient outcomes. The practice of clinical guidelines, including the management of anticoagulation therapy and the assessment of fracture risk in osteoporotic patients, emphasizes the importance of a carefully planned approach in decision-making. Routine screening for hematologic disorders facilitates the early detection of high-risk patients, enabling early intervention that can prevent complications intraoperatively. Furthermore, collaboration among multidisciplinary teams of professionals guarantees that a patient's every need for health is met and ultimately leads to an environment of safety and effectiveness for surgical intervention. As innovations are continued to be practiced in both hematology and surgical nursing, a focus on practice development and education will remain essential in the process of delivering the most optimal patient outcomes achievable in surgical care.

KEY TERMS FROM THIS CHAPTER

- Complete blood count (CBC)
- Hematocrit
- Platelet count
- Prothrombin time (PT)
- Thalassemia
- Leukemia
- Hemophilia
- Bone marrow biopsy
- Immunosuppression
- Hemoglobin
- White blood cells (WBC)
- Coagulation profile
- Anemia
- Sickle cell disease
- Lymphoma
- Thrombocytopenia
- Blood transfusion
- Anticoagulant therapy

CRITICAL THINKING QUESTIONS

1. **Which laboratory test is commonly used to assess a patient's oxygen-carrying capacity?**
   a. Prothrombin time (PT)
   b. Hematocrit (Hct)
   c. Platelet count
   d. Erythrocyte sedimentation rate (ESR)
2. **A patient with iron-deficiency anemia is most likely to present with which symptom?**
   a. Jaundice
   b. Bradycardia
   c. Fatigue and pallor
   d. Cyanosis of the lips
3. **Which hematologic disorder involves the destruction of red blood cells faster than they can be produced?**
   a. Aplastic anemia
   b. Hemolytic anemia
   c. Leukemia
   d. Thrombocytopenia
4. **In a patient with thrombocytopenia, which complication is the nurse most concerned about?**
   a. Hypertension
   b. Bleeding and bruising
   c. Fever and chills
   d. Weight gain
5. **Which of the following is a key nursing responsibility during a blood transfusion?**
   a. Administer the blood rapidly within 15 minutes
   b. Monitor the patient's blood glucose level
   c. Check vital signs before, during, and after transfusion
   d. Warm the blood to room temperature in a microwave

Short Answer Questions

1. What is the normal function of hemoglobin in the blood?
2. Name two common signs of anemia.
3. What is thrombocytopenia, and why is it clinically significant?
4. Which lab test helps assess clotting function?
5. List two causes of iron-deficiency anemia.
6. Describe the nursing assessment and care for a patient with low hemoglobin and hematocrit levels.
7. Explain the pathophysiology, symptoms, and nursing management of sickle cell anemia.
8. Discuss the precautions a nurse should take when caring for a patient with thrombocytopenia.
9. Describe the types of leukemias and their general impact on hematologic function.
10. Explain the nursing responsibilities during and after a blood transfusion, including possible transfusion reactions.

Answers to Critical Thinking Questions

1. (b); 2. (c); 3. (b); 4. (b); 5. (c).

REFERENCES

1. Allard, S., Anagnou, N., Andolfo, I., Andrau, M., et al. (2016). The European Hematology Association roadmap for European hematology research: A consensus document. https://core.ac.uk/download/79516495.pdf (accessed on 30th June 2025).
2. Atyea, A., Hussein, S., Mehany, M., Morsy, A., et al. (2018). Mortality prediction among critically ill patients during intensive care unit stays at Assuit University Hospital. https://core.ac.uk/download/234692469.pdf (accessed on 30th June 2025).
3. Bavendam, T., Dicianno, B. E., Dosa, N. P., Gomez-Lobo, V., et al. (2017). Research needs for effective transition in lifelong care of congenital genitourinary conditions: A workshop sponsored by the National Institute of Diabetes and Digestive and Kidney Diseases. https://core.ac.uk/download/161627514.pdf (accessed on 30th June 2025).
4. Buigues, C., Navarro-Martínez, R., Sánchez-Martínez, V., Serrano-Carrascosa, M., Rubio-Briones, J., & Cauli, O. (2020). Interleukin-6 and lymphocyte count associated and predicted the progression of frailty syndrome in prostate cancer patients undergoing antiandrogen therapy. *Cancers, 12*, 1716–1716. https://doi.org/10.3390/cancers12071716 (accessed on 30th June 2025).
5. Buscemi, C., & Milanes Villa, Y. (2022). Improving clinicians' knowledge of thromboelastographic: A quality improvement project. https://core.ac.uk/download/548486092.pdf (accessed on 30th June 2025).
6. Callahan, M. F., Mikhailov, T., O'Brien, M., Rice, M., et al. (2019). Creation and implementation of a pediatric advanced practice nurse critical care fellowship program. https://core.ac.uk/download/288816871.pdf (accessed on 30th June 2025).
7. Chimbira, W., Crawford, H., Gupta, S., Legg, M., et al. (2001). Acute lung injury in pediatric intensive care: Course and outcome. https://core.ac.uk/download/pdf/8715345.pdf (accessed on 30th June 2025).
8. Copeland, L. I. B. T., James, D., Duinkerken, M. S. I., Kelsey, G., et al. (2019). Jefferson Digital Commons quarterly report: October–December 2019. https://core.ac.uk/download/286097805.pdf (accessed on 30th June 2025).
9. Cox, A. J. (2016). The effects of iron deficiency anemia and iron supplementation in pregnancy. https://core.ac.uk/download/58827031.pdf (accessed on 30th June 2025).
10. Delaney, A., Kritsotakis, E. I., Horner, K., Kitchen, S., Sedcole, J., Baxter, T., Maclean, R. M., et al. (2025). High prevalence of platelet function disorders in women referred for surgical management of refractory heavy menstrual bleeding. *Haemophilia: The Official Journal of the World Federation of Hemophilia*. https://www.semanticscholar.org/paper/5bd94b977cbe9a173939e5513b893b49b2918cbd (accessed on 30th June 2025).
11. Deutsch, A., Dever, J., Gage, B., Garfinkel, S., et al. (2012). Post-acute care payment reform demonstration: Final report Volume 3 of 4. https://core.ac.uk/download/230872866.pdf (accessed on 30th June 2025).
12. Donnell, S. (2017). Meta-regression: Prognostic models as objective predictors of mortality among ICU cancer patients. https://core.ac.uk/download/235238285.pdf (accessed on 30th June 2025).

13. Eslami, A. A., Khayri, F., Masoudi, R., Rabiei, K., et al. (2014). Sleep quality and spiritual well-being in hemodialysis patients. https://core.ac.uk/download/143841276.pdf (accessed on 30th June 2025).

14. Hartanti, N., Wardoyo, E., & Sugiarto, S. (2025). Nursing care for patients with post debridement diabetic ulcers with moist wound healing innovation interventions at General Ahmad Yani Hospital, Metro City. *INDOGENIUS*. https://www.semanticscholar.org/paper/5cd361f8f53d97e21117c85f775c922eaeaadc1b (accessed on 30th June 2025).

15. Haynes, A. (2020). Assessing nurse practitioners' knowledge and clinical practice with regard to the oral-systemic link. https://core.ac.uk/download/368327433.pdf (accessed on 30th June 2025).

16. Hu, J., Zhou, C., Feng, L., & Yang, Y. (2024). An evidence-based nursing practice affects stress state, coagulation, complications and quality of life in patients with upper gastrointestinal bleeding in the emergency department: A retrospective observational study. *BMC Gastroenterology, 24*. https://www.semanticscholar.org/paper/77cbd3f07810238f4c101e956172861af1739746 (accessed on 30th June 2025).

17. John, M., Ely, E. W., Halfkann, D., Schoen, J., Sedemund-Adib, B., Klotz, S., Radtke, F., et al. (2017). Acetylcholinesterase and butyrylcholinesterase in cardiosurgical patients with postoperative delirium. *Journal of Intensive Care, 5*. https://www.semanticscholar.org/paper/9b6ab1ec5484fa30d4ee1ad6ad5b48fc627401d0 (accessed on 30th June 2025).

18. Kleinpell, R., Grabenkort, W. R., Boyle, W. A., Vines, D., & Olsen, K. M. (2021). The Society of Critical Care Medicine at 50 years: Interprofessional practice in critical care: Looking back and forging ahead. *Critical Care Medicine, 49*, 2017–2032. https://doi.org/10.1097/ccm.0000000000005276 (accessed on 30th June 2025).

19. LeBoff, M. S., Greenspan, S. L., Insogna, K., Lewiecki, E. M., Saag, K. G., Singer, A., & Siris, E. S. (2022). The clinician's guide to prevention and treatment of osteoporosis. *Osteoporosis International, 33*, 2049–2102. https://doi.org/10.1007/s00198-021-05900-y (accessed on 30th June 2025).

20. Matsui, T., Shoji, M., Watanabe, N., Yoshino, K., et al. (2017). Transactions of The Showa University Society: The 335th meeting. Serum level on admission is a useful predictor for treatment response in patients with acute pulmonary thromboembolism sodium bicarbonate-ascorbic acid combination for prevention in undergoing. https://www.semanticscholar.org/paper/5f05805ec68b72ff08e047000132ec81b9c61dc4 (accessed on 30th June 2025).

21. Pierpont, M. E., Brueckner, M., Chung, W. K., Garg, V., Lacro, R. V., McGuire, A. L., Mital, S., et al. (2018). Genetic basis for congenital heart disease: Revisited: A scientific statement from the American Heart Association. *Circulation, 138*. https://doi.org/10.1161/cir.0000000000000606 (accessed on 30th June 2025).

22. Quan, M., Wang, X., Gong, M., Wang, Q., Li, Y., & Jia, J. (2023). Post-COVID cognitive dysfunction: Current status and research recommendations for high-risk population. *The Lancet Regional Health–Western Pacific, 38*, 100836–100836. https://doi.org/10.1016/j.lanwpc.2023.100836 (accessed on 30th June 2025).

23. Ramer, L., Hunt, P., Ortega, E., Knowlton, J., Briggs, R. P., & Hirokawa, S. (2015). Effect of intravenous (IV) assistive device (VeinViewer) on IV access attempts, procedural time, and

patient and nurse satisfaction. *Journal of Pediatric Oncology Nursing, 33*, 273–281. https://doi.org/10.1177/1043454215600425 (accessed on 30th June 2025).

24. Riba, M. B., Donovan, K. A., Andersen, B. L., Braun, I., Breitbart, W., Brewer, B. W., Buchmann, L., et al. (2019). Distress management, Version 3.2019, NCCN clinical practice guidelines in oncology. *Journal of the National Comprehensive Cancer Network, 17*, 1229–1249. https://doi.org/10.6004/jnccn.2019.0048 (accessed on 30th June 2025).
25. Shenoy, E. S., Macy, E., Rowe, T. A., & Blumenthal, K. G. (2019). Evaluation and management of penicillin allergy. *JAMA, 321*, 188–188. https://doi.org/10.1001/jama.2018.19283 (accessed on 30th June 2025).

IMMUNE SYSTEM DISORDERS AND ALLERGIC REACTIONS

6

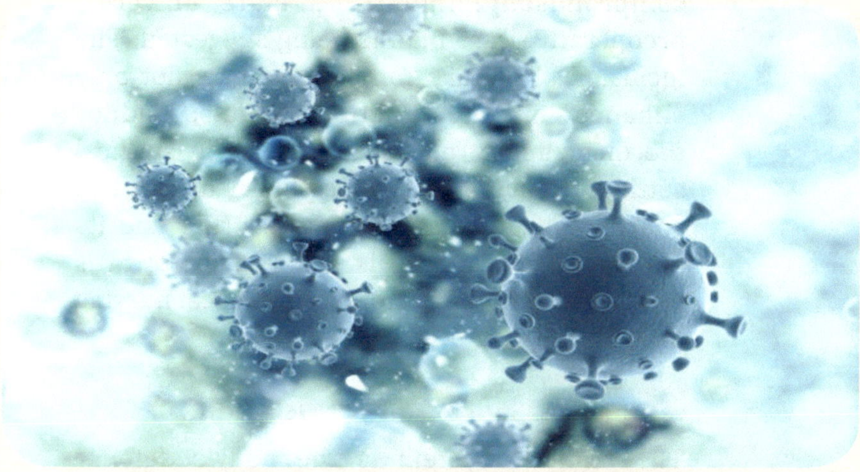

LEARNING OBJECTIVES

After studying this chapter, you will be able to:

1. Understand the immune system
2. Explain the common immune system disorders
3. Discuss the allergic reactions in surgical patients
4. Focus on role of surgical nurses in managing immune disorders
5. Learn about preoperative considerations for patients with immune disorders
6. Evaluate the postoperative care for patients with allergic reactions

Introduction

The study of immune system disorders and allergic reactions is a significant area of research in the field of surgical nursing. It is necessary to learn about these disorders comprehensively because they not only impact the overall well-being of the patients but also have a tremendous influence on the success of the surgery. The primary function of the immune system is to defend the body against pathogens; nevertheless, hypersensitivity or dysfunctions can lead to disorders, making surgery more complicated. High levels of allergic reactions and immune-related disorders, highlight the necessity for surgical nurses to possess deep knowledge in this subject. Through the targeting of mechanisms and risk factors associated with such disorders, surgical nursing can be adapted to incorporate preventive and response measures that enhance patient safety and the effectiveness of surgery (Burns et al., 2019). The inclusion of research evidence on the mechanisms of hypersensitivity reactions provides significant information about managing allergic diseases within the framework of surgery. Among some of the risk factors for developing allergies are genetic factors and environmental influences. With allergic responses often occurring during surgery or post-operative treatment, nurses must be trained to recognize and counteract such effects.

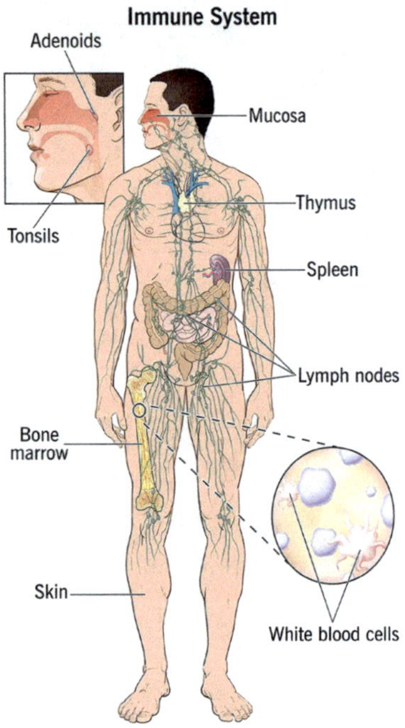

Figure 6.1. Immune system function.

Source: https://my.clevelandclinic.org/-/scassets/images/org/health/articles/immune-system.jpg.

Researchers indicate that having knowledge of how immune responses are coordinated enables surgical teams to adopt evidence-based decision-making approaches on perioperative care. Additionally, the development of evidence-based practices, such as preoperative allergen avoidance or the selective use of antihistamines, can also enhance patient well-being and overall rates of surgical success (Burns et al., 2019). In addition, new developments of how food elements affect immune response also emphasize the requirement of a more integrated methodology for the care of patients in surgical nursing. Studies have shown that dietetic therapy can affect immune function and potentially benefit patients with allergies by enhancing their overall response to surgical stress. Through stratifying studies of the food's immune-modulating activity in various patient groups, including hypersensitivity and compromised immunity, a more universal preoperative care plan is being suggested. The inclusion of dietary components may not only enhance immune function but also reduce the incidence of allergic reactions in surgical settings. Hence, an interdisciplinary descriptive conceptualization of immune disorder and its management strategy is a key step towards optimizing patient outcomes in surgical nursing practice (Figure 6.1).

Definition of the Immune System

The immune system is the body's defense against foreign materials and pathogens and is responsible for maintaining homeostasis. The immune system consists of an intricate array of cells, tissues, and organs that identify and destroy potential attackers in the form of bacteria, viruses, and even cancer cells. The system operates via two mechanisms: innate immunity, an immediate, nonspecific reaction to pathogens, and adaptive immunity, which is slower but a much more specific reaction that accumulates memory against previously encountered pathogens. This is a sophisticated interaction between heterogeneous immune cells and biochemical mediators and is necessary for optimal function, particularly in surgical nursing, where patients may develop compromised immunity via stressors such as anesthesia or surgery. Furthermore, recent research has highlighted the potential of food components to modulate immunity, and it has been shown that not only does the immune system become shaped by inherent determinants, but it could also be influenced by extrinsic factors such as diet. Research findings indicate that food could enhance innate and adaptive immunity, which would be beneficial, especially in patients. For example, patients undergoing surgery and those with allergic reactions can achieve improved immune function with a certain diet regimen. By sorting studies according to people's health status, obviously, nutritional interventions can normalize immune functions and thus potentially overcome the risks of allergic reactions and enhance postoperative recovery. According to these findings, surgical nurses should consider the nutritional status of patients as an essential component for deciding overall immune health (Kaminogawa et al., 2004). In addition to immune response modulation through nutrition, awareness of certain treatment side effects, such as those related to cancer treatment, is also crucial in cases involving immune system disorders. For this reason, children with acute lymphoblastic leukemia have several characteristics of adverse effects of treatment that weaken immune function, and they need to be in a coordinated system of care. The research has proved acute toxic effects, such as hypersensitivity and pancreatitis, that show the necessity for an explicit definition of such effects to have successful management and coordination of research (Attarbaschi et al., 2016). The relevance of these findings also extends to surgical nursing, where recognizing immunocompromised conditions is crucial in preventing complications, managing allergic reactions, and achieving improved patient outcomes. Therefore, an in-depth knowledge of the immune system is not only necessary for efficient surgical practice but also for improving the integrative care of patients with immune disorders.

Importance of the Immune System in Surgical Nursing

The immune system plays a vital role in surgical nursing because it greatly influences patient outcome in terms of prevention during and after surgery. There is a need for an effective immune response to prevent infections, manage inflammation, and facilitate wound healing. Every surgery carries a risk of exposing the underlying tissues to pathogens, hence the need for the immune system to eliminate these harmful threats. Surgical nurses' success is typically due to their patients' baseline immunity status; patients with compromised immune systems may experience increased rates of infection and delayed healing. Consequently, surgical nurses must be vigilant in monitoring patients for signs of immune dysregulation and adjusting their perioperative care strategies appropriately. For instance, preoperative assessment should include finding out patients' immune statuses, such as ~~by~~ taking history for immune disorders or requesting laboratory tests to be available for surgery. Moreover, understanding immune system disorders and their repercussions is necessary for surgical nursing practice. Patients with conditions such as allergies, asthma, or autoimmune disease might pose specific challenges to surgery. For example, as identified in the findings of a study measuring existing health conditions among adolescents in a quasi-military program, allergies were among the most prevalent health conditions (n = 170) among the participants. This highlights the need for surgical nurses to receive proper training in managing allergic reactions among patients during surgery, particularly in those with known sensitivities. Developing comprehensive care plans that consider such conditions enables surgical nurses to reduce risk, creating a safer operating environment adequately. One can observe from this that awareness of the intricacies of the immune system directly impacts surgical nurses' strategies for caring for the patient pre-, intra-, and post-operatively. Education and advocacy for the immune system also largely contribute to improving patient outcomes for surgical nursing. Preparation on the part of nurses with knowledge about immune response mechanisms would enhance their ability to educate patients and families on the importance of maintaining a healthy immune system, particularly during the perioperative period. Strategies such as promoting vaccinations, educating patients on optimal nutrition, and encouraging optimal hydration can empower patients to take action to optimize their immune function pre-operatively. Furthermore, if operating room nurses understand how immune system disorders lead to complications, they can better argue for patient resources and care programs. Such a global view enhances the nurse practice and patient safety, ultimately leading to better outcomes from surgeries. The application of immune system knowledge in surgical nursing is not only a best practice; it is also essential for comprehensive care and improved patient outcomes (Figure 6.2).

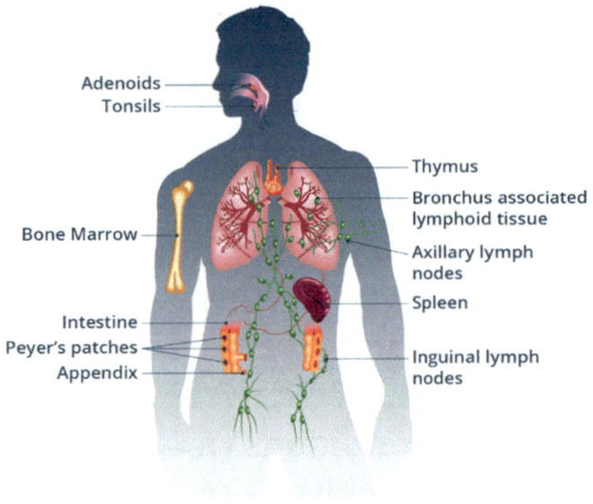

Figure 6.2. Immune system.

Source: https://media.healthdirect.org.au/images/inline/original/organs-of-the-immune-system-cc9363.png.

Overview of Immune System Disorders and Allergic Reactions

The immune system plays a vital role in maintaining homeostasis and protecting the body from infection; however, when it fails, it can cause a host of disorders, including allergies and autoimmune diseases. Allergic reaction refers to the immune system responding hypersensitively to usually harmless substances called allergens. Such allergens can vary from pollen and dust mites to food and drugs that cause an abnormal immune reaction. Symptoms can manifest in various ways, including respiratory issues, cutaneous reactions, or gastrointestinal distress. Additionally, the increasing prevalence of allergies, particularly among children, underscores the need to investigate the underlying mechanisms that make individuals susceptible to such hypersensitivity reactions. An in-depth understanding of the dynamic interactions between genetic, environmental, and immunological factors is essential for surgical nursing professionals to identify, prevent, and manage potential allergic reactions in surgical patients (Burns et al., 2019). Investigating mechanisms that control hypersensitivity reactions reveals complex interactions within the immune response. Between innate and adaptive immunity, the latter is particularly relevant to allergic disease because it is associated with the production of IgE antibodies against the allergen. Re-exposure triggers the release of histamines and other inflammatory mediators by IgE antibodies, leading to acute allergic reactions. In surgery, awareness of these mechanisms is of the most tremendous significance because these influence preoperative assessment and postoperative management. ~~It~~ also needs to understand how the underlying immune disorders can complicate surgical outcomes, for example, by increasing the risk of infections and delaying wound healing. The surgery nursing staff should be trained to identify symptoms of allergic reactions and act quickly to prevent complications. This knowledge not only enhances patient safety but also improves overall surgical success rates (Burns et al., 2019). Furthermore, recent studies have placed greater importance on the contributions made by nutrition to immune modulation, particularly in relation to hypersensitivity responses. Foods are found to exert a positive influence on immune processes, with the potential to reduce symptoms of allergic responses. Recent studies have categorized this research into three groups:

healthy individuals, hypersensitive patients, and immunocompromised patients, including those undergoing surgery. Current evidence suggests that diet has a significant influence on innate and acquired immunity, supporting the body's ability to combat allergies and other diseases. In operating room nursing, supportive diets that enable immune function can be a significant part of integrative patient care. By integrating food immune-modulating information into practice, nursing professionals can better prepare patients for surgery and promote recovery by reducing the frequency of allergic reactions and related complications.

6.1. Overview of the Immune System

Learning Outcome

1. Describe the components of the immune system
2. Focus on functions of the immune system
3. Learn about types of immune responses

The immune system is a complex system of cells, tissues, and organs that work in concert to defend the body against pathogens such as viruses, bacteria, and other toxic substances. The immune response is essentially separated into innate and adaptive immunity at its core. Innate immunity is the initial line of defense, utilizing physical barriers such as the skin and mucous membranes, and employing immune cells like phagocytes that respond to infection rapidly and nonspecifically. Adaptive immunity is acquired gradually and involves specialized lymphocytes, such as B cells and T cells, which create immunological memory. This double aspect of the immune system makes room for a subtle response to one specific threat, highlighting its role not only in preserving health but also in the possibility of pathology of the immune system that may disrupt homeostasis and initiate an allergic reaction, exceedingly relevant to the field of surgical nursing. Immunological disease occurs when the balance is disrupted within the immune response, creating conditions that can severely compromise patient health. For instance, allergy is a misplaced immune reaction to otherwise harmless substances, and autoimmunity is the attack of the body on its own cells. Such dysregulations can complicate surgery, as patients with compromised immune systems may experience heightened susceptibility to infections or hyperinflammatory responses. Therefore, understand the pathophysiology of these disorders to properly screen patients preoperatively and monitor them postoperatively for complications.

Furthermore, advances in immunotherapy, such as for peanut allergies, highlight efforts at enhancing allergic reaction effects and patient outcomes (Rauscher et al., 2015). The role of surgical nursing in managing patients with compromised immune systems also underscores the importance of ongoing training and education. In acknowledging the increasing number of allergies among diverse patient populations, nurses must be prepared to identify early warning signs of perioperative complications associated with these conditions. Resources such as the Iowa Board of Nursing's newsletters are significant in keeping nurses up-to-date on best practices when caring for patients with these complexities (N/A, 2017). Intermingling knowledge of the immune system and its disorders in the surgical patient care can enhance patient safety and improve successful surgical outcomes. Such an integrated strategy benefits individual patients and contributes to a more comprehensive understanding of immune system disorders, thereby improving public health responses to these pervasive diseases (Figure 6.3).

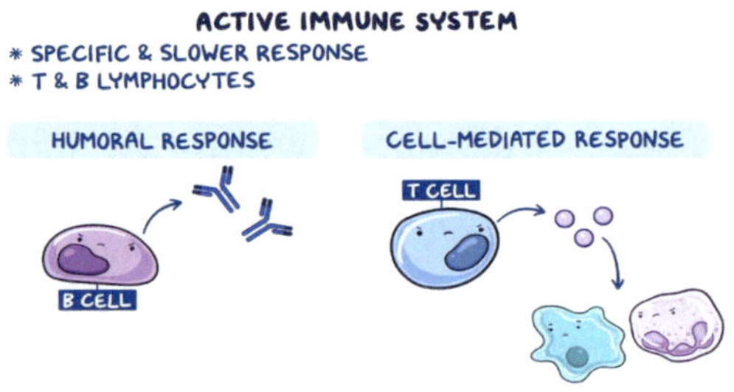

Figure 6.3. Innate and adaptive immunity.

Source: https://www.osmosis.org/_next/image?url=https%3A%2F%2Fd16qt3wv6xm098.cloudfront.net%2FpdATKH6yQMi2ZxgCEJY1wPMtQyqoV8P1%2F_.jpg&w=3840&q=75.

6.1.1. Components of the Immune System

The immune system is a highly complex network that has a variety of components that work together to protect the body from foreign substances and pathogens. White blood cells are among these components, which are essential as individual entities such as lymphocytes, neutrophils, and macrophages all have specific tasks to accomplish. Lymphocytes are critical for adaptive immunity, which recognizes specific antigens and reacts with tailored responses. Neutrophils and macrophages, as part of the innate immune system, serve as the body's first line of defense by engulfing and killing invading microbes. It is critical to know these cellular processes in surgical nursing, particularly because patients with immune disorders have varying reactions to surgery, which can complicate healing and recovery. The role of antibodies is another essential aspect of the immune system, facilitating a specific response to infections. Produced primarily by B cells, antibodies bind to and neutralize foreign antigens, marking them for destruction by other immune cells. The humoral response is particularly applicable in situations of allergic reactions, in which the immune system is inadvertently sensitized to harmless substances, such as pollen or pet dander. Understanding the mechanisms of antibody production and how they relate to hypersensitivity is essential for surgical nurses to recognize that allergy-susceptible patients are more likely to experience complications related to anesthesia and wound healing. Additionally, these facts can inform the development of preoperative protocols that prioritize patient safety by considering potential allergic reactions. A second significant element of the immune system is the intricate interaction among the numerous disparate immune elements, including cytokines, which are signal proteins that enable immune cells to communicate with each other. Cytokines play a crucial role in regulating immune responses, modulating immune responses, and controlling cellular interactions during both acute and chronic immune responses. Dysregulation of cytokine production can cause potentially deadly immune disorders, such as allergies and autoimmune disease. Surgical nurses should identify this interaction. They can effectively handle patients with such disorders, particularly during and after the operating room. In-depth knowledge of the components and interactions within the immune system enables healthcare professionals to provide more precise interventions, thereby minimizing the risk of complications from allergic reactions and optimizing patient outcomes in the operating room.

6.1.2. Functions of the Immune System

The immune system plays a crucial role in defending the body against pathogens, including bacteria, viruses, fungi, and parasites. Its primary functions are the detection and killing of these foreign organisms, which is attained through a sophisticated machinery of cells, tissues, and organs. Among the most significant components are white blood cells, including lymphocytes and phagocytes, which collectively regulate immune responses. When they encounter pathogens, these immune cells trigger a cascade of responses that lead to the production of antibodies and the activation of numerous immune pathways. Not only do they identify and kill foreign invaders, but in the process, they generate immunological memory, which enables the body to respond more easily to subsequent exposure. These systems are crucial for general well-being, and failure in such a system will result in immune-mediated disease or allergic reactions that severely compromise a patient's quality of life. In surgical nursing, it is essential to understand the functions of the immune system, particularly in addressing postoperative complications that may result from an altered immune response. Surgical operations inherently compromise the body's defense system, making patients susceptible to infection and other immunologic complications. In addition, patients with compromised immune status, either due to pre-existing conditions or through surgical excision, are at risk for hypersensitivity reactions. These reactions can be manifest as mild allergic reactions to anaphylactic shock. Therefore, operating room nurses should be sufficiently trained in recognizing signs of impaired immune status and allergic reaction, with provision of immediate intervention for optimized health protection. This requires a sufficient understanding of the immune system's mechanisms and determinants, such as environmental sensitization noted in the literature, that influence individual patient responses (Burns et al., 2019). Current evidence highlights the significant role that diet plays in immune function, which is of considerable concern in surgical nursing. The role of nutrition in modulating the immune response should be considered, as certain foods have been shown to enhance both innate and acquired immunity. For instance, nutrients in various foods have been shown to increase phagocytic activity and enhance T cell responses, thereby boosting the immune status of patients. This is particularly critical in the postoperative phase, where immune enhancement is crucial for a successful recovery. Furthermore, managing potential food sensitivities and allergies is crucial in operating room nursing to prevent exacerbating the patient's allergic reaction. Evidence-based guidelines, based on new findings, not only aim to optimize nutritional interventions but also emphasize observing the manner in which nutritional interventions actually help in managing immune functions (Kaminogawa et al., 2004) (Figure 6.4).

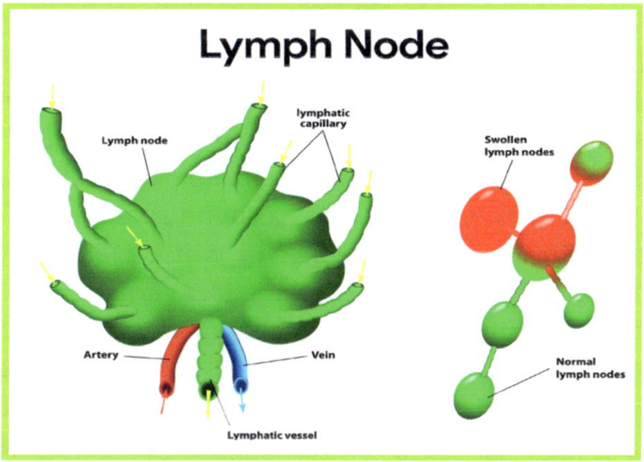

Figure 6.4. Lymph node.

Source: https://nurseslabs.com/wp-content/uploads/2017/08/Lymph-Node-Lymphatic-System-Anatomy-and-Physiology.png.

6.1.3. Types of Immune Responses

The immune system comprises innate and adaptive immunity that function synergistically to protect the body against pathogens. Innate immunity is the primary defense, employing physical barriers such as the skin and mucosal membranes, as well as immune cells like macrophages and neutrophils. They respond rapidly to infection through a non-specific mechanism of pathogen-associated molecular pattern recognition. In contrast, adaptive immunity elicits a more specific response involving lymphocytes, such as B cells and T cells. The antibodies produced by B cells are specifically tailored to act against the particular antigens. In contrast, T cells orchestrate and regulate the immune response, directly killing infected host cells. Understanding these two fundamental types of immune responses is essential in surgical nursing, especially in caring for patients with immune disorders and allergic reactions since these can complicate recovery and predispose patients to infections. In the event of an allergic reaction, the immune response becomes overreactive, resulting in hypersensitivity. Allergens, generally harmless substances, can trigger a powerful immune response in vulnerable individuals, resulting in diseases such as allergic rhinitis, asthma, or food allergies. Such an uncontrolled immune reaction is largely made possible by Immunoglobulin E (IgE), which binds to allergens and triggers the release of histamines and other inflammatory mediators from mast cells. The consequences of such reactions can be anything from bothersome to fatal. Surgical nursing has an obligation to remain aware of such responses because the care of allergic patients may require preoperative assessment and vigilant surveillance of allergens throughout surgery. Immune responses' understanding with respect to surgical management is crucial to patient safety and successful outcomes. Furthermore, the aging population also presents specific challenges regarding immune responses, particularly in allergic conditions. With increasing age, the human immune system also undergoes changes, which may increase susceptibility to allergic reactions. Not only do older patients bear a history of allergies, but their declining immunological power also complicates pre-existing conditions. With rising pollution and food contamination, these allergic reactions tend to be aggravated as well, because elderly people are more likely to be sensitive due to the overall weakening of their immune systems with age. Evidence suggests that physiological changes, such as chronic inflammation and shifts in cytokine profiles, exacerbate the complexity of treating allergies in this group. Hospital operating room nurses need to keep abreast of the complexity of these age-related immune responses in order to offer proper care and prevent adverse outcomes in patients presenting with allergic conditions in old age (Bonini et al., 2017; Rauscher et al., 2015) (Figure 6.5).

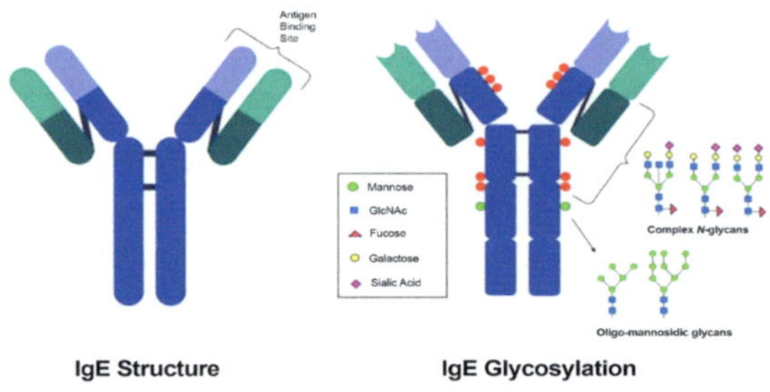

Figure 6.5. Immunoglobulin-E-IgE-structure-and-functions.

Source: https://microbenotes.com/wp-content/uploads/2018/07/Immunoglobulin-E-IgE-Structure-and-Functions.jpeg.

Test Your Knowledge

1. What is the main function of white blood cells in the immune response?
2. How does the body recognize and respond to foreign antigens?

6.2. Common Immune System Disorders

Learning Outcome

1. Explain the autoimmune diseases
2. Define the immunodeficiency disorders
3. Discuss the hypersensitivity reactions

The immune system is highly evolved to defend against pathogens, but its breakdown can lead to a range of disorders that heavily impact patient care in surgical nursing. Autoimmune disorders, allergy, and immunodeficiency disorders are some of the most prevalent immune system disorders. Autoimmune disorders, in which the immune system mistakenly attacks the body's own tissues, can manifest as diseases such as rheumatoid arthritis and lupus. These conditions are particularly challenging in the operating room, since they are associated with chronic inflammation and altered healing. Understanding the pathophysiology of such conditions plays a central role for surgical nurses as they prepare to address and manage complications in patients who exhibit immune dysregulation, thereby delivering the best possible outcome with minimal complications. Allergies are another very prevalent type of immune system disease, wherein hypersensitivity is elicited by what is otherwise innocuous substance. Allergic reactions can be as subtle as sneezing and itching or as severe as anaphylaxis, an immediate, life-threatening situation. Among children's populations, there has been a rising concern about the rise in food allergy, hay fever, and eczema, most of the time with environmental and genetic links (Burns et al., 2019). Surgical nurses should be highly attentive to these allergies, particularly in preoperative assessments, as undiagnosed sensitivities may complicate anesthetic and surgery procedures. By remaining vigilant and taking precautions against allergies, surgical nursing professionals can contribute significantly towards improving the quality of care and the safety of patients. Immunodeficiency disorders, whether primary or secondary, further complicate the scenario of immune system disorders. Primary immunodeficiencies describe inherited defects in immune function that lead to an increased susceptibility to infections. Secondary immunodeficiency, however, is often a result of external factors, such as infection (e.g., HIV), malnutrition, or the action of certain drugs (e.g., corticosteroid therapy for prolonged periods). Immunocompromised patients have a higher risk of surgical complications, where observing strict protocols becomes essential to prevent infection (N/A, 1986). Identification of such conditions facilitates preoperative planning and postoperative adjustments in care by surgical nurses, who have to implement proper precautions and interventions to benefit vulnerable patients. The convergence of these common immune system disorders with surgical nursing practices emphasizes the need for complex and multifaceted patient care approaches.

6.2.1. Autoimmune Diseases

Autoimmune diseases pose a significant challenge in surgical nursing practice, as they involve a complex interaction between the immune system and the body's own tissues. In autoimmune diseases, the body's immune system mistakenly identifies normal cells as foreign pathogens and initiates an attack on them, resulting in inflammation and tissue damage. Examples are rheumatoid arthritis, lupus, and multiple sclerosis with various pathophysiological mechanisms. These conditions also make it difficult to manage surgically, as patients may experience altered immune reactions and delayed healing. It is also essential that the requirements and threats of such patients be familiar to surgical nurses, including higher rates of infection and slower healing because of the inherent autoimmune reactions. These are essential to consider in maximizing surgical function and holistic treatment ~~to~~ for patients. Autoimmune conditions often require a multidisciplinary approach that incorporates pharmacological, physical, and psychological therapies. Immunosuppressive therapy is also commonly utilized to suppress the autoimmune reaction, but comes with potential risks such as increased infection risk, leading to a significant challenge in the perioperative setting. Other challenges may include fatigue and chronic pain, which can complicate recovery and overall well-being. Surgical nurses must be knowledgeable of these complexities to provide specialized care that enhances the patient's recovery and diminishes the impact of such chronic illness. Increased awareness of the psychological factors, such as anxiety and depression, concerning chronic autoimmune disease, is critical in the formulation of holistic care. The new field of immunotherapy presents novel prospects for treating autoimmune diseases, underscoring the importance of further research and clinical trials in this area. As explained, regulatory T cells (Tregs) play a crucial role in maintaining tolerance and preventing the onset of autoimmunity. New protocols for Treg expansion create novel therapeutic opportunities for treating autoimmune diseases, as expanded Tregs are capable of effectively modulating immunity and inducing self-antigen tolerance. The impacts of such therapies would greatly enhance the success of surgery by mitigating the inflammatory responses that hinder healing (Bluestone et al., 2005). Additionally, understanding the psychological and physiological impacts on autoimmune patients can inform more comprehensive care models for surgical nursing (Segev et al., 2014). Acting on such knowledge, surgical nurses can play a crucial role in improving patient outcomes for those with autoimmune diseases (Figure 6.6).

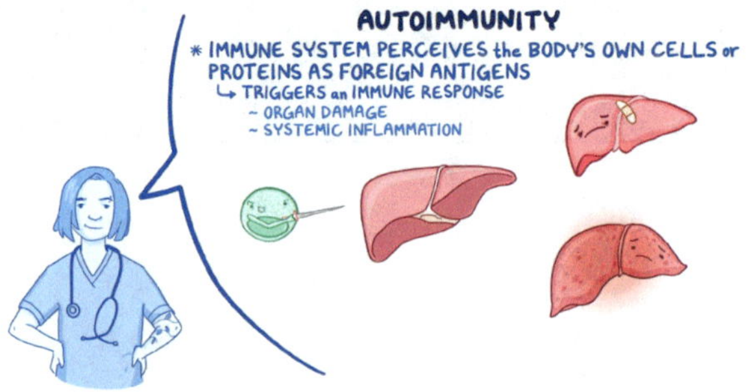

Figure 6.6. Autoimmunity.

Source: https://d16qt3wv6xm098.cloudfront.net/Tqv4Y01jSk_F_BbXrWBLXfLaTQaco0oW/_.jpg.

6.2.2. Immunodeficiency Disorders

Immunodeficiency disorders are among the most significant challenges in surgical nursing as they impair the body's ability to respond effectively to infection. Immunodeficiency disorders are classified into primary and secondary types. Primary immunodeficiencies, which are typically genetic in nature, affect the major components of the immune system, such as B and T lymphocytes, resulting in persistent infections and increased susceptibility to diseases. Secondary immunodeficiencies are induced by external factors, including chemotherapy, malnutrition, or diseases like HIV, that can severely damage the immune system. Surgical nurses need to understand these classifications due to the risk factors presented by patients during pre-operative workups, surgery, and post-operative care, necessitating an expert regimen of patient treatment for their compromised immune systems. Surgical plans for treating patients with immunodeficiency disorders entail a coordinated approach that involves intensive pre-surgical evaluation and deliberate surgical planning. The healthcare team must assess the extent of immunodeficiency by reviewing lab findings indicative of immune status to provide the most beneficial treatment regimen. Prophylactic antibiotics and other interventions may be necessary to avoid infection that could complicate the recovery process. In addition, surgical procedures can be altered to minimize bleeding and infection risks, designed according to the needs of the patient. Enhanced post-operative care protocols, like more cautious infection monitoring and careful wound care, are unavoidable to minimize complications to which these compromised patients will be vulnerable because of their compromised immune systems. Lastly, recent research has shown the role of nutrition in modulating immune function, particularly for immunocompromised patients. Studies demonstrate that certain dietary manipulations can enhance immune function, potentially normalizing immune mechanisms in immunocompromised hosts. As mentioned, foods play a beneficial role in modulating innate and acquired immunity, affecting such parameters as NK cell activity and T cell response (Kaminogawa et al., 2004). For operating room nurses, this translates into an increasingly holistic approach to patient care, with nutritional assessment and care integrated into the overall treatment protocol. Proper nutrition can have a twofold function in improving outcomes from surgery while mitigating complications from existing immunodeficiencies, underscoring the necessity for balanced care plans that consider both surgical and dietary considerations (Vykhrystenka et al., 2008) (Figure 6.7).

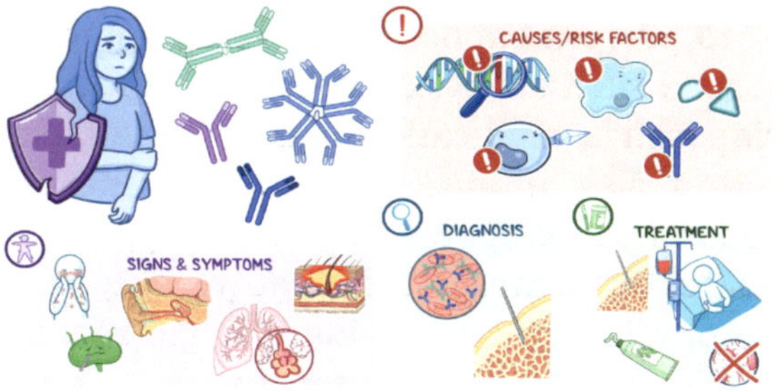

Figure 6.7. Immunodeficiency disorders.

Source: https://osmose-it.s3.amazonaws.com/Bh_IYcu3TQWR-Z-XYD-XKiz9RPiMvwJb/_.png.

6.2.3. Hypersensitivity Reactions

The basis of hypersensitivity reactions lies in the essential significance of the perception of immune mechanism concepts, notably in surgical nursing. Hypersensitivity reactions are undesirable immune responses that result in tissue damage or impairment. The classification of hypersensitivity reactions into four groups—Type I (immediate), Type II (antibody-dependent), Type III (immune complex-dependent), and Type IV (delayed-type)—helps to understand the mechanisms of allergic reactions. Type I hypersensitivity, for example, is hyperreactivity to environmental allergens with presentations ranging from mild (e.g., rhinitis) to lethal anaphylactic reactions. These reactions and their presentations must be recognized by surgical nurses to implement appropriate, timely, and effective interventions, especially when patients may be at risk of exposure to potential allergens during surgery. An awareness of the mechanisms, therefore, can prevent and treat hypersensitivity reactions in the operating room. One of the most crucial factors influencing susceptibility to hypersensitivity reactions is the mix of genetic and environmental factors. It has been observed that children are particularly susceptible to hypersensitivity, and various studies have identified genetic inheritance and environmental sensitization as potential causative factors for the development of allergies. This growing incidence of pediatric hypersensitivity makes early detection and intervention important. As Burns et al. (2019) expound, knowing these risk factors and their association with immune function will enable surgical nurses to anticipate possible complications. Because operating rooms inadvertently expose patients to allergens, awareness of demographic patterns and hypersensitivity risk factors is essential to improve patient outcomes and safeguard patient safety during surgery. In addition to identifying hypersensitivity reactions, therapeutic management strategies tailored to unique patient situations must be incorporated into operating room nursing practice. This requires awareness of the various hypersensitivity reaction types and their applications in clinical practice. For instance, early intervention and appropriate pharmacological management, including the use of antihistamines or epinephrine, are critical in anaphylaxis. Moreover, patient education plays a crucial role in preventing and managing hypersensitivity reactions, particularly in individuals with a known history of allergies. Nurses must engage patients in learning about their illnesses and preparation for potential allergic reactions during surgeries. By converting this knowledge into practice, surgical nurses can make significant contributions to enhancing patient care and safety, as they play an active role in both preoperative and postoperative settings (Burns et al., 2019). This holistic care for immune system disorders attests to the need for continuous education and sensitization in the dynamic setting of allergic reactions in surgical nursing (Figure 6.8).

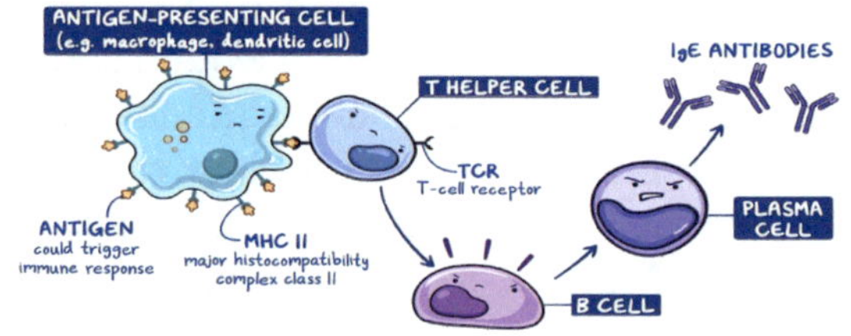

Figure 6.8. Hypersensitivity reactions.

Source: https://www.osmosis.org/_next/image?url=https%3A%2F%2Fd16qt3wv6xm098.cloudfront.net%2F7HfIE8beQBufvC4bj2zjQilDRjuCL2Hq%2F_.jpg&w=3840&q=75.

Test Your Knowledge

1. What is the difference between an autoimmune disorder and an immunodeficiency disorder?
2. How does HIV affect the body's immune system?

6.3. Allergic Reactions in Surgical Patients

Learning Outcome

1. Explain the types of allergic reactions
2. Define the symptoms and signs of allergic reactions
3. Describe the impact of allergies on surgical outcomes

Allergic reactions of patients undergoing surgery are a highly troublesome problem in surgical patient care and nursing. The body's reaction to allergenic substances by the immune system can lead to a variety of complications intraoperatively and postoperatively, making clinical management more difficult and prolonging recovery time. Allergic reactions vary in severity from insignificantly localized reactions to potentially fatal anaphylaxis, which requires immediate medical intervention. Operating room settings tend to present exposure to multiple potential allergens such as latex gloves, antiseptics, and perioperative medications. Identifying allergic reaction risk in patients through intensive preoperative screening is vital for preventing adverse outcomes. With knowledge of the pathophysiology underlying allergic reactions and the use of preventive methods, nurses can effectively mitigate the risks associated with operative procedures, thereby enhancing patient safety and overall surgical outcomes. The nurse's surgical responsibility for managing allergic reactions extends beyond preoperative assessment to include astute observation during the operation. Continuous observation of patients for signs of an allergic reaction is essential, especially as anesthesia and surgical techniques continue to evolve. For instance, administration of certain anesthetic drugs and adjuvant medications has been associated with hypersensitivity reactions, necessitating familiarity with their pharmacologic properties. Additionally, effective intraoperative communication among the surgical team will ensure averted delayed response in case of an allergy. Adopting procedure protocols in the process of identifying and responding to operating room allergic reactions will not only improve patient safety but also enable nurses to respond in a timely and effective manner. Such proactive management of allergies is a testament to the importance of education and training in operating room nursing practice. Postoperative care is also relevant in managing allergic reactions among surgical patients.

During postoperative periods, continual observation for any emergent allergic reactions in patients as they recover from surgery and anesthesia is necessary. These reactions may arise at various times and need continuous observation by nursing personnel. Awareness of cross-reactive potential among different allergens is particularly relevant in this context, especially when patients are initiated on novel medications or encounter various materials in their postoperative environment. Moreover, deployment of a holistic discharge plan that takes into account allergy awareness—e.g., potential manifestations of allergic reaction and medication directions—can influence patient outcomes immediately. By focusing on the entire surgical continuum, from preoperative assessment to postoperative care, nurses can be at the center of preventing anaphylactic reactions and maintaining the health of surgical patients despite their weakened immune systems (Figure 6.9).

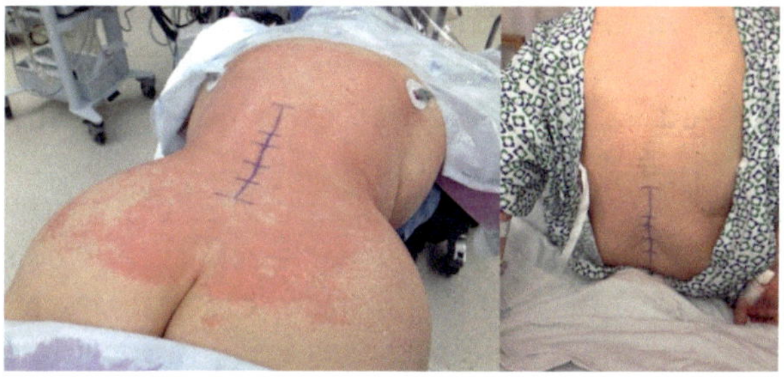

Figure 6.9. Allergic reactions in surgical patients.

Source: https://casereports.bmj.com/content/casereports/2015/bcr-2015-209660/F1.large.jpg.

6.3.1. Types of Allergic Reactions

Allergic reactions are classified into four broad categories based on their underlying immunological mechanism. Type I hypersensitivity, also known as immediate hypersensitivity, is a hyperactive immune reaction triggered by allergens such as pollen, food, or insect stings. This type is responsible for the production of Immunoglobulin E (IgE) antibodies, which bind to mast cells and basophils upon initial exposure. Re-exposure leads to the rapid release of histamines and other inflammatory mediators, which cause reactions like hives, asthma, or anaphylaxis. This occurs in a matter of minutes, underscoring the importance of discovering and controlling these reactions, particularly in a surgical setting where patients may experience adverse reactions to anesthetics or antiseptics, thus necessitating preoperative screening measures to reduce risk. Type II hypersensitivity, in contrast to the immediate nature of Type I, is cytotoxic in nature. In this type, the antibodies, usually IgG or IgM, are directed against specific cells, causing their killing. Classic examples include autoimmune hemolytic anemia and transfusion reactions, in which the patient's immune system mistakenly identifies foreign red blood cells as harmful. In the context of the operating room, an understanding of Type II reactions is crucial, especially where transfusions are involved, with an accent on blood type and cross-matching procedures. Secondly, disease-afflicted patients with autoimmune conditions open themselves up to such reactions, necessitating thorough preoperative testing to guide anesthetic and surgical interventions properly. Type III hypersensitivity involves reactions mediated by immune complexes that occur when antibodies and antigens interact to form complexes, inducing inflammation. This type can be observed in conditions such as serum sickness and certain types of vasculitides. The tissue deposition of the immune complexes leads to inflammation and tissue damage. About surgery, it is relevant to be cognizant of the potential for Type III reactions, particularly in patients receiving antibody therapy or with autoimmune diseases, because inflammatory reactions complicate postoperative recovery. Finally, Type IV hypersensitivity or delayed-type hypersensitivity results from T cells rather than antibodies and is more likely to result in dermatitis and transplant rejection.

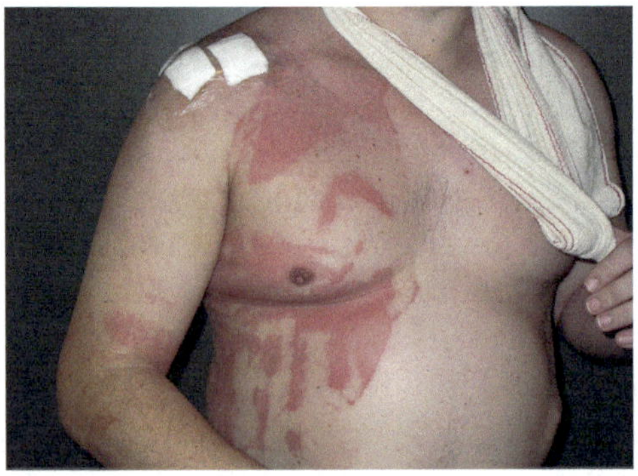

Figure 6.10. Acute skin lesions after surgical procedures.

Source: https://static.elsevier.es/multimedia/15782190/0000010400000009/v1_201310240051/S1578219013002084/v1_201310240051/en/main.assets/gr3.jpeg.

This complexity further underscores the necessity for proper patient evaluation and tailored perioperative care plans to prevent and treat any allergic reactions that may occur with surgical interventions (Figure 6.10).

6.3.2. Symptoms and Signs of Allergic Reactions

Allergic reactions are an indication of an inappropriate immune response to usually harmless substances referred to as allergens. The signs can be highly diverse, depending on the individual and the type of allergen. Urticaria (hives) and eczema are typical cutaneous signs that develop due to inflammation and vasodilation resulting from the release of histamine. The signs in the respiratory system may also arise, such as nasal congestion, sneezing, and wheezing due to bronchoconstriction and production of mucus. Gastrointestinal symptoms also occur, as nausea, vomiting, or diarrhea. Such presentations serve to emphasize the multifaceted nature of allergic reactions and the importance of attentive observation in surgical situations, where early detection of such symptoms can have significant consequences for patient safety and outcome. Of particular concern is anaphylaxis, a severe and potentially lethal allergic reaction that demands urgent treatment. Symptoms tend to develop rapidly, typically within minutes of the affected person being exposed to an allergen. The initial symptoms can vary from shortness of breath, swelling of the throat and tongue, and acute loss of blood pressure, which then progresses to shock. Other manifestations could include abdominal discomfort and cutaneous signs such as generalized urticaria. Prompt recognition and intervention are crucial, particularly in surgical nursing, since the anxiety induced by anaphylaxis complicates anesthesia and surgery management. Nursing practice is not only effective when acute symptoms are recognized, but also when emergency measures to maintain the patient's safety are initiated. Such measures can involve the administration of epinephrine and the prompt activation of emergency response teams. The implications of this sensitivity are far-reaching. In addition, surgical allergic reactions can be managed by taking a detailed history of the patient's medical history and identifying suspected allergens. Preoperative assessment should include thorough questioning about known allergies, past reactions to drugs, foods, and environmental allergens. This is important in preventing surgical and postoperative allergic reactions. Systematic education and communication among the healthcare professionals can facilitate an active allergy response in surgical nursing. Success can imply the initiation of open procedures for record-keeping and communication of allergies so that the healthcare team can be alerted to allergy risks. Overall, extensive knowledge of signs and symptoms of allergic reactions is crucial for enabling surgical nurses to enhance patient care and thereby maximize surgical outcomes.

6.3.3. Impact of Allergies on Surgical Outcomes

Allergic effects on surgical results are a critical consideration in surgical nursing, and an allergic reaction can complicate perioperative and postoperative treatment. Allergies, particularly drug, anesthetic, or operating materials allergies, might lead to increased morbidity due to increased risk of hypersensitivity reactions such as anaphylaxis with fatal consequences. Additionally, allergic responses may prolong recovery periods by causing further inflammation or complications, such as infection.

Nurses must be mindful when taking thorough patient histories to identify possible allergens so that ~~allergic~~ patients will require special strategies in anesthetic management and in operative planning according to their unique sensitivities. Knowledge of the patient's allergic profile thus becomes essential in maximizing surgical outcomes and preventing unnecessary risks. Besides, the prevalence of allergies is substantial in specific groups, which alters the typical reaction to surgical intervention. Children, for instance, have shown escalating rates of allergies, as indicated by a growing literature on immune-mediated hypersensitivity among the pediatric population (Burns et al., 2019). This rising prevalence has the connotation of necessitating sophisticated preoperative assessment about the special vulnerabilities of young patients, who may exhibit unpredictable allergic reactions. Surgeons and nurses must collaborate to develop tailored care plans that accommodate these allergies, possibly by selecting allergy tests or desensitization protocols prior to surgery.

These pre-emptive strategies are vital for improving both short-term surgical outcomes and long-term patient well-being, demonstrating the significance of individualized nursing care in the operating room. Finally, the recognition of the role of allergies in the success of surgery has expanded to evaluating necessary changes to accepted procedures and protocols within surgical settings. Incorporating current recommendations, such as the Pre-Participation Physical Evaluation guidelines for detecting prevalent health disorders, including allergies, plays a vital role in effectively addressing patients' requirements (Doughty et al., 2014). Through objective screening for allergy, doctors are not only able to ascertain patients' fitness for surgery but also significantly minimize the possibility of serious adverse events. Such improvements in the assessment of health history are intended to ensure that states of allergy are incorporated into the overall surgical plan. Thus, heightened awareness and understanding of the role of allergies within the operating room ultimately lead to optimized patient safety, reduced rates of complications, and improved recovery trajectories (Figure 6.11).

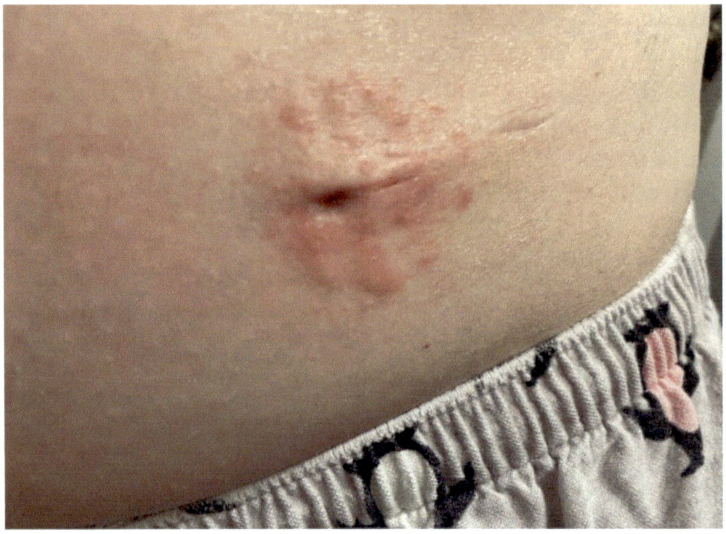

Figure 6.11. Allergies on surgical outcomes.

Source: https://www.newyorkliposuction.com/wp-content/uploads/2024/10/idxehox7qe6a1-1024x768.jpg.

Test Your Knowledge

1. What are common signs of an allergic reaction that nurses should monitor for during surgery?
2. Why is it important to review a patient's allergy history before administering anesthesia?

6.4. Role of Surgical Nurses in Managing Immune Disorders

Learning Outcome

1. Identify the assessment and identification of immune disorders
2. Define the patient education and counseling
3. Describe the collaboration with interdisciplinary teams of immune disorders

The role of surgical nurses in managing immune disorders is becoming increasingly critical in healthcare today, particularly due to the complexity of surgical procedures and the higher complication risks associated with patients who have compromised immune responses. Surgical nurses must have in-depth knowledge of the immune response in order to effectively monitor and provide care for operating patients. This includes identifying any underlying immune disorders and adjusting patient management policies as needed to minimize risks during and after surgical procedures. They also have the duty of educating patients regarding their condition, the nature of any suggested procedure, and potential allergic reactions or complications, thereby establishing a knowledgeable and empowered patient relationship that can significantly impact outcomes in recovery. Furthermore, operating room nurses play an essential part in the implementation of evidence-based practice that is highly vital in the prevention of transfusion complications during surgery, particularly among patients who have immune disorders. Blood transfusion usually is necessary but comes with inherent risks, particularly in immunocompromised patients. Studies show that despite strict clinical precautions, errors in the transfusion process can cause patients significant harm. Operating room nurses have the mandate to strictly adhere to procedures that ensure the identification of the correct blood unit for a specific patient and monitor for adverse effects throughout the process. The application of technological innovations, such as barcoding systems on patient identifiers, is an efficient measure in mitigating the risk of transfusion errors to guarantee increased patient security throughout blood product surgical procedures (Vasiliki, 2011). In addition to direct patient care, surgical nurses play a crucial role in advocating for policies and protocols that promote safety and efficacy in surgeries involving patients with immune disorders. They collaborate closely with multidisciplinary teams, including surgeons, anesthesiologists, and pharmacists, to ensure holistic care approaches that address the complex needs of these patients. Operating room nurses help create pathways of care to outline specific interventions aimed at reducing the risks of surgical site infections, allergic reactions, and other complications related to the immune system. Ongoing professional development and active engagement in research on immune disorders form the core prerequisites for operating room nurses, whereby updated knowledge will allow them to implement best practice and adapt new technologies, improving surgical care for patients with immune system disorders and related allergic reactions (N/A, 1986) (Figure 6.12).

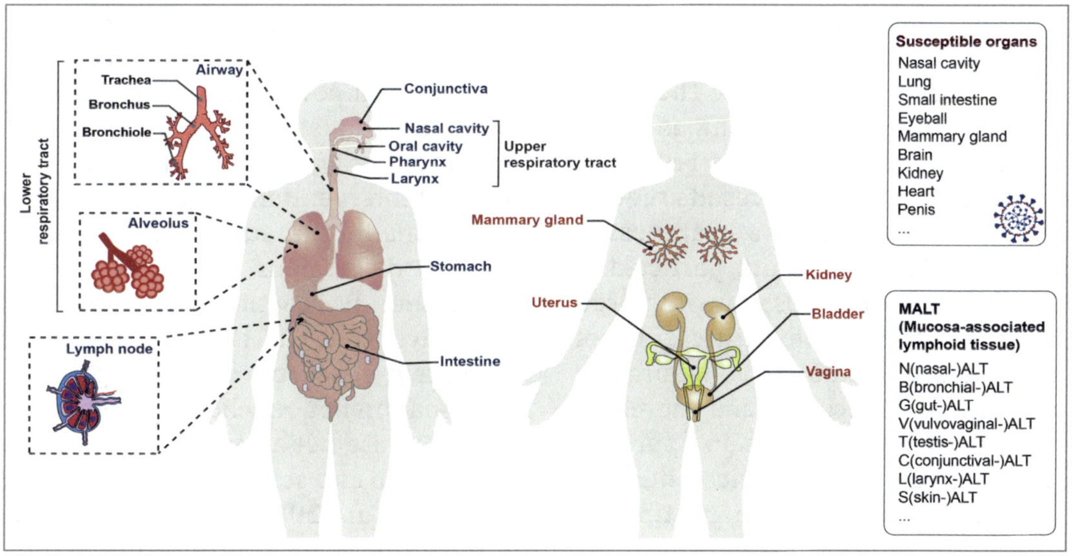

Figure 6.12. Mucosal immune response.

Source: https://media.springernature.com/full/springer-static/image/art%3A10.1038%2Fs41392-024-02043-4/MediaObjects/41392_2024_2043_Fig1_HTML.png.

6.4.1. Assessment and Identification of Immune Disorders

The diagnosis and assessment of immune disorders require extensive familiarity with the immune system's intricate processes, as well as the complex factors that may be implicated in dysregulation. Proper assessment begins with a detailed patient history, during which physicians obtain information on family history, past allergic episodes, and environmental exposures that may lead to potential hypersensitivity disorders. Clinical examinations typically involve a physical examination, along with laboratory tests, to determine abnormal immune responses. According to existing studies, a sharp rise in pediatric allergies necessitates an in-depth analysis of the environmental, genetic, and immunologic determinants for hypersensitivities. Examples such as environmental sensitization and genetic heredity are significant determinants of allergy development, underscoring the need for proper assessment protocols to identify these risk factors early in the patient's trajectory (Burns et al., 2019). Laboratory examinations are an essential component of the immune disorder evaluation process, giving vital information about various immune parameters. Blood work, such as complete blood counts (CBC), immunoglobulin levels, and allergen-specific testing, helps clinicians diagnose autoimmune diseases and allergies. These are complemented by diagnostic imaging and skin tests that further define an immune response. The clinical implications of these results require not only clinical expertise but also awareness of the patient's general state of health, particularly in surgical patients with possibly impaired immune status. Effective identification of immune disorders depends on collaboration between clinicians and specialists and, therefore, there is a need for a multidisciplinary approach to improving outcomes in surgical nursing (Vasiliki, 2011). In addition, the continuous advancement of technology is also significant to the improvement in the evaluation and identification of immune disorders. Advances, such as extensive genomic assessment and superior immunoassays, have enabled doctors to transcend conventional methods of evaluation. These technologies help accurately identify specific immune disorders, enabling the design of targeted treatment protocols. For instance, the increasing application of personalized medicine in immunology holds promise to design individualized care plans based on the patient's own immune environment. With continued study revealing the intricacies of immune pathology, operating room nurses must keep pace with new technologies and methods. This data not only maximizes their assessment abilities but also ensures that patients receive effective, timely treatments, particularly those prescribed to meet their unique immune needs (Vasiliki, 2011; Burns et al., 2019).

6.4.2. Patient Education and Counseling

Patient education and counseling are significant roles in surgical nursing, particularly when handling immune system ailments and allergies. Effective communication between patients and healthcare providers maximizes treatment compliance and success. By informing patients accurately about their conditions, nurses can empower them to take a more active role in their care. This empowerment is especially important for individuals with allergies, as education regarding triggers and symptoms can lead to prompt intervention and effective management. Additionally, the educational process should include discussions of risk factors associated with allergic reactions, including hereditary and environmental factors, as noted in recent pediatric research. The integration of this information not only helps patients learn about their disease but also encourages the proactive prevention and self-management of the disease (Burns et al., 2019). Patient education is not merely the delivery of information; it involves developing patient-specific counseling plans that respond to patients' unique needs. In operating room nursing, working with the complexities of immune system dysfunctions requires an integrative approach that tackles the individual needs of each patient. Personalized education can include the creation of customized plans of action for managing allergic reactions, with emphasis on avoiding familiar allergens and recognizing anaphylaxis onset. Beyond that, engagement in decision-making strengthens trust and increases the possibility of compliance with future medical advice. Evidence suggests that actively engaged patients in their treatment plans tend to experience better health outcomes and a higher quality of life (Burns et al., 2019). Thus, surgical nurses must prioritize patient-centered education and counseling to facilitate the effective management of immune disorders affecting the immune system. Counseling for potential allergic reactions is also crucial in preoperative care, particularly for hypersensitive patients. Understanding that operations have the potential to expose patients to various allergens—such as latex or specific medications—is a core reason why preoperative education is essential. Nurses are responsible for conducting thorough assessments to learn about past allergic responses and inform patients about the potential impact on their surgical procedures.

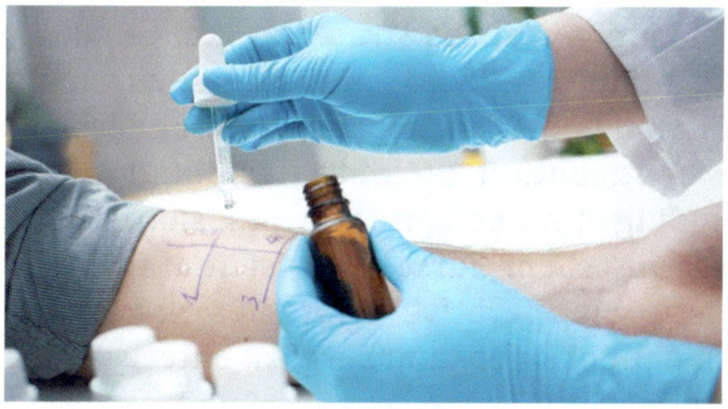

Figure 6.13. Allergy and immunology.

Source: https://cdn.castleconnolly.com/dims4/default/406557f/2147483647/strip/true/crop/1000x563+0+0/resize/840x473!/quality/90/?url=http%3A%2F%2Fcastle-connolly-brightspot.s3.us-east-1.amazonaws.com%2Fdf%2Fa7%2F3432d4134088bf7add8ac125dbc1%2Fpillar-allergy-immunology-49-1200x675.jpg.

Educating patients on the significance of reporting allergies makes them aware of the critical elements of their health and safety. Also, the introduction of successful counseling methods can reduce anxiety associated with the surgical procedure as well as emphasize the need for adherence to sequential preoperative protocols. The ultimate goal is to develop a shared environment that prioritizes patient safety and enables individuals to manage their health issues effectively (Figure 6.13).

6.4.3. Collaboration with Interdisciplinary Teams

Effective collaboration with multi-disciplinary teams is critical in the management of immunological system disorders and allergic reactions in surgical nursing. Surgical nurses can handle patients with complex requirements due to their medical histories, particularly those with food allergies or immunological disorders. Collaboration with nutrition specialists, allergists, psychologists, and other experts allows surgical nurses to design detailed care plans that address the complex issues presented by these disorders. This team-based approach ensures that all aspects of a patient's health are considered, leading to improved outcomes. The integration of multiple professional opinions not only enhances the quality of care but also provides a comprehensive picture of a patient's condition, allowing for tailored interventions to manage both physical and psychological aspects of surgical treatment. The complex nature of allergic reactions and immune disorders necessitates ongoing communication and coordination between team members. For instance, children with Avoidant/Restrictive Food Intake Disorder (ARFID) can require the intervention of multiple experts. Pediatric nurses collaborate with mental health professionals to implement Cognitive Behavioral Therapy (CBT) and Family-Based Therapy (FBT), and also nutritionists to ensure food restrictions are managed accordingly. Such collaboration is crucial to effectively guide families through the process of managing allergies while maintaining optimal nutrition. Incorporating psychological care into surgical nursing practice benefits not only the patient but also comforts families, making the surgical process and recovery more straightforward. Interdisciplinary practice also facilitates the development of clinical guidelines that suit individual patient needs with immune disorders and allergies. Healthcare professionals can utilize shared platforms that consolidate best practices across the professions to close care gaps and enhance patient safety. For example, treatment protocol standardization that considers medications and interventions across specialties can significantly mitigate risks of allergic reactions during surgery. As highlighted in current literature, the role of specialists in complementary pediatrics, i.e., surgical and psychosocial professionals, plays a pivotal role in creating evidence-based interventions to meet the particular needs of pediatric patients presenting allergic reactions and immune system issues (N/A, 2021; Bosco et al., 2024). Overall, therefore, this kind of interdisciplinary collaboration is essential in delivering whole-person care and enables the overall vision of maximizing patient well-being within surgical settings.

Test Your Knowledge

1. How can surgical nurses help prevent infection in immunocompromised patients?
2. What precautions should a surgical nurse take when caring for a patient with an autoimmune disorder?

6.5. Preoperative Considerations for Patients with Immune Disorders

Learning Outcome

1. Describe the preoperative assessment protocol
2. Define the medication management and adjustments;
3. Discuss the infection control measures

Preoperative care of patients with immune disorders is vital during preparation for surgery and for optimal outcomes. These patients vary in their response to surgical stress and need a tailored preoperative assessment. Care should be taken in their history, including that of the specific immune disorder, any related comorbidities, and previous medication history. For instance, medical patients under immunosuppressive therapy ~~may be~~ are at a higher risk of infections or complications from the operative procedure. Surgeons will need to create individualized strategies that can include drug modification to minimize such risks or immunomodulation before surgery. Furthermore, the contribution of multidisciplinary teams, including immunologists, anesthesiologists, and operating room nurses, is essential to prepare holistic preoperative strategies that balance both patient safety and surgical efficacy equally. Besides drug management, preoperative teaching is a pillar of improving outcomes among patients with immune disorders. Patients might have fear-related issues with underlying diseases, which could undermine their preparedness for surgery. Effective communication of the surgery process, associated risks, and post-operative care can diminish fear and improve compliance with preoperative treatment. Apart from that, it can also enhance the patient's immunity by educating patients on the importance of maintaining their own health through a healthy diet and compliance with any prescribed immunoenhancing interventions. Shared decision-making with the patient promotes a sense of empowerment, which in turn leads to increased satisfaction and adherence to the surgery. Thus, preoperative education sessions should include holistic teaching components to address both physical and psychological care. Finally, patients with immune disorders should be tested preoperatively to evaluate potential allergic reactions, as these can significantly influence surgical planning and care. A thorough history of previous allergic reactions, including both medication and environmental triggers, can inform the selection of anesthetic agents and perioperative medications to minimize the risk of a reaction. The surgical team must be prepared to implement procedures for the early detection and management of potential allergic reactions, as these are likely to lead to significant complications.

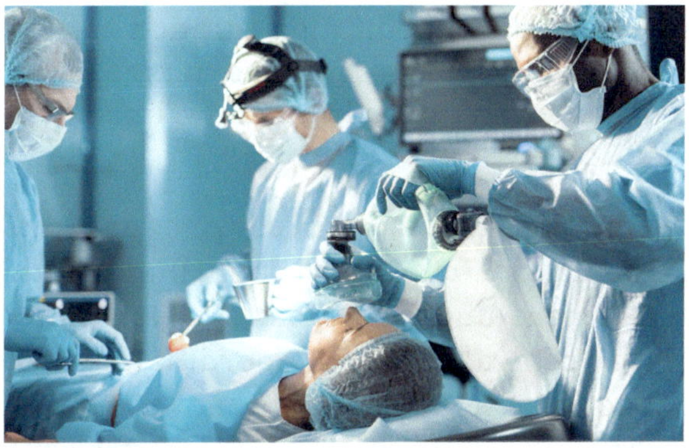

Figure 6.14. Anesthesiology.

Source: https://external-content.duckduckgo.com/iu/?u=https%3A%2F%2Fwww.jeffersonhealth.org%2Fcontent%2Fdam%2Fhealth2021%2Fimages%2Fphotos%2Fstock%2Fpeople%2Fclinical%2Fanesthesia-operating-room-team.jpg&f=1&nofb=1&ipt=e9e213c8bca9ef146f87ece6f3236716c012c0755fd6983977738d115f80bccc.

Through the integration of allergy tests into preoperative assessment, healthcare providers can enhance patient safety and optimize surgical outcomes. Effective management of immune disorders and allergies is an ongoing process, and continuous surveillance in the perioperative period is warranted to address emergent matters promptly, ultimately advancing the specialization of surgical nursing practice in vulnerable populations (Figure 6.14).

6.5.1. Preoperative Assessment Protocols

Preoperative assessment policies play a very crucial role in surgical nursing, particularly in the management of patients with immune disorders or allergies. Not only do these policies help evaluate the overall health of patients, but they also identify potential complications that may arise during and after surgery. A practical preoperative assessment includes a thorough medical history, evaluation of the patient's immune status, and examination of any current allergies. This information enables anesthesiologists and surgeons to tailor anesthetic techniques and operative procedures to minimize risk. Furthermore, careful attention to pre-existing diseases, such as asthma or autoimmune disorders, is capable of avoiding significant intraoperative and postoperative complications that threaten patient recovery and wound healing, therefore optimizing surgical outcome. Of all immune system diseases, a stringent preoperative evaluation is paramount. This involves familiarizing oneself with the patient's status, for instance, whether they are immunocompromised or have experienced hypersensitivity reactions. Protocols should encompass an interdisciplinary process in which surgical teams collaborate with specialists to plan the safest operative approaches. For instance, patients with a history of anaphylaxis may require some preoperative medication to prevent allergy reactions in the course of surgery. Additionally, it is imperative to evaluate immunomodulatory therapy because such drugs significantly contribute to the modulation of the body's response to surgical stress. By embracing risk assessment using well-documented protocols, nurses can implement planned interventions aimed at reducing complications, such as postoperative infections resulting from poor immune responses. Additionally, the significance of preoperative protocols extends to the treatment of postoperative complications, such as edema, which may be exacerbated in patients with underlying allergic conditions. Recent research has shown that the interaction between edema and surgical outcomes underscores the importance of systematic patient assessment before any surgery. Proper documentation of a patient's baseline health enables the evaluation of changes after surgery, directing appropriate intervention in the case of undeserved edema or inflammatory responses. Preventive measures, such as controlling fluid intake and administering anti-inflammatory medication, can further minimize these phenomena. Thus, the utilization of robust protocols not only facilitates the enhancement of surgical proficiency but also the comprehension of preoperative elements that influence the trajectory of recovery and patient safety overall (Andreani et al., 2016; da Silveira et al., 2018).

6.5.2. Medication Management and Adjustments

Effective management of drugs is vital in surgical nursing, particularly for the treatment of immune system disorders and allergic states. Patients with immune system disorders and allergic patients tend to have complex drug histories that need careful assessment of their pharmacotherapeutic needs. Evaluation of the effectiveness and side effects of the medication is also critical, particularly because the patient may be on corticosteroids or immunosuppressants that alter immune responses and surgical outcomes. As highlighted by some studies, comprehensive medication management encompasses not only the proper selection of medications but also ongoing modifications in relation to the patient's individual physiological responses and surgical requirements. Careful monitoring ensures that perioperative drug-induced adverse effects, such as heightened allergic reactions, are evaded and better patient outcomes are guaranteed (Cairns et al., 2022). Dosage adjustments are usually necessary in response to unexpected patient reactions throughout the perioperative period. In surgical practice, this involves the ability to immediately adjust dosages or switch drugs when encountering allergies or complications resulting from a patient's underlying immune condition. For instance, if the operating patient is having an allergic response to a routine anesthetic, there will be a need to halt the agent or administer an alternative immediately. Changes such as these are not only important in managing the immediate clinical problem but also require a proper understanding of the patient's medical history and drug interaction, since any modification may have adverse impacts on the patient's immune system. Appropriate and pre-emptive medication titration can lead to better surgical outcomes and minimize risks for postoperative complications (Witmanowski et al., 2019).

Furthermore, interprofessional collaboration is crucial for optimal medication management during surgery. Surgical nurses play a central role in coordinating with anesthesiologists, pharmacists, and physicians to ensure complete understanding and optimization of every area of a patient's medication regimen. This collaboration helps identify patient allergies, assess drug interaction risks, and determine the need for alternative treatments, all of which are crucial when treating patients with compromised immune systems. Further, continuous education of nurses regarding the latest advancements in drug selection and drug protocols can enhance the quality of treatment provided to such patients. By progressing interdisciplinarity, surgical nursing can improve medication management significantly, resulting in better, safer, and more efficient care for patients with immune system illnesses and allergic reactions (Cairns et al., 2022).

6.5.3. Infection Control Measures

Practicing infection control precautions form a part of surgical nursing, particularly keeping in mind the vulnerability of patients with immune disorders as well as allergic patients. The operating suite, where invasive procedures are performed, demands strict conformity to procedures that minimize the risk of pathogen spread. Hand washing, the use of personal protective equipment (PPE), and proper sterilization of equipment are the necessary pillars of infection control. Such practices not only protect the operating team but also their patients, particularly those whose immunity may already be compromised. Implementation of these measures is crucial in preventing postoperative complications and improving overall patient outcomes, thereby confirming the need for vigilance and adherence to current guidelines throughout the surgical process. Furthermore, understanding the specific risks associated with both immune system disorders and allergic reactions can inform the development of tailored infection control strategies. For instance, patients with compromised immune function may experience heightened susceptibility to hospital-acquired infections, making it imperative that surgical teams incorporate enhanced surveillance and rapid response protocols. This includes monitoring for the development of infection during the postoperative period and also adjusting antibiotic prophylaxis based on the patient's medical history. In addition, the reduction of exposure to allergens within the operating room environment for patients with known allergies is imperative. Through the provision of a sterile and allergen-free environment, surgical nurses can provide assurance that minimizes inflammatory reactions, which may complicate healing, thereby enhancing the operative experience to be safer. Lastly, continuous training and education in infection control procedures among surgical nursing staff is critical to the prevention of the evolving threats posed by infectious agents and patient vulnerability. Up-to-date knowledge on evolving pathogens, resistance, and emerging infection control technologies enables surgical nurses to remain proactive in guarding their patients' health. This vigilance is particularly relevant because studies, such as one demonstrating immune modulation via relaxation, highlight the intimate interaction between mental processes and immune function (Albaladejo-Blázquez et al., 2014). Therefore, combining holistic care with rigorous infection control practices can lead to improved recovery patterns for immune-compromised patients, ultimately benefiting from enhanced levels of care in surgical nursing (N/A, 1986) (Figure 6.15).

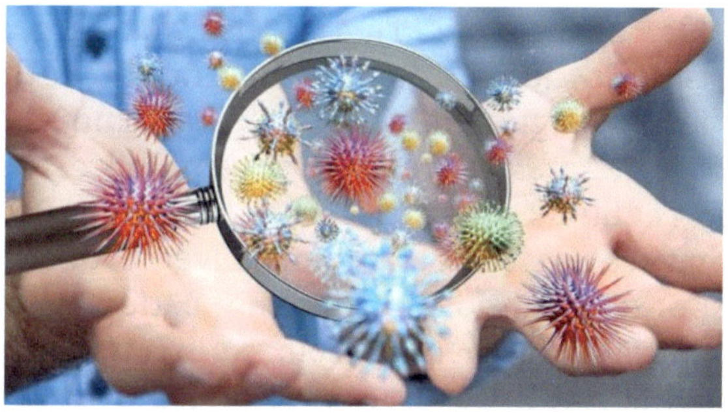

Figure 6.15. Infection prevention.

Source: https://www.belmatt.co.uk/wp-content/uploads/2020/09/infection_control-639x357.jpg.

Test Your Knowledge

1. Why is it important to assess immune function before surgery in immunocompromised patients?
2. What special precautions should be taken during the preoperative period for patients with autoimmune diseases?

6.6. Postoperative Care for Patients with Allergic Reactions

Learning Outcome

1. Describe the monitoring for allergic reactions
2. State the management of allergic symptoms
3. Know the documentation and reporting procedures

Postoperative care of patients with allergic reactions is a complex phenomenon that requires a thorough understanding of both surgical and immunological elements affecting recovery. Postoperative patients may experience allergic reactions that complicate their recovery and overall healing process. Nursing staff are key to observing signs that could indicate an allergic reaction, such as rash, swelling, or shortness of breath. Prompt recognition and intervention are critical, as the response to allergens can rise to more severe complications, such as anaphylaxis. This implies that surgical nursing practice should include thorough patient allergic assessments before and after surgery. Successful postoperative practices may also require consultation with medical teams to mitigate risk factors for adverse allergic responses, additionally ensuring patient safety and optimal recovery outcomes. Nutrition plays a crucial role in postoperative care, particularly in patients with hypersensitivity reactions. It has been demonstrated that nutrients influence the immune function, and hence must be regulated in postoperative patients. Certain foods with established immune-modulating properties can facilitate postoperative recovery, particularly in patients who have suffered from hypersensitivity or autoimmune diseases. Personalized meal plans to remove allergens and add immunostimulatory foods can contribute to recovery, reduce inflammation, and enhance overall health. It not only addresses the acute allergic reaction but also has a positive effect on patients' overall well-being in the long term since adequate postoperative nutrition can restore immune mechanisms disrupted by allergies or surgical stress. Hence, nutritional aspects become enable a smoother recovery process. Emotional and psychological treatment are also essential for managing patients who experience allergic reactions after surgery. Stress from surgery, coupled with the presence of allergic complications, can significantly influence a patient's emotional well-being. Nurses play a crucial role in creating a caring atmosphere that fosters both physical and emotional healing. They should communicate with patients, enlightening them about allergic reactions and reassuring them about their care plan and expected outcomes. Encouragement by doctors can also help patients express their concerns and symptoms more effectively. This model of postoperative care integrates so effectively as it not only reduces anxiety but also empowers patients in their health. The synergy of effective medical management with psychotherapy can yield enhanced recovery outcomes and a better quality of life among individuals with allergic reactions following surgery (Figure 6.16).

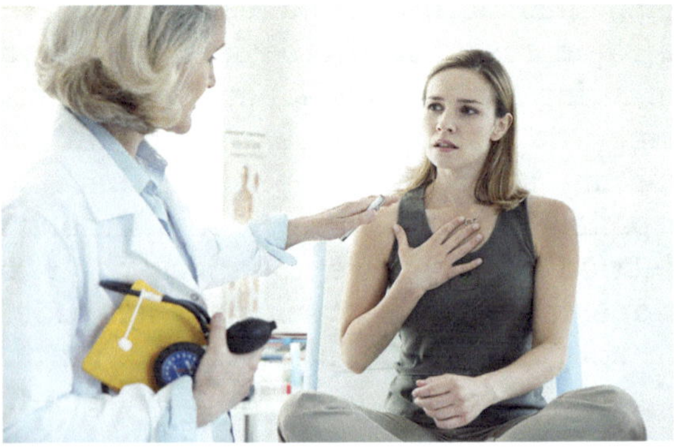

Figure 6.16. Allergy treatments.

Source: https://www.australianallergycentre.com.au/wp-content/uploads/2019/04/treatment.jpg.

6.6.1. Monitoring for Allergic Reactions

Surveillance of allergic reactions is a must in surgical nursing for patient safety and well-being. This includes vigilant observation for signs of hypersensitivity after and during surgeries, particularly in patients with known allergy histories or those under the influence of certain allergens. Nurses are responsible for identifying early signs of allergic reactions and understanding how these signs can manifest through skin effects, breathing problems, or gastrointestinal issues. By having high sensitivity and conducting adequate preoperative assessments, surgical nurses can effectively reduce risks associated with allergic reactions. This process not only builds confidence in patients but also enhances general surgery outcomes via the prevention of complications that may arise due to undiagnosed allergic reactions. Moreover, the work of the surgical nurse is not confined to mere observation alone; it encompasses extensive documentation and immediate intervention when an allergic response is noted. For instance, if a patient is exhibiting signs of anaphylaxis, immediate intervention is essential. This may involve administering immediate medication, such as epinephrine, in conjunction with supportive care interventions to stabilize the patient. Efficient communication among the operating team and other health practitioners is also critical at this time. By developing collaborative practice, nurses ensure that the entire team is well-informed and can effectively manage potential allergic reactions, thereby improving patient safety. Incorporating evidence-based alerting protocols for monitoring allergic reactions further enhances the nursing function of preventing adverse effects of immune disorders on the immune system in surgical settings. The presence of allergies, particularly in children, adds to the complexity involved in monitoring allergic reactions in operating room nursing. Rising pediatric hypersensitivity, as documented in recent studies, makes comprehending risk factors concerning allergic reactions increasingly important. Sensitization in the environment, genetic predisposition, and a history of allergic reaction are all factors that may contribute to an increased risk. By educating patients and their families about such factors, surgical nurses can enhance preoperative care and predict potential allergic reactions even before they occur. Continuous monitoring and education are integral to the process of preventing hypersensitivity reactions that could lead to serious complications in younger patients. These issues are not only discussed in informing present-day surgical practice but also echo the need for ongoing study within the topic area, as outlined in contemporary literature on pediatric allergy and its role in surgical nursing (N/A, 1986; Burns et al., 2019) (Figure 6.17).

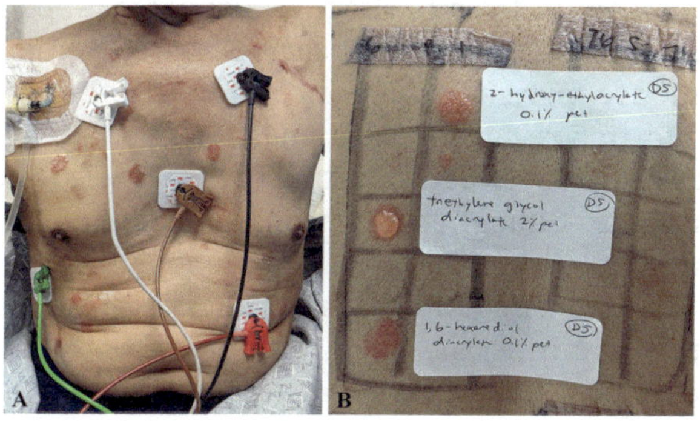

Figure 6.17. (A) Allergic contact dermatitis to electrocardiogram electrodes in a patient undergoing continuous cardiac monitoring prior to heart transplantation. (B) Patch testing after discharge revealed strongly positive reactions to multiple acrylates, which were confirmed to be present in the electrodes.

Source: https://www.researchgate.net/publication/362480564/figure/fig1/AS:11431281107228858@1670987751319/A-Allergic-contact-dermatitis-to-electrocardiogram-electrodes-in-a-patient-undergoing.jpg.

6.6.2. Management of Allergic Symptoms

The management of allergic reactions is a crucial area of surgical nursing, particularly considering the potential for adverse reactions to occur during and after surgery. Management of allergies necessitates knowledge of the patient's specific allergic reactions and appropriate intervention measures. One of the primary interventions involves the use of antihistamines that can alleviate symptoms by disrupting histamine activity in the body. Corticosteroids may also be employed to reduce inflammation in severe allergic reactions. Tailor-made treatment regimens are essential, considering the patient's history of allergic reactions and medication. Implementing proactive practices, such as preoperative assessment that identifies likely allergens, can significantly enhance patient safety and deliver an effective management plan in the course of surgical care. Surgical nursing practice more and more directs its attention to education regarding the management of allergic reactions between healthcare providers and patients. Education is essential in enhancing patient understanding of the potential allergens they may encounter during their treatment. Staff training is also necessary; medical personnel should be adequately trained in the spectrum of allergic reactions, ranging from minor to significant anaphylaxis. Adherence to standardized protocols of allergy management in operating rooms ensures that everyone can respond suitably and promptly. In addition, patient education on signs and symptoms of allergic reactions can empower individuals to play an active role in engaging with healthcare providers. These educational programs ultimately lead to earlier diagnosis and treatment of allergic reactions, thereby enhancing surgical success and safety in patients (Burns et al., 2019). To further enhance the management of allergic symptoms, the existence of multidisciplinary teams is crucial. This multidisciplinary approach involves collaborative effort by allergists, surgical staff, and nursing staff in creating individualized care plans. Regular interdisciplinary sessions could facilitate the sharing of patient allergy data and the identification of the at-risk population for allergic reactions during surgery. Improved strategies in management can be offered by advances in molecular immunology, as future therapies could target the mechanisms of allergic reactions. Conducting and reviewing research on risk factors for the development of allergic manifestations, especially in children, would provide the foundation for designing preventive interventions. With an increasing understanding of allergic reactions, surgical nursing must adapt and integrate new evidence-based practices into its practice to enhance patient care and outcomes (N/A, 1986).

6.6.3. Documentation and Reporting Procedures

Effective reporting and documentation procedures are essential for realizing patient safety and enhancing quality care in surgical nursing, particularly in cases involving immune system diseases and allergic reactions. Accurate documentation facilitates efficient information sharing among healthcare providers, thereby reducing the likelihood of medical errors in transfusion procedures and other critical interventions. For instance, close familiarity with the patient's relevant medical history, including specific allergies and immune responses, enables the nursing staff to anticipate potential complications most likely to arise from surgery. In this way, this anticipation proves invaluable in creating a tailored care plan that responds to the specific needs of every patient, allowing for appropriate precautions to be taken before, during, and after surgical procedures. Moreover, the applicability of documentation extends beyond actual patient interaction; it underlies responsibility and compliance with present policies. Operating room nurses have an obligation to document transfusion processes in detail, including verifying patient identification and tracking the administration of blood components. Practitioner failure is reported to be responsible for most transfusion errors, according to studies, underpinning the need for systematic and methodical reporting procedures (Vasiliki, 2011). With the adoption of advanced documentation practices, such as the use of electronic health records and standardized forms, surgical nurses are able to effectively prevent errors and consequently enhance patient safety and quality of care. Moreover, such practices will assist in guaranteeing compliance with legal and regulatory requirements, which are key in any healthcare setting. In addition to standard documentation, the utilization of technology has significantly transformed reporting procedures in surgical nursing. Innovations like barcode medication administration systems enhance the accuracy of drug administration and patient identification, greatly reducing the risk of adverse events (Vasiliki, 2011). In addition, continued education on emerging technologies and best practices is essential for nursing professionals to stay current with the latest developments that can be used to improve care delivery. These learning materials not only keep nurses up to date on procedural updates but also reiterate the importance of adhering to meticulous documentation protocols. In general, by adopting both cutting-edge and traditional reporting methods, operating room nursing can seamlessly navigate the technicalities of immune system diseases and allergic reactions, ultimately resulting in improved patient outcomes.

Test Your Knowledge

1. What are the key nursing interventions after a patient experiences an intraoperative allergic reaction?
2. Why is ongoing monitoring necessary in the postoperative period for patients with a history of allergies?

SUMMARY

It is crucial for surgical nurses to comprehend immune diseases and allergic processes because they have a significant bearing on patient outcomes. The sophisticated processes involved in the immune system, particularly hypersensitivity reactions, highlight how surgical nurses must grasp the intricacy of allergic reactions. With continued medical research, particularly for child allergy and risk factors such as genetic preconditions and environmental etiology, surgical specialists have to stay abreast with the current state of these fields. Overall knowledge enables nurses to anticipate potential complications from allergic reactions that may occur during and after surgery. Increased vigilance equips healthcare professionals to advocate for personalized interventions that mitigate risk, underscoring the nursing role in promoting patient care and safety during surgical operations (Burns et al., 2019). Moreover, the imperative to improve transfusion practices within the surgical environment cannot be overemphasized. Safety of blood transfusion is directly proportional to the efficiency of surgical nursing, in which strict observation at every step of the whole process of transfusion becomes of great concern. At various levels, errors can occur, and therefore, sharp vigilance by nurses is essential to ensure that the correct blood components are administered to the correct patients. Introduction of new technologies, such as barcode systems, becomes essential to minimize risk and maximize patient safety. This technology innovation within healthcare not only facilitates the transfusion process but also enhances the nurses' ability to monitor and respond to complications promptly. Continuous training on transfusion risks equips nurses with the competencies necessary to advance practice results and outcomes of patients (Vasiliki, 2011). Finally, the development of surgical nursing relative to immune system illness and allergic conditions should occur with ongoing research and development of evidence-based practice. Addressing the complexity of patient care relative to allergic reactions is essential in improving surgical outcomes. With ongoing advancements in surgical intervention, the practice of nursing must be proactive in researching new treatment modalities and advocating for patients' issues within the perioperative environment. The convergence of clinical practice in immune dysfunction and allergy, informed by current evidence, will foster an integrated model of surgical nursing that emphasizes patient safety, quality care, and desirable outcomes. The commitment to acquire and apply such ideas reflects the dynamic nature of surgical nursing practice and its pivotal position in patient-centered healthcare (Vasiliki, 2011; Burns et al., 2019).

One of the most important aspects of surgical nursing is understanding the subtleties of immune system diseases and their impact on patient care. These diseases have the potential to result in grave complications during surgery, primarily due to their effects on wound healing and infection susceptibility. Acute lymphoblastic leukemia provides a perfect illustration of the intricate relationship between surgical risk and immunocompetence. While survival rates for such patients have improved, they typically suffer from severe toxic effects related to treatment procedures; these include conditions such as pancreatitis and neuropathy, which complicate postoperative recovery and necessitate strict preoperative screening (Attarbaschi et al., 2016). Recognizing the specific consequences of these conditions, thus, facilitates surgical nurses in managing the risks to be effectively overcome. Also, allergic reactions are another added layer of complexity in the area of immune system disease that surgical nurses face. Allergies can trigger a mild reaction to anaphylactic shock that is potentially fatal. Operating room settings are particularly vulnerable to allergic reactions because patients are exposed to potential allergens within surgical equipment or medications. The pathophysiology of allergic responses in such instances is most commonly based on hypersensitivity reactions that can prove pivotal in disrupting surgery. For example, anaphylactic attacks under anesthesia can rapidly lead to harmful consequences, which is why in-depth patient history assessment is necessary (Segev et al., 2014). Recognition of these risks enables surgical nursing professionals to implement preventive measures, such as preoperative screening for allergens and establishing emergency protocols for the efficient management of severe reactions. Furthermore, the convergence of immune response with psychological factors also holds significant importance in influencing patient outcomes, underscoring the necessity of holistic nursing care. Distress has been established to be linked with compromised immune function, impacting surgical patients, most especially those with chronic immune disorders. Surgical nurses should therefore be attuned to the psychological aspect of their patients' health, promoting a supportive environment that facilitates psychological resilience. Supportive care can alleviate stress, potentially augmenting global immune capacity and healing. As outlined in care manuals for ailments such as psoriasis, having an immunologic impact, it is crucial in surgical nursing to understand the interaction between emotional health and immune disorders (Segev et al., 2014). This holistic strategy is crucial for optimizing patient outcomes in surgical settings with immune-mediated complications.

KEY TERMS FROM THIS CHAPTER

- Acquired immunodeficiency syndrome (AIDS)
- Allergen
- Allergy testing
- Anaphylaxis
- Antibody
- Antigen
- Autoimmune disease
- Cytokines
- Desensitization therapy
- Histamine release
- Human immunodeficiency virus (HIV)
- Hypersensitivity reaction
- Immunodeficiency
- Immunoglobulins
- Immunosuppressive therapy
- Mast cells
- Opportunistic infections
- Rheumatoid arthritis

CRITICAL THINKING QUESTIONS

1. **Which of the following is a characteristic feature of anaphylaxis?**
   a. Localized skin rash
   b. Mild nasal congestion
   c. Sudden drop in blood pressure and airway obstruction
   d. Gradual increase in white blood cells
2. **What is the primary role of antibodies in the immune system?**
   a. Produce hormones
   b. Transport oxygen
   c. Identify and neutralize foreign substances
   d. Break down carbohydrates
3. **Which immune disorder is characterized by the body attacking its own tissues?**
   a. Anaphylaxis
   b. Immunodeficiency
   c. Autoimmune disorder
   d. Allergic rhinitis
4. **What is the first-line treatment for severe allergic reaction (anaphylaxis)?**
   a. Antihistamines
   b. Corticosteroids
   c. Epinephrine injection
   d. Oxygen therapy
5. **Which of the following conditions is considered an immunodeficiency disorder?**
   a. Systemic lupus erythematosus
   b. Rheumatoid arthritis
   c. HIV/AIDS
   d. Asthma

Short Answer Questions

1. What is the role of the immune system in the human body?
2. Define an autoimmune disorder with one example.
3. What is anaphylaxis, and why is it a medical emergency?
4. Name two common triggers of allergic reactions.
5. What is the function of immunoglobulin E (IgE) in allergies?
6. Explain the pathophysiology, clinical signs, and nursing management of anaphylactic shock.
7. Describe the differences between primary and secondary immunodeficiency disorders with examples.
8. Discuss the nursing assessment and intervention for a patient with systemic lupus erythematosus (SLE).
9. Explain the mechanisms and treatment options for allergic reactions.

Answers to Critical Thinking Questions

1. (c); 2. (c); 3. (c); 4. (c); 5. (c).

REFERENCES

1. Attarbaschi, A., Barzilai, S., Escherich, G., Frandsen, T. L., et al. (2016). Consensus definitions of 14 severe acute toxic effects for childhood lymphoblastic leukemia treatment: A Delphi consensus. https://core.ac.uk/download/42370388.pdf (accessed on 30th June 2025).
2. Bluestone, J. A., Bonyhadi, M. L., Earle, K. E., Liu, W., et al. (2005). *In vitro* expanded human CD4+CD25+ regulatory T cells suppress effector T cell proliferation. https://core.ac.uk/download/323073865.pdf (accessed on 30th June 2025).
3. Bonini, M., Canonica, G. W., Del Giacco, S., Gangemi, S., Lombardi, C., Minciullo, P. L., et al. (2017). Allergic diseases in the elderly: Biological characteristics and main immunological and non-immunological mechanisms. https://core.ac.uk/download/80193935.pdf (accessed on 30th June 2025).
4. Bosco, V., Giordano, V., Guillari, A., Mercuri, C., Nocerino, R., Rea, T., & Simeone, S. (2024). Development and management of avoidant/restrictive food intake disorder and food neophobia in pediatric patients with food allergy: A comprehensive review. https://core.ac.uk/download/636830095.pdf (accessed on 30th June 2025).
5. Burns, H. (2019). The development of hypersensitivity reactions in the pediatric population: A review. https://core.ac.uk/download/213464303.pdf (accessed on 30th June 2025).
6. Cairns, C., & Kang, K. (2022). *National Hospital Ambulatory Medical Care Survey: 2019 Emergency Department Summary Tables.* https://doi.org/10.15620/cdc:115748 (accessed on 30th June 2025).
7. Kalbermatter, C., Fernandez Trigo, N., Christensen, S., Ganal-Vonarburg, S. C. (2021). Maternal microbiota, early life colonization and breast milk drive immune development in the newborn. *Frontiers in Immunology, 12.* https://doi.org/10.3389/fimmu.2021.683022 (accessed on 30th June 2025).
8. da Silveira, J. S. Z., de Almeida Barbosa Mello, M., Valente, A. C. B., Yaedu, R., et al. (2018). Edema management in oral and maxillofacial surgery. https://core.ac.uk/download/322439968.pdf (accessed on 30th June 2025).
9. Doughty, M. W. (2014). Determining the health problems of Alaska Military Youth Academy participants. https://core.ac.uk/download/162576817.pdf (accessed on 30th June 2025).
10. Witmanowski, H., & Błochowiak, K. (2019). The whole truth about botulinum toxin–A review. *Advances in Dermatology and Allergology, 37,* 853–861. https://doi.org/10.5114/ada.2019.82795 (accessed on 30th June 2025).
11. Kaminogawa, S., & Nanno, M. (2004). Modulation of immune functions by foods. https://core.ac.uk/download/pdf/3552804.pdf (accessed on 30th June 2025).
12. Kyriazi, V. (2011). Enhancing transfusion safety: Nurse's role. https://core.ac.uk/download/pdf/27030705.pdf (accessed on 30th June 2025).
13. Pirazzini, M., Rossetto, O., Eleopra, R., & Montecucco, C. (2017). Botulinum neurotoxins: Biology, pharmacology, and toxicology. *Pharmacological Reviews, 69,* 200–235. https://doi.org/10.1124/pr.116.012658 (accessed on 30th June 2025).
14. Obielak, I. D. (2024). Opieka pielęgniarska nad dzieckiem po zabiegu usunięcia migdałka gardłowego i migdałków podniebiennych. https://core.ac.uk/download/636386258.pdf (accessed on 30th June 2025).

15. Pisani, S. (2010). The nurse of the Mediterranean. https://core.ac.uk/download/46602269.pdf (accessed on 30th June 2025).
16. Rauscher, B. (2015). Use of immunotherapy in the treatment of peanut allergies in the pediatric population. https://core.ac.uk/download/58826198.pdf (accessed on 30th June 2025).
17. Segev, E. (2014). Psoriasis in chronic and acute patients: A comprehensive care guide for practicing nurses. https://core.ac.uk/download/268095402.pdf (accessed on 30th June 2025).
18. Vykhrystenka, L. R., & Yanchanka, U. V. (2008). *Handbook of Clinical Immunology*. https://core.ac.uk/download/80151571.pdf (accessed on 30th June 2025).
19. Wolfgram, A. M. (2011). Interoperative pain management: Attenuating postoperative pain in paramedic patients. https://core.ac.uk/download/567882351.pdf (accessed on 30th June 2025).

7

MUSCULOSKELETAL ASSESSMENT AND MANAGEMENT OF TRAUMA

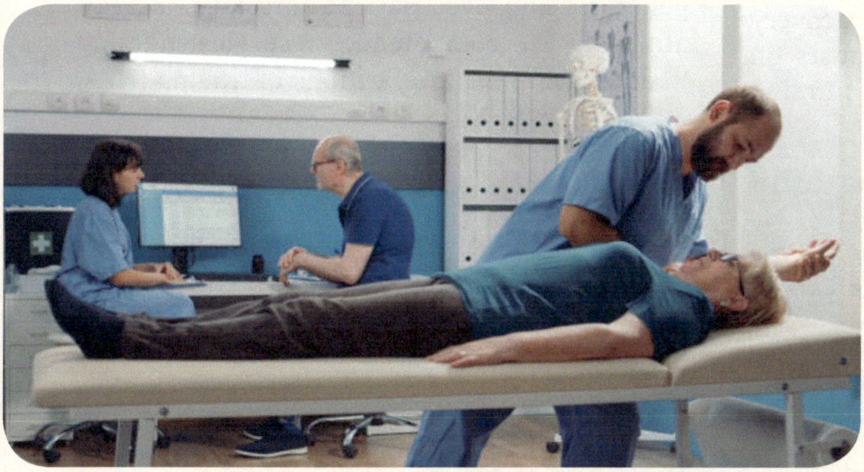

LEARNING OBJECTIVES

After studying this chapter, you will be able to:

1. Understand the anatomy and physiology of the musculoskeletal system
2. Explain the types of musculoskeletal traum
3. Discuss the assessment techniques in musculoskeletal trauma
4. Focus on pain management strategies
5. Learn about surgical interventions for musculoskeletal trauma
6. Evaluate the rehabilitation and recovery of the musculoskeletal system

Introduction

Surgical practice in nursing has a vital component in the assessment and management of musculoskeletal trauma. In healthcare settings, especially in surgical units, the importance of a thorough musculoskeletal assessment cannot be overstated. The initial evaluation not only aids in the detection of injuries such as fractures, dislocations, and soft tissue damage but also plays a significant role in the decision-making process for interventions. As musculoskeletal trauma forms a large percentage of injuries, surgical nursing is charged with a complex range of work that relies on accurate assessments and efficient management strategies. Understanding the mechanisms of injury and the complexity of musculoskeletal anatomy, surgical nurses excel at facilitating maximum patient outcomes while navigating the often unpredictable nature of trauma (N/A, 2023). In addition to direct assessment of musculoskeletal injuries, surgical nursing involves implementing management programs that are essential for patient recovery.

Effective management programs should not only address short-term physical needs following an injury but also consider long-term rehabilitation elements. This interdisciplinary aspect emphasizes the importance of collaboration among health providers, including surgeons, physical therapists, and pain management specialists. Each contributes unique expertise to the surgical team, contributing to the overall quality of patient care. Following established clinical guidelines and policies can also make a very significant contribution to the recovery trajectory of patients, with an emphasis on evidence-based practice in surgical nursing (Glikson et al., 2021).

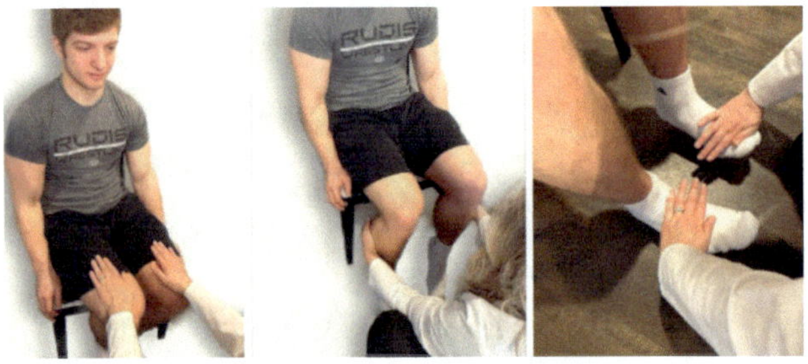

Figure 7.1. Musculoskeletal assessment in nursing skills.

Source: https://external-content.duckduckgo.com/iu/?u=https%3A%2F%2Fwtcs.pressbooks.pub%2Fapp%2Fuploads%2Fsites%2F29%2F2020%2F09%2FAssessing-for-Equal-Strength-in-Lower-Extremities-1024x451.png&f=1&nofb=1&ipt=111bc6c7a0ff9c1f5d859990654cc994d54608454f1bfdc5e1330c7b55bcf253.

Such collaboration ensures that surgical nurses are extremely well-equipped to deal with trauma management complexity. Appreciation for the broader ramifications of treating musculoskeletal trauma extends beyond direct clinical intervention and intersects with public health and safety initiatives. Rising trends in trauma-related injuries have raised demands for holistic evaluation of prevention strategies, compelling healthcare stakeholders to place on the back burner the investigation of incidence patterns and outcomes. Technological gains in surgical techniques, imaging modalities, and novel rehabilitation strategies all play essential roles in redefining musculoskeletal practice. Further, consideration of patient education and self-management arises as an underlying aspect of trauma recovery, acknowledging the need for engagement of patients in their own healing. Lastly, improvement of a sound appreciation of musculoskeletal assessment and management generates improved patient outcomes, thereby affirming the competence of surgical nursing in addressing the implications of trauma (N/A, 2023) (Figure 7.1).

Definition of Musculoskeletal Trauma

Musculoskeletal trauma is an array of injuries to bones, muscles, tendons, ligaments, and related soft tissues. It may occur secondary to acute insults like falls, motor vehicular accidents, or sports injuries to result in fractures, sprains, or strains. The challenge in the management of musculoskeletal trauma is not merely the injury itself but its impact on the functional capacity and quality of a patient's life. An understanding of the biomechanics of injury is necessary for effective diagnosis and management, as surgical nursing involves a holistic approach to meeting the patient's short-term and long-term needs. Effective assessment of musculoskeletal trauma is essential as misdiagnosis leads to suboptimal care and prolonged recovery. Hence, the definition of musculoskeletal trauma provides a significant foundation for surgical nursing practice and trauma management protocols. Optimal management of musculoskeletal trauma is both surgical and non-surgical, depending on the nature of the injury and the patient's circumstances. Non-operative treatment usually relies on immobilization, physical therapy, and pain relief, which are crucial for maximum recovery and the best prevention of complications. Surgical care, on the other hand, is necessary in the presence of significant fractures, dislocations, or when non-operative care fails to yield a satisfactory result. The understanding of musculoskeletal trauma dynamics, as highlighted by contemporary guidelines, informs these treatment methods in surgical nursing. For instance, the cautious method outlined in pertinent guidelines emphasizes the need for clinicians to balance the rate of treatment with the precision of diagnostic tests, thereby delivering comprehensive care pathways for patients with musculoskeletal trauma (Glikson et al., 2021). The process of evaluation is pivotal in deciding the appropriate intervention for musculoskeletal trauma. A comprehensive clinical assessment in terms of physical examination and imaging studies has to be done by the health workers to determine the level of injury. In surgical nursing, it is essential to be committed to ongoing education about evolving evaluation tools and techniques. Growing consciousness around fracture risk scores, as in various guidelines, can also affect treatment of at-risk groups, such as older adults or those with osteoporosis (Compston et al., 2017). Thus, characterization of musculoskeletal trauma is not merely the identification of injuries but is a holistic approach of practical assessment, management, and rehabilitation programs, ultimately resulting in the restoration of patients' functional capacity and overall health outcomes within a surgical environment (Figure 7.2).

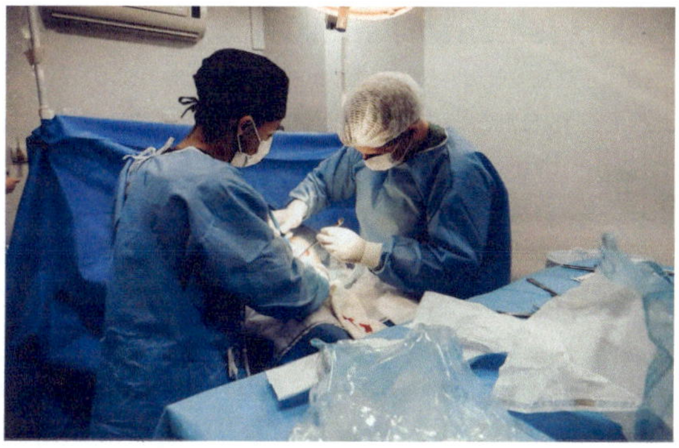

Figure 7.2. Trauma in surgical nursing.

https://nightingale.edu/_resources/images/blog/trauma-nurse-vlarge.jpeg.

Importance of Assessment in Surgical Nursing

The inherent contribution of evaluation in surgical nursing cannot be overstated, especially in the management of musculoskeletal trauma. In-depth evaluations enable nurses to identify potential complications and tailor individualized care plans accordingly. A standard for monitoring recovery patterns in patients is established through the initial evaluation, thereby informing surgical procedures and postoperative regimens. Proper management of conditions such as potential fractures or soft tissue injuries ensures that nursing interventions are preventative rather than responsive, making significant contributions to patient outcomes. Identification of underlying conditions like osteoporosis, which can go undetected until diagnosis of a fracture, is also important. For instance, any fracture patient aged 50 years and beyond is already at a high risk for future events, indicating the need for a practical assessment strategy to prevent a vicious cycle of recurring injuries (LeBoff et al., 2022). This shows the need for detailed assessments in guiding clinical decision-making in surgical nursing. Moreover, the assessment process offers a robust framework for patient education and engagement. Surgical nursing extends beyond bodily procedures; it also involves educating patients to promote better compliance with prescribed therapies. For instance, following a systematic assessment, nurses need to educate patients about the risk of osteoporosis, the relevance of pharmacological treatment, and lifestyle changes, including increased calcium and vitamin D intake, weight-bearing exercise, and fall prevention (LeBoff et al., 2022). Through integrating assessment results in teaching materials, nurses can improve the awareness of patients regarding their health status and, in turn, their adherence to the treatment plan and preventive interventions. This educational role in assessment serves to underscore the multidisciplinary nature of surgical nursing, where healthcare workers collaborate with patients to empower them throughout their healthcare journey, thereby ensuring more effective clinical outcomes. Moreover, ongoing reevaluation is critical in the realm of surgical nursing, as it plays a significant role in determining recovery dynamics. Continued assessment of musculoskeletal integrity, coupled with careful monitoring of pain levels, range of motion, and functional capacity, can guide early intervention and necessary modifications to treatment protocols. For instance, the model by the ESC Guidelines emphasizes ensuring that decision-making is informed by ongoing patient assessment, integrating clinical interventions with evolving health statuses. This process of cycles reinforces the therapeutic alliance, as patients feel they are being heard and their treatment is in reaction to their states. Responsiveness has the potential to establish an environment where surgical complications are minimized and recovery trajectories are optimized. Ultimately, the importance of a scientific and formal approach to assessment in surgical nursing is aligned with improved patient outcomes and holistic healthcare delivery.

7.1. Anatomy and Physiology of the Musculoskeletal System

Learning Outcome

1. Describe the components of the musculoskeletal system;
2. Focus on functions of bones, muscles, and joints;
3. Learn about common injuries and their impact on function.

The musculoskeletal system is a vital component of the human body, comprising bones, muscles, tendons, ligaments, and joints. All of them play a vital role in support, stability, and motion. The bones provide a rigid, immobile structure, which encloses delicate organs and serves as levers facilitating motion when muscles contract. Fibrous tissue muscles are charged with generating force and accommodating a spectrum of motions, from the most rudimentary gestures to the most complex athletic accomplishments. Joints, at which bones meet, rely on the tensile strength of cartilage and synovial fluid to facilitate smooth motion and to absorb shock. Surgical nursing relies on a thorough understanding of this anatomy as a foundation for assessing trauma, developing interventions, and implementing effective rehabilitation methods. Physiology within the musculoskeletal system is similarly complicated and is biochemical as well as mechanical processes necessary for the maintenance of homeostasis and facilitation of movement. Muscle contractions are initiated through a series of neuromuscular functions, where nervous system stimuli trigger muscle fibers to become shorter. Not only does this contraction permit voluntary movement, but it also stabilizes joints throughout dynamic motion. In addition, the integrity of the musculoskeletal system also depends on various other systems in the body, including the hormonal and circulatory systems, which control the delivery of nutrients and waste removal. Such physiological interactions are significant when it comes to deciding trauma because changes can result in the occurrence of complications such as muscle atrophy or impaired healing in surgical situations (Pan et al., 2022). In the management of musculoskeletal trauma, extensive assessments are needed to identify the extent of injuries and devise a tailored treatment protocol. Traumatic injury, such as a fracture or soft tissue injury, can cause alterations in the anatomy and physiological function of the affected region. Oral and craniomaxillofacial injuries are particularly the best example of the intricacy of treating musculoskeletal trauma due to interference with such vital functions as speech, mastication, and respiration. Operating room nursing must provide a precise assessment to prevent complications such as airway obstruction and long-term injury. The use of evidence-based practice in the management of trauma—supported by technological advances such as virtual surgical planning—transforms the process of management and improves recovery outcomes (Pavani et al., 2016). Knowledge of the anatomy and physiology of the musculoskeletal system thus forms a precondition for effective surgical care and patient management (Figure 7.3).

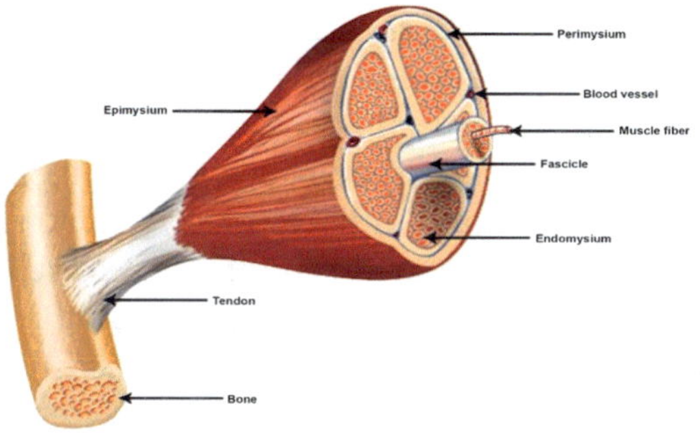

Figure 7.3. Anatomy and physiology of the musculo-skeletal system.

Source: https://nursesrevisionuganda.com/wp-content/uploads/2023/03/Anatomy-skeletal-muscle.jpg.

7.1.1. Components of the Musculoskeletal System

The musculoskeletal system comprises a highly complex interplay of bones, muscles, cartilage, tendons, and ligaments, all of which contribute to mobility, structural support, and the protection of vital organs. The bones supply the structure with its framework, securing it in place and facilitating movement through their joints. The skeletal system is not merely passive but plays an active role in metabolic processes, including the production of blood cells and the storage of minerals such as calcium and phosphorus. In addition, muscles—subclassified into skeletal, smooth, and cardiac—are critical in effecting movement through contraction and relaxation. The interaction among these components is crucial; for instance, tendons connect muscles to bones, facilitating movement, while ligaments stabilize joints. Understanding of this integrated system is a requirement for surgical nursing, as it enables practitioners to diagnose and treat trauma effectively within this system. Cartilage, a vital component of the musculoskeletal system, is a resilient yet flexible tissue that serves several important functions. It acts as a cushion in joints, reducing the friction between bones as they move, which is necessary for joint function and health. Cartilage is also very critical in bone development and growth, particularly in children, where it continually ossifies to form mature bone structures. Cartilage degeneration, as prevalent in degenerative diseases such as osteoarthritis, leads to significant loss of function and more pain, therefore necessitating comprehensive assessment and management interventions in surgical nursing. The treatment of cartilage disorders by the organizations may involve both conservative and surgical options, like arthroscopy or joint replacement, ensuring the imperative need for a detailed understanding of cartilage's role within the musculoskeletal system. In addition to the crucial need for complex structures and muscles, the musculoskeletal system also relies on sufficient connective tissues, such as tendons and ligaments, to support stability and enable movement. Tendons are fibrous cord tissue that join muscles to bones, and ligaments join bones to bones, where they form joints, providing stability and strength. Their tears or sprain can seriously impact a patient's mobility and require immediate assessment and intervention. Surgical nursing will need to be at the forefront in examining the severity of such injuries and how they are managed. This may include physical therapy, surgical reconstruction, and rehabilitation to regain function. Surgical nurses must be well-versed in anatomy and physiology of ligaments and tendons since the information forms the basis of clinical judgment and postoperative care, ultimately translating to patient outcomes in trauma management.

7.1.2. Functions of Bones, Muscles, and Joints

The human musculoskeletal system is an intricate network of bones, muscles, and joints, each serving a crucial role in the body's overall physiology and movement. The bones are the structural framework that keeps the body in shape, houses essential organs, and facilitates movement by their articulation at joints. The bones also serve as a reservoir for minerals, particularly calcium, which is used in various cellular processes. This mineral storage gains additional significance in the context of diseases like osteoporosis, in which lower bone density translates to increased risk of fractures. As literature also discusses, osteoporosis, if not treated, can create a cycle of recurrent fractures, suggesting that constant monitoring of bone status is essential for preventive and curative nursing practice in operating theatres (LeBoff et al., 2022). Muscles, which are attached to bones by tendons, are responsible for generating forces for movement. Muscles are categorized into three types: skeletal, smooth, and cardiac, of which skeletal muscles are an important part in voluntary movements and joint stabilization. Physical activity decreases with age, resulting in muscle atrophy and impaired muscle function. This may lead to severe impairment of mobility and independence in older individuals. It is also crucial to engage in systematic exercise programs, as studies have concluded that exercise can slow the age-related decline in muscle mass and strength (Izquierdo et al., 2021). For this reason, understanding the functional mechanics of muscles is vital for nurses who are engaged in rehabilitation programs aimed at restoring mobility and mitigating the risks of complications resulting from prolonged immobility after traumatic injuries. Joints are the significant points of intersection for bones, allowing multiple movements required for most daily tasks. Joint design and structure vary to support various motions, such as flexion, extension, and rotation, depending on the type of joint—synovial, fibrous, or cartilaginous. Proper joint maintenance is essential, considering the importance of trauma. Joint injuries can lead to severe pain and impaired function and thus need thorough assessment and intervention strategies. Based on knowledge of joint biomechanics as well as on the potential effects of trauma on joint function, nurses can adopt more effective care regimens, thus enhancing the recovery outcomes and improving patients' quality of life following injury (LeBoff et al., 2022) (Figure 7.4).

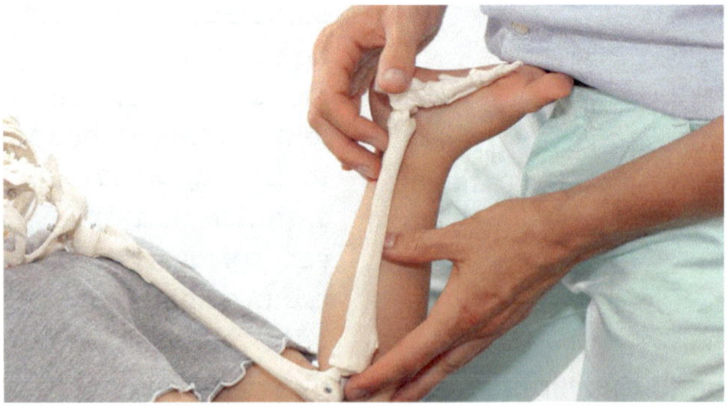

Figure 7.4. Functions of the skeletal system.

Source: https://vervecollege.edu/wp-content/uploads/2023/06/Skeletal-System.jpg.

7.1.3. Common Injuries and Their Impact on Function

In surgical nursing, routine musculoskeletal trauma assessment and management are of paramount significance as functional ability is significantly influenced by these injuries. Fractures, sprains, and strains commonly result in restricted mobility and altered patterns of physical functioning. For instance, a broken limb can initiate prolonged immobilization, which not only may trigger muscle wasting but also may postpone recovery of surrounding tissues. This functional impairment extends beyond mere pain and restriction, as it can have a direct impact on a patient's overall quality of life. Early recognition and proper management are thus paramount, allowing healthcare providers to institute rehabilitation interventions that focus not only on physical rehabilitation but also on functional recovery. This emphasizes the importance of multidisciplinary intervention in optimizing treatment outcomes for these injuries. Osteoporosis is also a prevalent disorder that causes fractures, particularly in older groups, and adds significantly to functional impairments. Commonly referred to as a silent disease, osteoporosis is rarely identified until a fracture occurs, and vertebral fractures specifically add increased risks of subsequent injuries. The presence of such fractures can exact severe functional consequences, including decreased autonomy and increased reliance on caregivers for daily functioning. Notably, a new fracture in an individual 50 years of age and older is a very predictive finding for subsequent increase in fracture risk and deserves early intervention to avoid future repeat events and maximize functional status. Careful use of effective antifracture medications and lifestyle modification is essential to interrupt the revolving door of repeat fractures and accompanying disability (LeBoff et al., 2022). Within the integrated management of musculoskeletal injuries, surgical nursing experts need to integrate knowledge from established guidelines in a way that informs practice. The European Society of Cardiology (ESC) guidelines emphasize the importance of personalized treatment plans in addressing the unique health needs of each patient. They must evaluate the patient's functional status, injuries, and overall condition, as well as their current comorbidities. Through rigorous assessment protocols, it becomes possible to implement an effective and patient-friendly treatment plan that places equal importance on rehabilitation and educational components, which can help avert fractures and maximize recovery. These interventions not only align with best clinical practices but also maintain the health-giving purposes of healthcare providers in safeguarding the functional well-being of patients against the damaging effects of common musculoskeletal injuries (Glikson et al., 2021).

Test Your Knowledge

1. What is the primary function of skeletal muscles in the human body?
2. How do bones and joints work together to enable movement?

7.2. Types of Musculoskeletal Trauma

Learning Outcome

1. Explain the fractures: classification and types
2. Define the soft tissue injuries: strains and sprains
3. Discuss the dislocations and their implications of musculoskeletal trauma

Musculoskeletal trauma constitutes a broad spectrum of injuries to bones, joints, and soft tissues, thereby placing a heavy demand on surgical nursing experts. The most common among them are fractures, which can be classified into closed, open, and stress fractures. Closed fractures do not penetrate the skin, whereas open fractures extend through the skin, exposing bone and thereby increasing the risk of infection. Furthermore, stress fractures result from repeated force, and this is most frequently noticed in athletes or those with high-impact exercise. Understanding such distinctions is crucial in facilitating targeted assessments and interventions. Proper classification of fracture types not only aids in the development of effective treatment plans but also facilitates accurate estimations of patient recovery time, with the surgical nurse's role being crucial in tracking and coordinating the healing process throughout the patient's trajectory. A second critical category of musculoskeletal injury is that of joint injuries, specifically sprains and dislocations. Overstretching and tearing of ligaments, typically resulting from sudden blows or twists, constitute a sprain. Dislocations occur when bones in a joint become displaced, resulting in severe pain and potential immobilization. These injuries have long-term implications if not adequately diagnosed and treated, and can predispose patients to recurrent instability or osteoarthritis. Surgical nursing plays a key role in the assessment of such injuries and the use of standardized scales to measure the stability and function of the joints. Moreover, coordination of wound care and rehabilitation following injuries relies on a complete understanding of the traumatic events to obtain optimal patient outcomes, again stressing the importance of training surgical nurses in the nuances of joint trauma. Soft tissue injury, including contusions and torn tendons, is another part of musculoskeletal trauma that is paramount to surgical nursing. Contusions tend to result from blunt force trauma, which in turn creates localized bruising and swelling, while tendon tears can result from acute or chronic overload syndromes. Both conditions require intensive examinations to assess their severity and causative factors, with direct implications for treatment modalities. Accurate diagnosis of soft tissue injury is vital in providing the proper management program with elevation, immobilization, and possibly surgery based on the severity and nature of the tears. Nurses should also be adequately equipped with knowledge on instructing patients on rehabilitation processes, aimed at regaining lost function and preventing possible injury, as early intervention has been shown to significantly improve overall recovery and rehabilitation among patients experiencing musculoskeletal trauma, according to research on effective recovery processes (Glikson et al., 2021; LeBoff et al., 2022) (Figure 7.5).

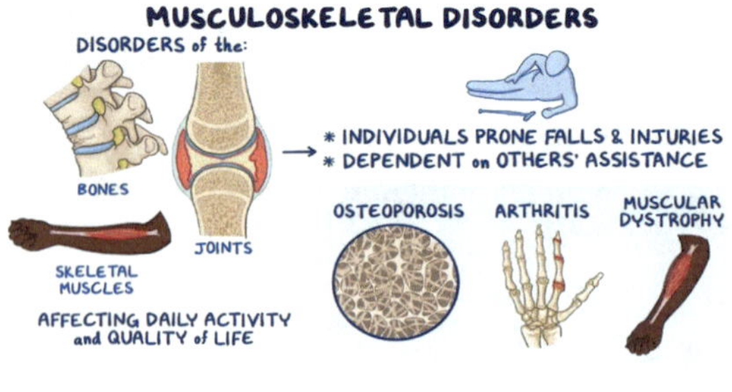

Figure 7.5. Musculoskeletal disorders.

Source: https://www.osmosis.org/_next/image?url=https%3A%2F%2Fd16qt3wv6xm098.cloudfront.net%2FKc3MmY9jQ5ui6rTjO90S3auNRqm6PgUR%2F_.jpg&w=3840&q=75.

7.2.1. Fractures: Classification and Types

The pattern of the fracture is a crucial consideration in the management of musculoskeletal injuries, particularly in surgical nursing. Fractures fall under two broad categories: closed fractures and open fractures. Closed fractures result when the skin is intact, while open fractures, also known as compound fractures, occur when the skin is open and the bone is visible, with a higher risk of infection. Identification of these differences is essential, as they dictate an immediate assessment and treatment plan that is required for the best recovery. Open fractures, for example, tend to require more urgent surgery to prevent complications than closed fractures, illustrating how effective classification is in trauma care. A good classification system facilitates smooth communication among healthcare professionals and informs clinical decision-making, ultimately enhancing patient outcomes and enabling comprehensive care. Also, there are numerous types of fracture classifications, with each being devised to address specific areas regarding the nature of the fracture. One of the most popular ones is the AO classification system, which divides fractures into their anatomic site and complexity and provides an excellent understanding of treatment and prognosis. Fractures may also be classified based on morphology, including transverse, oblique, spiral, and comminuted fractures. These variations not only determine the immediate treatment protocol but also the estimated recovery times and rehabilitation methods. Accurate classification of fractures is essential for documentation and research, as demonstrated in studies correlating fracture classification with post-operative treatment, which show how findings from such data enhance surgical outcomes and optimize trauma procedures (Abdulaziz et al., 2017). In the practice of surgical nursing, understanding the classification of fractures is key to the delivery of efficient musculoskeletal assessment and management. Classification of fractures informs practitioners about the possible need for operative management, such as internal Columbia spine fractures, or nonoperative management mechanisms such as immobilization. In addition, proper documentation of fracture type is necessary when evaluating trauma patients, as it can influence the decision-making process for resource allocation in trauma programs. For instance, administrative use of databases such as All Patient Refined Diagnosis-Related Groups (APR-DRG) has been examined for its ability in trauma case identification; however, studies reveal that these systems would underreport less severe fractures, a consideration that might skew hospital utilization measures. This could affect practice in care (Askegard-Giesmann et al., 2017). Thus, a clear understanding of fracture classifications not only enhances the care of individual patients but also the system of trauma care in surgical nursing.

7.2.2. Soft Tissue Injuries: Strains and Sprains

An understanding of soft tissue injury, specifically strains and sprains, is essential within the context of musculoskeletal examination and management in operating room nursing. Strains are caused by overstretching or tearing muscle fibers or tendons as a result of sudden movement or force. Sprains, on the other hand, are the overstretching or tearing of ligaments, which hold bones together at a joint. These types of injury can lead to disabling functional impairment and swelling, usually accompanied by pain and bruising. Hospital settings where physical effort is the standard have the highest incidence of such injury, for example, in many work environments. High-quality injury prevention and rehabilitation practices are crucial in mitigating disabling effects to facilitate patient recovery and care, and evidence-based practice is critical in surgical nursing. Treatment of sprains and strains largely depends on the accuracy of assessment techniques. Physicians must be able to identify the grade and intensity of the injury to implement the correct treatment protocol. The initial phase of treatment typically involves implementing the RICE method—rest, ice, compression, and elevation—to reduce pain and swelling. This is then complemented by further interventions, such as physical therapy and, where appropriate, surgery, depending on the severity of the injury. Furthermore, more recent studies suggest that prevention, particularly ergonomic interventions, can effectively reduce the incidence of soft tissue injuries in most occupational groups, stressing the worth of active participation in managing musculoskeletal health in the operating room (N/A).

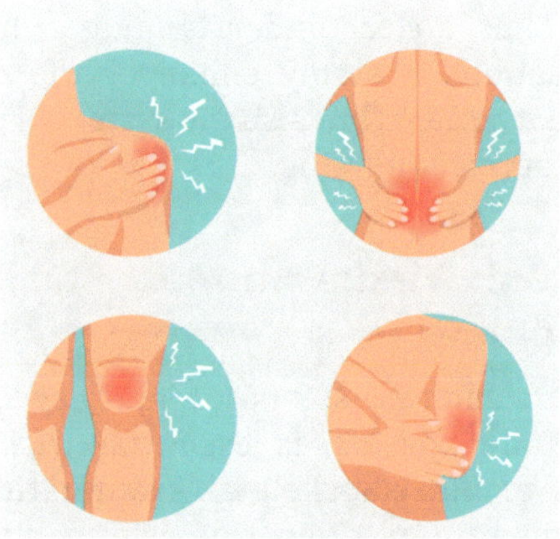

Figure 7.6. Soft tissue injuries.

Source: https://images.ctfassets.net/eexbcii1ci83/54WslpdtlshBhD5Q6DshOv/ad00a42d6393f2a51988b058ec9eb3f2/What_are_the_types_of_soft_tissue_injuries.png.

In addition, the epidemiology of musculoskeletal injuries within targeted populations, including elite athletes, highlights the complexities of addressing the efficient prevention of strains and sprains. Evidence suggests that these injuries not only hinder performance but also have long-term physical and psychological implications for athletes (Polo et al., 2023). Economic considerations are equally relevant, affecting the overall financial health of sports organizations and professional athletes. By comprehensively understanding the causative factors of such traumas and their impact on both physical function and psychological health, surgical nurses can effectively assist athletes and patients through individualized rehabilitation and recovery strategies. This multidisciplinary technique enhances the quality of care provided and is a subset of the broader ambition of musculoskeletal assessment in surgical nursing (Figure 7.6).

7.2.3. Dislocations and Their Implications

Dislocations are a general category of musculoskeletal trauma, wherein the joint surfaces are completely divided. Dislocations typically occur in major joints, such as the hip, knee, and shoulder, and result in acute pain, swelling, and impairment of the involved limb. Dislocations have significant implications beyond merely physical complaints and can affect a patient's mobility and quality of life. Prompt dislocation management and identification are integral components of surgical nursing because delayed action may result in chronic instability, ligament injury, and repeated dislocations. The challenge, hence, lies in early reduction of dislocated joints that will prevent long-term complications and enhance rehabilitation in the process, emphasizing the need for thorough musculoskeletal assessment in trauma care. Dislocation management is a complex process involving both surgical and non-surgical approaches, which are tailored to the severity and nature of the dislocation. The initial treatment can include a reduction procedure in which the dislocated joint is reduced or replaced into its normal position. Reduction is then followed by close observation and inspection to determine any associated injury, such as fractures or nerve damage. In children, dislocation implications may be added to by growth problems that have the potential to affect joint stability and healing (As et al., 2014). Surgical intervention will be necessary in those cases with joint instability or osseous damage, which is frequently present with recurrent dislocations. Therefore, surgical nursing also makes a critical contribution to pre-operative assessment, post-operative care, and educating patients about rehabilitation processes. Understanding the broader impacts of dislocations facilitates the establishment of comprehensive treatment plans that address both the short-term and long-term demands of recovery. After dislocation, patients might suffer from immobilization and rehabilitation for an extended period, which could lead to psychosocial problems like anxiety and frustration due to limited mobility. ~~Surgical nursing staff~~ Nursing intervention and support can promote patient compliance with rehabilitation exercises, ultimately resulting in improved outcomes (Aagesen et al., 2017). Moreover, educating the patient in prevention strategies, such as strengthening the surrounding muscles and refraining from high-risk activities, can minimize the chance of recurrent dislocations. Overall, the implications of dislocations in trauma care emphasize the importance of integrated care, which combines both clinical acumen and patient-centered care into the process of musculoskeletal assessment and management.

Test Your Knowledge

1. What is the difference between a sprain and a strain?
2. How can a fracture be identified through clinical assessment?

7.3. Assessment Techniques in Musculoskeletal Trauma

Learning Outcome

1. Explain the patient history and symptom evaluation
2. Define the physical examination methods
3. Describe the diagnostic imaging and its role within musculoskeletal assessment

Accurate assessment techniques in musculoskeletal trauma are of the most significant concern to surgical nursing since they have a direct impact on treatment plans and, indirectly, on patient outcomes. Accurate history-taking is the foundation of a proper assessment, whereby the nurse or clinician obtains essential information concerning the mechanism of injury, symptoms, and limitation of functioning. This accurate documentation enables the identification of individual patterns of injury, particularly in cases of fracture or soft tissue injuries. The evaluation must extend beyond a thorough physical examination, including visual and palpation inspections for tenderness, deformity, or swelling. The use of standardized assessment tools, such as the Visual Analog Scale (VAS) for pain, facilitates a more objective evaluation of the patient's condition, while also allowing for regular patient-reported outcome measures that are crucial for tracking recovery and therapeutic efficacy. In addition to visual and manual examination techniques, radiological assessments play an essential role in the diagnosis of musculoskeletal trauma. Techniques such as X-rays, CT scans, and MRIs prove helpful in providing clues about the integrity of bones and the tissues surrounding them, thereby facilitating the diagnosis of fractures, dislocations, and occult injuries. Radiological imaging is an adjunct to clinical assessment, enabling surgical nurses to provide precise differential diagnoses and tailor management plans to meet the specific needs of patients. Technological advances in imaging, combined with existing standards for interpreting scan results, further emphasize the importance of a multidisciplinary team in managing complex musculoskeletal trauma. It is essential that practicing nurses stay current with the latest protocols and best evidence-based practices for the appropriate use of these assessment tools in their practice settings.

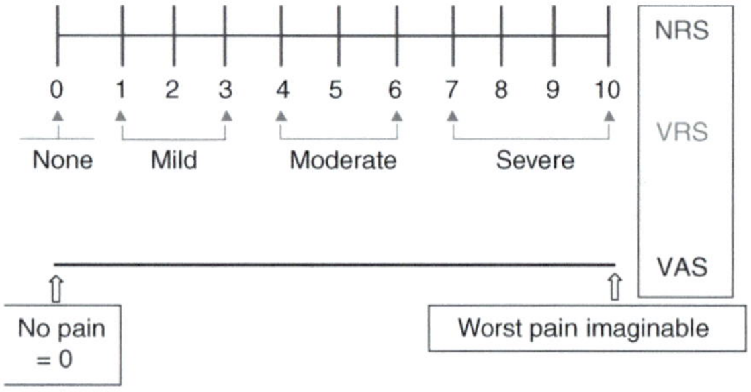

Figure 7.7. Visual analog scale (VAS) for pain.

Sourcehttps://www.bjanaesthesia.org/cms/10.1093/bja/aen103/asset/836a050b-7ce4-4346-9c9f-a7ead8a6e1dc/main.assets/gr1_lrg.jpg.

The integration of assessment tools must also consider the physiological implications of musculoskeletal trauma, particularly within populations who have varying bone density and health status, like the geriatric population with osteoporosis. According to the Clinicians Guide published by the Bone Health and Osteoporosis Foundation, the diagnosis of previous conditions is extremely important because they significantly influence treatment outcomes and the management of fracture risk (LeBoff et al., 2022). Furthermore, the European Society of Cardiology guidelines emphasize that clinical staff professionals are obligated to apply professional judgment grounded in concrete patient conditions, which is particularly relevant in the case of trauma assessment (Glikson et al., 2021). Thus, operating room nurses not only need to be skilled at performing thorough assessments of musculoskeletal trauma but also in actively applying this knowledge in advance to prevent complications and maximize recovery through focused prevention measures and education tailored to the individual patient's case (Figure 7.7).

7.3.1. Patient History and Symptom Evaluation

Obtaining a complete patient history and symptom evaluation is a crucial part of musculoskeletal examination in surgical nursing. Obtaining a full patient history encompasses questioning not only the current symptoms but also previous medical illness, lifestyle, and family history. All these factors have the potential to play a mammoth role both in diagnosis and management plans. For instance, a patient with musculoskeletal pain is likely to have a history of osteoporosis. This condition is subclinical until the development of a fracture, which may increase their risk of fracture (LeBoff et al., 2022). Identifying these risk factors allows healthcare professionals to determine the underlying causes and direct interventions in order to minimize the risk of future injury and maximize patient outcomes in general. As an additional factor, the cluster of various symptoms, including intensity and duration of pain and any resultant functional impairment, aids in charting an individualized pattern of care essential for attaining optimal post-surgical recovery. Symptom evaluation also examines the nature of the pain, acute or chronic, and identifies its location, quality, and any factors that relieve or aggravate it. This comprehensive process allows surgical nurses to differentiate between various musculoskeletal conditions. For example, a patient with prior vertebral fracture must be monitored carefully for signs of additional trauma and fragility fractures, as these fractures are strongly related to elevated future fracture risk (LeBoff et al., 2022). Wherever a fracture is detected, evaluation of accompanying signs such as swelling, instability, or immobility is critical. Such subtle symptom assessment not only guides acute management but also informs long-term management strategies, which include both drug treatments and lifestyle modifications, thereby establishing an overall care plan. Additionally, the use of evidence-based guidelines in patient assessment enhances surgical nursing practice. Healthcare professionals are encouraged to adopt systematic approaches that integrate clinical acumen and today's leading research data, taking into account patient variations. This two-pronged approach facilitates a comprehensive and informed understanding of a patient's condition. For example, in patients aged 50 years and above who come with an acute fracture, a rigorous evaluation for osteoporosis should be undertaken due to the heightened risk associated with age (LeBoff et al., 2022). When performed in an organized fashion, thorough history taking and symptom evaluation not only facilitate the appropriate diagnosis and management of musculoskeletal trauma but also allow healthcare practitioners to provide individualized preventive measures against potential future musculoskeletal complications, which, in the long term, is beneficial for improved quality of care.

7.3.2. Physical Examination Methods

The effectiveness of the physical examination methods in musculoskeletal examination plays a crucial role in surgical nursing, particularly in the treatment of trauma. A thorough physical examination allows medical professionals to correctly diagnose injuries, assess the severity of musculoskeletal pathologies, and determine the appropriate intervention methods. A complete physical exam typically includes inspection of the affected area, assessment of range of motion, and palpation to identify tenderness, swelling, or deformity. Apart from this, the use of objective measurements, such as measurement of strength and neurologic examinations, can provide us with more information regarding the patient's status. These tests can often lead the practitioner to make immediate clinical decisions, particularly when it comes to surgical interventions. These aids facilitate communication among surgical teams and nursing staff, ensuring that the patient's course of treatment is well-documented and comprehensible to everyone on the healthcare team. Also, specific examination techniques specialized to trauma injuries enhance diagnostic sensitivity and patient safety. These include the utilization of imaging modalities, which have been determined to be essential in corroborating observations of a physical nature. Techniques such as X-rays, MRIs, and ultrasounds can help delineate the extent of soft tissue and bone injuries, which may not be accessible through physical examination. However, it is also necessary to consider the risks of such tests, especially on vulnerable groups, e.g., pregnant patients where fetal safety is of utmost concern (Madkhali et al., 2024). Regarding this, the inclusion of multidisciplinary staff, such as obstetricians and radiologists, can optimize the diagnostic process while maintaining a focus on the fetus's health. This collaboration highlights the significance of interdisciplinary teamwork in surgical care and trauma management. Care after trauma is not all about initial examination and intervention; it requires constant monitoring and pain management as well as postoperative recovery management. Effective nursing practice integrates the findings of physical examinations to guide postoperative pain management interventions (Lestari et al., 2023). These include ongoing evaluation of the degree of pain, state of functional mobility, and potential complications of the surgery. With these assessment tools, nursing professionals can individualize pain management protocols, leading to improved patient comfort and recovery. Interventions such as guided imagery, patient education, and rest advocacy have the potential to influence recovery outcomes. Lastly, thorough physical examinations, coupled with postoperative management interventions, validate the holistic nature of surgical nursing in musculoskeletal trauma recovery.

7.3.3. Diagnostic Imaging and Its Role

The use of diagnostic imaging in musculoskeletal assessment has a pivotal role in the treatment of trauma, especially within surgical nursing practice. Imaging modalities such as X-rays, magnetic resonance imaging (MRI), and computed tomography (CT) scans provide indispensable information about the integrity of bones and soft tissues. These imaging modalities are vital in the detection of fractures—particularly in the presence of osteoporosis, a frequent condition that considerably increases the risk of fractures in elderly patients. Clinical practice must lay the most significant emphasis on early diagnosis of such fractures, as highlighted by the establishment that any fracture in individuals over 50 years signifies a heightened risk of future complications (LeBoff et al., 2022). This unique function of diagnostic imaging not only facilitates immediate management but also directs long-term care strategies critical to preventing repeated injury among the frail population. Diagnostic imaging is greater than fracture detection; it is an essential tool for the formulation of comprehensive treatment approaches. To put things into perspective, imaging assessment may help elucidate the extent of soft tissue damage that accompanies fractures, something of value in planning for and intervening during surgery. Imaging enables surgical personnel to assess other concerns, such as joint alignment and potential nerve or vascular compromise, thereby allowing for more precise surgical methods. This is particularly vital in the context of the prevalence of complicated injuries in trauma environments, where accurate imaging can clarify present pathologies that might otherwise go undetected. The application of advanced imaging modalities enables surgeons to individualize their interventions according to the unique needs of each patient, thereby enhancing both operative and postoperative outcomes. Furthermore, diagnostic imaging is of importance in the ongoing monitoring and assessment of treatment outcomes in nursing. Post-surgical imaging may be employed to evaluate the healing process, with the interventions being effective against the initial injury and no complications such as malunion or nonunion of fractures occurring. This continuous evaluation is particularly crucial among high-risk patient groups, such as those with diseases like osteoporosis, where therapeutic compliance may be uncertain (Glikson et al., 2021). By systematically integrating imaging into follow-up, clinicians can make evidence-based choices that support the principles of effective and safe patient care. Overall, an emphasis on diagnostic imaging during musculoskeletal trauma evaluation encourages an aggressive process of patient care that is essential for the prevention of long-term morbidity in trauma.

Test Your Knowledge

1. What does the acronym "CMS" stand for in musculoskeletal assessment?
2. Why is comparing both limbs significant during trauma evaluation?

7.4. Pain Management Strategies

Learning Outcome

1. Identify the pharmacological interventions of musculoskeletal trauma
2. Define the non-pharmacological approaches to musculoskeletal trauma
3. Describe the multimodal pain management

Effective pain management methods are crucial in the event of musculoskeletal examination and trauma care for surgical nursing. They not only minimize immediate discomfort but also support general recovery by enabling patients to be more actively involved in rehabilitation. The pharmacological approach is commonly a mixture of nonsteroidal anti-inflammatory drugs (NSAIDs) and opioid analgesics, which are used to manage various levels and types of pain. New guidelines emphasize the importance of having individually tailored pain management plans based on patients' history, present health, and the potential hazards of specific drugs. With fractures caused by osteoporosis, for example, immediate assessment and effective treatment are necessary because untreated pain can increase functional impairment as well as predispose to subsequent injury, indicating that interventions that reduce pain but also enhance quality of life as well as mobility in trauma patients are required (LeBoff et al., 2022). In addition to pharmacologic treatment, non-pharmacologic interventions have to be integrated into ~~surgical~~ nursing care for trauma. Physical therapy, acupuncture, and cognitive-behavioral therapy have been found to reduce pain and improve patient outcomes. These interventions can have the ability to treat the multifaceted nature of pain, particularly in chronic pain or post-operative conditions. Taking a multimodal pain management strategy—one that combines pharmacologic as well as non-pharmacologic interventions—ensures a more comprehensive care effort. For instance, early mobilization and low-intensity exercises following surgery may not only reduce dependence on pain medicines but also improve recovery and reduce the rate of immobilization complications (Glikson et al., 2021). Lastly, ongoing education and information exchange between healthcare professionals and patients are central to the success of pain management strategies. Operating room nurses play a central role in regularly evaluating patients' levels of pain and adjusting care plans as needed, as well as educating and empowering patients to take an active role in their own care. By actively involving patients in consultations about their pain and wishes, professionals can create a collaborative partnership more likely to yield beneficial results. Furthermore, knowledge of up-to-date evidence-based guidelines for treating chronic pain and newer therapy modalities serves to optimize individualized approaches. These kinds of discussions not only support adherence to directed treatments but also alleviate concerns regarding medicines and treatments, and hence, patients become more engaged in their healing process (LeBoff et al., 2022).

7.4.1. Pharmacological Interventions

In musculoskeletal trauma treatment, pharmacological therapy plays an essential role in the alleviation of pain, reduction of inflammation, and recovery of the patient. Nonsteroidal anti-inflammatory drugs (NSAIDs) are usually employed as the first course of treatment due to their capacity to ease pain and swelling in the case of acute injury. Opioids may also be given in cases of severe pain, particularly following surgery. However, the risk of dependency and side effects needs close observation and early substitution with less potent analgesics. The appropriate choice and utilization of these pharmacological tools have the ability to influence a patient's entire course of recovery, and well-structured pharmacological management is a characteristic of surgical nursing care. Recent evidence suggests that integrating non-pharmacologic interventions with pharmacologic interventions is associated with better outcomes in musculoskeletal rehabilitation. For example, the amalgamation of manual therapy with pharmacotherapy has been revealed to bring significant pain and functional mobility gains in situations like congenital muscular torticollis (CMT) among children. The cervical rotation and the improvement in head posture when two interventions are used together were reported in CMT's systematic review, highlighting the importance of a multidisciplinary intervention strategy (Antares et al., 2025). These findings support collaboration between surgical nursing and physiotherapists, as well as other allied health professionals, to formulate multidisciplinary, individually tailored treatment regimens that effectively address both functional rehabilitation and pain management. As a supplementary component of a postoperative maximization strategy for scoliosis surgery correction, pharmacologic treatment is not unwelcome in rehabilitation nursing. Effective pain management by drugs has the ability to make major contributions to patient engagement in the rehabilitation program, thus resulting in more effective mobility and functionality. Delivery of a rehabilitation nursing intervention that incorporates both drug and non-drug interventions, such as instructional intervention to equip patients with greater knowledge of the disease, is vital (Sousa et al., 2024). This holistic approach not only aids in physical rehabilitation but also enables patients to become more independent, thereby improving their quality of life after surgical intervention. With the ongoing advancement in surgical nursing practice, the integration of pharmaceutical management in the holistic treatment of musculoskeletal injury remains an integral part of effective patient care.

7.4.2. Non-Pharmacological Approaches

In musculoskeletal trauma assessment and management, non-pharmacological interventions play a critical role in optimizing patient outcomes. These include physical therapy, occupational therapy, and lifestyle modifications for improved mobility and pain relief. The interventions have been found to significantly decrease the requirement for pharmacologic pain medication and, therefore, lower the incidence of side effects and drug interactions. With increased recognition of musculoskeletal diseases, the inclusion of non-pharmacological measures, such as customized exercise regimens and ergonomic modifications, is essential. This shift not only fosters physical rehabilitation but also promotes psychological healing, necessitating an integrated approach to patient care within the field of nursing. Physical therapy, being one of the foundations of non-pharmacologic measures, addresses restoring movement and function following trauma or surgery. Individualized exercise programs, guided by licensed physical therapists, help patients regain strength and range of motion, as well as manage pain. Such interventions can be helpful in orthopedic recovery or for trauma patients, as they involve progressive adaptation based on their specific demands. Occupational therapy complements this by helping patients accommodate themselves to daily activities and optimizing their quality of life. Both therapies focus on empowering the patient in their recovery process, informing and empowering them, which can lead to improved adherence to treatment plans and better outcomes, aligning with the clinical goals of nursing interventions. In addition to therapeutic modalities, lifestyle modifications provide a crucial component of non-pharmacological intervention in the treatment of trauma. Suggestions such as dietary advice to help strengthen bones, as well as weight-bearing activities, have been effective in preventing subsequent complications and promoting recovery. For example, proper consumption of calcium and vitamin D is essential for managing diseases such as osteoporosis, which, if not managed, leads to fractures and additional trauma. Additionally, strategies to prevent falls are vital among vulnerable groups, especially the elderly. Emphasizing these lifestyle changes as part of an extensive management plan accentuates the importance of multidisciplinary collaboration among medical practitioners. Because of this, ~~operating room~~ nurses play a crucial role in informing patients about non-pharmacological interventions, as they also contribute to long-term musculoskeletal health and patient energy, which supports the overarching objective of quality trauma care (Glikson et al., 2021; LeBoff et al., 2022).

7.4.3. Multimodal Pain Management

The application of multimodal pain management is critical in surgical nursing, particularly in the management of musculoskeletal trauma. The approach involves the use of multiple analgesic modalities to enhance pain relief with less dependence on opioids, which are burdensome with heavy side effects and risks. The combination of non-opioid analgesics, such as acetaminophen and ibuprofen, with local anesthetics enables healthcare providers to manage pain through various mechanisms, thereby rendering enhanced analgesia. For instance, constant infusion of local anesthetic close to incisions during surgery has proven to lower postoperative pain effectively while allowing reduced doses of opioids, which aligns with current trends in pain management protocol. Such techniques not only lead to improved patient outcomes but also allow for increased mobility and shorter hospital stays, making it imperative to form a comprehensive pain management plan in surgery for musculoskeletal disorders. In the postoperative environment, nurses play a key role in ensuring multimodal pain management regimens. They ensure that pain levels are assessed, local anesthetic infusions are administered correctly, and patients are educated on reporting any adverse effects. For instance, local anesthetic infusions are beneficial for providing prolonged analgesia but carry cardiotoxic and neurotoxic risks that need to be carefully monitored. The regular assessments allow for early identification of side effects, ensuring patient comfort and safety. Additionally, integrating patient education into the nurse's practice enables a deeper understanding of treatment protocols. Patients are more likely to be active participants in their care when they are informed about their analgesic regimen, as well as the justification for using a multimodal regimen, thus encouraging an environment of support among healthcare providers and patients during recovery. Improvement of pain management techniques within the operating room also reflects the increased knowledge about opioid stewardship. Since the increasing use of opioids has become more common to cause complications, routine implementation of a switch towards single-agent opioid therapy instead of combination therapy is taking place. Research has shown that postoperative pain management through single-agent prescription of opioids can readily maximize pain relief while minimizing risks related to polypharmacy. For example, opioids like oxycodone are being favored more ~~now,~~ with their strength without the hassle of drugs that have a combination of opioids with acetaminophen or ibuprofen. Not only does this trend align with public health goals of minimizing opioid abuse and dependence, but it also imposes the commitment to go forward with evidence-based practice in surgical nursing.

Test Your Knowledge

1. What is the role of non-pharmacological methods in managing acute pain?
2. Why is regular pain assessment important in planning effective pain management?

7.5. Surgical Interventions for Musculoskeletal Trauma

Learning Outcome

1. Describe the indications for surgical management for musculoskeletal trauma
2. Define the common surgical procedures for musculoskeletal trauma
3. Discuss the postoperative care and monitoring for musculoskeletal trauma

Surgical interventions for musculoskeletal trauma are pivotal in the management of complex injuries that threaten the structural support and function of the damaged structures. The procedures focus on anatomical reconstruction and optimizing healing conditions to facilitate rehabilitation. Screw and plate internal fixation, external fixator appliances, and bone grafting are some of the common surgical interventions used in severe fractures to aid in healing. These interventions are not only necessary for fracture fixation but also for the treatment of ligamentous injury or joint instability, which may be a result of trauma. Through judicious use of surgical intervention methods, healthcare providers are able to enhance patients recovery and days of function significantly, which emphasizes the importance of global surgical assessment and management in musculoskeletal trauma care. The use of advanced imaging technologies, such as MRI and CT scans, hugely improved the accuracy of musculoskeletal injury diagnosis and thereby the planning and execution of surgical procedures. Precise imaging enables surgical teams to visualize the degree of soft tissue engagement and select the most effective approach to intervention. Furthermore, measurable evaluation, as documented in current nursing practices, can optimize postoperative recovery and follow-up. Evidence suggests that complication rates can be reduced and patient outcomes overall improved by following structured follow-up care (Tan et al., 2025). Postoperative care should not be overemphasized, as reasonable control early after surgical intervention can influence long-term functionality and return to work among trauma patients. In addition to the technological modalities of operations, there is increasing interest in the role of nursing care during the preoperative, intraoperative, and postoperative phases in surgical nursing for musculoskeletal trauma. Multidisciplinary measures for care, which include risk assessments and patient-specific education, have been shown to enhance patients' adherence to recovery plans and decrease risk for complications during recovery. As evident in recent studies, patients who receive enhanced nursing interventions exhibit higher levels of satisfaction and lower rates of adverse events (Zhang, 2025). The strategy highlights the importance of syncretizing surgical technique proficiency with precise nursing management to achieve the best outcomes for musculoskeletal trauma patients. This synergy is necessary in optimizing recovery, durability, and functionality of the musculoskeletal system post-surgery.

7.5.1. Indications for Surgical Management

Surgical intervention for musculoskeletal trauma is typically reserved when non-surgical treatment cannot yield satisfactory outcomes. It can occur in fractures with evidence of malalignment or instability, where surgery is necessary to achieve proper alignment and restore functionality. For example, osteoporotic fracture patients, particularly those above the age of 50 years, can have a high risk for further fractures if primary injuries are not adequately addressed. Surgical fixation through internal fixation or arthroplasty is crucial in such situations to prevent a cycle of recurrent fractures and enhance mobility, thus mitigating the threat of long-term disability and premature death from poorly managed conditions such as osteoporosis (LeBoff et al., 2022). Therefore, early detection of such indications is crucial for optimal patient benefit in surgical nursing.

Apart from mechanical instability, surgery is indicated in the presence of massive soft tissue damage or complicating factors such as compartment syndrome, which compromises blood supply and tissue viability. In pressure within the muscle compartments due to trauma, emergency fasciotomy surgery must be performed to alleviate the condition to prevent permanent loss of function (Glikson et al., 2021). Surgical treatment is decided following thorough evaluation, i.e., clinical examination and imaging reports that detail the degree of trauma and complications. The patient's general condition, age, and comorbidities are also highly critical factors in deciding surgical selection, emphasizing the need for a multidisciplinary approach in trauma management. Effective management of these indications can lead to improved recovery patterns and reduced hospital stays. Finally, surgery can become necessary in instances of chronic pain and dysfunction that do not respond to conservative modalities such as physical therapy, medications, or corticosteroid injections. Diseases like severe osteoarthritis will eventually necessitate total joint arthroplasty if quality of life is significantly compromised. Understanding how to transition from conservative to surgical means requires ongoing musculoskeletal assessment and patient education regarding alternative options for preventing complications and achieving successful pain control (LeBoff et al., 2022). Being proactive using early surgery can result in good outcomes, such as improved joint function and pain relief, and thereby play its role in the broader goals of surgical nursing for trauma. Lastly, careful consideration of these surgical indications enables medical providers to provide effective, patient-centered care.

7.5.2. Common Surgical Procedures

In orthopedic care of musculoskeletal trauma, routine operations are the cornerstone in restoring function and eliminating pain. Of all the surgical procedures, total hip replacement (THR) is one of the most frequently performed orthopedic surgeries. THR is generally reserved for individuals with severe degeneration of the hip joint due to osteoarthritis or trauma. Patients after THR have, in the past, been instructed to follow particular hip precautions and use aids like raised toilet seats and furniture risers. These interventions have been employed to mitigate the risk of complications, particularly dislocations, during the postoperative period. A recent British survey of physiotherapists and occupational therapists revealed that an overwhelming majority refer to these interventions on a routine basis, while there is some variation in the duration they support them, highlighting the importance of postoperative care practice standardization in surgical nursing (Drummond et al., 2016). However, another significant common surgical intervention is arthroscopy, which is frequently used to diagnose and treat various joint disorders, most notably those of the knee. This minimally invasive technique enables direct visual inspection of joint structures and provides access for the use of specialized tools to repair issues such as meniscal damage, loose fragments, and cartilage lesions. One advantage of arthroscopic surgery is that it involves less recovery time compared to open procedures, which aligns with the trend toward more outpatient procedures. In the evaluation of the musculoskeletal system, the ability to perform arthroscopic interventions has revolutionized the treatment process, as patients experience less postoperative pain and regain function more quickly. This new advancement requires ongoing education and training of surgical nursing professionals to realize optimal patient outcomes and adherence to evolving best practices for preoperative and postoperative care. Furthermore, piriformis syndrome is another condition for which surgical treatment can be considered. Although typically treated conservatively, when severe enough, they can require surgical release of the piriformis muscle to alleviate pressure on the sciatic nerve. This procedure, while less common than THR or arthroscopic surgery, enforces the importance of complete musculoskeletal examinations. A good diagnosis is imperative, as it can determine whether piriformis syndrome or another similar condition, such as sciatica from herniated discs or spinal stenosis (Chantraine et al., 2010), is present. As operating room nurses, knowledge of these differences and surgical indications ensures an exhaustive process in patient management that meets the best trauma management. Development in surgery demands that nursing practitioners remain updated and adaptable in managing musculoskeletal trauma.

7.5.3. Postoperative Care and Monitoring

Postoperative monitoring and management are critical elements in the care of patients undergoing musculoskeletal surgery, such as hip and knee arthroplasties. Effective postoperative management begins with vigilant monitoring of patients' vital signs and the condition of their wounds for recognizing any impending complications, such as infections or hemorrhage. Nurses play the core role in this area, using assessment tools to track patients' responses to surgical interventions. By way of pain intensity monitoring, multimodal pain treatment strategies are needed to minimize narcotic dependence. Not only do these practices enhance patient comfort, but they also minimize risks associated with opioid use and align with national guidelines advocating multispectral approaches to pain care (Hsu et al., 2019). The integration of a repertoire of physical, cognitive, and pharmacological interventions augments the recovery trajectory as a whole, promoting optimal outcomes in patients. Pharmacological interventions enhance the overall recovery trajectory, promoting maximum benefits. The role of education to foster postoperative recovery cannot be overstated. Educating patients through tailored interventions promotes their self-efficacy in pain management and postoperative care behaviors. Studies show that patients who engage with educational materials—i.e., educational DVDs featuring self-efficacy activities—report greater satisfaction and better pain management outcomes during their hospital stay (Allegrante et al., 2016). Empowering patients to participate in their healing process is central, as it enhances their sense of agency and responsibility, and thus, compliance with prescribed care regimes. Therefore, integrating these educational elements into the postoperative period not only facilitates more effective pain control but also enhances overall recovery rates and provides a solid foundation for patient education within surgical nursing. Finally, continuing observation and revision of postoperative care plans are necessary to address changing patient needs in the aftermath of surgical interventions. Regular observation enables the tailoring of interventions based on the response to surgery, thereby accelerating recovery and minimizing complications. For instance, implementing evaluation protocols that evaluate pain, mobility, and psychological status may direct timely adjustment of pain management strategies, supposedly with reduced narcotic needs, as suggested by Hsu et al., (2019). Furthermore, feedback mechanisms used to track patient improvement provide nursing personnel with the necessary information to optimize care protocols. This closed-loop model of care enhances not only patient safety but also fosters the culture of ongoing improvement in surgical nursing that ultimately leads to improved outcomes for patients undergoing musculoskeletal surgery.

Test Your Knowledge

1. What is the purpose of internal fixation in the treatment of fractures?
2. How does postoperative care support recovery after orthopedic surgery?

7.6. Rehabilitation and Recovery

Learning Outcome

1. Describe the importance of rehabilitation in recovery
2. Define the physical therapy techniques
3. Identify the patient education and self-management

The process of recovery and rehabilitation following musculoskeletal trauma is a vital aspect of surgical nursing that necessitates a multidisciplinary approach. Effective rehabilitation targets not only physical recovery but also the psychological needs of the patient. In the aftermath of surgical management of conditions such as multi-ligament knee injuries (MLKIs) or complex limb fractures, it is imperative to implement an official rehabilitation program targeting specific needs. This is typically initiated during the acute phase, with a focus on reducing pain, controlling inflammation, and promoting mobilization. With advancing healing, rehabilitation enables strengthening and functional movement through progressive exercise programs, providing patients with enough capacity to return to their usual activities. Such comprehensive rehabilitative schemes significantly decrease the risk of arthrofibrosis complications and enable better recovery times and outcomes for patients (Sleem et al., 2025). Rehabilitation schemes with complex limb fractures become even more complicated because they often entail coordination among various specialists, like orthopedic, vascular, and plastic surgeons. Rehabilitation interventions should incorporate both functional training and psychosocial support to effectively address the multifaceted problems these patients face. Because limb salvage can lead to longer recovery times and more complications, a thoughtful decision-making process should be utilized in developing a plan that is harmonious with the patient's functional abilities and quality of life standards. Programs such as the Mangled Extremity Severity Score (MESS) can help determine the most suitable method of treatment, whether limb salvage or amputation is desired, and thus tailor rehabilitation programs that work towards regaining mobility and independence (Koshy et al., 2025). Ultimately, the rehabilitation process after surgical treatment of musculoskeletal trauma is one of what determinants of optimal patient outcome and satisfaction. This procedure emphasizes education, adherence to rehabilitation protocols, frequent assessment, and modifications reflecting patient improvement and participation. With persistent encouragement and interaction from the healthcare staff, as patients transition from postoperative care to rehabilitation, their compliance and motivation are significantly impacted. With continuous support and therapeutic guidance, patients can expect to experience greater strength, stability, and confidence in their recovery. This focus on holistic rehabilitation not only aids in recovery from the physical component but also aids in mental resilience, enabling a person to regain a sense of normalcy and well-being following trauma (Sleem et al., 2025).

7.6.1. Importance of Rehabilitation in Recovery

Rehabilitation is a significant component of recovery from musculoskeletal trauma and plays a substantial role in patient outcomes. Effective rehabilitation programs are initiated to restore function, enhance mobility, and abolish pain, which are critical components for patients who undergo surgical interventions. Sticking to a formal rehabilitation routine allows patients to become more stable and stronger in the injured areas, which is particularly important for those who have undergone surgery such as joint reconstruction or reductions of fractures. For instance, patients receiving treatment for central hip dislocations in conjunction with knee trauma benefit significantly from the use of progressive weight-bearing therapy and function-based movement in individually tailored rehabilitation interventions, which complies with the best practices of surgical nursing practice. Therefore, not only does rehabilitation help patients overcome physical limitations, but also address their psychological well-being, encouraging them to resume their recovery process. Proper execution of rehabilitation also reduces the potential for postoperative complications, hence emphasizing its worth in surgical nursing practice. Following surgery, such as a ventral slot procedure for intervertebral disc herniation, the patient may present with variable clinical signs that require close monitoring and management. Rehabilitation is not merely passive recuperation, but rather demands active initiative and ongoing monitoring of improvement on the part of the patient. Interventions such as pain management, bladder management, and guided exercise instructions facilitate maximum recovery. The integration of patient education into rehabilitation enables patients to gain a better understanding of their conditions and adhere to prescribed interventions, thereby significantly enhancing outcomes in rehabilitation. Rehabilitation thereby becomes a mainstay in managing musculoskeletal trauma, establishing a link between surgical intervention and the return of the patient to normal activities. Lastly, the long-term success of the rehabilitation process depends on the application of a multidisciplinary system with ongoing assessment and revision of recovery objectives. In complex situations, such as those involving multiple injury patients, the need for regular reevaluation of the rehabilitation program is highlighted. When complications like avascular necrosis occur as a byproduct of surgeries, as in patients undergoing recovery from traumatic injuries, rapid revisions of rehabilitation processes are warranted. These problems of instability or pain can be solved by way of specific exercises and modalities to prevent further compromise of function, thus improving the quality of life for the patient. This requirement for adaptability highlights the role of rehabilitation within the overall management of trauma, enabling patients to achieve their optimal potential after surgery and reducing the risk of complications that may complicate recovery (Jaques, 2024; Khan et al., 2024).

7.6.2. Physical Therapy Techniques

Physical therapy interventions play a significant role in musculoskeletal assessment and management of trauma in surgical nursing. Physical therapy is meant to facilitate recovery and restore function after injury or surgery and therefore is an essential part of postoperative care. Of the procedures utilized, therapeutic exercises, manual therapy, and modalities play a very critical role. Therapeutic exercises are designed to improve strength, flexibility, and range of motion to attain independence and restore activities of daily living. Manual therapy involves the application of hands-on techniques like mobilization and manipulation of soft tissues and joints to alleviate pain and improve mobility. Utilizing these techniques, physical therapists can effectively tailor rehabilitation programs to each patient's specific injuries and procedures, thereby achieving optimal recovery outcomes. The implementation of evidence-based physical therapy interventions is critical in an attempt to treat trauma-related musculoskeletal dysfunctions effectively. Invention of newer therapeutic technologies, including electrical stimulation and ultrasound therapy, has also enhanced rehabilitation by facilitating tissue repair and alleviating pain. These modalities serve as adjuncts to exercise-based treatments, particularly in those patients experiencing significant discomfort or delayed healing. Furthermore, implementation of a multidisciplinary care model necessitates coordination among physical therapists, surgical teams, and nurses. The clinicians' combined experience ensures comprehensive patient care that addresses every aspect of rehabilitation, from physical therapy to emotional support throughout the healing process. As a result, evidence-based physical therapy techniques not only improve functional recovery but also create an enabling environment that raises patient compliance and engagement. In addition to standard physical therapy techniques, education and self-management procedures are equally vital in musculoskeletal recovery after trauma.

Through ergonomic education, activity modification, and lifestyle modifications, patients are typically taught to prevent re-injury and promote long-term health. This educational component enables patients to take charge of their rehabilitation process and practice compliance with home exercise regimen orders and lifestyle changes. Moreover, the integration of prevention measures, such as fall prevention attempts, is particularly vital for elderly individuals at higher risk of fractures due to osteoporosis, based on clinical guidelines (LeBoff et al., 2022).

Such broad frameworks ensure that the role of physical therapy is emphasized as a first choice of intervention in recovery processes, ultimately leading to better patient outcomes and less healthcare costs spent on complications from inappropriate rehabilitation. Secondly, adherence to the ESC Guidelines (Glikson et al., 2021) ensures that nursing staff are well-versed in the emerging best evidence for the diagnosis and treatment of musculoskeletal trauma, thereby ensuring the maximum effectiveness of treatment protocols.

7.6.3. Patient Education and Self-Management

Effective patient education is a foundation of self-management, and this is particularly significant in the context of musculoskeletal examination and trauma care in surgical nursing. Patient education about their conditions enables them to appreciate the pathophysiology involved, hence empowering them to make informed health choices. For instance, osteoporosis patients may not have any idea about how much more vulnerable they become to subsequent fractures following a first event. By conveying the importance of monitoring and anticipation management, operating room nurses have a significant impact on a patient's trajectory regarding their health condition. Moreover, an informed patient is more likely to adhere to treatment strategies, including pharmacologic therapy to prevent fractures. This active role is priceless in avoiding the individual and economic consequences of untreated osteoporosis and other musculoskeletal conditions (LeBoff et al., 2022).

Self-management programs extend beyond medication adherence to include lifestyle modifications critical to musculoskeletal health. Conditioning through exercise regimens tailored to each patient's unique needs can have a profoundly life-transforming effect on results. According to current evidence, integrating regular physical activity maintenance can temper the decline spirals resulting from aging and long-term disease, facilitating a vision of fostering sustainable health (Izquierdo et al., 2021). They must be instructed on the types of exercises that would benefit them, such as weight-bearing exercise to improve bone density and muscle strength. In addition, heightened awareness of the detrimental effects of a sedentary lifestyle to musculoskeletal function underscores the patient's necessity for physical activity.

Planned exercise programs can be both prophylactic and therapeutic, underscoring the importance of ongoing patient education for physical activity (Izquierdo et al., 2021). Furthermore, patient education needs to include fall and nutrition prevention to promote comprehensive self-management. Patients require adequate calcium and vitamin D intake to maintain bone health, and many are unaware of the types of foods or supplements to consume. Furthermore, educating patients about the risks of falls—especially those with osteoporosis—can be of significant benefit to both safety and well-being. Implementing fall prevention strategies, such as adapting to the environment and engaging in balance exercises, will help patients maintain their independence while reducing the risk of injuries. As nurses ~~in the operating room~~, fostering a culture of continuous learning not only empowers patients but also equips them with the competencies needed for effective self-management, ultimately enhancing the quality of their lives (LeBoff et al., 2022).

Test Your Knowledge

1. Why is early mobilization necessary in the rehabilitation process after musculoskeletal surgery?
2. How can nurses support patients in adhering to their rehabilitation plans?

SUMMARY

Management of musculoskeletal trauma as a surgical nursing procedure is a vital and multidisciplinary one. Successful assessment measures and timely interventions are key to achieving optimal patient outcomes. With the use of evidence-based practices, surgical nurses can provide accurate diagnoses, initiate appropriate treatment protocols, and play a crucial role in a patient's rehabilitative process. The inclusion of comprehensive assessments, such as visual assessments and functional evaluations, is significant in identifying underlying reasons that cannot be directly observed. With the development of solid knowledge and skills in musculoskeletal anatomy and injury mechanisms, surgical nurses can further their potential to manage traumatic injury effectively. Additionally, an appreciation of implications from conditions like osteoporosis is imperative when dealing with musculoskeletal trauma. In particular, preventing fractures in susceptible populations, particularly among the elderly, should be an utmost priority due to their susceptibility to fractures. As mentioned, osteoporosis may not be diagnosed until a fracture occurs, leading to a chain of consequences that can severely reduce the quality of life for such individuals (LeBoff et al., 2022). Therefore, operating room nurses should be aware of these risks and encourage proper screening and education regarding fracture prevention, monitoring, and requirements for pharmacological interventions as indicated. Ultimately, adherence to established guidelines and ongoing professional development are crucial factors in ensuring the quality of musculoskeletal trauma care. The ESC Guidelines emphasize the importance of integrating clinical judgment with evidence-based knowledge and guidelines from recognized health authorities (Glikson et al., 2021). This continuous, evidence-based practice enables surgical nurses to manage complex clinical scenarios effectively while maintaining the highest quality standards of care. Finally, creating a sense of teamwork between healthcare professionals, patient education, and applying an integrative approach will give surgical nursing the power to enhance the results in musculoskeletal trauma cases greatly. As progress is made within the field, ongoing evaluation of practice and outcomes is crucial to enhancing the overall quality of care in surgical environments.

The assessment of musculoskeletal trauma is critical in surgical practice as it determines appropriate management avenues for patients. A thorough evaluation includes understanding the mechanism of trauma, conducting an extensive physical examination, and utilizing advanced imaging modalities to determine the extent of damage. This multimodal approach not only aids in the diagnosis of fractures, soft tissue injuries, and dislocations but also enables the surgical nurse to formulate an optimal treatment plan that may include non-surgical interventions. The leading indicators in assessment are swelling, range of motion, and pain, which, when taken together, direct clinical decision-making. Furthermore, the introduction of evidence-based practice, as noted in recent literature, ensures assessments are patient-centered and systematic to increase further the overall success of trauma care in surgical environments (N/A, 2023). Musculoskeletal injury management varies based on severity and patient factors such as comorbidities and age. Surgical intervention may be warranted for acute dislocations or fractures and can range from open reduction and internal fixation to arthroscopy. When considering older adults, frailty is a crucial factor, as it can complicate both recovery and the surgical procedure (Maltese et al., 2020). Surgical nurses play a pivotal role in preoperative education and postoperative care, ensuring that patients understand their treatment options and adhere to rehabilitation protocols. This multifaceted approach not only emphasizes the importance of surgical techniques but also underscores the nurse's role in holistic patient care, promoting optimal outcomes and minimizing complications post-surgery. Furthermore, the role of continuous education and training for surgical nurses in musculoskeletal trauma cannot be overstated. Continuous updating of knowledge regarding the latest advances in surgical techniques, imaging modalities, and rehabilitation protocols is essential to enhance the level of care provided to patients. The complexity of musculoskeletal injuries necessitates that surgical nurses receive comprehensive theoretical education, as well as practical training. Continuing professional development, workshops, and the application of current evidence are essential for building and enhancing assessment and management practices. With a culture of learning, surgical nursing can not only enhance clinical competencies but also emphasize patient-centered care, which will ultimately improve recovery pathways and outcomes, as well as patient quality of life (N/A, 2023).

KEY TERMS FROM THIS CHAPTER

- Cast care
- Crepitus
- External fixation
- Immobilization
- Musculoskeletal trauma
- Open reduction internal fixation (ORIF)
- Pain assessment
- Range of motion (ROM)
- Skeletal muscle injury
- Strain
- Compartment syndrome
- Dislocation
- Fracture
- Muscle strength grading
- Neurovascular assessment
- Orthopedic surgery
- Physical rehabilitation
- RICE protocol (Rest, Ice, Compression, Elevation)
- Sprain
- Swelling and ecchymosis

CRITICAL THINKING QUESTIONS

1. **What is the primary purpose of performing a neurovascular assessment in a patient with a limb injury?**
   a. To evaluate kidney function
   b. To assess bowel sounds
   c. To check circulation, sensation, and movement
   d. To monitor vital signs
2. **Which of the following findings requires immediate attention in a patient with a suspected fracture?**
   a. Mild swelling
   b. Redness around the injury
   c. Absent distal pulses
   d. Pain relieved with rest
3. **What is the most common symptom of a musculoskeletal injury?**
   a. Fever
   b. Pain
   c. Hypertension
   d. Headache
4. **Which of the following is a priority nursing action for a patient with a suspected spinal cord injury?**
   a. Encourage the patient to sit up
   b. Immobilize the spine and keep the patient flat
   c. Apply heat to the spine
   d. Check vision regularly
5. **The "RICE" method for initial trauma management stands for:**
   a. Rest, Ice, Compression, Elevation
   b. Rest, Intake, Cold, Exercise
   c. Raise, Ice, Cast, Exercise
   d. Range of motion, Ice, Cast, Elevate

Short Answer Questions

1. What are the main components of a neurovascular assessment?
2. Name two common signs of a bone fracture.
3. Define the "RICE" method used in initial injury care.
4. What is the purpose of immobilization in musculoskeletal trauma?
5. List two complications of untreated musculoskeletal trauma.
6. Describe the nursing assessment of a patient with a suspected limb fracture, including priority checks.
7. Explain the pathophysiology, signs, and emergency management of compartment syndrome.
8. Discuss the role of imaging and diagnostic tools in musculoskeletal trauma evaluation.
9. Outline nursing interventions and patient education following a cast application.
10. Describe the phases of bone healing and nursing support provided during recovery.

Answers to Critical Thinking Questions

1. (c) 2. (c) 3. (b) 4. (b) 5. (a).

REFERENCES

1. Zaremski, J. L., Diamond, M. C., Aagesen, A., Casey, E., Davis, B., Ellen, M., Mautner, K., McInnis, K., Nichols, J., Rao, A., & Krabak, B. (2017). Musculoskeletal and Sports Medicine Physical Medicine and Rehabilitation Curriculum guidelines. *PM&R, 9*(12), 1244–1267. https://doi.org/10.1016/j.pmrj.2017.07.006Abdulaziz, M., Alaleet, W., Al Ghamdi, N. S. M., AlHaddad, E. M. M., et al. (2017). Fracture classification associated with the orthopedic trauma. https://core.ac.uk/download/234692177.pdf (accessed on 30th June 2025).
2. Aishat, M., Segovia, A., Campbell, T., Williams, L., Reyes, K., Hamby, T., Farbo, D., et al. (2025). Quality improvement project to change prescribing habits of surgeons from combination opioids such as hydrocodone/acetaminophen to single-agent opioids such as oxycodone in pediatric postop pain management. *Anesthesia Research.* https://www.semanticscholar.org/paper/c59972598f72bc01bf009f45b722c3dd78a0f281 (accessed on 30th June 2025).
3. Allegrante, J. P., Apfelbaum, J. L., Archer, K. R., Australian Orthopedic Association, Avins, A. L., Caesar, R. R., et al. (2016). Pre-operative self-efficacy education vs. usual care for patients undergoing joint replacement surgery: A pilot randomized controlled trial. https://core.ac.uk/download/76982232.pdf (accessed on 30th June 2025).
4. Almazán Polo, J., García Pérez de Sevilla, G., González-de-la-Flor, Á., López-López, D., et al. (2023). Prevalence, diagnosis and management of musculoskeletal disorders in elite athletes: A mini-review. https://core.ac.uk/download/595770886.pdf (accessed on 30th June 2025).
5. Antares, J. B., Jones, M. A., Chak, N. T. N., Chi, Y., Li, H., Li, M., Chan, E. Y. W., et al. (2025). Efficacy of non-surgical, non-pharmacological treatments for congenital muscular torticollis: A systematic review and meta-analysis. *BMC Musculoskeletal Disorders, 26.* https://www.semanticscholar.org/paper/82a48e1b5f3ffe1af2989171ff501b7ddbeb1a62 (accessed on 30th June 2025).
6. Askegard-Giesmann, J., Benneyworth, B., Hackworth, J., Rouse, T. M., et al. (2017). The trauma registry compared to all patient refined diagnosis related groups (APR DRG). https://core.ac.uk/download/129149052.pdf (accessed on 30th June 2025).
7. Chantraine, A., Hulbert, A., Ku, A., Miller, A., Filler, A. G., Freiberg, A. H., Freiberg, A. H., et al. (2010). The clinical features of the piriformis syndrome: A systematic review. https://core.ac.uk/download/2780274.pdf (accessed on 30th June 2025).
8. Chen, J., & Hou, F. (2023). Unmet needs for healthcare. *Health at a Glance.* https://doi.org/10.1787/c122a43b-en (accessed on 30th June 2025).
9. Compston, J., Cooper, A., Cooper, C., Gittoes, N., Gregson, C. L., Harvey, N. C., Hope, S., et al. (2017). UK clinical guideline for the prevention and treatment of osteoporosis. *Archives of Osteoporosis, 12.* https://doi.org/10.1007/s11657-017-0324-5 (accessed on 30th June 2025).
10. Constantin, M. (2022). Romanian Congress of Physical Medicine and Rehabilitation and Balneology, Slănic Moldova / Techirghiol, 03–10 September 2022–Congress abstracts. *Balneo and PRM Research Journal, 13,* 510–510. https://doi.org/10.12680/balneo.2022.510 (accessed on 30th June 2025).
11. Cox, F. (2025). How to administer a local anesthetic infusion for pain management. *Nursing Standard (Royal College of Nursing (Great Britain): 1987).* https://www.semanticscholar.org/paper/a9501a5ee89a1cf04d7d265f720ea4ab8d41b522 (accessed on 30th June 2025).

12. Drummond, A., Lucas, B., Higgins, B. T., Restrepo, C., Sorbie, C., Sackley, C. M., Jones, C. A., et al. (2016). UK survey of occupational therapists and physiotherapist's experiences and attitudes towards hip replacement precautions and equipment. https://core.ac.uk/download/41994520.pdf (accessed on 30th June 2025).

13. Glikson, M., Nielsen, J. C., Kronborg, M. B., Michowitz, Y., Auricchio, A., Barbash, I. M., Barrabés, J. A., et al. (2021). 2021 ESC guidelines on cardiac pacing and cardiac resynchronization therapy. *European Heart Journal, 42*, 3427–3520. https://doi.org/10.1093/eurheartj/ehab364 (accessed on 30th June 2025).

14. Hsu, J. R., Jahangir, A. A., Miller, A. N., Mir, H. R., et al. (2019). Confronting the opioid crisis: Practical pain management and strategies: AOA 2018 critical issues symposium. https://core.ac.uk/download/286537307.pdf (accessed on 30th June 2025).

15. Izquierdo, M., Merchant, R. A., Morley, J. E., Anker, S. D., Aprahamian, I., Arai, H., Aubertin-Leheudre, M., et al. (2021). International exercise recommendations in older adults (ICFSR): Expert consensus guidelines. *The Journal of Nutrition, Health & Aging, 25*, 824–853. https://doi.org/10.1007/s12603-021-1665-8 (accessed on 30th June 2025).

16. Jaques, R. (2024). Nursing care of the recumbent canine patient after ventral slot surgery. *Veterinary Nursing Journal.* https://www.semanticscholar.org/paper/58ca07b717114ec0f158f5749430289236e02f99 (accessed on 30th June 2025).

17. Khan, A. Q., Abbas, M., Agrawal, P., Anwer, A., Firoz, A., & Harun, F. (2024). From trauma to triumph: Navigating the complexities of a central hip and ipsilateral knee dislocation with associated fractures. *Journal of Orthopedic Case Reports, 14*, 118–124. https://www.semanticscholar.org/paper/eea80c1c70283bc923f2d00ab57a0fad146e7503 (accessed on 30th June 2025).

18. Koshy, D. I., Koshy, D., & Ishaku, Z. (2025). Assessment and decision-making in complex limb fracture management. *Cureus, 17*. https://www.semanticscholar.org/paper/c4ffa5b04413e5c5988d4da9b83a6f3fc9414671 (accessed on 30th June 2025).

19. Lamont, T. (2021). *Making Research Matter.* Policy Press eBooks. https://doi.org/10.56687/9781447361176 (accessed on 30th June 2025).

20. LeBoff, M. S., Greenspan, S. L., Insogna, K., Lewiecki, E. M., Saag, K. G., Singer, A., & Siris, E. S. (2022). The clinician's guide to prevention and treatment of osteoporosis. *Osteoporosis International, 33*, 2049–2102. https://doi.org/10.1007/s00198-021-05900-y (accessed on 30th June 2025).

21. Lestari, H., Purwanti, L., & Andayani, S. (2023). Asuhan keperawatan pada pasien post operasi apendiktomi dengan masalah keperawatan nyeri akut. *Health Sciences Journal.* https://www.semanticscholar.org/paper/0c4797c70fec604687de51da3ce571400c731a4b (accessed on 30th June 2025).

22. Madkhali, N. A. M., Alsomali, M. Y., Al-Dosari, Y. N. M., AlHarbi, S. T. A., Alruwaili, S. T. F., Alahdal, A. A. M., Almutiri, G. H. D., et al. (2024). A comprehensive multidisciplinary strategy for the management of musculoskeletal fractures throughout pregnancy: Evaluation, treatment, and maternal-fetal considerations. *Journal of Eco Humanism.* https://www.semanticscholar.org/paper/1fadbcf125a68de23b44a434dd67281b5ece527b (accessed on 30th June 2025).

23. Maltese, G., Corsonello, A., Di Rosa, M., Soraci, L., Vitale, C., Corica, F., & Lattanzio, F. (2020). Frailty and COVID-19: A systematic scoping review. *Journal of Clinical Medicine, 9*, 2106–2106.

https://doi.org/10.3390/jcm9072106 (accessed on 30th June 2025).

24. Pan, Y., Zhu, H., & Hou, L. (2022). Epidemiological analysis and emergency nursing care of oral and craniomaxillofacial trauma: A narrative review. *Annals of Palliative Medicine, 11*(4), 1518–1525. https://www.semanticscholar.org/paper/05c11de4428993c6f8d80e68f7e40ee75e4c76cb (accessed on 30th June 2025).

25. Pavani, M., Fonseca, L. F., & Conchon, M. F. (2016). Thirst in surgical patients: Perceptions of the nursing team in inpatient units. *Journal of Nursing UFPE Online, 10*, 3352–3360. https://www.semanticscholar.org/paper/7b1c41214be605f210aba1e3ab634ea3e746553f (accessed on 30th June 2025).

26. Sleem, B., Nassar, J. E., Tollefson, L. V., & LaPrade, R. F. (2025). Management and reconstruction strategies for multifilament knee injuries: Advances in diagnosis, surgical techniques, and rehabilitation. *Journal of Arthroscopic Surgery and Sports Medicine.* https://www.semanticscholar.org/paper/5bf47900219fcacaad50716ac268029a3f648c56 (accessed on 30th June 2025).

27. Sousa, L., Raposo, C., Guerra, N., Faleiros, F., Albuquerque, G., & Severino, S. (2024). Rehabilitation nursing care for a patient undergoing corrective surgery for scoliosis: Case report. *Salud, Ciencia y Technology.* https://www.semanticscholar.org/paper/3ebc37823985fdf1b4a78d5b83c2efa68878f217 (accessed on 30th June 2025).

28. Tan, X. Q., & Huang, X. L. (2025). Effects of postoperative quantitative assessment strategy-based nursing in patients with colorectal cancer. *World Journal of Gastrointestinal Surgery, 17.* https://www.semanticscholar.org/paper/b6e11a1b3ad3fdf32bcf81d43dd26e4ebc9fc729 (accessed on 30th June 2025).

29. van As, À. B., van Dijk, M., Mevius, H., Numanoglu, A., et al. (2014). The management of pediatric polytrauma: Review. https://core.ac.uk/download/43313566.pdf (accessed on 30th June 2025).

30. Zhang, Q. (2025). Effectiveness of nursing risk management in surgical nursing care for head and neck tumors. *Advanced Journal of Nursing.* https://www.semanticscholar.org/paper/2fef3f0a49ee5e3d4985e8d95f0c47560b9f41e8 (accessed on 30th June 2025).

GASTROINTESTINAL FUNCTION: DISORDERS AND THERAPEUTIC MANAGEMENT FOR NURSING

8

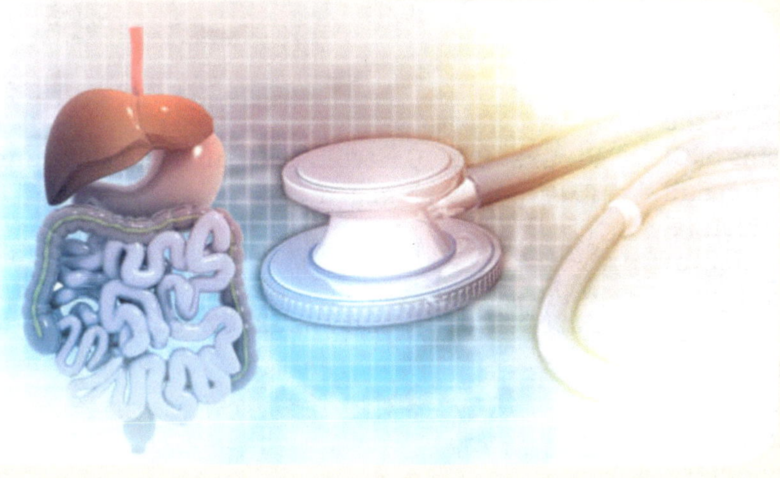

LEARNING OBJECTIVES

After studying this chapter, you will be able to:

1. Understand the common gastrointestinal disorders
2. Explain the pathophysiology of gastrointestinal disorders
3. Discuss the diagnostic approaches in gastrointestinal disorders
4. Focus on therapeutic management strategies
5. Learn about nursing interventions in gastrointestinal care
6. Evaluate the challenges in gastrointestinal nursing

Introduction

The gastrointestinal (GI) system plays a vital role in the proper functioning of the human body by facilitating the digestion, absorption, and excretion of waste products. The GI system comprises diverse organs, including the esophagus, stomach, intestines, liver, and pancreas, which collectively constitute the GI tract. This sensitive group of organs plays a crucial role in metabolizing food into energy. The process is initiated through mechanical digestion, which occurs through chewing, followed by chemical digestion, facilitated by acids and enzymes. The substances absorbed primarily in the small intestine provide cellular activities with essential ingredients, while the large intestine concentrates waste for excretion. Awareness about the coordinated functions and controlling mechanisms of this system is crucial to nursing practice, particularly because many gastrointestinal conditions can compromise these essential processes and create profound health consequences for patients. The intricate nature of GI function also incorporates intrinsic and extrinsic mechanisms that influence its functioning. Neural and hormonal regulations are crucial in coordinating the interplay between different components of the GI tract to have effective digestive mechanisms and nutrient absorption. An example would be the enteric nervous system, which is autonomous but also communicates with the central nervous system, controlling motility and secretions. Furthermore, diseases such as inflammatory bowel disease, irritable bowel syndrome, and gastrointestinal infections can disrupt these balancing processes, producing symptoms like discomfort, malnutrition, or systemic illness. Therefore, nurses should possess an idea of the pathological and physiological mechanisms of GI function since this aids in the identification and management of such common gastrointestinal illnesses. Therapeutic management of gastrointestinal disorders is guided by an overarching approach that often encompasses both pharmacological and non-pharmacological interventions. Recommendations from guidelines, such as those of the Enhanced Recovery After Surgery (ERAS) Society, emphasize the benefits of multimodal care pathways for the attainment of optimal patient outcomes with and after surgical procedures of the GI tract (Gustafsson et al., 2018). These routes encompass selective diet modifications, pain relief, and the use of specific medications to promote gastrointestinal wellness, as is the case with GI functions, which are complex and interrelated. Furthermore, treatment of psychosocial issues, patient counseling, and lifestyle modification can empower patients to become self-managers of their own healthcare, culminating in improved outcomes. Such intensive management strategies emphasize the importance of understanding gastrointestinal function, enabling nurses to provide appropriate and individualized patient care, regardless of the diverse GI disorders (Figure 8.1).

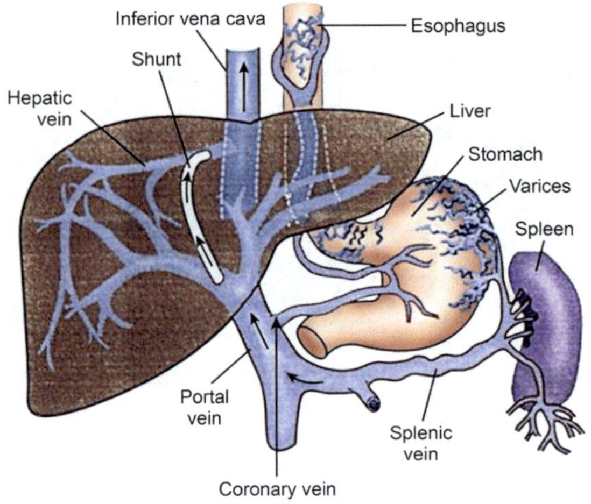

Figure 8.1. Gastrointestinal Disorders and Therapeutic Management.

Source: https://clinicalgate.com/wp-content/uploads/2015/03/F00022Xf022-002-9780323074612.jpg.

Overview of the Gastrointestinal System

The GI system is responsible for a person's overall health and well-being, as it is a complex system that facilitates digestion, absorption, and elimination. The GI system comprises a multitude of vital components, including the mouth, esophagus, stomach, small intestine, large intestine, rectum, and anus, all of which work together to facilitate the complex process of breaking down food and absorbing nutrients. The system begins in the mouth, where food is digested by enzymes present in saliva, and food then travels through the esophagus into the stomach. Food is further digested by gastric juices here before it is passed to the small intestine to absorb nutrients. The large intestine manages waste material for expulsion. Anatomy and physiology knowledge of the system is vital because dysfunctions will lead to severe health issues that must be well-managed through therapeutic intervention in nursing. Several gastrointestinal disorders can have a profound impact on a patient's life. Such conditions comprise the gastroesophageal reflux disease (GERD), irritable bowel syndrome (IBS), inflammatory bowel diseases (IBD) such as Crohn's disease and ulcerative colitis, and cancers of the gastrointestinal system of various sorts. All of these diseases have unique symptomatic characteristics, which most often lead to complex management strategies. For example, although GERD is characterized mainly by reflux and heartburn, IBD offers a very diverse array of symptoms, including abdominal pain, diarrhea, and weight loss. Also, illnesses such as gastric cancer complicate management due to late diagnosis and treatment complexity. Nursing specialists must be proficient in symptom detection, holistic assessment, and implementation of effective interventions to alleviate pain and improve gastrointestinal health in ailing patients, hence the necessity for in-depth GI system knowledge. The treatment of gastrointestinal illnesses is always therapeutic and must be conducted on a multidisciplinary level, utilizing both pharmacological and non-pharmacological interventions. Nurses the act as the intermediary, counseling the patients regarding lifestyle modification that can decrease symptoms, such as diet, management of stress, and medication compliance. In more significant illnesses like IBD, specific therapies through the use of biologic drugs may be used to manage inflammation as well as bring about remission. Additionally, palliative management methods, particularly in treating late-stage cancers like gastric cancer, are inevitable in enhancing the quality of life through the relief of pain and other distressing symptoms. Through improvements in healthcare, patient-centered care for gastrointestinal management is becoming clearer, and thus close coordination between healthcare providers is inevitable to ensure the best results for patients with GI disorders (Figure 8.2).

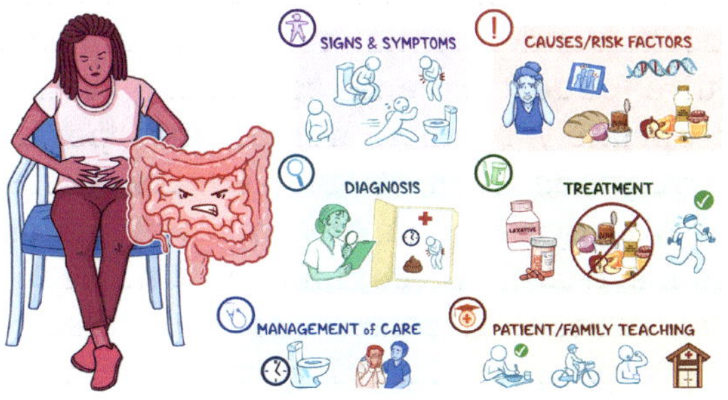

Figure 8.2. Irritable bowel syndrome (IBS).

Source: https://osmose-it.s3.amazonaws.com/mu4szL_FRZK0aAYkbsiIlxQZTtmqRkyi/_.png.

Importance of Gastrointestinal Health

The gastrointestinal (GI) system is important to overall wellness by digesting food, supporting immune function and influencing psychological well-being. A well-functioning gastrointestinal tract ensures the effective breakdown of food, absorption of nutrients, and elimination of waste required for homeostasis in the body. Moreover, there exists a multifaceted relationship between mental and gastrointestinal health; malfunction in the gut may lead to psychological states such as depression and anxiety. There is evidence to support this claim, and it has been proven that treating gastrointestinal illness can directly correlate with improved mental health. Thus, GI health maintenance is imperative not only for physical but also mental well-being, emphasizing the importance of holistic nursing care that addresses both aspects of health. In nursing, awareness of the importance of gastrointestinal health is crucial in assessing risks and planning interventions. Nurses are at the point of patient contact, so have a solid understanding of common GI disorders and their impact on global health. IBS, IBD, and gastrointestinal infections are disorders that can significantly impact the quality of life of patients and exhibit a diverse range of signs and symptoms beyond the gastrointestinal tract. Furthermore, the complexities involved in managing such disorders, such as nutritional restriction and potential nutritional imbalance, require educating and counseling patients appropriately by their nurses. Incorporating interventions such as biofeedback therapy for bowel dysfunction can empower patients, enhance treatment compliance, and lead to improved health outcomes, thereby underscoring the pivotal role nurses play in promoting gastrointestinal health (Chelvanayagam et al., 2012). Lastly, gastrointestinal well-being also comes into play in the control of comorbidities, e.g., late-life depression (LLD), which tends to complicate the clinical presentation in older adults. The interaction between gastrointestinal upset and mental illness can be a vicious cycle, further exacerbating each condition that requires a multidisciplinary team. The presence of gastrointestinal conditions renders the clinical presentation of LLD complex and, hence, it is crucial for clinicians, such as nurses, to recognize and screen out older adults for these dual issues. The timely detection of gastrointestinal-related symptoms may lead to more targeted interventions addressing the physical as well as psychosocial components of health, thereby optimizing patient care and outcomes. Ultimately, an integrative approach to gastrointestinal health can be a keystone for improving not just GI function but also the psychological well-being of patients (Declercq et al., 2018).

Role of Nursing in Gastrointestinal Care

Patient management and assessment are also critical in gastrointestinal nursing. Nurses often the first to attend to patients with gastrointestinal issues, so they must be able to conduct comprehensive assessments. They are taught to identify signs and symptoms of various gastrointestinal disorders, including irritable bowel syndrome, inflammatory bowel disease, and gastroesophageal reflux disease. By utilizing their clinical skills and knowledge, nurses can effectively collect patient histories, conduct physical examinations, and interpret valid laboratory test results. This grounding in care is the first assessment on which care is subsequently based, allowing for proper interventions and referrals as needed. Also included in the assessment process is education regarding lifestyle changes that benefit the gastrointestinal tract, thereby allowing patients to become active partners in their own care. Aside from evaluation, nursing interventions are crucial in treating gastrointestinal diseases. Nurses adopt personalized plans of care that not only control the physical state but also the emotional well-being of patients.

This holistic approach involves the use of medications, nutritional management, and psychoeducation to lessen the fear most associated with gastrointestinal disease. For instance, biofeedback has been implemented as a conservative management to address bowel dysfunction and demonstrated ways in which nurses could become engaged in therapeutic modalities beyond routine pharmacotherapy (Chelvanayagam et al., 2012). Nurses are advocates for patients and assist with relaying the patient's needs to other healthcare providers, ensuring an integrated approach to treatment.

The ability to provide individualized care not only enhances health outcomes but also improves the patient experience overall. The nursing role also expands to patient education, in which nurses educate patients with information they need concerning their gastrointestinal health. Education is vital, as many patients with gastrointestinal diseases often have misconceptions about their conditions that can undermine treatment regimens. By educating patients about their ailments and therapies to which they can be subjected, nurses can play a role in minimizing the risk of complications as well as promoting healthier living. The significance of this is most evident in treating late-life depression, which can be a secondary development of chronic gastrointestinal illness. Nurses have to watch for psychological distress within the elderly person, as gastrointestinal complaints can mask underlying mental illness (Declercq et al., 2018). By integrating mental health assessment into routine nursing assessments, they can enhance detection and treatment earlier, resulting in an overall improved practice of gastrointestinal care.

8.1. Common Gastrointestinal Disorders

Learning Outcome

1. Describe the gastroesophageal reflux disease (GERD)
2. Focus on inflammatory bowel disease (IBD)
3. Learn about irritable bowel syndrome (IBS)

Of the common gastrointestinal disorders, constipation is a widespread issue, particularly in care homes. The condition can be distressing to the patients if left untreated, often leading to more complex health issues in the future. Early detection is critical in treatment; if constipation is identified early, interventions can remain uncomplicated and cost-effective. Delayed recognition, however, may require multifaceted interventions that consume a significant amount of medical resources and incur additional expenses for nursing staff. A good understanding of the primary causes of constipation, ranging from dietary factors to decreased mobility, enhances nurses' effectiveness in using appropriate preventive interventions tailored to individual needs, thereby improving patient outcomes. Furthermore, the use of a 'red flag' table can equip medical professionals with the resources to recognize constipation as a red flag symptom for more serious underlying conditions, allowing proactive clinical management strategies (Lee et al., 2016). Irritable bowel syndrome (IBS) is another common gastrointestinal illness that has a significant impact on quality of life in patients. Characterized by symptoms such as abdominal pain, bloating, and alteration of bowel habits, IBS presents both diagnosis and treatment difficulties. Nursing interventions are often implemented through patient education, including dietary modification and stress management techniques, both of which are crucial to symptom management. Recent studies have investigated the efficacy of nurse-administered cognitive behavior therapy (CBT) as a potential IBS intervention, with its ability to reallocate nursing duties away from routine medical practice. As this research indicates, patient nonadherence to treatment can be traced back to preconceived notions about the treatment approach, thereby necessitating proper communication techniques on the part of ~~nurses~~ in order to promote compliance. Through the establishment of ~~empathetic~~ therapeutic relationships, nurses can help foster increased participation and adherence to management regimens, ultimately optimizing the care experience for IBS patients (Callaghan et al., 2017). Additionally, knowing the simple mechanisms underlying gastrointestinal illnesses, such as gastroesophageal reflux disease (GERD), is essential to nursing management. GERD is characterized by ~~normal~~ abnormal retrograde movement of gastric acid into the esophagus, with resultant symptoms of heartburn and regurgitation. In affected patients, lifestyle interventions such as nutritional adjustments, weight control, and positioning maneuvers are typically recommended as first-line interventions. Nurses play a pivotal role in teaching patients about these accommodations, with an emphasis on the importance of individualized care plans tailored to diverse needs and precipitating factors. Pharmacologic interventions may also be necessary in more severe cases, underscoring the importance of comprehensive evaluations to inform clinical decisions. By educating patients with relevant information and resources, nurses have the potential to significantly contribute to the management of GERD by enhancing patient compliance and overall health outcomes. Research and education in these areas are therefore crucial to successful practice in gastrointestinal health (Figure 8.3).

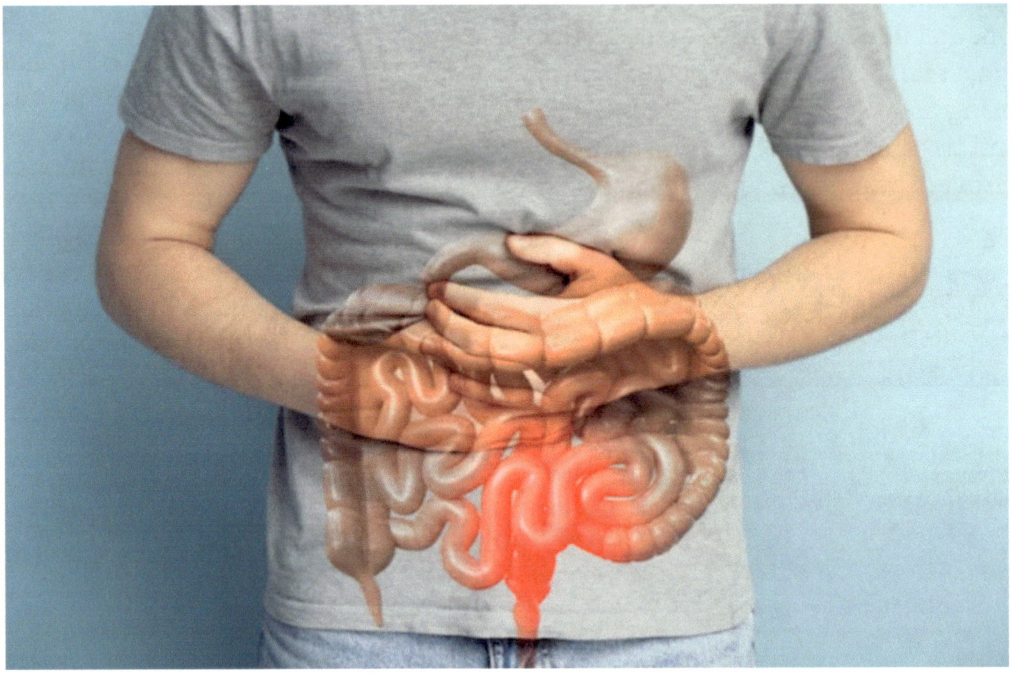

Figure 8.3. Importance of early detection and treatment of gastrointestinal disorders.

Source: https://drramchandrasoni.in/wp-content/uploads/2024/01/Treatment-of-Gastrointestinal-Disorders-Dr-Ram-C-Soni.png.

8.1.1. Gastroesophageal Reflux Disease (GERD)

Gastroesophageal reflux disease (GERD) emerges as one of the most common gastrointestinal diseases affecting millions of people across the globe. Characterized by the abnormal retrograde flow of stomach contents into the esophagus, GERD classically presents with heartburn, regurgitation, and dysphagia. GERD, if not treated, can lead to serious complications like erosion of the esophagus, stricture, and even Barrett's esophagus, which is an antecedent of esophageal cancer. In practice, primary care providers play a significant role in the diagnosis and management of GERD, ensuring that patients receive appropriate treatment. Evidence-based practice guidelines, such as those published by the American College of Gastroenterology (ACG), are necessary to mitigate the adverse effects of the disease on patient health (Fernando et al., 2022). The aggressive management of GERD includes lifestyle modifications and prudent use of pharmacologic therapy to enhance outcomes. Treatment for GERD focuses on lifestyle modifications and pharmacologic treatment. Effective measures include weight loss advice, avoidance of trigger foods, and nighttime head positioning, which collectively can alleviate symptoms in many patients. Pharmacological treatment is typically an eight-week course of proton pump inhibitors (PPIs), which have been proven to suppress acid secretion from the stomach and to reduce symptoms rapidly. Compliance with ACG guidelines ensures that individualized therapy schedules are correctly implemented and allows for referral to a specialist promptly if conservative treatment proves insufficient (Fernando et al., 2022). Moreover, early intervention and frequent monitoring can prevent the onset of serious complications such as esophageal strictures or chronic esophagitis. Application of these practices in the clinic itself demonstrates the significant role played by nursing professionals in the proper management of GERD. Complementary to conventional modalities, there is growing interest in the role of alternative and complementary medicines, particularly herbal medicines, in the management of GERD. Since approximately 80% of the global population utilizes some form of traditional medicine, the popularity of herbal products often relates to their perceived safety and tolerability compared to synthetic medications. Added to this is the economic aspect of herbal therapy, making it an attractive choice for patients with gastrointestinal manifestations, like GERD. While anecdotal evidence supports the efficacy of certain herbs, it is essential that medical practitioners examine the scientific literature behind these therapies and not interfere with regulated medical treatment. Thus, understanding the interaction between mainstream and complementary practices can enhance the quality of patient care, offering a more thorough perspective on the management of GERD and gut health (Figure 8.4).

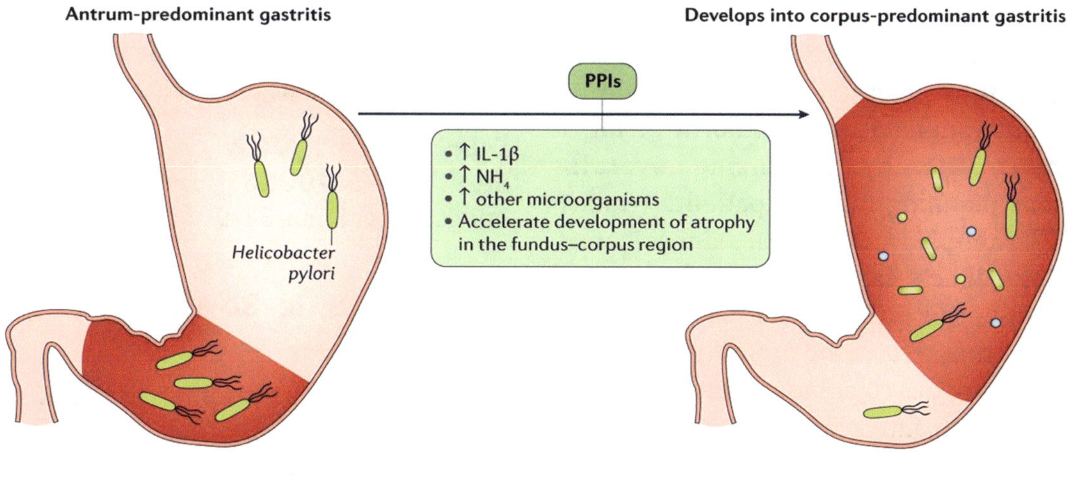

Figure 8.4. Proton-pump inhibitors.

Source: https://media.springernature.com/lw1200/springer-static/image/art%3A10.1038%2Fnrgastro.2017.117/MediaObjects/41575_2017_Article_BFnrgastro2017117_Fig3_HTML.jpg.

8.1.2. Inflammatory Bowel Disease (IBD)

Inflammatory bowel disease (IBD), with conditions such as Crohn's disease and ulcerative colitis, is a significant issue in gastrointestinal disease. Contributed by gastrointestinal tract chronic inflammation, IBD leads to incapacitating symptoms that, in turn, disrupt a patient's quality of life. The pathogenic mechanisms leading to IBD are multifaceted, involving genetic predisposition, environmental triggers, and an abnormal immune response. Recent evidence supports a strong link between diet and the onset of IBD, with the suggestion that nutrition is an important modifiable risk factor and therapeutic management aspect. As noted, the comprehensive review by the

D-ECCO working group elucidates that diet plays a crucial environmental role in the pathogenesis of IBD, speculating that dietary exposures are partially responsible for the increasing prevalence of the disease (Allan et al., 2017). Treatment modalities in IBD management are quite different, from drug therapies to dietary modification and nutrition support interventions. In particular, management of IBD is a multifaceted intervention that involves the use of immunosuppressive drugs, biologics, and nutrition specially tailored for each individual.

There is increasing evidence to indicate that dietary treatment ~~can not~~ ~~only~~ should be employed as induction ~~but~~ and also as maintenance therapy of IBD, representing an interesting prospect for patients who want to utilize or add on pharmaceutical treatments. Nutritional assessment should be incorporated into practice, as it can reveal a patient's nutritional status and inform dietary management, thereby enhancing overall management planning for IBD patients (Allan et al., 2017). Non-pharmacological management, such as biofeedback, has also been effective in the management of bowel dysfunction in IBD. This conservative treatment approach utilizes behavioral techniques to enhance bowel control and alleviate gastrointestinal discomfort. The published literature assessing biofeedback in IBD patients has been encouraging, particularly for individuals with comorbid conditions like anorexia nervosa, which is traditionally common in IBD patients. According to reports, a high incidence of such comorbidities favors holistic management approaches that incorporate psychological and behavioral interventions alongside conventional therapies. In light of the requirement for a holistic approach, nursing professionals need to be well-versed in various therapeutic modalities, as mentioned above, to facilitate maximum patient benefit in IBD management (Figure 8.5).

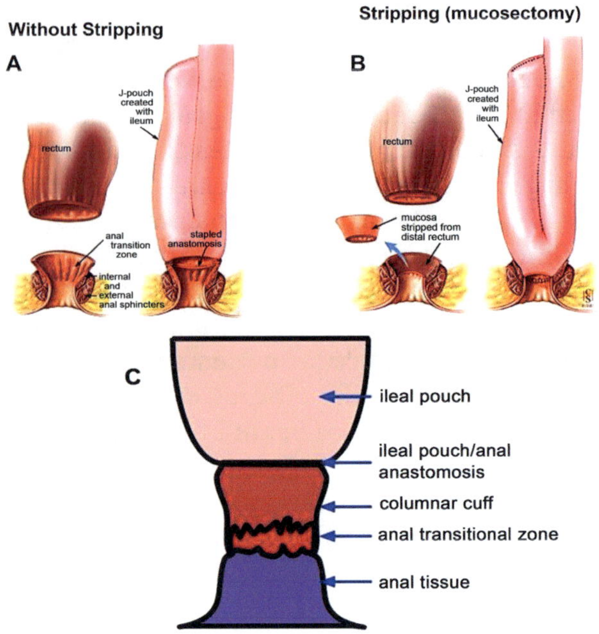

Figure 8.5. Inflammatory bowel disease: clinical diagnosis and surgical treatment.

Source: https://www.mdpi.com/medicina/medicina-58-00567/article_deploy/html/images/medicina-58-00567-g001.png.

8.1.3. Irritable Bowel Syndrome (IBS)

Irritable bowel syndrome (IBS) is a prevalent gastrointestinal disorder that has a broad symptom profile, including abdominal discomfort, bloating, and alterations in bowel movements such as constipation and diarrhea. The etiology of IBS is multifactorial in nature, with the disorder's expression being influenced by genetic, psychological, and nutritional factors. An understanding of these complexities is essential for nurses in our role to provide holistic care in the therapeutic management of IBS. A thorough assessment, including an accurate patient history and a detailed description of symptoms, enables a personalized strategy, ensuring that the care plan aligns with the individual needs of each patient. The significance of effective symptom management cannot be overstated, as the well-being of IBS patients can be profoundly affected, necessitating an interprofessional approach comprising dietetic modification, pharmacological treatment, and psychosocial intervention. As far as therapeutic management is concerned, evidence indicates that psychological therapy, such as cognitive behavioral therapy and hypnotherapy, has a significant role to play in the management of IBS. Evidence has confirmed that hypnotherapy, in addition to routine medical treatment, leads to substantial improvements in quality of life and symptoms of patients with this condition. Specifically, the effectiveness of psychological treatments has been established in clinical trials, where the treatment performed favorably compared to medical interventions without such methods. Secondly, the symptoms of pain and distress have been reduced, and the psychological quality of life of patients has been enhanced, indicating the need to address the emotional aspects of IBS for the provision of integral care. As nurses utilize such treatment methods, they must also be sensitive to the psychological aspects of IBS and integrate these into the treatment protocols for optimal patient outcomes (Pour-Dehkordi et al., 2016). Another promising avenue within the treatment model of IBS is the "gold standard" position of biofeedback therapy in treating bowel dysfunction. This technique employs behavioral techniques to enhance self-regulation of physiological processes, thereby empowering patients to exert greater control over their symptoms. A retrospective review of patients on biofeedback yielded promising results, suggesting its utility as an adjunctive therapy in patients with IBS. While not effective in all patients, biofeedback training may be helpful in those patients whose symptomatology is stress- and anxiety-sensitive. By incorporating biofeedback and other adjunct therapies into mainstream treatment models, nursing clinicians can provide an enhanced and more holistic model of IBS management. Additionally, measuring the efficacy of these interventions contributes to a dynamic presentation of IBS management and aids in justifying individualized care plans based on each patient's specific circumstances (Chelvanayagam et al., 2012).

Test Your Knowledge

1. What are typical symptoms of gastroesophageal reflux disease (GERD)?
2. How does irritable bowel syndrome (IBS) differ from inflammatory bowel disease (IBD)?

8.2. Pathophysiology of Gastrointestinal Disorders

Learning Outcome

1. Explain the mechanisms of disease development
2. Define the impact of lifestyle factors on gastrointestinal function
3. Discuss the genetic predispositions and environmental triggers

Pathophysiology of GI diseases encompasses a wide range of biological and physiological mechanisms that disrupt the usual digestive functions. The conditions have more than one etiology, including genetic disposition, inflammatory reactions, and alterations in intestinal microbiota. For instance, diseases like IBD are characterized by the occurrence of chronic inflammation following an inappropriate immune response, leading to severe mucosal damage and compromised gut permeability. Similarly, functional disorders such as irritable bowel syndrome (IBS) result from dysregulation of gut motility and visceral hypersensitivity and generate symptoms of abdominal pain and changed bowel habits. Nursing professionals need to understand the complex interplay of these factors, as it has a direct impact on patient management interventions aimed at alleviating symptoms and restoring gastrointestinal function. Aging anorexia (AA) is another significant issue among the GI conditions, mainly in older adults. The illness typically manifests as decreased appetite secondary to several determinants, including sensory impairments, depression, and social isolation. AA has far-reaching consequences, as it also poses greater risks of malnutrition, frailty, and unhealthy outcomes, thereby influencing overall quality of life. Evidence has established that treating AA through interventions tailored to individual needs is effective in improving nutritional status and weight, as demonstrated by meta-analytic results showing increases in energy intake and weight control (Donini et al., 2018). For nurses, recognizing the symptoms of AA is essential in creating comprehensive care plans that incorporate nutritional interventions to enhance the health and quality of life in older patients with the condition. Late-life depression (LLD) can complicate the course of gastrointestinal disease, contributing to the burden of care in patients. The condition is frequently underdiagnosed in the elderly due to overlapping somatic symptoms, such as gastrointestinal distress, nausea, and anorexia. The intricate interconnection between LLD and GI disorders is highlighted by the bidirectionality of their pathophysiology, in which depression can potentially induce changes in gut motility and secretion, and gastrointestinal symptoms can potentially contribute to the psychological severity of depression (Declercq et al., 2018). Therefore, the role of psychological assessment and intervention within a multidisciplinary strategy is critical in nursing practice. By utilizing screening tools and integrating mental health care into the management of GI disorders, nurses can significantly improve patient outcomes and quality of life in older adults (Figure 8.6).

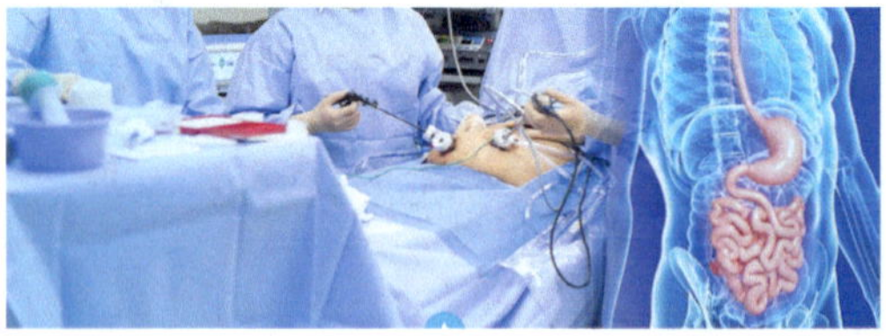

Figure 8.6. Gastroenterology surgery.

Source: https://www.irishospital.co.in/wp-content/uploads/2021/05/Gastroenterology-GI-Surgery.jpg.

8.2.1. Mechanisms of Disease Development

The pathogenesis of gastrointestinal (GI) diseases can be attributed to various mechanisms that constitute the pathophysiology of these diseases. One such underlying mechanism involves dysregulation of ~~the gut's~~ digestive system's defense barriers, e.g., the mucosal layer and tight junctions between epithelial cells. If the barriers are compromised, they can lead to increased intestinal permeability, also known as leaky gut. This permeability allows antigens and toxins to enter the systemic circulation, inducing inflammatory reactions that exacerbate disease mechanisms, such as gastroesophageal reflux disease (GERD) and inflammatory bowel disease (IBD). Additionally, interactions between genetic, environmental, and lifestyle factors play a significant role in causing and exacerbating these GI diseases. Understanding this complex interaction is critical in nursing practitioners as it dictates therapeutic interventions that re-establish mucosal integrity and regulate inflammation, thus improving patient outcomes of GI disorders, as demonstrated in Hunt et al. (2017). Another critical mechanism of disease establishment in the gastrointestinal tract is the dysregulation of the microbiome, which has significant impacts on health and disease states. Dysbiosis, or dysregulation of the gut microbiota, has been associated with the pathogenesis of numerous GI disorders, such as irritable bowel syndrome (IBS) and colorectal cancer. The microbiota interacts with the ~~guts~~ gastrointestinal immune system, producing short-chain fatty acids and other metabolites that affect intestinal health and inflammation. A disrupted microbiome can lead to a decrease in anti-inflammatory bacteria, resulting in a pro-inflammatory environment that can exacerbate symptoms and disease progression. Thus, therapeutic management often includes probiotics or other therapies aimed at rebalancing the microbiome. Nurses must be familiar with these microbial interactions and their implications for patient instruction and care planning, particularly when writing orders for dietary modifications or adjunctive therapies to effectively treat disorders, as outlined in Hunt et al. (2015). Lastly, disease initiation mechanisms in gastrointestinal illnesses are typically moderated by environmental factors such as diet, stress, and drug consumption. High-fat diets, for example, may increase the risk for GERD, leading to esophagitis and, in more serious cases, Barrett's esophagus. Psychological stress, however, can also contribute significantly to GI function, which may lead to such presentations as dyspepsia or exacerbation of a disorder such as IBD. Drugs, particularly the nonsteroidal anti-inflammatory drugs (NSAIDs), can interfere with the gastric mucosal barrier to result in ulceration. These etiologic considerations highlight the importance of thorough patient evaluation by nursing personnel, which will enable them to review lifestyle behaviors, monitor dietary interventions, and advise on stress management. By controlling these multifactorial variables, nurses play a significant role in the prevention and therapeutic management of gastrointestinal illness, finally affecting patient adherence to treatment regimens and global health outcomes, as depicted in the holistic strategies outlined in Hunt et al. (2015, 2017).

8.2.2. Impact of Lifestyle Factors

The dialogue between lifestyle determinants and gut function is no longer a controversial issue and is now widely accepted as a major determinant of the etiology and management of many gastrointestinal disorders. Nutritional lifestyle, physical activity, and psychosocial stressors are all pivotal in characterizing gut health. A diet rich in fat and low in fiber, for instance, is associated with a disturbed gut microbiome that leads to dysbiosis, which can drive the development of diseases such as irritable bowel syndrome (IBS) and inflammatory bowel disease (IBD). Additionally, physical inactivity exacerbates metabolic dysregulation, which is associated with gastrointestinal symptoms. As medical practitioners, nurses are obligated to emphasize nutrition and physical exercise as key factors in therapeutic interactions, not just compliance with medication, but also overall lifestyle modifications that promote gastrointestinal health and patient outcomes. Therefore, lifestyle factors need to be tackled appropriately for optimal management and prevention in clinical practice, particularly through nursing interventions. Psychological stress is also a significant lifestyle factor that affects gastrointestinal function, which is an interaction of complex mind-gut relationships essential for patient care. Chronic stress can induce activation of neuroendocrine pathways, which lead to alterations in gut motility and increased visceral hypersensitivity, which can potentially play a role in exacerbating gastrointestinal illness. Such interactions suggest that psychological well-being is crucial for maintaining gastrointestinal health, as stressed patients may become more sensitive to gastrointestinal disturbances. This association highlights the importance of incorporating stress-reduction interventions, such as cognitive behavioral therapy, mindfulness techniques, and counseling, into patient treatment plans when attending to patients presenting with gastrointestinal symptoms. By understanding the impact that psychological stress has on the gut, nursing clinicians can create a more holistic approach to treatment that cares for both mental and physical health, thereby improving patient outcomes. Furthermore, the gut microbiome serves as an interactive interface between lifestyle and gastrointestinal physiology, reflecting the complex relationship between diet, lifestyle, and gut health. Increasing evidence suggests that lifestyle factors, such as diet and exercise, can have direct effects on gastrointestinal microbiota composition and its far-reaching implications for overall health and disease risk. For example, the intake of fruits, vegetables, and whole grains provides a healthy microbiome, whereas the consumption of sugars and processed foods can negatively impact gut bacteria diversity. The study reveals that lifestyle patterns also predispose individuals to gastrointestinal complications and cognitive impairment in older age, further indicating the need for early dietary interventions (Nohesara et al., 2024). By educating patients about the role of gut microbiome health, nursing professionals can play an integral part in preventing and controlling gastrointestinal diseases through lifestyle changes, promoting an integrated approach to health (Figure 8.7).

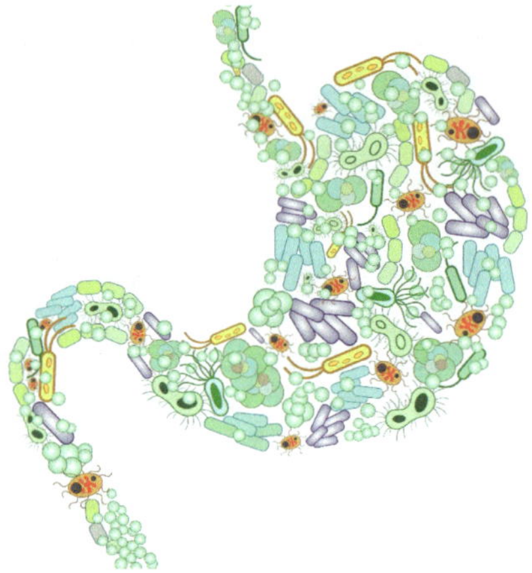

Figure 8.7. Gut dysbiosis and IBS.

Source: https://magazineup.com/wp-content/uploads/2021/02/gut_bugs.original-2048x2048.jpg.

8.2.3. Genetic Predispositions and Environmental Triggers

The interaction between genetic vulnerabilities and environmental triggers has significant implications for understanding gastrointestinal illnesses. Genetic factors contribute to an individual's susceptibility to ailments such as inflammatory bowel disease (IBD), where genetic factors may influence the severity and progression of symptoms. For instance, specific polymorphisms in genes that regulate immune response and gut flora may predispose an individual to such illnesses. However, genetic propensity is insufficient in explaining the full spectrum of disease expression; environmental factors, such as diet, drugs, and stress, also play a significant role. Through the investigation of both environmental variables and genetic markers, healthcare practitioners are better equipped to tailor treatment approaches, thereby contributing to improved patient outcomes. Environmental provocation can come in a variety of forms, with diet representing a primary precipitating factor for gastrointestinal disorders. For example, diets high in fat and high sugar intake have been associated with increased inflammation and severity of symptoms in patients with IBD. Additionally, psychosocial factors such as stress and anxiety can potentially be accelerators for worsening of the conditions. A study found that IBD patients had a strong association between dietary impact awareness and symptom control, where improved dietary knowledge led to quality-of-life improvements (Abdu et al., 2024). This reinforces the need for healthcare providers to incorporate both genetic susceptibility and environmental factors into management strategies for treatment, with dietary education being a key component. Additionally, interactions among genetic predispositions, environmental triggers, and inflammatory responses can explain why certain patients develop more severe gastrointestinal disorders than others. It has been shown through research that individuals with specific personality types, with greater emotional instability being an example, will have more intense symptoms as a result of psychosomatic responses. Comorbid individuals with IBD have been observed to express more emotional distress and physical discomfort, thus underscoring the complexity of such interactions (Gheonea et al., 2024). This also underlines the importance of an overall approach in nursing care that is not merely responsive to the genetic basis but also actively seeks to override environmental stressors and psychological disturbances in patients. With this holistic management strategy, nursing professionals can considerably increase the therapeutic success in gastrointestinal disease cases.

Test Your Knowledge

1. How does inflammation contribute to the development of Crohn's disease?
2. What is the underlying pathophysiology of peptic ulcer disease?

8.3. Diagnostic Approaches in Gastrointestinal Disorders

Learning Outcome

1. Explain the clinical assessment and patient history
2. Define the laboratory tests and imaging studies in assessing gastrointestinal disorders
3. Describe the endoscopic procedures and their significance for gastrointestinal disorders

With the intricate nature of gastrointestinal disease, diagnostic approaches play a pivotal role in deciding successful treatment directions. Physicians utilize a variety of diagnostic modalities, ranging from patient history and physical examination to efficacious imaging modalities and laboratory studies. Effective diagnosis begins with a diagnostic history that explores dysphagia, heartburn, and abdominal pain, which are typically manifestations of underlying gastrointestinal illness. Aids such as symptom questionnaires can assist in calculating the frequency and severity of symptoms, but knowledge of regional epidemiology is essential in determining the relevance of these symptoms for each disorder. The application of endoscopic methods, including esophagogastroduodenoscopy (EGD), plays a central role in visualizing internal structures and procuring biopsies, thereby facilitating diagnosis and treatment optimization in alarm features such as dysphagia or gastrointestinal bleeding (Hunt et al., 2017). When diagnosing gastrointestinal disorders, the relationship between clinical assessment and diagnostic machinery cannot be downplayed. Non-invasive tests, including upper gastrointestinal barium studies, provide valuable information on structural derangement but have their limitations when contrasted with endoscopy. In the last decade, advances in imaging technology, particularly in modalities such as CT and MRI, have greatly helped explain complex disorders, including Crohn's disease and cancer. These technologies provide wide panoramic views that inform management strategies tailored to the specific requirements of a patient. Moreover, laboratory tests, for example, fecal infection or inflammatory marker tests, enhance the diagnostic process by providing a biological context. However, context-specific management principles are necessary to guide the interpretation of these tests, particularly in regions where the prevalence of gastrointestinal disease is highly heterogeneous (Hunt et al., 2017). Apart from that, evidence-based guidelines for the confirmation of diagnostic practices are essential for proper treatment. The World Gastroenterology Organization's (WGO) guidelines advocate systematic management through diagnostic cascades that are patient-centered care and resource-oriented management of gastrointestinal disease. The hierarchical system emphasizes appropriate, resource-sensitive management strategies that address the divergent capacities of health systems globally. For instance, in settings where the availability of advanced diagnostic tests is limited, empirical treatment approaches may be more desirable than invasive testing, provided that patient care is made available and yet effective. Ultimately, by synthesizing various diagnostic methodologies and tailored management plans, healthcare providers can optimize patient outcomes for gastrointestinal disease maximally while addressing both clinical needs and systemic concerns of nursing practice (Hunt et al., 2017) (Figure 8.8).

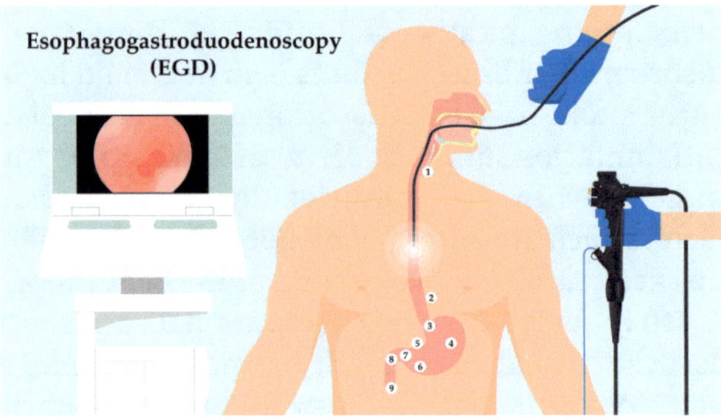

Figure 8.8. Sequential landmarks during EGD..

Source: https://www.researchgate.net/publication/376801525/figure/fig1/AS:11431281214392307@1703506911751/Sequential-landmarks-during-EGD-Utilizing-an-endoscope-to-traverse-the-upper-GI-tract.png.

8.3.1. Clinical Assessment and Patient History

Prompt clinical assessment and careful patient history are the cornerstone of treating gastrointestinal (GI) disease. A thorough patient history enables clinicians to identify symptoms that may indicate underlying disease. Patient interviews typically yield a wealth of information, with food and dietary practices, lifestyle, and family health patterns being significant determinants of gastrointestinal function.

Nurses are instructed to appreciate the significance of these facts, since they not only affect diagnosis but also guide treatment plans. By systematically collecting a patient's history, including prior gastrointestinal issues, medications, and psychosocial factors, the nursing staff establishes a foundation for patient-specific care and reaffirms their understanding of the entire patient within the context of their disease. In assessing patients with gastrointestinal complaints, the importance of some symptoms often takes center stage. Critical symptoms such as abdominal pain, change in bowel habits, and weight loss must be attentively documented to affect subsequent investigation and management. For instance, awareness of how often and in what fashion bowel movements occur can give rise to conditions ranging from irritable bowel syndrome to more sinister pathologies. Clinical tools, including physical examinations and laboratory tests, complement the patient history and contribute to the diagnostic process. Interdisciplinary consultation is important; nurses play a key role in informing physicians and dietitians of important observations. As a result, extensive clinical assessment not only assists in the diagnosis but also in the formulation of extensive therapeutic plans according to individual patients' circumstances. A few of the gastrointestinal diseases, such as myofascial pelvic pain (MFPP), underscore the intricacy of patient assessment and the necessity of a multidisciplinary team. MFPP itself is often underdiagnosed due to overlapping symptoms and relative lack of awareness on the part of healthcare professionals.

The typical presentations include discrete myofascial trigger points within pelvic floor musculature that have the capacity to produce referred pain within adjacent areas. Hence, a thorough history of the patient, including chronic pelvic pain complaints, can enlighten about such myofascial conditions so appropriate management steps can be taken with such biofeedback and physical therapy modalities. Also, the implementation of inter-disciplinary teams is critical because practical treatment approaches are contingent on the convergence of different health professionals coming together to manage the physical as well as the psychological components of GI disorders, finally delivering enhanced patient outcomes (Chelvanayagam et al., 2012; Katzman et al., 2012).

8.3.2. Laboratory Tests and Imaging Studies

Laboratory testing is essential in the assessment of gastrointestinal disorders, which is crucial for accurate diagnosis and effective therapeutic management in nursing practice. Comprehensive blood studies, such as complete blood counts, liver function tests, and specific marker studies, play a crucial role in identifying conditions like liver cirrhosis, pancreatitis, and infections. For instance, abnormal liver enzymes might imply hepatic impairment, while specific serologic testing identifies autoimmune gastrointestinal disease. In addition, stool tests play a critical role in the etiologic diagnosis of infectious conditions, such as bacterial gastroenteritis or parasitic diseases, revealing pathogens that significantly influence patient outcomes. By traversing such intricate test protocols, laboratory intelligence ensures prompt interventions. Therefore, reading competency in these tests is essential for nursing professionals to provide quality care tailored to the individual patient's specific needs. Along with laboratory tests, imaging studies are helpful tools in evaluating gastrointestinal function and detecting abnormalities in anatomical structure. Techniques such as ultrasound, computed tomography (CT), and magnetic resonance imaging (MRI) provide non-invasive methods for viewing the gastrointestinal tract. These imaging modalities can detect serious pathologies, including malignancies, obstructions, and inflammatory conditions like Crohn's disease or ulcerative colitis. Furthermore, higher-level imaging provides valuable information about the functionality of various organs involved in digestion, which aids in differential diagnosis. For instance, CT scans are especially helpful in examining appendicitis, and MRIs will provide better liver and pancreatic abnormality visualization. Due to the multiple applications and meanings of these imaging studies, nursing practitioners should collaborate with radiographic experts to ensure that correct interpretation and resultant management plans are aligned with diagnostic findings. The integration of laboratory studies and imaging studies yields a common framework for managing gastrointestinal illnesses in nursing. This interdisciplinary approach presents a comprehensive understanding of the patient's disease, enabling precise therapeutic interventions. Nursing practice requires nursing practitioners to have a keenly sensitive understanding of the dynamic interplay between test findings and clinical findings, as conditions can change rapidly. For example, newer imaging test findings may require revisiting previous laboratory test findings to refine the diagnosis and tailor treatment plans. The subtleties of conditions like infective endocarditis, where discrimination of pathogenesis from associated gastrointestinal symptoms is crucial, justify the use of an interprofessional practice environment. With the growing complexity of healthcare, nurses possessing extensive knowledge of imaging and laboratory procedures are well-positioned to provide support for effective patient care routines, ultimately leading to desirable health outcomes and optimized recovery patterns among patients with gastrointestinal impairment (Baddour et al., 2015; Pascarella et al., 2020) (Figure 8.9).

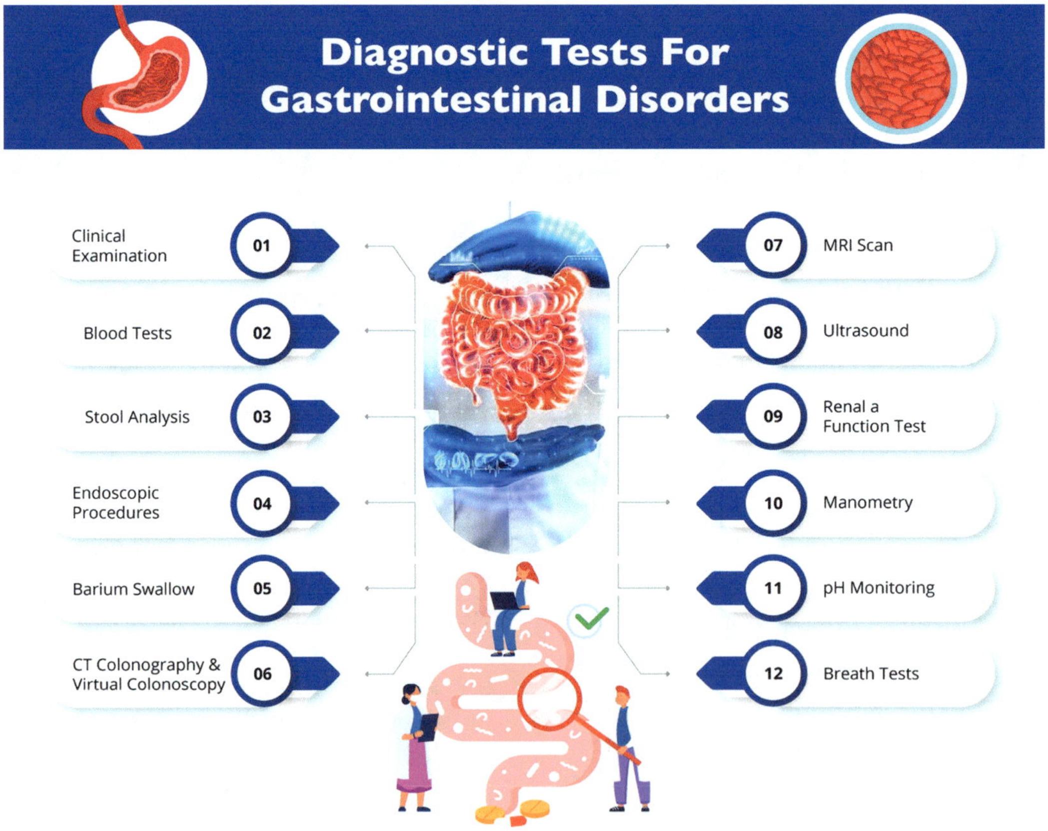

Figure 8.9. Diagnostic tests for gastrointestinal disorders.

Source: https://images.ctfassets.net/eexbcii1ci83/7ve6grc8ek4EYSrLoTDRJ/ddfb6e24f2332bbd1643b3417f549361/Diagnostic_Tests_For_Gastrointestinal_Disorders.jpg.

8.3.3. Endoscopic Procedures and Their Significance

Endoscopic procedures form the nucleus of diagnosis and treatment of gastrointestinal diseases, with therapeutic and diagnostic benefits having a profound effect on patient care. Therapeutic as well as diagnostic benefits of minimally invasive endoscopic procedures like esophagogastroduodenoscopy (EGD) and colonoscopy allow healthcare professionals to see the gastrointestinal tract endoscopically. Visualization facilitates the detection of abnormalities, such as lesions, polyps, and other pathologies, that may not be diagnosed by imaging tests like X-rays or CT scans. Additionally, the ability to harvest biopsy samples during these processes provides crucial diagnostic information for diseases such as cancer or inflammatory bowel disease (IBD). Through the integration of endoscopy into clinical practice, nursing clinicians can offer a rapid and reliable method of treating patients, ultimately leading to improved outcomes in individuals afflicted with gastrointestinal disease.

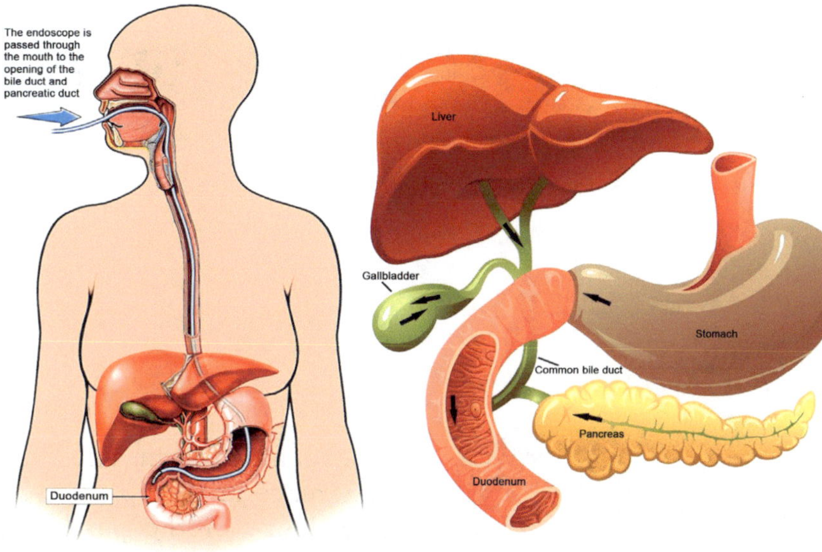

Figure 8.10. Endoscopic retrograde cholangio-pancreatography (ERCP).

Source: https://www.sages.org/wp-content/uploads/2015/03/SAGES-PI-ERCP.png.

The function of endoscopic procedures extends beyond mere diagnosis; besides that, they entail therapeutic interventions with the potential to alleviate symptoms or treat underlying conditions. For instance, through ERCP, medical professionals can treat obstruction or gallstones of the biliary tree and hence prevent further complications. Furthermore, endoscopic procedures enable interventions such as ablation of precancerous lesions, strictures dilatation, or stenting, thus enhancing the quality of care offered to patients. The capability to perform such interventions within a single visit not only reduces the need for more invasive interventions but also reduces the time to recovery for patients. As such, it is of the highest priority that nursing practitioners understand the multifaceted applicability of endoscopic procedures because it has a direct impact on treatment planning and the provision of care strategies. Some clinical advantages aside, endoscopic procedures also have significant roles to play in patient education and empowerment in the clinical setting. As patients become better educated about their conditions and the interventions involved, they can take active roles in their care decisions. It is the responsibility of the healthcare providers, particularly nurses, to play a vital role in the educational process by providing descriptive feedback about the procedure, its indications, and potential risks and benefits. Involving patients in discussions about their treatment enhances knowledge acquisition, reduces anxiety, and makes them feel in control of their health. Moreover, dedicated endoscopy units, which ensure high standards of quality, ensure that patients receive comprehensive care throughout their treatment procedure (Allum et al., 2018). With the global population aging and the rising incidence of gastrointestinal disorders, ongoing education and training in endoscopic procedures will remain a priority for nurses (Blasi et al., 2017). This integrated model of care not only benefits patients but also fosters improved health outcomes in various populations (Figure 8.10).

Test Your Knowledge

1. What is the purpose of an endoscopy in diagnosing GI disorders?
2. How can stool tests help identify gastrointestinal infections?

8.4. Therapeutic Management Strategies

Learning Outcome

1. Identify the pharmacological treatments for gastrointestinal (GI) disorders
2. Define the dietary modifications and nutrition therapy
3. Describe the surgical interventions and their indications in gastrointestinal disorders

Therapeutic management of GI diseases demands a multifaceted, holistic approach that integrates clinical management with patient-centered intervention. Nurses play a pivotal role in delivering these interventions, including not only drug regimens but also lifestyle interventions and emotional support. Effective education and counseling empower patients to implement self-management techniques, thereby promoting adherence to therapeutic regimens. Moreover, knowledge of the particular background of each patient, including psychological, social, and cultural factors, is critical. This aligns with findings from more recent research, which indicate that integrating knowledge and training for common mental disorders has a significant influence on the effectiveness of chronic disease care in primary healthcare (Beaudin et al., 2025). Thus, the collaboration of nurses and patients, facilitated by effective educational measures, leads to improved quality of life and health outcomes for patients with GI disorders. Dietary and lifestyle modifications play a crucial role in the therapeutic management of GI disorders. There is evidence to suggest that lifestyle changes through diet can play a vital role in alleviating symptoms associated with diseases such as gastroesophageal reflux disease (GERD) and inflammatory bowel disease (IBD) (Chughtai et al., 2024). Patients need to be encouraged by nurses to adopt personalized diets that minimize irritants and optimize nutrient absorption to manage their condition. Furthermore, health education about good lifestyle practices, such as physical activity and stress reduction, cannot be overlooked in providing overall well-being and disease avoidance.

The biopsychosocial model emphasizes the importance of addressing both physiological and psychological aspects of well-being, underscoring the need for integration among healthcare professionals to effectively apply these management strategies. By prioritizing diet and lifestyle interventions, nursing interventions can effectively enhance patient care holistically that empowers patients and optimizes their health status. The integration of new therapeutic developments in GI disorder management has the potential to advance patient outcomes significantly. The latest evidence highlights the gut microbiome's role in regulating gastrointestinal disorders, introducing microbiome-guided treatments that promise to transform therapeutic models (Chughtai et al., 2024). Nurses must keep abreast of such developments and incorporate them into patient education and care strategies. Interprofessional collaborative approaches involving dietitians, psychologists, and other healthcare professionals ensure that all aspects of a patient's condition are considered. These holistic strategies not only optimize the effectiveness of treatment but also reflect the imperative necessity of continual research in this field to extend patient benefits and reduce the cost of GI diseases. By promoting cooperation and synergizing new treatments, nursing care can be a key factor in overcoming the complexities of gastrointestinal health care (Figure 8.11).

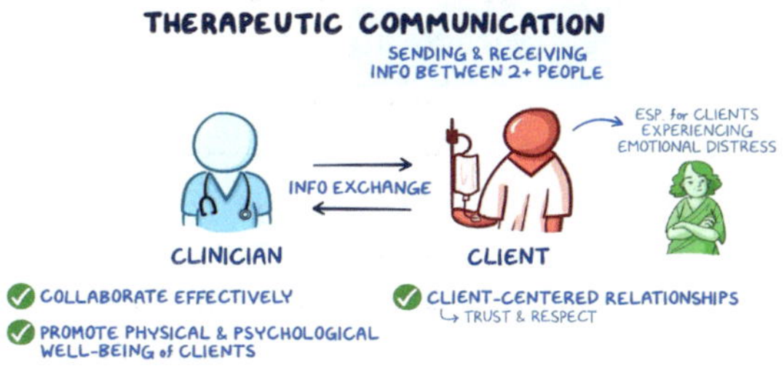

Figure 8.11. Therapeutic communication in nursing.

Source: https://www.osmosis.org/_next/image?url=https%3A%2F%2Fd16qt3wv6xm098.cloudfront.net%2F2q44BeQbTZOiugskwY7RM_ieR32zdcp0%2F_.jpg&w=3840&q=75.

8.4.1. Pharmacological Treatments

Pharmacological intervention in GI diseases is crucial for symptomatic relief and improvement in patients' quality of life. Frequent use is prevalent among proton pump inhibitors (PPIs), H2 receptor antagonists, and prokinetic drugs, which are used to treat disease conditions such as gastroesophageal reflux disease, peptic ulcers, and gastroparesis. PPIs, such as omeprazole, reduce gastric acid secretion effectively, thereby providing relief and facilitating mucosal healing. At the same time, prokinetic agents, such as metoclopramide, enhance gastric motility, thereby alleviating symptoms of delayed gastric emptying. Their use and surveillance are significant because their side effects may include enhanced risk of infection or electrolyte imbalance, particularly in elderly patients with associated illness. Thus, pharmacologic interventions have the obligation to weigh therapeutic efficacy against safety considerations, ensuring that pharmacologic treatments bring maximum benefit to the overall health status of the patient. In addition to acid-related disorders, pharmacologic treatment plays a decisive role in managing anorexia of aging (AA), which can severely affect gastrointestinal function and produce frailty in elderly groups. The use of appetite promoters, such as megestrol acetate or dronabinol, has proven successful in enhancing food intake and nutritional status in this population. Evidence has shown that these drugs can achieve remarkable gains in body weight and energy intake because they act on the multi-factorial basic etiologies of AA, i.e., depression and taste and smell sensory deficits (Donini et al., 2018). Thus, the strategic use of pharmacological therapies can reverse the adverse effects of malnutrition and enhance overall health. Nurses are obligated to consider every patient's distinct needs and maximize therapeutic effectiveness by prioritizing pharmacological interventions that best suit their particular condition. Integrating pharmacological treatments into the comprehensive care of gastrointestinal disorders is optimally achieved through an interdisciplinary collaboration among physicians, nurses, and nutritionists. Good communication among health team members ensures that patients receive comprehensive care that not only addresses pharmacological but also dietary and lifestyle modifications that support the gastrointestinal tract. For instance, dietary modifications aside from medication could include supplementing fiber to treat constipation or adjusting the frequency of meals to ease digestion. Moreover, screening for illnesses such as late-life depression (LLD), which is an aggravating factor in GI disorders, is vital for early care and treatment (Declercq et al., 2018). Adopting a holistic approach that encompasses both pharmacological treatment, dietary changes, and psychosocial intervention enables healthcare providers to offer a more effective treatment option that enhances gastrointestinal function in patients.

8.4.2. Dietary Modifications and Nutrition Therapy

In managing gastrointestinal disorders, nutrition therapy and dietary modification play a significant role in influencing patient outcomes. Such therapy plays a critical role in managing disorders such as inflammatory bowel disease (IBD), irritable bowel syndrome (IBS), and celiac disease, whose symptoms can critically impair daily functioning. Nutritional modification may involve the elimination of the irritant or allergen, such as gluten in the case of celiac disease, or the addition of fiber and probiotics to ensure intestinal balance. Nutrition therapy also helps balance macronutrient intake according to individual requirements, which is especially critical for patients experiencing malnutrition due to chronic gastrointestinal discomfort. The addition of nutritional interventions allows a comprehensive approach to treatment, ultimately leading to better patient adherence to medical regimens and improved quality of life in patients with gastrointestinal disorders. Use of nutrition therapy is not a matter of simply modifying diets, but rather a comprehensive assessment of a patient's nutritional status and the implementation of evidence-based practice. For healthcare practitioners, it is crucial to identify the specific dietary deficiencies associated with gastrointestinal diseases in order to develop effective interventions. For instance, ~~malabsorption~~ patients with malabsorption issues will require tailored supplementation to provide vital nutrients that they will be lacking as a consequence of their condition. Additionally, continued education on healthy eating habits and eating patterns can enable patients to actively participate in managing their own health. The use of documents like food diaries can assist in tracking and adjusting diet plans to help ensure that nutritional strategies are aligned with clinical outcomes. The inclusion of nutrition therapy in the therapeutic regimen is hence essential to help promote effective self-management in patients. Secondly, the impact of lifestyle modifications, such as organized exercise and dietary intervention, demonstrates the synergistic effects of a healthy lifestyle on GI health. Regular physical exercise has been found to improve gastrointestinal function through enhanced motility and reduced stress, which can exacerbate conditions like IBS. The interconnectedness of nutrition, exercise, and gastrointestinal well-being underscores the importance of a holistic approach in treating such disorders. Preventative measures, such as promoting balanced diets consisting of whole foods and reducing processed foods, can significantly lower the risk of developing gastrointestinal disorders. Through an understanding of the intricate relationship between diet, exercise, and overall health, nurses are ideally suited to advocate for holistic treatment programs incorporating both nutritional therapy and lifestyle modification that result in better health outcomes and improved patient quality of life (Figure 8.12).

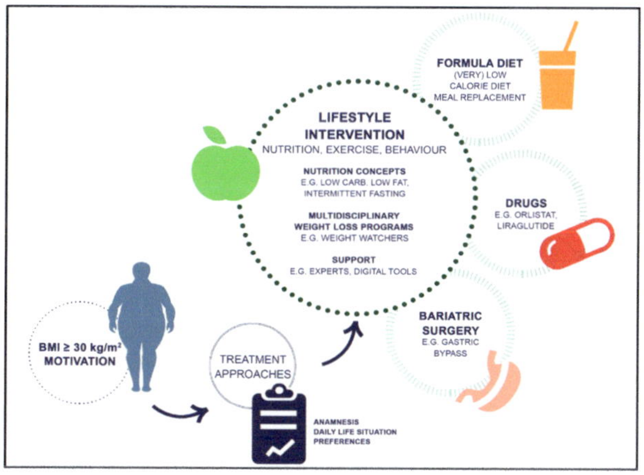

Figure 8.12. Dietary modifications and nutrition therapy.

Source: https://pub.mdpi-res.com/nutrients/nutrients-14-00169/article_deploy/html/images/nutrients-14-00169-g001.png?1640870579.

8.4.3. Surgical Interventions and Their Indications

Understanding the indications for surgical treatment of gastrointestinal diseases is important to the practice of nursing, particularly in acute care. Surgical intervention is generally indicated when nonsurgical treatment cannot alleviate severe illness, such as catastrophic lower GI bleeding or neoplastic tumors. For instance, in the case of gross lower GI bleeding that conditions like diverticular disease could cause, surgical intervention can become unavoidable when non-operative investigative techniques like CT angiography are unable to identify the source of bleeding. A good example was a patient who had recurrent bleeding and ultimately required an emergency right hemicolectomy following failure of conservative measures. This case emphasizes the importance of early surgical referral to minimize risks of blood loss and to repair underlying anatomical defects as with less common diseases like colonic submucosal lipomas, as is discussed in the literature at present (Dadigamuwage et al., 2025).

The efficacy of various surgical techniques, including minimally invasive surgery, also warrants significant attention regarding gastrointestinal disease. Evidence-based nursing care in the ~~guise~~ form of Enhanced Recovery After Surgery (ERAS) protocols has gained increasingly prominent roles in maximizing postoperative outcomes. The protocols have been found to provide particularly valuable benefits in the scenario of endoscopic management of early-stage gastrointestinal tumors. Randomized controlled trials have found that ERAS-based nursing care is associated with lower complications and shorter hospital stays, as well as higher patient satisfaction and quality of life. For example, patients cared for according to ERAS protocols had fewer Comprehensive Complication Index (CCI) scores and improved functional recovery as evaluated using tools such as the Six-Minute Walk Test (6MWT) (Shen et al., 2025). All this demonstrates the strong support for incorporating ERAS protocols into nursing practice to achieve optimal surgical outcomes, emphasizing the need for continuous education and adherence to these innovative care practices within clinical settings. Finally, the postoperative management of surgery involves complexities that must be addressed through a multidisciplinary process, encompassing both physical and psychological recovery. Complications such as thromboembolic conditions and infections contracted in the hospital environment are likely, necessitating close observation within the postoperative environment. The case of a patient developing pulmonary embolism after surgery, for instance, emphasizes the need for integrated postoperative care alongside surgical intervention. According to ERAS protocols, nursing interventions such as early mobilization and fluid hydration play a significant role in reducing these complications and promoting patient recovery. Improved communication between surgical teams and nurses enables healthcare practitioners to better anticipate and manage risk factors, ultimately resulting in improved patient outcomes and optimal recovery in patients undergoing surgical interventions for gastrointestinal disorders (Dadigamuwage et al., 2025; Shen et al., 2025) (Figure 8.13).

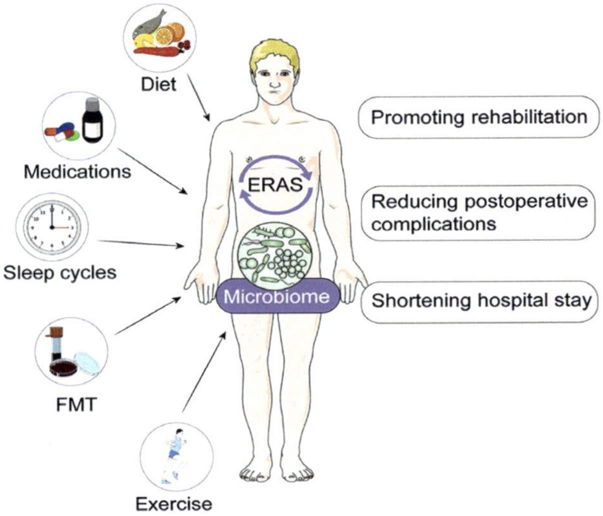

Figure 8.13. Exploring the roles of intestinal flora in enhanced recovery after surgery.

Source: https://ars.els-cdn.com/content/image/1-s2.0-S2589004223000366-fx1.jpg.

Test Your Knowledge

1. How do proton pump inhibitors (PPIs) help manage acid-related gastrointestinal disorders?
2. Why is dietary modification necessary in the treatment of irritable bowel syndrome (IBS)?

8.5. Nursing Interventions in Gastrointestinal Care

Learning Outcome

1. Describe the patient education and counseling in gastrointestinal disorders
2. Define the monitoring and assessment techniques in gastrointestinal disorders
3. Discuss the collaboration with interdisciplinary teams in gastrointestinal disorders

Effective nursing interventions in GI management are significant in the handling of various disorders affecting the gastrointestinal (GI) system. The interventions play a key role in improving outcomes for patients and comprise a broad range of measures targeting specific conditions such as gastroesophageal reflux disease (GERD), inflammatory bowel disease (IBD), and acute gastric bleeding. The biopsychosocial model is significant because it integrates medical management with dietary modifications, psychological treatment, and lifestyle modifications, thereby addressing not only the physiological factor but also the psychological and social determinants of health. This holistic approach addresses the need for understanding the interface between the gut microbiome and these diseases, with emphasis on patient education and interprofessional practice in optimizing treatment efficacy and overall gastrointestinal health (Chughtai et al., 2024). Nursing involvement throughout the acute phases, such as with acute gastric bleeding (AGB), also underscores the direct influence of nursing interventions on clinical outcomes. Studies have demonstrated that extensive nursing interventions have a far-reaching influence on a patient's recovery pattern. Patients, for instance, who receive tailored nursing intervention in the form of individualized plans, closer monitoring, and early patient education experience more rapid hospital discharge rates and lower mortality rates than those patients not receiving such interventions. Studies demonstrate that such patients demand fewer blood transfusions and experience fewer postoperative complications. These findings underscore the importance of integrating evidence-based, structured nursing protocols in acute GI cases, affirming the significant role nurses play in ensuring improved quality of care (Yuan et al., 2024). It is vital to continue educating and training nursing staff to ensure proper management of GI care. This includes maintaining abreast with current evidence-based intervention practices in GI disorders and associated nursing interventions. Regular professional practice sessions can help nurses enhance their skills in patient assessment, implementing interventions, and evaluating care interventions.

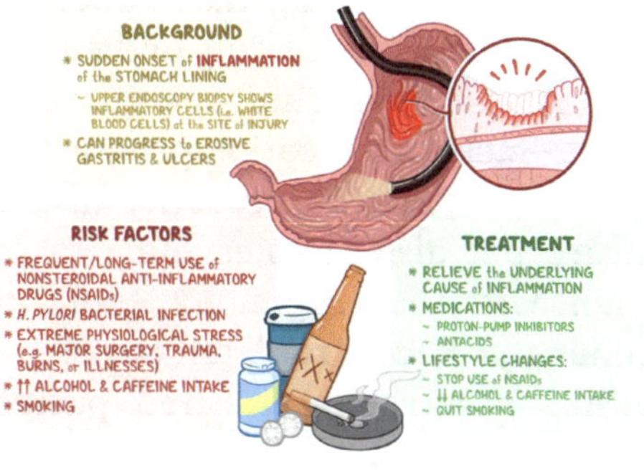

Figure 8.14. Acute gastritis causes, symptoms and diagnosis.

Source: https://www.osmosis.org/_next/image?url=https%3A%2F%2Fd16qt3wv6xm098.cloudfront.net%2F_vZaEoLmTSqaEUmdNldfRSACQ7yspi_L%2F_.png&w=1920&q=75.

Furthermore, communication between the healthcare members is enhanced to help nurses work with other professionals effectively, further improving the patient's health trajectory. The evolving nature of GI disease necessitates a commitment on the part of nurses to lifelong learning, enabling them to provide high-level, interdisciplinary care while adapting to the complex challenges presented by these diseases. Through commitment to ongoing educational growth and teamwork, nurses can significantly enhance the quality of treatment in the area of gastrointestinal health (Chughtai et al., 2024) (Figure 8.14).

8.5.1. Patient Education and Counseling

Education and counseling appropriate type for the patient are also of critical significance in managing gastrointestinal diseases, with a significant role in determining the success and satisfaction of treatment. Nurses play a crucial role in educating patients about the nature of these diseases, their symptoms, and the available therapeutic options. Nurses can help patients understand their misconceptions and phobias while fostering an open communication setting, thereby ensuring that patients have a comprehensive understanding of their condition and the rationale behind specific treatment strategies. Such an education program not only prepares patients to be proactive in their own healthcare but also enables them to be more compliant with their regimens. Additionally, as the Enhanced Recovery After Surgery (ERAS) guidelines illustrate, informed patients are more likely to adhere to preoperative and postoperative care instructions, which in turn provides better overall surgical outcomes in gastrointestinal cases (Gustafsson et al., 2018). The incorporation of technology in patient education also enhances the efficiency of counseling, facilitating engagement and improving memory. Electronic media such as mobile health applications provide patients with convenient access to educational material addressing their specific gastrointestinal issues. Such technologies can be used as adjuncts to traditional counseling interventions, providing reminders for drug compliance and diet alerts at the appropriate times. While current mobile interventions have yielded limited benefits, as highlighted by Free and colleagues, the potential for robust high-quality trials remains strong (Free et al., 2013). In applying these technologies, nurses must continually assess their effectiveness to ensure that patient education remains aligned with advances in healthcare technology. Ultimately, patient education and counseling for gastrointestinal illnesses seek to enhance patient self-management and quality of life. By equipping carers with the necessary skills and knowledge, patients can be empowered to manage the complexities of their disease. By adopting a patient-centered approach, not only is anxiety averted, but also behavior changes are motivated that minimize symptoms and generally improve health. Together with the evolving nursing practice, the combination of evidence-based practice and empathetic communication shall remain a signature of effective patient education. Emphasizing well-informed decision-making is at the core of empowering patients, ultimately leading to improved therapeutic outcomes and an efficient healthcare delivery system.

8.5.2. Monitoring and Assessment Techniques

Effective monitoring and assessment techniques are essential components of nursing management of gastrointestinal disorders. Nurses must use various techniques to evaluate patients' gastrointestinal function in a systematic and logical manner. This begins with an extensive health history, facilitating easy identification of symptoms such as cramping, altered bowel function, or hematochezia. The process of evaluation typically involves physical examinations, including inspection, palpation, percussion, and auscultation, which enable nurses to detect swelling, tenderness, or unusual sounds within the abdomen. Coupled with diagnostic imaging and laboratory tests, these evaluations contribute to the development of a patient-specific care plan. By implementing evidence-based practices, nurses can deliver targeted interventions for specific gastrointestinal complaints, thereby ensuring improved patient outcomes within a structured system, as seen in guidelines such as the ERAS protocol (Gustafsson et al., 2018). In addition to standard checks, monitoring processes in gastrointestinal treatment must also include the use of modern technology. Technological advancements, such as electronic health records (EHRs), enable improved longitudinal patient information tracking, allowing nurses to recognize trends in gastrointestinal symptoms and therapeutic effects more easily. Point-of-care technology, such as bedside ultrasound machines, also enables real-time measurements, which can be potentially life-saving in acute clinical situations. The integration of telehealth services has become increasingly pertinent in the treatment of patients who have chronic gastrointestinal disorders, such that ongoing monitoring of symptoms and interventions can be implemented remotely. All of these technological advancements contribute to enabling an active approach to managing the gastrointestinal tract, emphasizing the ongoing collection and evaluation of patient data to inform clinical decision-making and therapeutic interventions (Baddour et al., 2015). Most importantly, patient assessment of gastrointestinal disease requires a multidisciplinary approach with strong emphasis placed on communication between healthcare professionals. Integration with dietitians, pharmacologists, and specialists ensures the comprehensive consideration of all gastrointestinal health factors in the assessment. Nurses have to be constantly updated with new assessment techniques and best practices. Their adoption of team-based models of care not only enhances the sensitivity of evaluations but also fosters global management plans that are responsive to the multifaceted needs of patients. With the integration of guidelines such as those provided by the American Heart Association in relation to management frameworks, nurses are in a position better to fit monitoring and evaluation strategies into different patient profiles. This emphasis on collaboration and evidence-based recommendations ultimately leads to improved-quality care and better outcomes for patients with gastrointestinal disease (Gustafsson et al., 2018) (Figure 8.15).

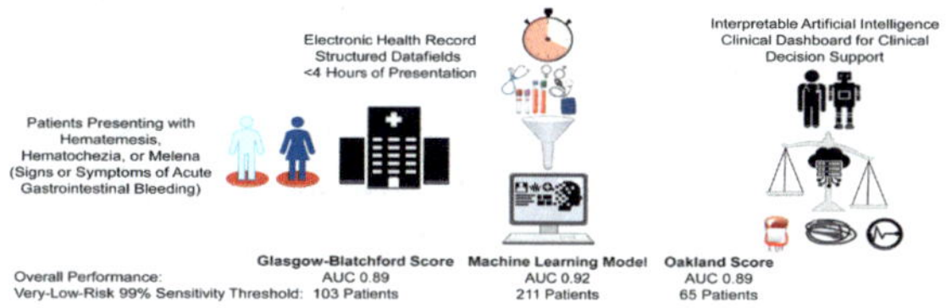

Figure 8.15. Electronic health records (EHR).

Source: https://www.gastrojournal.org/cms/10.1053/j.gastro.2024.06.030/asset/773eab5e-e3ed-47c7-9f32-1f5ce04adb3b/main.assets/ga1_lrg.jpg.

8.5.3. Collaboration with Interdisciplinary Teams

Successful interdisciplinary working is crucial to the management of GI disorders, as these conditions often require multidisciplinary treatment. Nursing specialists are key to this team's effectiveness, liaising with physicians, dietitians, pharmacists, and mental health specialists to create holistic treatment plans tailored to the individual patient's needs. Each practitioner has a specialist contribution to assist with the overall management of GI disorders. For instance, nutritionists provide key evidence for nutrition management in diseases such as inflammatory bowel disease or celiac disease, while pharmacists play a crucial role in medication management and monitoring of side effects. By utilizing open communication and shared decision-making among healthcare team members, nursing professionals can ensure that treatment plans remain patient-centered, thereby enhancing health outcomes and patient satisfaction. The implementation of interdisciplinary teams also mirrors best practices observed in successful healthcare models, particularly in chronic disease management. The successful transition of pediatric patients to adult care for chronic conditions, such as Type 1 diabetes, is an exemplary success story attributed to interdisciplinary practice, yielding positive outcomes. Research indicates that collaborative efforts involving patients and healthcare providers in transition processes lead to improved health status and glycemic control (Bagnall et al., 2013). Adopting such practices in cases of GI disorders leads to timely intervention, the avoidance of complications, and the sustainability of long-term management practices, which are crucial in conditions related to gastrointestinal function. Furthermore, demands for evidence-based practice in nursing require strengthening interdisciplinary collaboration in care paradigms. Studies indicate that interdisciplinary approaches enhance the efficacy of diagnostic methods and therapeutic interventions on complex states, including autism spectrum disorders (Barrientos-Figueroa et al., 2020). In the context of gastrointestinal function, interdisciplinary collaborations can maximize disease assessment and management in conditions such as gastroesophageal reflux disease (GERD) or irritable bowel syndrome (IBS), leading to more accurate diagnosis and tailored treatment regimens. As nursing practitioners increasingly adopt collaborative approaches, they not only enhance the value of the care offered but also take center stage as pivotal players in an integrated healthcare system, providing holistic and coordinated care to patients.

Test Your Knowledge

1. What nursing interventions help manage nausea and vomiting in patients with GI disorders?
2. How can nurses support patients with altered bowel elimination?

8.6. Challenges in Gastrointestinal Nursing

Learning Outcome

1. Describe the management of chronic conditions
2. Define the addressing patient compliance and adherence
3. Identify the navigating cultural and socioeconomic factors of gastrointestinal disorders and their therapeutic management

In gastrointestinal practice nursing, practitioners have to deal with a very complex set of problems caused by the very complicated interactions of gastrointestinal diseases. The sophisticated anatomy and physiology of the gastrointestinal tract require a thorough understanding of the pathophysiology of various conditions, including inflammatory bowel disease, irritable bowel syndrome, and gastrointestinal cancers. Nurses are invited to be alert, observing the delicacy of each patient's presentation to ensure addressing individualized care. The dynamic nature of symptoms, combined with the psychological and emotional burden of these illnesses on patients, compels nursing professionals to undertake whole-person evaluation and communication. The application of evidence-based guidelines ensures the adoption of effective therapeutic management strategies; however, variations in patient reactions render it challenging, thereby increasing the need for continued training and modification in nursing practice.

Furthermore, the problem of gastrointestinal nursing is made complex by the requirement of interprofessional collaboration. Nurses must collaborate with gastroenterologists, dietitians, and other healthcare professionals to develop comprehensive care plans tailored to the complex needs of patients. Failure in communication or coordination among healthcare team members can lead to fragmented care, which is particularly detrimental in the management of chronic gastrointestinal disease. Findings from high-quality randomized controlled trials report the value of structured multidisciplinary care to enhance patient outcomes and satisfaction (N/A, 2012). Practical limitations like limited time, staffing issues, and patient acuity can, however, hinder effective collaboration, resulting in possible gaps in patient care and patient education. Apart from interprofessional challenges, gastrointestinal nurses must also contend with the ethical challenges that accompany the treatment of diseases that are highly stigmatized in society, e.g., inflammatory bowel disease or hepatitis. The patients usually suffer discrimination or ignorance at the hands of society, which makes them feel ashamed and isolated and may deter them from seeking treatment. Nurses are obligated to represent these individuals, who, in addition to receiving proper medical therapies, require emotional care. A greater emphasis on evidence-based practice in nursing highlights the need to incorporate patients' experiences and societal determinants into care plans, making treatment more sympathetic in nature (Perk et al., 2012). These integrated management approaches can empower patients to take an active role in their care, ultimately enhancing compliance and health outcomes, thus solving a central problem in gastrointestinal nursing.

8.6.1. Managing Chronic Conditions

Management of chronic diseases, particularly those affecting the gastrointestinal (GI) tract, requires an interdisciplinary approach that encompasses medical management, lifestyle modification, and patient education. Chronic GI diseases such as irritable bowel syndrome (IBS) and inflammatory bowel disease (IBD) demand that nurses adopt a holistic approach that acknowledges the complex relationship between the physiological and psychological factors. Good management practice must not just address the physical symptom but also the psychosocial impact experienced by patients. By adopting evidence-based interventions, including dietary and pharmacological interventions, nurses can empower patients to effectively manage their conditions. Nurses must have knowledge regarding current guidelines and practice because nurses play a central coordinating role in care coordination and providing integrated support to the patient through their chronic GI diseases (Cosman et al., 2014). Besides, educating the patient about the disease cannot be overemphasized in the management of chronic GI illnesses. Nurses must involve patients in education about the nature of the disease, treatment, and potential complications. By ensuring patients understand their treatment regimen and the importance of compliance, clinicians can significantly improve health outcomes. Furthermore, the application of motivational interviewing principles enables patients to identify their own health goals, thereby creating an enabling atmosphere vital for the effective management of chronic disease. The application of technology, such as telehealth, can also enhance patient access to clinicians and facilitate continuous monitoring of their condition. Moreover, nurses' educational interventions are key to reconceptualizing patient compliance and participation in the management of chronic gastrointestinal illness (N/A, 2012). Finally, management of chronic diseases involves continuous monitoring and evaluation of treatment plans to see whether they remain effective and appropriate for patients' evolving needs. Routine follow-ups enable nurses to monitor the effectiveness of therapies provided and adjust them as needed.

Such assessments usually involve reporting changes in symptoms, medication side effects, and changes in lifestyle or diet. A patient-centered approach involves encouraging patients to report new issues early, which promotes cooperation between the patient and healthcare provider. The inclusion of evidence-based assessment ensures that interventions align with the most current best practices in chronic disease care, leading to improved patient satisfaction and health outcomes. In summary, the management of chronic gastrointestinal disease requires a commitment to ongoing evaluation, patient education, and the promotion of multimodal care strategies (Cosman et al., 2014) (Figure 8.16).

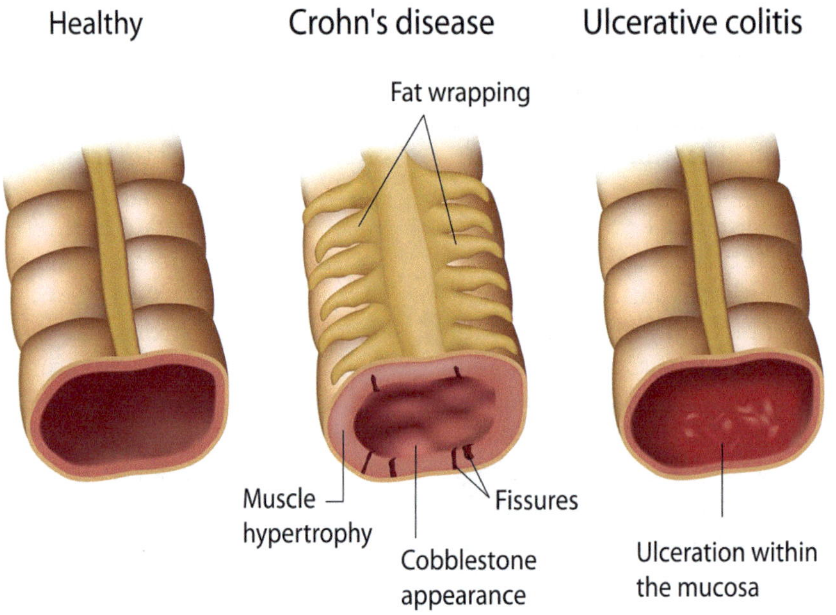

Figure 8.16. Chronic inflammatory bowel disease (IBD) nursing care plan & management.

Source: https://www.rnpedia.com/wp-content/uploads/2015/09/Inflammatory-bowel-crohns-ulcerative-colitis.jpg.

8.6.2. Addressing Patient Compliance and Adherence

In clinical practice, patient compliance and adherence management are most critical, even more so when dealing with gastrointestinal function disorders. Proper adherence not only controls the therapeutic regimen but also helps to sustain patients' overall state of health and well-being. Understanding the psychological and physiological determinants that influence compliance is crucial for nurses, as the determinants might vary significantly from one patient to another. Through proper education and communication with patients, nurses can empower patients to be active partners in their own care and hence potentially manage symptoms of gastrointestinal disease. Through the employment of motivational interviewing techniques and a relationship of trust, nurses can assess potential barriers to compliance and thus deliver effective interventions that address the patient's individual circumstances more fundamentally. Secondly, compliance is also greatly affected by patients' understanding of the disease and prescribed treatment. Education programs that simplify complex medical data produce a significant effect on compliance. Applying teach-back methods, where patients are instructed to explain their understanding of the treatment plan, can demystify what otherwise would be obscure. Approaches such as pictures and instructions can also aid understanding, enabling patients to actively engage in therapy. With gastrointestinal illness, one must also control the potential side effects of drug treatment, for instance, those for treating pain, as they deter patients from following therapy. As indicated in current studies, making patients feel informed and supported in monitoring their treatment will result in good compliance and a better health status (Ballet et al., 2016). Apart from education and support, an effective support environment is required to enhance compliance among gastrointestinal disorder patients. The interaction of healthcare providers not only entails but also extends to familial and social support networks. Multidisciplinary collaboration among mental health care workers, dietitians, and pharmacists can develop a comprehensive plan for patient care that encompasses not only physical treatment but also the emotional aspects of compliance. Nurses play a crucial role in facilitating this coordination, ensuring that patients receive comprehensive care tailored to their specific needs. Additionally, special-needs patients may require taking additional considerations due to past systemic afflictions or medication therapies, which exacerbate gastrointestinal complications. By the use of holistic management strategies, considering these, healthcare workers can significantly improve patient compliance, thereby enhancing the therapeutic effects of interventions (Allocca et al., 2018).

8.6.3. Navigating Cultural and Socioeconomic Factors

It is essential to comprehend the role of cultural and socioeconomic factors in the context of gastrointestinal diseases and their management. Individuals from diverse backgrounds are likely to approach healthcare with a blend of beliefs, practices, and behaviors influenced by their cultural contexts. For example, patients may have diverse interpretations of gastrointestinal symptoms due to cultural explanations that guide their perception of sickness.

Additionally, socioeconomic status significantly impacts access to healthcare resources, which can influence outcomes in gastrointestinal diseases. A person with lower socioeconomic status may be hindered by such factors as limited health education, limited access to quality nutrition, and lack of frequent health care. Hence, knowledge of these dimensions is essential for nurses, who must tailor their assessments and interventions to meet the cultural and socioeconomic needs of their patients to maximize overall health outcomes (Shuja, 2025). Moreover, the complex interplay between mental health and gut function, particularly in poor communities, demands cultural sensitivity. It would appear from evidence that economic disparities possess the ability to worsen mental illness, thus enhancing the prevalence of gastrointestinal illnesses. Too much stress and anxiety, which are generally prevalent among socioeconomically weaker sections, will precipitate or exacerbate symptoms such as irritable bowel syndrome (IBS) and functional dyspepsia. Nursing practice then has to consider both mental illness and culture, adopting a holistic perspective that acknowledges the patient's actual experiences. For instance, education on diet and stress coping should be responsive to the eating habits and availability at the local level. The integration of these factors in care will enable nurses to work more efficiently in handling the multiple interplays among gastroenterological disorders, cultural identity, and mental health, ultimately leading to enhanced therapeutic management

(Pereira et al., 2025). Moreover, stigma surrounding mental illness and gastrointestinal disease also differs significantly across cultural environments, something to which nurses must approach with sensitivity. In most communities, particularly those of a more conservative mindset, mental illness can be stigmatized as something shameful, where individuals show fewer symptoms or do not present at all. Additionally, cultural beliefs regarding gastrointestinal disease also seem to affect symptom reporting and health-seeking attitudes and, consequently, patient compliance with necessary interventions. Hence, nursing practitioners must develop a safe therapeutic environment where patients feel at ease discussing their problems. With the help of culturally competent communication strategies, such as active listening and compassionate interaction, stigma can be mitigated, and a deeper trust between healthcare providers and patients is fostered. Lastly, by addressing cultural and socioeconomic determinants of care, nurses can ensure comprehensive management of gastrointestinal illnesses and thus improve patient outcomes (Shuja, 2025) (Figure 8.17).

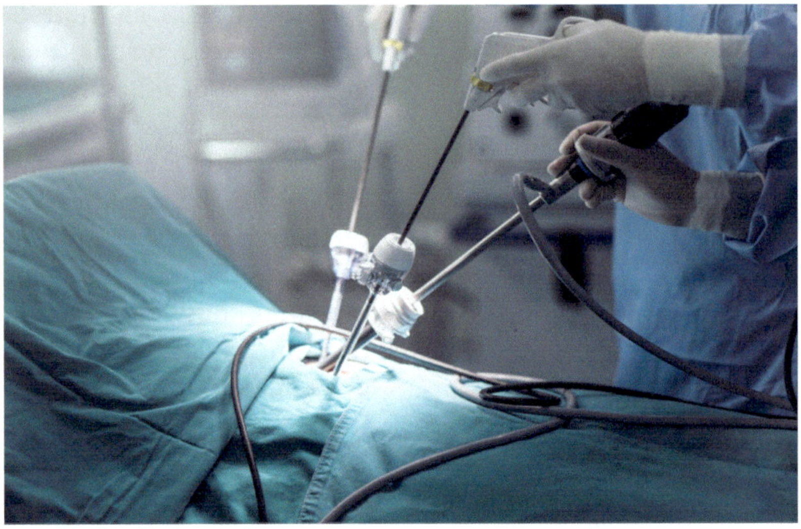

Figure 8.17. Laparoscopic gastrointestinal surgery.

Source: https://sydneygutclinic.com/wp-content/uploads/2022/03/shutterstock_1380842939.jpg.

Test Your Knowledge

1. What are common challenges nurses face when managing patients with chronic gastrointestinal disorders?
2. How can nurses address patient anxiety related to invasive GI procedures?

-

SUMMARY

The complexity of GI disorders necessitates an all-rounded treatment approach and management. Many treatments and therapies are needed to manage diseases such as irritable bowel syndrome (IBS), inflammatory bowel disease (IBD), and functional gastrointestinal disorders. The nursing team plays a vital role in monitoring patient improvement and creating individualized care plans that incorporate both pharmacological and non-pharmacological interventions. For instance, the use of biofeedback has been noted as an effective conservative management approach for bowel dysfunction, emphasizing the importance of nurses staying current with emerging treatment techniques that can optimize their patients' outcomes (Chelvanayagam et al., 2012). This kind of integrative practice not only optimizes patient quality of life but also fosters a collaborative practice culture among healthcare providers dedicated to advancing GI health. In addition, evidence-based practice should form the foundation of therapeutic care for gastrointestinal diseases. Systematic reviews, and in particular maternal medicine systematic reviews, highlight a stark difference in research quality present, necessitating more robust studies to be integrated into clinical guidance. It is vital that nursing practitioners access good-quality, methodologically sound literature in order to guide practice and deliver patient care grounded on the most recent available evidence (Conde-Agudelo et al., 2007). The increased use of research evidence in nursing practice is expected to enhance decision-making processes, leading to improved management of gastrointestinal disorders. With the advancement of nursing education, there will be a need to focus on staying current with new treatments and evidence-based practices. Lastly, proper communication between patients and nursing personnel is crucial in the management of gastrointestinal disorders. Treatment is contingent on a patient's understanding of their illness, adherence to treatment protocols, and open communication of information regarding their symptoms and fears. Nurses need to utilize their empathy and compassion skills to establish patient trust, thereby enabling them to implement more integrated care interventions. Furthermore, by adopting a patient-centered approach, nurses can empower patients to be active participants in managing their GI health. This interdependent dynamic not only increases compliance with treatment but also enhances the overall effectiveness of therapeutic interventions, establishing a synergistic relationship that ultimately benefits both healthcare providers and patients in the context of gastrointestinal care.

Gastrointestinal disease is a serious issue within the nursing practice and therefore warrants an extensive knowledge of its management. Certain conditions, such as Zieve's syndrome, emphasize the importance of proper diagnosis and the need for early intervention. Zieve's syndrome is characterized by a characteristic triad of presentations — hemolytic anemia, cholestatic jaundice, and transient hyperlipidemia — especially in alcoholics. The diagnostic problems are typically compounded by other autoimmune disorders, requiring thorough evaluation and serial examinations. Such conditions cannot be treated holistically unless the significance of lifestyle adjustments, such as alcohol avoidance, is also addressed in addition to treatment interventions (Zalavadiya et al., 2024). Another important gastrointestinal condition gaining more attention is eosinophilic gastrointestinal disorders (EGIDs), more notably eosinophilic esophagitis (EoE). This is caused by a disease in the gut, which presents with dysphagia, vomiting, and abdominal pain. Clinical examination and biopsy findings of increased eosinophils are used to diagnose it. Different treatment modalities include food elimination diets and pharmacologic therapy, such as proton-pump inhibitors, topical corticosteroids, and biologics, that are aimed at reducing inflammation and eosinophil counts. Recent advancements in standardized measures for evaluating the outcomes of treatment reflect the ongoing efforts to refine the quality of treatment administered to EoE patients. These developments not only aid in refining clinical practice but also reflect a growing awareness and understanding of the pathophysiology of EGIDs (Pesek et al., 2022). The incorporation of nursing science in gastrointestinal disease management ensures improved patient outcomes through a multidimensional process. In Zieve's syndrome and EoE, symptom identification and understanding of the underlying pathophysiologic process are essential factors in successful treatment planning. Nurses play a pivotal role in patient education, guiding individuals towards lifestyle modifications and adherence to therapeutic processes. The instructions regarding varying treatment protocols, ranging from dietary changes to pharmacological interventions, underscore the need for a multidisciplinary approach among nurses. Continuing to develop professionally in the field of gastrointestinal disease prevention will enable nurses to provide empathetic evidence-based care, as well as ensure they are continuously involved in research and debate concerning research and innovation in therapeutic management (Pesek et al., 2022; Zalavadiya et al., 2024).

KEY TERMS FROM THIS CHAPTER

- Antiemetic therapy
- Bowel obstruction
- Constipation
- Diarrhea
- Gastroenteritis
- Hepatitis
- Irritable bowel syndrome (IBS)
- Nausea and vomiting
- Parenteral nutrition
- Surgical resection
- Appendicitis
- Cirrhosis
- Crohn's disease
- Endoscopy
- Gastroesophageal reflux disease (GERD)
- Inflammatory bowel disease (IBD)
- Nasogastric tube
- Pancreatitis
- Peptic ulcer disease
- Ulcerative colitis

CRITICAL THINKING QUESTIONS

1. **Which of the following is a common symptom of gastroesophageal reflux disease (GERD)?**
   a. Lower back pain
   b. Burning sensation in the chest (heartburn)
   c. Difficulty urinating
   d. Joint stiffness
2. **Which dietary recommendation is appropriate for a patient with peptic ulcer disease?**
   a. High-fat meals at bedtime
   b. Caffeinated beverages
   c. Bland, non-irritating foods in small frequent meals
   d. Spicy and acidic foods
3. **Which condition involves inflammation of the appendix and usually requires surgical removal?**
   a. Diverticulitis
   b. Appendicitis
   c. Gastritis
   d. Cholecystitis
4. **What is a priority nursing concern for a patient with prolonged vomiting and diarrhea?**
   a. Joint pain
   b. Fluid and electrolyte imbalance
   c. Visual disturbances
   d. Skin irritation
5. **Which of the following medications is commonly used to treat constipation?**
   a. Omeprazole
   b. Loperamide
   c. Docusate sodium
   d. Ranitidine

Short Answer Questions

1. What is the function of the gastrointestinal (GI) system?
2. Name two common symptoms of peptic ulcer disease.
3. What is GERD, and how is it typically managed?
4. List two complications of prolonged vomiting and diarrhea.
5. What dietary advice is given to a patient with irritable bowel syndrome (IBS)?
6. Describe the pathophysiology, clinical signs, and nursing care of a patient with appendicitis.
7. Discuss the assessment, diagnostic tools, and nursing interventions for a patient with gastrointestinal bleeding.
8. Explain therapeutic management strategies for inflammatory bowel diseases (Crohn's disease and ulcerative colitis).

Answers to Critical Thinking Questions

1. (b) 2. (c) 3. (b) 4. (b) 5. (c).

REFERENCES

1. Abdu, L. A., Mohamed, M. A., & Hussein, A. H. (2024). Effect of Learning Package on Knowledge, Symptoms Severity and Quality of Life for Patients with Inflammatory Bowel Disease. *South Eastern European Journal of Public Health*, 1243–1263. https://doi.org/10.70135/seejph.vi.2029Ajani, J. A., D'Amico, T. A., Bentrem, D. J., Chao, J., Cooke, D. T., Corvera, C. U., Das, P., et al. (2022). Gastric cancer, version 2.2022, NCCN clinical practice guidelines in oncology. *Journal of the National Comprehensive Cancer Network, 20*, 167–192. https://doi.org/10.6004/jnccn.2022.0008 (accessed on 30th June 2025).
2. Allan, P., Fiorino, G., Gatti, S., Gerasimidis, K., et al. (2017). Research gaps in diet and nutrition in inflammatory bowel disease. A topical review by D-ECCO Working Group (Dietitians of ECCO). https://core.ac.uk/download/84340703.pdf (accessed on 30th June 2025).
3. Allocca, G., Menozzi, G., Battista, G. B., F., M., et al. (2018). Oral malodor in special care patients: Current knowledge. https://core.ac.uk/download/159636738.pdf (accessed on 30th June 2025).
4. Allum, W., Alsina, M., Andritsch, E., Ba-Ssalamah, A., et al. (2018). ECCO essential requirements for quality cancer care: Esophageal and gastric cancer. https://core.ac.uk/download/157587654.pdf (accessed on 30th June 2025).
5. Baddour, L. M., Wilson, W. R., Bayer, A. S., Fowler, V. G., Tleyjeh, I. M., Rybak, M. J., Baršić, B., et al. (2015). Infective endocarditis in adults: Diagnosis, antimicrobial therapy, and management of complications. *Circulation, 132*, 1435–1486. https://doi.org/10.1161/cir.0000000000000296 (accessed on 30th June 2025).
6. Bagnall, A., Day, R., & Kime, N. H. (2013). Systematic review of transition models for young people with long-term conditions: A report for NHS Diabetes. https://core.ac.uk/download/29018738.pdf (accessed on 30th June 2025).
7. Ballet, S., De Baerdemaeker, A., Hoogenboom, R., Madder, A., et al. (2016). Controlled-release of opioids for improved pain management. https://core.ac.uk/download/84045024.pdf (accessed on 30th June 2025).
8. Barrientos-Figueroa, L. (2020). Analyzing the triad diagnosis requirement for autism in Arkansas. https://core.ac.uk/download/322958889.pdf (accessed on 30th June 2025).
9. Beaudin, J., Chouinard, M., Hudon, É., & Hudon, C. (2025). Factors and strategies influencing integrated self-management support for people with chronic diseases and common mental disorders: A qualitative study of Canadian primary care nurses' experience. *Journal of Advanced Nursing.* https://www.semanticscholar.org/paper/cca55f419a7a92e78685dd9c0e06982d24b691e1 (accessed on 30th June 2025).
10. Blasi, P., Bonacucina, G., Cespi, M., Ferrara, A., et al. (2017). Oral drug therapy in elderly with dysphagia: Between a rock and a hard place! https://core.ac.uk/download/pdf/84497287.pdf (accessed on 30th June 2025).
11. Callaghan, P., Dainty, A., Fox, M., Holtham, E., et al. (2017). The feasibility of nurse-delivered, low-intensity cognitive behavioral therapy for irritable bowel syndrome. https://core.ac.uk/download/148791607.pdf (accessed on 30th June 2025).
12. Chelvanayagam, S., Collins, B., Duncan, J., O'Brien, T., et al. (2012). Uncovering anorexia nervosa in a biofeedback clinic for bowel dysfunction. https://core.ac.uk/download/20321227.pdf (accessed on 30th June 2025).

13. Chughtai, M. A., Kerimkulova, M. K., Mushtaq, O., Hagenahalli Anand, V., Rehman, A., Shehryar, A., Hassan, B., et al. (2024). Integrated approaches in the management of gastrointestinal disorders: A biopsychosocial perspective. *Cureus, 16.* https://www.semanticscholar.org/paper/6b7e7d3aaf4e22e506842c23dc4a07a9e032b26c (accessed on 30th June 2025).

14. Conde-Agudelo, A., Coomarasamy, A., Coomarasamy, A., Oxman, A. D., Oxman, A. D., Jadad, A. R., Dennis, C. L., et al. (2007). A review of the methodological features of systematic reviews in maternal medicine. https://core.ac.uk/download/pdf/18982.pdf (accessed on 30th June 2025).

15. Cosman, F., Jan de Beur, S. M., LeBoff, M. S., Lewiecki, E. M., Tanner, B., Randall, S., & Lindsay, R. (2014). Clinician's guide to prevention and treatment of osteoporosis. *Osteoporosis International, 25*, 2359–2381. https://doi.org/10.1007/s00198-014-2794-2 (accessed on 30th June 2025).

16. Dadigamuwage, S., Macaulay, A., & Jaufer, M. (2025). Massive lower gastrointestinal bleeding from colonic submucosal lipoma and diverticular disease: A rare case requiring surgical interventions and postoperative management challenges. *Cureus, 17.* https://www.semanticscholar.org/paper/86024e321291b3c39c873d161985f2b993558605 (accessed on 30th June 2025).

17. Declercq, T., Lemey, L., Petrovic, M., Tandt, L., et al. (2018). Late-life depression: Issues for the general practitioner. https://core.ac.uk/download/154408401.pdf (accessed on 30th June 2025).

18. Donini, L. M., Lenzi, A., Perna, S., Poggiogalle, E., Rondanelli, M., & Spadaccini, D. (2018). Are the therapeutic strategies in anorexia of ageing effective on nutritional status? A systematic review with meta-analysis. https://core.ac.uk/download/188830393.pdf (accessed on 30th June 2025).

19. Fernando, K. S., Harrelson, C. E., Jones, A. D., Rowley, M., et al. (2022). Management of gastroesophageal reflux disease (GERD) by primary care providers in Mississippi. https://core.ac.uk/download/618305445.pdf (accessed on 30th June 2025).

20. Free, C., Phillips, G., Watson, L., Galli, L., Felix, L., Edwards, P., Patel, V., et al. (2013). The effectiveness of mobile-health technologies to improve health care service delivery processes: A systematic review and meta-analysis. *PLoS Medicine, 10*, e1001363–e1001363. https://doi.org/10.1371/journal.pmed.1001363 (accessed on 30th June 2025).

21. Gheonea, D. I., Ionescu, E. M., Rada, C., Tieranu, M., et al. (2024). Inventario de personalidad de Freiburg en la enfermedad inflamatoria intestinal: Diagnóstico y necesidades psicoterapéuticas. https://core.ac.uk/download/596376496.pdf (accessed on 30th June 2025).

22. Gustafsson, U., Scott, M. J., Hübner, M., Nygren, J., Demartines, N., Francis, N., Rockall, T., et al. (2018). Guidelines for perioperative care in elective colorectal surgery: Enhanced recovery after surgery (ERAS®) Society recommendations: 2018. *World Journal of Surgery, 43*, 659–695. https://doi.org/10.1007/s00268-018-4844-y (accessed on 30th June 2025).

23. HasanPour-Dehkordi, A., Shahbazi, K., & Solati Dehkordi, S. K. (2016). Comparison of hypnotherapy and standard medical treatment alone on quality of life in patients with irritable bowel syndrome: A randomized control trial. https://core.ac.uk/download/143840502.pdf (accessed on 30th June 2025).

24. Hunt, B. J., Allard, S., Keeling, D., Norfolk, D. R., Stanworth, S., & Pendry, K. (2015). A practical guideline for the hematological management of major hemorrhage. *British Journal of Hematology, 170*, 788–803. https://doi.org/10.1111/bjh.13580 (accessed on 30th June 2025).
25. Hunt, R. H., Armstrong, D., Katelaris, P., Afihene, M., Bane, A., Bhatia, S., Chen, M., et al. (2017). World Gastroenterology Organization global guidelines. *Journal of Clinical Gastroenterology, 51*, 467–478. https://doi.org/10.1097/mcg.0000000000000854 (accessed on 30th June 2025).
26. Hyland, S. J., Brockhaus, K. K., Vincent, W. R., Spence, N. Z., Lucki, M. M., Howkins, M. J., & Cleary, R. K. (2021). Perioperative pain management and opioid stewardship: A practical guide. *Healthcare, 9*, 333–333. https://doi.org/10.3390/healthcare9030333 (accessed on 30th June 2025).
27. Izquierdo, M., Merchant, R. A., Morley, J. E., Anker, S. D., Aprahamian, I., Arai, H., Aubertin-Leheudre, M., et al. (2021). International exercise recommendations in older adults (ICFSR): Expert consensus guidelines. *The Journal of Nutrition Health & Aging, 25*, 824–853. https://doi.org/10.1007/s12603-021-1665-8 (accessed on 30th June 2025).
28. Katzman, W. B., & Pastore, E. A. (2012). Recognizing myofascial pelvic pain in the female patient with chronic pelvic pain. https://core.ac.uk/download/305124272.pdf (accessed on 30th June 2025).
29. LeBoff, M. S., Greenspan, S. L., Insogna, K., Lewiecki, E. M., Saag, K. G., Singer, A., & Siris, E. S. (2022). The clinician's guide to prevention and treatment of osteoporosis. *Osteoporosis International, 33*, 2049–2102. https://doi.org/10.1007/s00198-021-05900-y (accessed on 30th June 2025).
30. Lee, A. (2016). Identifying and managing constipation in older people. https://core.ac.uk/download/151161179.pdf (accessed on 30th June 2025).
31. Mohiuddin, A. K. (2019). Alternative treatments of minor GI ailments. https://core.ac.uk/download/327073474.pdf (accessed on 30th June 2025).
32. Nohesara, S., Abdolmaleky, H., Dickerson, F., Pinto-Tomás, A., Jeste, D. V., & Thiagalingam, S. (2024). Maternal gut microbiome-mediated epigenetic modifications in cognitive development and impairments: A new frontier for therapeutic innovation. *Nutrients, 16.* https://www.semanticscholar.org/paper/b42a036422b4fddd74021e05267ddf5ceb5dd8f8 (accessed on 30th June 2025).
33. Pascarella, G., Strumia, A., Piliego, C., Bruno, F., Del Buono, R., Costa, F., Scarlata, S., et al. (2020). COVID-19 diagnosis and management: A comprehensive review. *Journal of Internal Medicine, 288*, 192–206. https://doi.org/10.1111/joim.13091 (accessed on 30th June 2025).
34. Pesek, R., & Gupta, S. K. (2022). Is clinical trial data showing positive progress for the treatment of eosinophilic esophagitis? *Expert Opinion on Emerging Drugs, 27*, 225–227. https://www.semanticscholar.org/paper/b4f2789e6042ebe47d608201d2c1f70001bdab30 (accessed on 30th June 2025).
35. Shen, Y., Xi, Y., Xian Ru, L. G., & Liu, H. (2025). The impact of ERAS-based nursing interventions on postoperative complication management and prognosis in early gastrointestinal tumor endoscopic resection: A prospective randomized controlled study. *Langenbeck's Archives of Surgery, 410.* https://www.semanticscholar.org/paper/5bc8564ece32520e9818a1d9601baa9cd817ed9b (accessed on 30th June 2025).

36. Shuja, N. (2025). Unraveling the psychophysiological nexus–The impact of stress and mental health on chronic pain and gastrointestinal disorders. *Developmental Medico-Life-Sciences.* https://www.semanticscholar.org/paper/ef8b5b97ff5a26b832e8fd810d03d8ff9c730fa9 (accessed on 30th June 2025).

37. Stasevych, M., & Zvarych, V. (2023). Innovative robotic technologies and artificial intelligence in pharmacy and medicine: Paving the way for the future of health care—A review. *Big Data and Cognitive Computing, 7,* 147–147. https://doi.org/10.3390/bdcc7030147 (accessed on 30th June 2025).

38. Yuan, X., Yu, F., & Fu, S. (2024). Impact of professional nursing interventions on clinical outcomes in patients with acute gastric bleeding: A retrospective analysis. *Scientific Reports, 14.* https://www.semanticscholar.org/paper/672ab2d3f9746ab3fd7c03ea49d1bf3327dd76ae (accessed on 30th June 2025).

39. Zalavadiya, R., Bhatt, J., Nagori, I., Kagathara, N., & Neupane, S. (2024). An unusual case of Zieve's syndrome in a 36-year-old male with latent autoimmune diabetes of adult and disseminated intravascular coagulation. *Clinical Case Reports, 12.* https://www.semanticscholar.org/paper/10b90048d4a1652a6db12ee52cc3338278bdc290 (accessed on 30th June 2025).

ENDOCRINE DISORDERS AND DIABETES MANAGEMENT FOR NURSING

9

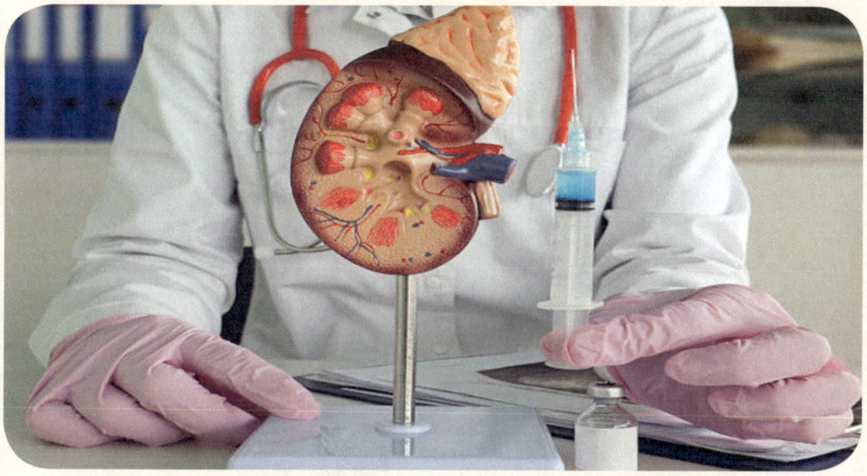

LEARNING OBJECTIVES

After studying this chapter, you will be able to:

1. Understand the types of endocrine disorders
2. Explain the pathophysiology of diabetes
3. Discuss the nursing assessment in endocrine disorders
4. Focus on diabetes management strategies
5. Learn about patient education and support
6. Evaluate the role of nurses in managing endocrine disorders

Introduction

The endocrine system plays a crucial role in maintaining homeostasis in the human body by regulating various physiological functions, including metabolism, growth, and reproduction. Endocrine disorders result from hormonal imbalance in their production, which could lead to multiple health issues. The disorders may be a result of genetic predispositions, autoimmune disease, or developmental anomalies, impacting individuals during their lifespan. Diseases such as diabetes mellitus, thyroid disease, and adrenal disease exemplify the complexity of endocrine impairment. Knowledge of these disorders is further emphasized in nursing because healthcare workers play a key role in diagnosis, treatment, and patient education related to endocrinological health. Diabetes mellitus, particularly Type II Diabetes, is a compelling case study in the study of endocrine disorders. Having previously been predominantly confined to adults, recent trends now indicate a concerning increase in its occurrence among children and hence the evolving epidemiological picture of this chronic condition. Given that heterogeneity of childhood Type II Diabetes is determined by both genetic elements as well as environmental factors, management and prevention calls for a multidimensional approach. Interventions targeting modifiable risk factors, such as obesity and unhealthy eating habits, are crucial in reducing the disease burden. The urgency for early screening and lifestyle intervention stems from the risk of advanced co-morbidities, including cardiovascular disease and renal disease, which can be linked to the development of diabetes in childhood, making it crucial for nursing intervention in patient education and guidance on lifestyle (Kapke et al., 2015). The economic burden of diabetes is much greater than individual morbidity, and it has extensive implications for health care systems nationwide.

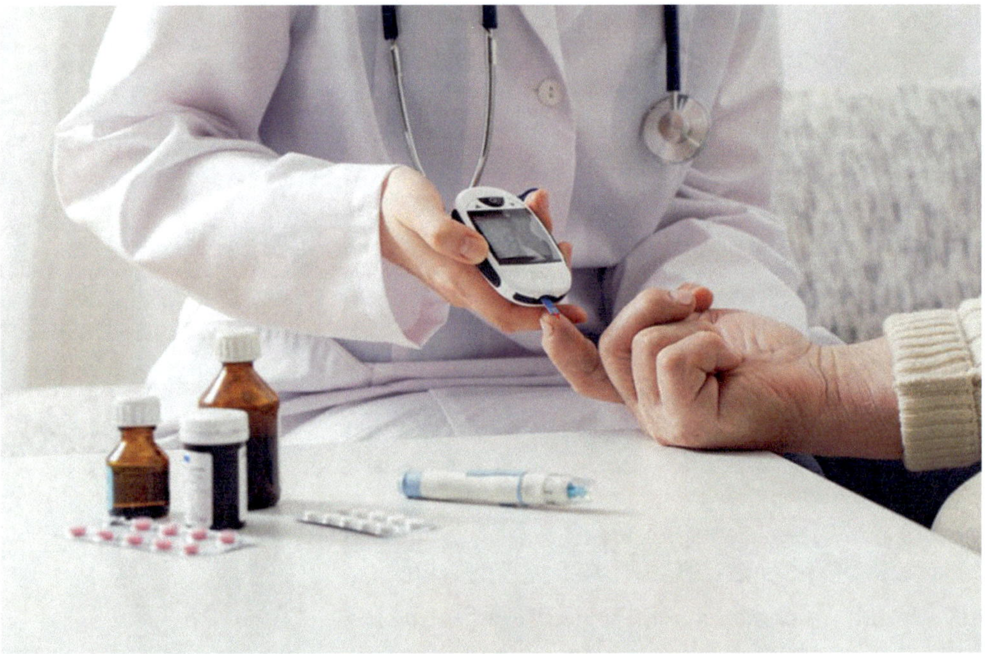

Figure 9.1. Endocrinology and diabetes.

Source: https://external-content.duckduckgo.com/iu/?u=https%3A%2F%2Fwww.shifa.com.pk%2Fwp-content%2Fuploads%2F2020%2F02%2FEndocrinology-980x653.jpg&f=1&nofb=1&ipt=b5745bb3e44c77658c04e0998a3984f316bc2f2fae4e5cc1986d2cb60716635a4.

Research has indicated that people with diabetescost healthcare approximately 2.4 times more than those who do not have the condition, which totals around $132 billion annually in direct and indirect expenses. This number not only illustrates the financial burden of the disease but also highlights the importance of early diagnosis and intervention strategies. Since nearly one-third of all individuals have undiagnosed diabetes, there is a requirement for physicians, including nurses, to expand patient outreach and screening activities. Due to the aging population and demographic changes, more efforts on endocrine disease prevention and control, such as diabetes, are required to minimize future healthcare expenses as well as overall public health results (Hogan et al., 2025) (Figure 9.1).

Definition and Overview of Endocrine Disorders

The endocrine system is an intricate set of glands that secrete hormones responsible for regulating a myriad of physiological processes, including metabolism, growth, and reproduction. Endocrine disorders arise when there is either over- or under-production of hormones, leading to grave medical issues. Diabetes mellitus, hypothyroidism, and polycystic ovary syndrome are a few of the many endocrine disorders. Diabetes, as the inadequate production or function of insulin or a dysfunction of glucose homeostasis, is particularly prevalent and requires intensive nursing care. For healthcare workers, being aware of the delicate balance in the endocrine system is essential as they are responsible for the diagnosis, treatment, and education of patients with these conditions, which can completely transform their quality of life and overall well-being. Polycystic ovary syndrome (PCOS) is a significant endocrine disorder that affects a large number of women and also has physical and psychological effects. Women with PCOS are likely to develop insulin resistance, which again aggravates their condition by making them more likely to develop type 2 diabetes and cardiovascular disease. The disorder is characterized by irregular periods, androgenic excess, and polycystic ovaries, which can cause infertility and metabolic disorders. Interventions to promote wellness in people with PCOS are a wellness-based, integrative intervention aimed at enhancing quality of life as well as health outcomes. Such a combined emphasis is especially relevant for nurses who will be attempting to manage not only the physiological impact of PCOS but also the emotional and psychological needs of their patients (Annagur et al., 2018). Apart from PCOS, childhood and adolescent HTN is now a significant public health condition among endocrine disorders. The increasing prevalence of HTN in youth is a significant danger, resulting in the looming cardiovascular disease epidemic. Having clear definitions and treatment plans is essential to effectively managing it. Existing literature suggests the need for comprehensive assessment tools that consider out-of-office blood pressures and cardiovascular clustering of risk factors. For nurses, acknowledgment of the impact of these factors is necessary for both diagnosis and intervention. With the adoption of newer guidelines and treatment regimens, nurses can facilitate early intervention and public health interventions for greater detection and control of hypertension among children (Agabiti-Rosei et al., 2016) (Figure 9.2).

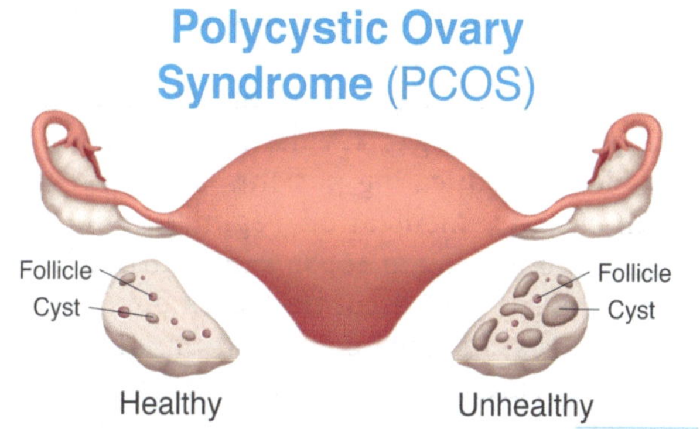

Figure 9.2. Polycystic ovary syndrome (PCOS).

Source: https://static.acne.org/ipb_uploads/monthly_2018_08/02-polycystic-ovary-syndrome-pcos.jpg.92a2e229cfe22f2517bda8879751c5d3.jpg.

Importance of the Endocrine System in Human Health

The endocrine system plays a crucial role in the overall well-being of human beings by regulating various physiological processes. It is made up of various glands that secrete hormones. The system is in charge of regulating metabolism, growth, and mood. Hormones are messengers that transfer vital information throughout the body to maintain homeostasis. An imbalance in hormone release can lead to several disorders, such as diabetes, thyroid conditions, and disorders of growth, which point towards the necessity of learning about this system if one is to manage health effectively. Most importantly in nursing, a comprehensive understanding of endocrine functions is essential, as nurses are often the first point of contact in identifying symptoms of hormonal imbalances. Understanding the endocrine system enables specialist treatments that can improve patient outcomes and provide control over chronic conditions like diabetes. Diabetes is ~~one of~~ the most ~~critical~~ common endocrine diseases that affects millions globally, thus complete nursing care is needed. The role of insulin, a pancreatic hormone, is key in controlling blood levels of glucose. In type 1 diabetes, the body does not produce insulin, whereas in type 2 diabetes, there is a resistance to insulin action, leading to high blood sugar levels. Nurses must be proficient in educating patients about lifestyle modifications, medication regimen, and self-glucose monitoring to ~~become in~~ control ~~of~~ their disease. Early and accurate treatments cannot be overstressed since complications that arise from unattended diabetes lead to unfavorable health status, including cardiovascular diseases and neuropathy. Therefore, education on the endocrine aspects of diabetes not only improves the quality of care administered by nurses but also empowers patients to actively participate in managing their health. Additionally, its interaction with other body systems highlights its importance in comprehensive healthcare. Stress, for instance, has a massive impact on hormones, disrupting body functions and even leading to long-term medical illnesses. As stated, across the lifespan, stress plays a core role in disease and health. Whereas it has been best proven that the brain regulates the different ways in which the body responds to these experiences, there is a lack of continuity between head-to-tail focus providers and head-down focus providers (Estrine et al., 2006). Nurses must offer psychosocial interventions for endocrine disorders by integrating mental health care into physical interventions. Furthermore, dietary concerns, particularly among the elderly, should not be taken lightly, as malnutrition exacerbates the complications caused by hormonal imbalances and weakens overall well-being, underscoring the need for a holistic care paradigm in nursing practice (Bordoni et al., 2015).

Prevalence and Impact of Endocrine Disorders

The prevalence of endocrine diseases, particularly diabetes mellitus, continues to rise globally, posing a significant public health threat. Current figures indicate that nearly 463 million adults have diabetes, a figure that is likely to increase in the coming decades. This bleak scenario is further compounded by the rise in the incidence of accompanying ~~endocrine~~ disorders such as obesity and metabolic syndrome, which complicate the management of diabetes. The overlap of these disorders points towards a coming epidemic that requires pressing attention from the medical community. The impact of endocrine disorders is not only on health ~~in form~~ but also imposes itself on healthcare systems and resources, necessitating a holistic approach to prevention and management. Nurses play a central role in this respect, connecting patient education with medical management to improve health outcomes and treatment compliance. The effect of endocrine disorders on maternal and neonatal well-being is most marked where pregnancies are complicated by disease, including gestational diabetes and hypothyroidism. Studies reflect that such endocrine disorders can lead to serious complications, including hypertensive disorders and preterm birth, with long-term effects on mothers and infants. As highlighted in recent evidence, multimodal care models that incorporate multidisciplinary approaches have been effective in overcoming these challenges, with findings indicating improved glycemic control and fewer adverse outcomes for both infants and mothers (Ullah et al., 2025). Such information highlights the importance of specialized management during pregnancy, ensuring that health professionals are coordinated in their approach to optimize the management of endocrine diseases. Greater sensitivity to such issues among nurses can lead to more targeted interventions that are vital to improving maternal and neonatal outcomes. Aside from physical health risk, endocrine disorders also affect mental health to a great extent. The co-occurrence of conditions such as diabetes and psychiatric illnesses, such as depression and anxiety, can hinder appropriate disease management via the health care system since it compromises the ability of patients to comply with treatment protocols. Mental health care, as an essential component of treatment for patients with endocrine illnesses, becomes integrated through behavioral interventions and support mechanisms aimed at alleviating distress and enhancing coping (Yelne et al., 2025). Thus, integrating mental health care into programs for diabetes care becomes a necessity. By addressing both the physical and psychological aspects of care, healthcare providers can enhance support to patients in self-care tasks, ultimately leading to improved quality of life and improved health outcomes. Blending physical treatment with mental wellness is essential, providing a complete approach needed to tackle the complexities of endocrine disorders.

9.1. Types of Endocrine Disorders

Learning Outcome

1. Describe diabetes mellitus: Type 1 and Type 2
2. Focus on thyroid disorders: hypothyroidism and hyperthyroidism
3. Learn about adrenal disorders: Cushing's syndrome and Addison's disease

Endocrine disorders are a group of illnesses resulting from imbalances in hormone production, affecting various bodily functions. Diabetes mellitus, thyroid disease, and adrenal insufficiency are the most prevalent types. Diabetes, a state of hyperglycemia due to a deficiency in insulin secretion or action, exists in two general forms: Type 1 and Type 2. Type 1 diabetes results from autoimmune destruction of the pancreatic beta cells and requires a lifelong need for insulin therapy. Type 2 diabetes is more likely to accompany lifestyle factors such as obesity and sedentary living, providing the potential for management with diet, exercise, and drugs. Recognition of the distinct mechanisms involved in these disorders is of the most critical concern in nursing practice, as each type demands distinct monitoring and intervention methods to optimize patient outcomes in diabetes effectively. Thyroid disease is a another category of endocrine diseases affecting primarily metabolism and energy regulation. Hyperthyroidism and hypothyroidism are conditions that arise due to an overactive or underactive thyroid gland, respectively. Hyperthyroidism, typically indicated by symptoms of weight loss, tachycardia, and nervousness, must be controlled and treated carefully, perhaps with antithyroid medication or radioactive iodine therapy. Conversely, hypothyroidism, presents with fatigue, weight gain, and depression, and requires hormone replacement therapy in the form of levothyroxine. The nurse's critical role includes educating the patient about symptoms and compliance with treatment, as well as monitoring thyroid hormone levels, which directly impact diabetic patients' glycemic control. Enhancing knowledge of these disorders not only improves nursing practice but also educates patients to be active participants in their own care. Adrenal insufficiency, specifically Addison's disease, is a significant endocrine disorder that affects the body's ability to respond to stress and fluid balance. This disorder is when the adrenal glands do not release enough cortisol and aldosterone, which results in hypotension, fatigue, and weakness. Nursing management of adrenal patients includes the identification of adrenal crises immediately, which are life-threatening and, in most cases, glucocorticoid treatment is necessary. It is also essential to understand the impact of immune-related adverse events (irAEs) on patients receiving immunotherapy, particularly on endocrine function. Guidelines for these irAEs promote multidisciplinary treatment, with an active role for nursing in patient education and symptom surveillance, further highlighting the necessity of having extensive knowledge of various endocrine disorders in the field of diabetes treatment (Schneider et al., 2021; LeBoff et al., 2022) (Figure 9.3).

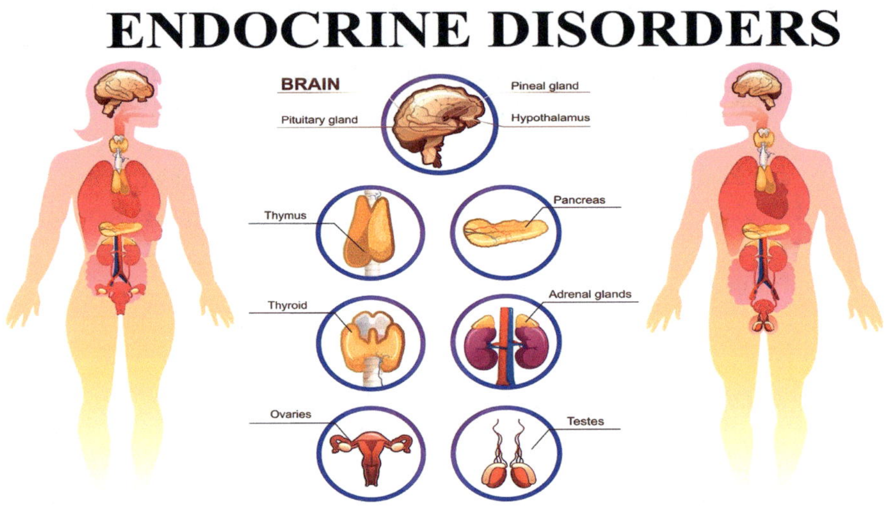

Figure 9.3. Types of endocrine disorders.

Source: https://easybiologynotes.com/wp-content/uploads/2024/11/Endocrine-disorders.jpg.

9.1.1. Diabetes Mellitus: Type 1 and Type 2

Diabetes Mellitus, Type 1 and Type 2, are significant public health concerns and critical to the study of endocrine disease. Type 1 diabetes is an autoimmune disorder with pancreatic beta-cell destruction, producing insulin-secreting cells, where patients need treatment with insulin for the rest of their lives. Type 2 diabetes often results from insulin resistance coupled with a relative insulin deficiency. Type 2 diabetes incidence rises with obesity, inactivity, and unbalanced diets in terms of lifestyle variables. Nurses must be able to identify these differences to tailor diabetes care regimens for their patients through a concentration on pharmacologic intervention, lifestyle modification, and patient education. The relationship between diabetes and other endocrine disorders should have greater visibility in diabetes care. A study comparing the prevalence of thyroid disorders in Type 2 diabetes patients revealed that large numbers of patients had disorders such as hypothyroidism and hyperthyroidism (Salimian et al., 2024). This finding points to the necessity of regularly screening Type 2 diabetes patients for thyroid disorders, given that thyroid disorders have a negative impact on glycemic control, as observed with their relation to raised glycosylated hemoglobin (HbA1c) levels. For the endocrinology practicing nurse, identification and treatment of such comorbidities are critical to promote patient outcomes, since overarching management strategies can optimize overall health upkeep methods for diabetic patients. Education and awareness of diabetes complications, such as osteoporosis, also illustrate the complexity of care for this endocrine disease. Research identifies that there is a staggering rate of Type 2 diabetic patients who do not have a sufficient degree of knowledge regarding osteoporosis. However, it is frequently common among them (Nasir, 2024). This inadequate knowledge highlights the importance of this area of education in empowering patients to maintain their health. For nurses, designing education materials that fill this knowledge gap can facilitate better self-care behavior, leading to greater patient adherence to treatment regimens. With advancements in diabetes care, the role of nursing professionals in educating and advocating for integrative health strategies becomes increasingly essential, ultimately aiming to reduce the overall burden of diabetic complications (Figure 9.4).

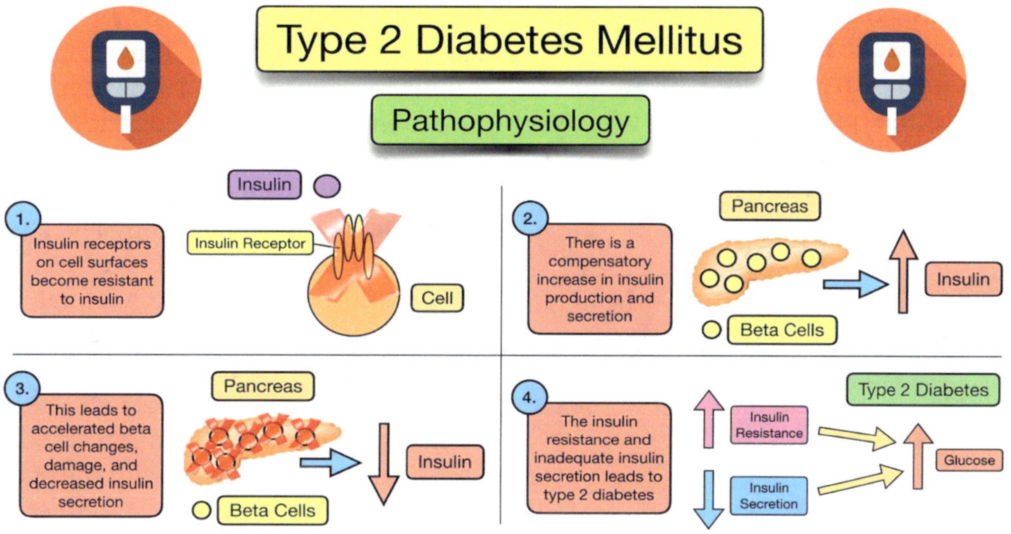

Figure 9.4. The types of diabetes mellitus.

Source: https://images.squarespace-cdn.com/content/v1/5e48489da899cd09424943db/efa0b7b7-8e01-4469-8961-c04a0128698b/diabetes-mellitus-type-2-pathophysiology-causes.jpeg.

9.1.2. Thyroid Disorders: Hypothyroidism and Hyperthyroidism

A nurse must understand thyroid conditions, such as hypothyroidism and hyperthyroidism, while dealing with endocrine disorders. Hypothyroidism is characterized by an underactive thyroid gland that cannot secrete sufficient thyroid hormones. The symptoms are fatigability, weight gain, and depression, all of which need careful assessment and appropriate lab tests to confirm diagnoses. Treatment usually consists of hormone replacement therapy with levothyroxine, and doses are changed based on regular monitoring of thyroid function tests. Adequate monitoring and communication regarding drug adherence are crucial parts of the nursing intervention to normalize the patient's metabolic processes and prevent complications. As patients with hypothyroidism may have comorbid conditions like diabetes, intense liaison with interprofessional teams is necessary for effective patient outcomes. Hyperthyroidism, however, involves excessive production of thyroid hormone, whose clinical presentation includes weight loss, palpitations, and increased anxiety. Such a state requires entirely different treatment, typically starting with antithyroid medication like methimazole or iodine-131 therapy. Patients need to be taught about potential side effects and the importance of maintain-the treatment schedule-as advised, as untreated hyperthyroidism may lead to severe complications, e.g., thyroid storm. Continuous monitoring of thyroid hormone levels is necessary to manage the condition effectively. Since hyperthyroidism has the potential to aggravate insulin resistance in diabetics, endocrine and metabolic management therapies are a part of nursing interventions to mitigate danger and optimize patients' quality of life. The compounded relationship between thyroid disease and diabetes control has some crucial implications for nursing practice.

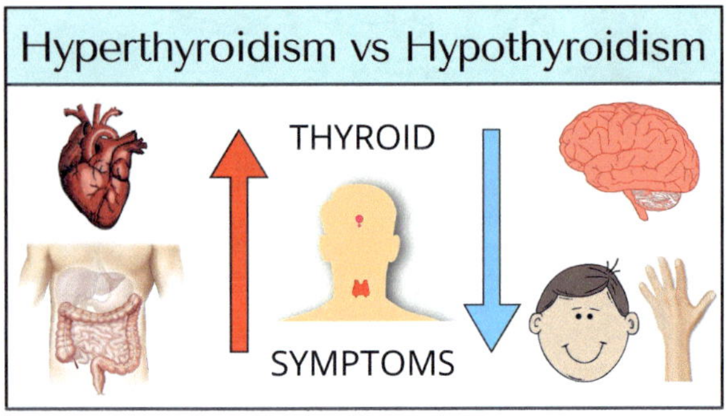

Figure 9.5. Hyperthyroidism vs hypothyroidism.

Source: https://i.ytimg.com/vi/47HYktFARww/maxresdefault.jpg.

Endocrine dysfunction, such as dysregulation of thyroid hormones, influences glycemic control. For instance, hypothyroid patients may become insulin-resistant and complicate diabetic control, and need very cautious therapeutic adjustment in the insulin regimen. Hyperthyroidism, by contrast, tends to produce variable blood glucose levels, necessitating that nurses take the initiative in monitoring patients and educating them about their condition. Moreover, the occurrence of such issues as COVID-19 emphasizes the importance of proper management of these endocrine conditions to prevent exacerbation in the event of systemic illness (Marazuela et al., 2020). An understanding of these dynamics allows nurses to provide successful, holistic care that both manages diabetes and thyroid function effectively, thereby resulting in improved patient outcomes (Schneider et al., 2021) (Figure 9.5).

9.1.3. Adrenal Disorders: Cushing's Syndrome and Addison's Disease

Adrenal disorders, in the form of Cushing's syndrome and Addison's disease, are ~~very real~~ issues in the field of endocrinology that call for in-depth knowledge by nursing practitioners. Cushing's syndrome is characterized by excess glucocorticoids on a chronic level, which could be due to any of a variety of etiologies, such as pituitary adenomas, adrenal tumors, or ectopic ACTH secretion. The clinical picture often includes obesity, hypertension, glucose intolerance, and characteristic skin changes, such as easy bruising and striae. Since many of these symptoms overlap with those of metabolic disease, early diagnosis and treatment are crucial. Nurses have a key role in observing patients for these hormonal imbalances and knowledge of their systemic effects, including the potential for diabetes to develop as an aftereffect of chronic hypercortisolism. Such observation allows for intervention at an early stage and possible alteration of treatment regimens to prevent subsequent health complications of Cushing's syndrome. On the other hand, Addison's disease or primary adrenal insufficiency presents with a unique constellation of clinical problems. The condition is characterized by the hyposecretion of adrenal hormones, specifically cortisol and aldosterone, resulting from damage to or autoimmune destruction of the adrenal glands. Its symptomatic presentation consists of weakness, weight loss, hyperpigmentation, and hypotension, capable of severely impairing quality of life. An understanding of the nuances of managing Addison's disease is essential for nursing personnel, particularly in developing an optimal regimen of glucocorticoid and mineralocorticoid replacement therapy. The patients must also be taught the importance of taking medication and monitoring for evidence of adrenal crisis, which is fatal if not addressed early. This wariness in management underscores the necessity of individualized management guidelines that target the specific presentations of hormonal deficiency. The overlap between adrenal diseases and diabetes is especially significant, as both share extensive pathophysiologic and treatment similarities. Endocrine disturbances secondary to Cushing's syndrome can lead to insulin resistance, which enhances the risk of diabetes in patients so affected. Patients with Addison's disease can have abnormal glucose metabolism, especially when under stress or during insufficient hormone replacement. This dualism emphasizes the necessity for nursing practitioners to possess a sound understanding of both endocrine disorders. Nurses must be proficient in blood glucose checking and counseling patients regarding lifestyle changes to aid in managing both diabetes and adrenal insufficiency. The ability to understand such complexities enables nurses to provide comprehensive care, improving outcomes for patients by addressing the multidimensionality of these endocrine disorders within the context of diabetes management.

Test Your Knowledge

1. What is the primary difference between type 1 and type 2 diabetes mellitus?
2. How does hypothyroidism affect the body's metabolism?

9.2. Pathophysiology of Diabetes

Learning Outcome

1. Explain the insulin production and function
2. Define the mechanisms of insulin resistance
3. Discuss the complications associated with diabetes

The pathophysiology of diabetes involves a complex interaction between metabolic derangements and chronic hyperglycemia, resulting from defects in insulin secretion, insulin action, or both. Type 1 diabetes is an autoimmune condition, and it leads to the loss of pancreatic beta cells and, therefore, severe impairment of insulin production. This necessitates therapy with exogenous insulin to prevent potentially life-threatening complications. Conversely, Type 2 diabetes, the prevalent type, arises essentially through the interplay of insulin resistance and resultant beta-cell deficiency. The insidiously developing form of Type 2 diabetes typically requires increasingly amplifying intervention to maintain glycemic control, illustrating the dynamic interplay between metabolic standards and endocrine function in this disease.

Understanding these mechanisms is essential for nursing clinicians who must recognize the varied presentations and etiologies of diabetes to deliver personalized, effective management plans to patients (Rizwan, 2025). In addition, the role of hormones in maintaining glucose homeostasis cannot be overstated, as changes in the endocrine system play a crucial role in the pathophysiology of diabetes. Insulin, secreted from the pancreas, facilitates glucose entry into cells; however, other hormones like glucagon, epinephrine, and cortisol counteract insulin's action, particularly during stress or starvation states. Dysregulation of this hormonal homeostasis may exacerbate hyperglycemia, creating an imminent challenge in diabetes management.

Also, conditions like Cushing syndrome and hypothyroidism can further affect glucose metabolism, creating additional obstacles to management by healthcare professionals. Given that the majority of these secondary endocrine disorders are usually associated with diabetes, nurses must be vigilant about assessing and managing the multifaceted implications of endocrine alterations (Ałczewska et al., 2025).

In the case of diabetic control, an understanding of its pathophysiology leads to more informed interventions regarding glycemic control and complications prevention. Effective nursing care must include rigorous screening for other endocrine disorders, as the presence of disorders like hypothyroidism or hormonal imbalance as a result of obesity can seriously compromise diabetic control. Furthermore, close patient education regarding lifestyle modification, medication adherence, and personal monitoring habits will also be essential in achieving effective management outcomes. Building a collaborative care model with the incorporation of dietitians, endocrinologists, and nursing practitioners is able to provide an all-encompassing approach that addresses both diabetes and related endocrine disease. Finally, understanding the complexities of diabetes pathophysiology enables nurses to provide dynamic care tailored to patients' needs (Rizwan, 2025) (Figure 9.6).

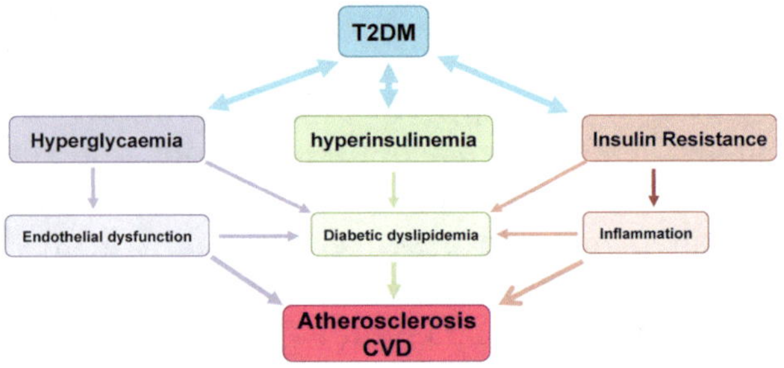

Figure 9.6. Diabetes mellitus type 1 pathophysiology.

Source: https://www.mdpi.com/ijms/ijms-21-06275/article_deploy/html/images/ijms-21-06275-g006.png.

9.2.1. Insulin Production and Function

Insulin production and function are integral parts of glucose metabolism and overall body homeostasis. Released by the beta cells of the pancreas, insulin is a peptide hormone that is responsible for regulating blood glucose levels. Following the ingestion of food, elevated glucose levels stimulate the release of insulin, which facilitates cellular glucose uptake and lowers blood sugar levels. Insulin also affects the muscle and liver to synthesize glycogen, providing a source of energy storage for future utilization. Insulin also inhibits gluconeogenesis and lipolysis, processes that increase blood glucose and fatty acid levels, respectively. The intricate interaction between insulin secretion and action is crucial to the maintenance of metabolic well-being, and abnormalities in this system can potentially induce frank endocrine disease, e.g., diabetes mellitus, and also metabolic syndrome-related complications. Insulin's action is not restricted to glucose metabolism alone but also affects lipid and protein metabolism. Insulin regulates the synthesis of lipids by stimulating the storage of fatty acids and glycerol for utilization in triglyceride synthesis while concurrently inhibiting lipolysis. In this regard, insulin helps reduce the concentration of free fatty acids in the blood, thereby lowering the risk of atherosclerosis and cardiovascular disease. Insulin stimulates protein synthesis by promoting the storage of amino acids in various tissues, resulting in muscle growth and repair. The hormone's multifaceted role emphasizes not only its importance in glucose homeostasis but also other metabolic processes. Any impairment in insulin production or function can lead to disorders such as hyperglycemia and, subsequently, the long-term effects of diabetes and cardiovascular disease. Efficient nursing care management of endocrine disorders is therefore required and relies on a thorough understanding of these roles.

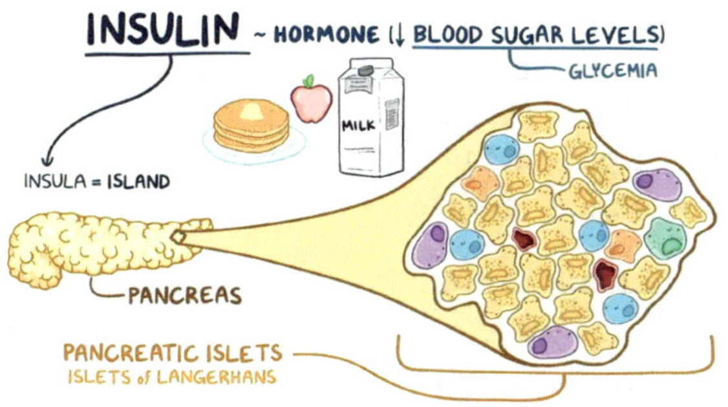

Figure 9.7. Insulin production and function.

Source: https://d16qt3wv6xm098.cloudfront.net/N54uUV6_Tuq-eNC2a36EF_lWS46veBJV/_.jpg.

Moreover, the connection of insulin secretion with other endocrine illnesses emphasizes the importance of integrated care interventions by nurses. For instance, Type 1 diabetes and Type 2 diabetes occur through different mechanisms of insulin deficiency or insensitivity. In Type 1 diabetes, there is an autoimmune response that leads to the breakdown of the pancreatic beta cells, culminating in an absolute lack of insulin. Conversely, Type 2 diabetes is generally characterized by insulin resistance, followed by a subsequent decrease in insulin secretion. Care management must respond to maintain glycemic control and avoid chronic hyperglycemia complications. Nurses must update themselves on insulin actions and the physiological consequences of endocrine dysregulation to deliver best-care services, employing evidence-based practice to manage associated disorders of health. This complete understanding of insulin production and operation ultimately supports enhanced patient outcomes of diabetes management and endocrine health (Petrakis et al., 2020; Schneider et al., 2021) (Figure 9.7).

9.2.2. Mechanisms of Insulin Resistance

The state of insulin resistance is a multifactorial metabolic state of decreased sensitivity of target tissues, such as muscle and fat, to insulin. The consequent impaired glucose uptake leads to an increased level of blood glucose. Etiological mechanisms are the cause of the pathogenesis of type 2 diabetes and are multifactorial in nature, including genetic, environmental, and lifestyle factors. In addition, the pathological accumulation of excess visceral fat has been described as a key cause of insulin resistance by releasing inflammatory cytokines and free fatty acids, which further disturb insulin signaling cascades. This series of events outlines the key connection between obesity and metabolic derangement, making specific interventions in diabetes treatment protocols essential (Schneider et al., 2021). The other important element of insulin resistance is the inflammatory process. It is a chronic low-grade inflammation that, in the majority of patients with obesity, is typically noted and has a central role in deranging the action of insulin. The adipose tissue, previously considered only as an energy depot, is currently known to be endowed with endocrine activity, releasing various pro-inflammatory cytokines such as TNF-alpha and interleukin-6. These cytokines interfere with insulin action by causing serine phosphorylation of insulin receptor substrate proteins, which finally results in blunting the metabolic effects of insulin. These observations point towards the importance of targeting inflammatory pathways in the management of endocrine disorders, particularly diabetic care in nursing practice (Gustafsson et al., 2018). In addition to inflammation and fat, oxidative stress has also emerged as a central feature in the development of insulin resistance. An excess of reactive oxygen species (ROS) is capable of inhibiting insulin action through damage to necessary cellular structures and fueling further inflammation. Mitochondrial dysfunction is invariably associated with increased levels of oxidative stress and has been linked to a reduced capacity for glucose oxidation. This disturbance creates a vicious cycle in which energy imbalance and insulin resistance feed into one another, amplifying the potential for developing type 2 diabetes. Importantly, awareness of these coupled mechanisms offers essential information to nursing practitioners when developing preventive and therapeutic interventions to reverse insulin resistance and improve metabolic health (Schneider et al., 2021) (Figure 9.8).

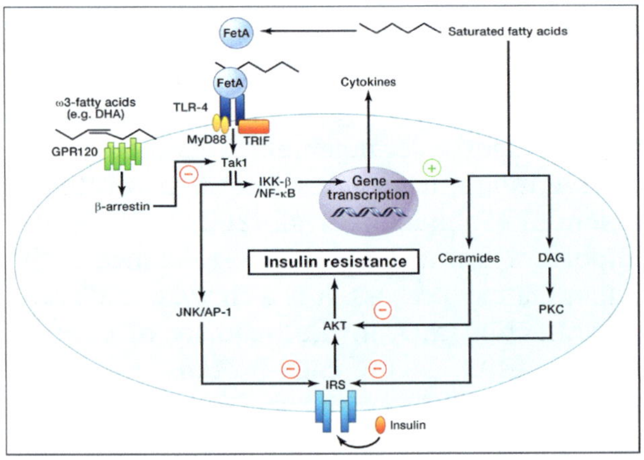

Figure 9.8. Mechanisms of insulin resistance.

Source: https://www.cell.com/cms/attachment/4b24d243-6686-449e-9b4c-cea0127809d5/gr2_lrg.jpg.

9.2.3. Complications Associated with Diabetes

Diabetes mellitus is a chronic endocrine disorder that can lead to a myriad of complications if not controlled well. The most significant complication is the progression into cardiovascular diseases, which are extremely prevalent among diabetic patients. Diabetic patients also have high lipid levels and hypertension, thus making their risk doubly greater for heart diseases. Moreover, glycemic control results in damage to the blood vessels, which is determinant of the microvascular complications, including retinopathy, nephropathy, and neuropathy. Such complications must be monitored and controlled by the nursing staff; therefore, diabetes education and intervention programs are indispensable in clinical practice (Dunger, 1998). In addition, the risk of neuropathy in diabetic patients poses major quality of life and management issues.

Neuropathy is nerve damage to the peripheral nerves that leads to numbness, pain, and tingling in the extremities. Not only does this affect mobility, but it also puts the patients at risk for injury to the feet and infections that can lead to severe complications such as amputations. Furthermore, autonomic neuropathy has the capability of making body functions dysfunctional, such that controlling blood pressure and digestion is problematic. Thus, nurses play a crucial role in educating patients about foot care and the importance of regular assessment to prevent long-term complications.

By prioritizing such care, healthcare providers can mitigate the dangers introduced by diabetic neuropathy and promote better patient outcomes (Oh, 1990). The additive effect of these complications requires a multi-dimensional approach to diabetes care, focusing on the delivery of care by interdisciplinary teams. Nurses should be trained with the knowledge and skills necessary for screening complications and working in coordination with physicians to achieve timely interventions. Lifestyle changes, including diet and exercise, are essential components of an overall diabetes management plan. Encouraging medication regimens as ordered and promoting patient involvement in self-care actions are crucial to preventing complications. By ensuring the proper use of these interventions, healthcare providers can enhance the well-being and overall health of individuals with diabetes, highlighting the significance of nursing interventions within the continuum of endocrine disorders and diabetes management (Dunger, 1998).

Test Your Knowledge

1. What causes insulin deficiency in type 1 diabetes mellitus?
2. How does insulin resistance contribute to the development of type 2 diabetes?

9.3. Nursing Assessment in Endocrine Disorders

Learning Outcome

1. Explain the patient history and symptoms evaluation in endocrine disorders
2. Define the physical examination techniques in endocrine disorders
3. Describe the laboratory tests and diagnostic procedures in endocrine disorders

The evaluation of endocrine disorders by nurses is necessary, as it serves as the foundation for effective care and patient outcomes. It begins with a complete history of the patient, in which the following are examined: familial patterns of endocrine disease, medications, and symptomatic presentation in terms of fatigue, weight change, and metabolic derangement. It is also necessary to evaluate lifestyle factors such as diet, physical exercise, and stress, which have a significant influence on endocrine function. Because of the complexity of the interrelation between various hormone systems, prompt detection of signs and symptoms can assist nurses in the identification of disorders, including diabetes mellitus, hypothyroidism, and hyperparathyroidism. Incorporating family genetic histories into the assessment also helps one understand potential hereditary endocrine issues, thereby promoting preventive management strategies. A comprehensive physical examination complements the primary history, assessing overall appearance and endocrine-specific indicators related to potential endocrine disturbances. Nurses should look for important signs, which are mostly endocrine-related and include alterations in skin, deviations in body mass index, and changes in cardiovascular status. For instance, results such as acanthosis nigricans could indicate insulin resistance in diabetics, while a ~~retarded~~ impaired wound healing could indicate a thyroid problem. Furthermore, blood pressure monitoring is also important as it can reveal unsuspected hormonal imbalances, particularly in the event of Cushing's syndrome or Addison's disease. Proper communication at this point is essential, through which nurses can establish rapport and make patients comfortable enough to give their experience unhesitatingly. The interaction establishes a platform that allows for more accurate assessment and individualized care plans. To further support nursing assessment in endocrine disorders, the correct laboratory and diagnostic tests are to be determined and interpreted. This entails familiarity with key indicators, such as blood glucose in diabetes, serum cortisol in adrenal insufficiency, and thyroid hormone levels in thyroid disorders.

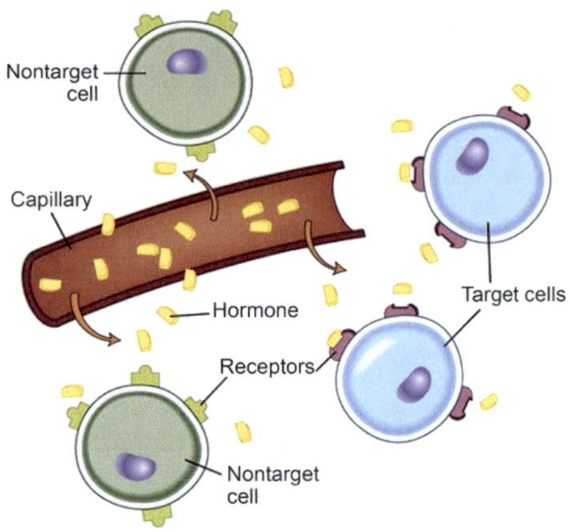

Figure 9.9. Nursing assessment endocrine system.

Source: https://nursekey.com/wp-content/uploads/2016/11/B9780323086783000484_f048-002-9780323086783.jpg.

The interpretation of these tests not only facilitates verification of the suspected diagnoses but is also very important in assessing the effectiveness of treatment and potential complications. For instance, regular HbA1c testing in diabetic patients can enable clinicians to tailor glycemic control treatment in a significant ~~way~~. Additionally, recent evidence from integrated care models has shown improved fetal and maternal outcomes in endocrine disorder-complicated pregnancies, emphasizing the contribution of a multidisciplinary approach to nursing assessments. With a whole-patient approach, nurses can give comprehensive evaluations that lead to best management and improved patient outcomes (Miao et al., 2024; Ullah et al., 2025) (Figure 9.9).

9.3.1. Patient History and Symptoms Evaluation

Evaluation of patient history is the core in endocrine disorder and diabetes care because it provides physicians with useful information ~~on~~ conering the patient's–state of health and individual risk factors. History includes– the initial start of diabetes, prior treatment, and comorbidities, all of which significantly influence patient outcomes. For instance, being aware of a patient's history of complications, such as neuropathy or retinopathy, helps in tailoring management plans. Accurate documentation of symptoms like polyuria, polydipsia, and lethargy gives a better picture of the severity of diabetes and its potential complications, which guides nursing interventions and treatment planning. Additionally, the evaluation may also encompass lifestyle factors, including diet and physical exercise, which are of paramount significance in devising a comprehensive management plan aimed at maximizing glycemic control and overall well-being. Besides a comprehensive patient history, symptom evaluation has a vital role to play in the day-to-day management of diabetes and other endocrine diseases. Symptoms such as nocturia, thirst, and undue fatigue must not only be identified but also assessed based on their onset, frequency, and severity to ensure that a greater understanding can be developed regarding how they represent the patient's health status. For example, deteriorating nocturia in a patient can indicate deteriorating glycemic control, for which their management must be re-evaluated on an emergency basis. Moreover, the presence of secondary symptoms, such as an unanticipated change in weight or mood alteration, may reflect the onset of complications or the need for modification of the treatment regimen. Through mindful observation of these symptoms, healthcare professionals can institute timely interventions, which ultimately lead to improved patient outcomes and better control of diabetes-related disorders. Integrative symptom assessment approaches further enhance knowledge of endocrine disorders when combined with traditional treatment methods. For instance, unifying classical medical perspectives with complementary therapies can lead to improved symptom management and patient satisfaction. In one case, the use of Ayurvedic principles along with conventional medical treatments resulted in significant symptom improvement for a long-standing diabetic patient who came with complications such as edema and lethargy (Farseena et al., 2025). In other cases where overlap between multiple conditions is encountered, as in electrolyte imbalances that occur together with diabetes, it becomes apparent that a holistic strategy is required to approach patient assessment and treatment. Here, multidisciplinary collaboration, involving input from nursing professionals and pharmacists, is imperative to guaranteeing successful outcomes, as evidenced in the handling of acute complications among the elderly via careful monitoring and treatment (Shah et al., 2024). Not only does such an integrative approach rectify immediate health problems—such as electrolytic imbalance—but it also guarantees long-term health by way of the comprehensive management of diabetes.

9.3.2. Physical Examination Techniques

Appropriate physical examination techniques are crucial when evaluating patients with diabetes and endocrine disorders. These techniques enable clinicians to identify signs and symptoms that may indicate underlying metabolic derangements. For instance, the patient's vital signs, skin, and body habitus upon examination can give important information regarding hormonal as well as glucose regulation. A thorough history, combined with a comprehensive patient examination, facilitates a comprehensive evaluation of the patient's current status and potential complications, such as neuropathy or retinopathy. Peripheral pulses and capillary refill time should be regularly monitored to detect vascular alterations secondary to diabetes. It is therefore essential that nursing professionals gaining experience in endocrine disorders are adequately competent in physical assessment skills, as this will equip them with the ability to make informed clinical choices based on what they actually observe. In diabetes management, certain physical examination maneuvers are crucial for monitoring disease progression and treatment outcomes. For instance, foot checks are necessary regularly to detect early neuropathy signs and avoid ulceration or risk of infection, which often complicates diabetes. One must screen regularly for calluses, skin integrity, and changes in sensation using monofilament or tuning fork tests. Moreover, monitoring body mass index (BMI) through clinical examination helps establish a sense of realization regarding the patients' nutritional status and potential weight-related metabolic complications. Since obesity is a key risk factor for type 2 diabetes, these measures are not only diagnostic but also learning experiences for patients to favorably influence self-management of the condition, along with lifestyle changes. The integration of holistic physical examination techniques into general nursing practice ensures that healthcare practitioners are competent to properly handle the complexities of endocrine disorders and diabetes care. By using these techniques, nurses can not only identify present complications but also risk factors for developing subsequent endocrine disturbances. Training nurses in physical examination skills assists in facilitating a more proactive approach to patient care. For instance, identification of evidence of hypertension or retinopathy on examination can initiate earlier referrals to specialist treatment, to avoid severe long-term complications. In addition, frequent use of physical examination skills promotes a culture of health awareness and attentiveness in nursing practice as a whole, ultimately leading to improved patient outcomes in the long-term care of endocrine and diabetes disorders (Figure 9.10).

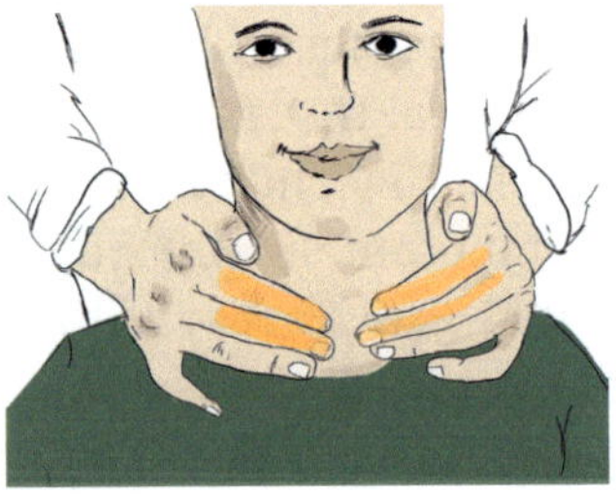

Figure 9.10. Endocrinology physical exam.

Source: https://endoconsult.b-cdn.net/wp-content/uploads/2019/04/thyroid-examination1-1024x819.jpg.

9.3.3. Laboratory Tests and Diagnostic Procedures

For diabetes and endocrine disease, laboratory analysis and testing are a priceless tool in the clinician's arsenal. Not only are they beneficial in establishing a diagnosis, but they are also critical in assessing the direction of the disease and the effectiveness of treatment. For instance, serum glucose tests can diagnose diabetes mellitus and aid in therapeutic interventions tailored to the patient through continuous monitoring. Additionally, endocrine hormone tests, such as for insulin, cortisol, and thyroid hormones, are incredibly beneficial in understanding the endocrine gland activities. These tests inform nursing interventions, enabling practitioners to manage patient care and treatment programs effectively. By using laboratory tests judiciously, healthcare professionals can provide comprehensive care for endocrine disorders, thereby enhancing patient outcomes and quality of life. Further, the application of sophisticated diagnostic procedures makes it feasible to enjoy the comorbidities of endocrine disorders in a superior manner, particularly for populations with associated conditions. An illustration is the presence of hypertension in children with endocrine disorders, which has been detected with higher risks for cardiovascular events as such subjects develop into adults. As outlined in the new guidelines, the inclusion of out-of-office blood pressure readings with routine checks enhances the accuracy of diagnosing hypertension in this population. Through this integrative strategy, nurses can take evidence-based action targeting not only blood glucose but also hypertension, a pertinent comorbidity. Thus, by examining various biomarkers and clinical markers, nursing practice can effectively address the complex impacts of endocrine illnesses on overall well-being. The intersection of autoimmune and endocrine diseases reveals further sophistications that need extensive laboratory research. For instance, a study highlighted the fact that women with fibromyalgia exhibit an increased prevalence of autoimmune and endocrine pathologies compared to their counterparts with chronic pain only. Specifically, thyroid disease was identified as having strong associations with fibromyalgia, implying an association that requires further investigation across clinical settings. Awareness of these crossover associations may guide nursing assessments that are sensitive to concurrent health conditions, allowing care to be better individualized. In addition, laboratory findings can initiate timely contemplation of lifestyle modification, patient education, and interprofessional referrals to ensure that care is maximized to manage the complex health needs of patients who have endocrine disorders as a component of their global health plans.

Test Your Knowledge

1. What signs and symptoms should nurses assess in a patient with hyperthyroidism?
2. Why is monitoring blood glucose levels significant in patients with diabetes?

9.4. Diabetes Management Strategies

Learning Outcome

1. Identify the lifestyle modifications: diet and exercise
2. Define the pharmacological interventions: insulin and oral medications
3. Describe the monitoring blood glucose levels

Effective management of diabetes intervention is crucial in controlling–the complications of this chronic disease. Multidisciplinary care, involving education, diet, and medical therapy, is critical in achieving optimal patient outcomes. Education empowers patients by optimizing diabetes knowledge, facilitating self-assessment of blood glucose, and providing assurance in following prescribed regimens. Additionally, healthcare professionals must emphasize the importance of regular physical activity and dietary modifications appropriate to the individual patient's requirements. This personalized therapy not only maintains blood glucose levels within the normal range but also reduces the risk of diabetic complications, thereby improving the quality of life for patients. Moreover, pharmacological therapy plays a significant role in controlling diabetes. Current strategies involve insulin therapy and various antidiabetic medications, with the goal of achieving maximum glycemic control. The selection of the drug should be made based on the individual's health profile, co-morbidities, and potential side effects. Individualization of the drug regimen will enhance compliance and effectiveness and improve outcomes in health. Regular peripheral and central blood glucose monitoring, as mentioned earlier, is a crucial aspect of evaluating the effectiveness of the management plan and making adjustments accordingly. By taking a holistic approach that incorporates both medical interventions and lifestyle changes, nurses also play a significant role in stabilizing diabetes in their patients. Beyond direct patient care, the financial burden of managing diabetes is also of grave concern to healthcare providers. The cost of diabetes is considerable, with direct medical expenses and lost productivity amounting to an estimated $327 billion annually in the United States, according to recent publications (N/A, 2018). It is for this reason that the provision of effective management strategies is necessary, not only to ensure optimal clinical gain but also to help reduce economic burdens for patients as well as the healthcare system. With the integration of economic considerations into care planning, nurses can potentially have more freedom to advocate for interventions based on both economic and clinical merit, and educate patients about the potential cost-effectiveness of preemptive diabetes care. With diabetes still on the rise, these actions will become increasingly critical, and nursing education and practice must adapt to address these escalating challenges (Figure 9.11).

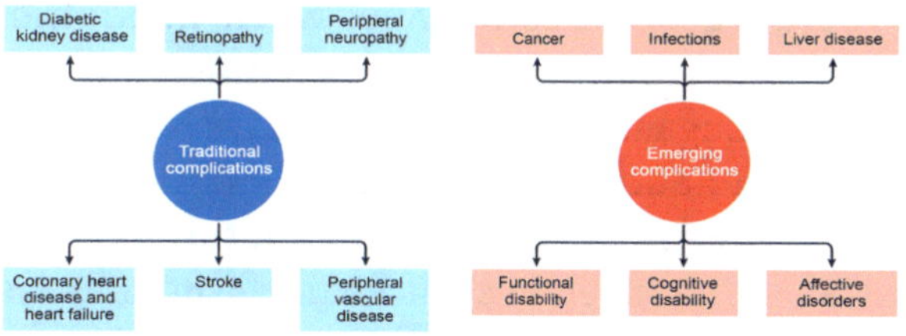

Figure 9.11. The burden and risks of emerging complications of diabetes mellitus.

Source: https://media.springernature.com/lw1200/springer-static/image/art%3A10.1038%2Fs41574-022-00690-7/MediaObjects/41574_2022_690_Fig1_HTML.png.

9.4.1. Lifestyle Modifications: Diet and Exercise

Dietary and physical exercise habits are critical factors in managing endocrine diseases ~~as well as~~ including diabetes. A balanced diet consisting of whole foods such as vegetables, fruits, whole grains, and lean proteins significantly impacts blood glucose levels as well as overall health. The dietary modifications enhance insulin sensitivity and regulate blood sugar levels. Moreover, the development of individualized meal plans can optimize nutritional value, taking into account patient preferences and medical background. By substituting low-glycemic index foods and reducing their intake of refined sugar and saturated fat, patients can create stabilizing environments for themselves. As a supplement, training in dietary portion control and careful eating habits can help patients develop healthier dietary lifestyles as part of their long-term self-management. In addition to dietary changes, daily physical exercise is also a crucial component in diabetes management and maintaining hormonal balance in the body. Physical exercise enhances the body's sensitivity to insulin and glucose, thereby lowering blood glucose levels and the likelihood of endocrine disorders and diabetes-related complications. Progressing to a minimum of 150 minutes of moderate aerobic activity per week, in addition to strength training, will yield significant health benefits. Engaging in physically active hobbies, in addition to addressing exercise limitations, not only promotes adherence to a routine regimen but also enhances overall health. Nurses must enact individualized strategies addressing the specific needs of those with exercise limitations. By cultivating a power-supportive climate that favors exercise, health care providers can promote sustainable lifestyle modifications that are an integral part of endocrine disease care, such as diabetes. Moreover, management of stress and lifestyle modification converge most powerfully in the context of endocrine disease. Stress has been shown to have documented physiological effects, including the release of cortisol, which can contribute to increased insulin resistance, as well as obesity and cardiovascular disease. Integrating stress-reduction techniques, such as mindfulness, meditation, and yoga, is crucial for developing a comprehensive approach to diabetes management. Recognizing the intricate dynamic interplay between mind and body enables healthcare practitioners to suggest holistic models of care that integrate stress management, as well as diet and exercise. Clinicians must also understand the particular challenge posed by chronic stress, which can undermine adherence to lifestyle change. In addressing these considerations, medical professionals can deliver a more rounded and realistic approach to the complexities of diabetes and endocrine diseases (Estrine et al., 2006; Agabiti-Rosei et al., 2016).

9.4.2. Pharmacological Interventions: Insulin and Oral Medications

Diabetes care, particularly in cases of endocrine disease, requires an in-depth understanding of pharmacological treatment, including insulin therapy and oral medications. Insulin, the hormone essential for secretion by the pancreas, plays a key role in glucose metabolism. In type 1 diabetes, insulin is the initial and often the sole type of therapy due to the absolute deficiency in endogenous insulin production. In type 2 diabetes, while oral medication is usually the first line of treatment, insulin treatment can be initiated if the glycemic control is poor. This multimodal approach is crucial to managing blood glucose and minimizing the risk of diabetes-related complications like cardiovascular disease, neuropathy, and nephropathy. Pharmacotherapy not only assists in the management of hyperglycemia but also contributes to improving the quality of life in these patients with chronic illness. Oral hypoglycemic medications, including various classes such as sulfonylureas, biguanides, and DPP-4 inhibitors, offer alternative options for glycemic control, particularly in the treatment of type 2 diabetes. All classes of drugs have different mechanisms, such as stimulating insulin secretion, sensitizing cells to insulin, or retarding glucose absorption from the intestine. Mechanisms of action not only inform us about their efficacy but also indicate how important treatment plans have to be individualized. For instance, metformin, a biguanide, is generally prescribed as a first-line drug for patients with Type 2 diabetes due to its capacity to reduce blood sugar and its very favorable safety profile. Understanding the pharmacokinetics and pharmacodynamics of these agents is crucial for nurses and prescribing practitioners to optimize patient education and drug administration, thereby enhancing compliance and therapeutic outcomes.

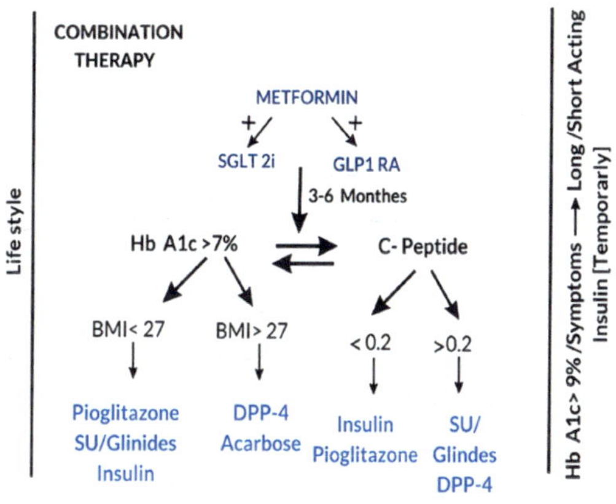

Figure 9.12. Drug therapies for diabetes.

Source: https://www.mdpi.com/ijms/ijms-24-17147/article_deploy/html/images/ijms-24-17147-g001-550.jpg.

For special populations such as pregnant women, particular concern for pharmacologic management is even more critical. Gestational diabetes mellitus (GDM) has certain nuances that require a tailored strategy to drug therapy. Insulin therapy is usually the preferred option due to its safety profile in both mother and fetus, exceptionally when oral drugs may be dangerous in terms of side effects. A recent review highlights the role of pharmacologic control of GDM and the optimization of medication management to enhance infant and maternal outcomes (Abdu et al., 2025). Moreover, the role of interprofessional healthcare teams, including pharmacists, is significant in monitoring medication therapy adherence and educating patients on the importance of pharmacological interventions (Upadhyay et al., 2025). Complete pharmaceutical care can notably reduce GDM-associated complications and maintain the importance of individualized treatment plans for diabetes management (Figure 9.12).

9.4.3. Monitoring Blood Glucose Levels

Blood glucose monitoring plays a crucial role in the management of endocrine diseases, particularly in diabetes, where blood sugar control is essential for preventing complications. Effective monitoring enables physicians to tailor treatment regimens based on the specific needs of patients. Regular monitoring of blood sugar levels can help identify trends that indicate a need for modification in medications, diet, or exercise. This is particularly urgent in conditions such as type 2 diabetes, where glucose management plans must be adaptive and responsive to changes in lifestyle or health status. The integration of technologies such as continuous glucose monitors and mobile health applications enhances the potential for real-time monitoring of these shifts, facilitating an active patient-nurse partnership in diabetes management with increased adherence and education. With this procedure, proper tracking is pivotal in improving the health condition of diabetic patients. The influence of educational interventions on blood glucose monitoring behavior is significant and cannot be overstated. Research has indicated that well-planned educational interventions, such as those based on King's Theory of Goal Attainment, have the potential to significantly enhance patients' knowledge about their condition and promote active self-management. Utilizing teach-back methods through digital technology not only provides patients with the information they need but also allows them to narrate their understanding, thereby reinforcing learning and alleviating anxiety about their condition. For instance, in a research study, these learning methods resulted in notable reductions in fasting plasma glucose and hemoglobin A1c among participants, along with decreased psychological distress related to hypoglycemia (Yan et al., 2024). By establishing a positive learning environment, nurses can empower patients to take control of their own health, demonstrating the power of education in diabetes management.

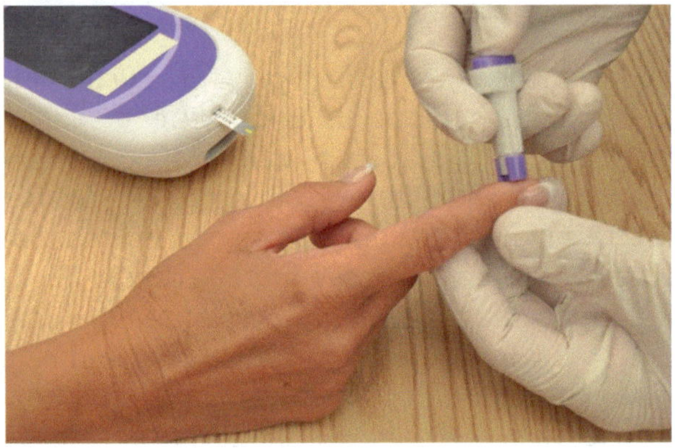

Figure 9.13. Monitoring blood glucose levels.

Source: https://wtcs.pressbooks.pub/app/uploads/sites/29/2020/11/DSC_1130-1-1024x678.jpg

Furthermore, the interaction between hormonal therapy and blood glucose monitoring makes diabetes management less mystical. Pharmacological treatments, such as the management of acromegaly with a somatostatin receptor agonist or a dopamine agonist, can have unwanted effects on glucose metabolism; therefore, close monitoring of blood glucose levels is necessary (Hasni et al., 2024).

For instance, a patient undergoing treatment for acromegaly may experience heightened fasting blood glucose levels as an adverse effect, which can lead to glucose regulatory complications.

This case points to the need for intense monitoring measures that address not just the direct consequences of diabetes drugs but also the effects of hormonal treatment. Given that nurses play a central role in this aspect of therapy, comprehension of the broader effects of endocrine diseases on glucose balance is essential to deliver effective nursing interventions and achieve optimal patient outcomes in diabetes therapy (Figure 9.13).

Test Your Knowledge

1. How does regular physical activity help in managing type 2 diabetes?
2. Why is blood glucose monitoring essential in insulin therapy?

9.5. Patient Education and Support

Learning Outcome

1. Describe the importance of patient education in diabetes management
2. Define the resources for patients and families
3. Discuss the strategies for effective communication with endocrine disorders and diabetes

Effective patient education and support are critical aspects ~~of~~ in the management of endocrine diseases, particularly diabetes. Nurses play a central role in fulfilling this educational role since they ~~take~~ assist patients through numerous treatment regimens and lifestyle modifications necessary for improved disease control. The education involved is comprehensive and goes beyond medication adherence education. It requires knowledge of diabetes pathophysiology, such as the role of glucose monitoring and the impact of diet and exercise on blood glucose levels. Central to such education is enabling patients to become capable of self-management, thereby creating a sense of responsibility and autonomy in the care process. Evidence shows that patient awareness of their condition can lead to improved health results and adherence to prescribed therapies, which in turn decrease the long-term effects of diabetes. The importance of ongoing support cannot be overstated within patient education. Continuing communication between healthcare professionals and patients provides a supportive environment that allows people to request explanations and question management plans. It fosters trust and helps patients report any adverse effects or issues they experience while implementing lifestyle changes or adhering to medication regimens. Ongoing follow-up visits by healthcare practitioners can reinforce education, adjust management as needed, and offer encouragement. Studies indicate that when patients feel nurtured, they are likely to embrace positive behavioral habits, therefore reducing risk factors related to diabetes complications such as cardiovascular disease or neuropathy. Furthermore, psychosocial issues related to diabetes care are part of the care provided to patients. Some patients have emotional problems such as depression and anxiety due to the burden of their diagnosis. Nurses must be aware of these issues and incorporate mental health resources into their patient education. Developing individualized care plans with psychosocial interventions can significantly enhance patients' quality of life. Engaging patients in support groups or educational workshops can foster a shared experience and promote community understanding. In addition, comprehensive guidelines indicate that physicians utilize multidisciplinary interventions within the management of both the physical and psychological components of endocrine illness. By ensuring that psychosocial needs are met, medical teams will be in a position to develop an integrated framework that not only addresses the medical aspects of diabetes treatment but also enhances patients' emotional well-being, thereby facilitating compliance with treatment and improving overall health outcomes.

9.5.1. Importance of Patient Education in Diabetes Management

Successful patient education is a cornerstone of diabetes care, as it empowers individuals to take responsibility for their own health. Diabetes, an endocrine chronic disease, necessitates that patients make choices about their way of life, medication compliance, and self-blood glucose monitoring. By informing patients about their condition, nurses can facilitate improved comprehension regarding diabetes management practices. This type of educational strategy is crucial, as it helps patients understand the role of diet, exercise, and medication in managing blood glucose levels, ultimately ensuring compliance with treatment. Moreover, well-educated patients are more likely to recognize symptoms of hypo- or hyperglycemia and respond accordingly, thereby avoiding complications associated with diabetes (Speiser et al., 2018). Additionally, individualized patient education can potentially lead to significant reductions in long-term healthcare costs associated with diabetes. Calculated in 2012 at $245 billion for diagnosed diabetes, both the medical care direct cost and lost productivity, the economic burden of poor control is substantial (N/A, 2013). Patient education courses that focus on general self-management skills can lead to reduced hospitalization rates and lower emergency room utilization, thereby alleviating the workload on healthcare resources. The integration of educational approaches with an orientation towards healthy lifestyle choices also promotes a preventive approach, leading to enhanced patient health outcomes and reduced healthcare expenses. Therefore, health systems that are interested in managing the economic and health implications of diabetes should invest in quality patient education programs a policy priority. In conclusion, the roles played by healthcare professionals in offering effective patient education cannot be exaggerated. The majority of patient education about diabetes is carried out by nurses, who are critical of patients and the complexity of their treatment regimens. Their ability to communicate effectively and provide tailored education based on individual patient needs can contribute to better understanding and management of the disorder. This tailored method not only improves patients' clinical outcomes but also their quality of life, since informed patients are more content with their care. Involving patients in their own education makes them responsible for their health, which is crucial in the treatment of diabetes, a chronic illness. Therefore, enhancing the educational quality of nurses in managing diabetes becomes crucial to improve patient outcomes and cope with the multifaceted nature of this endocrine disease (Figure 9.14).

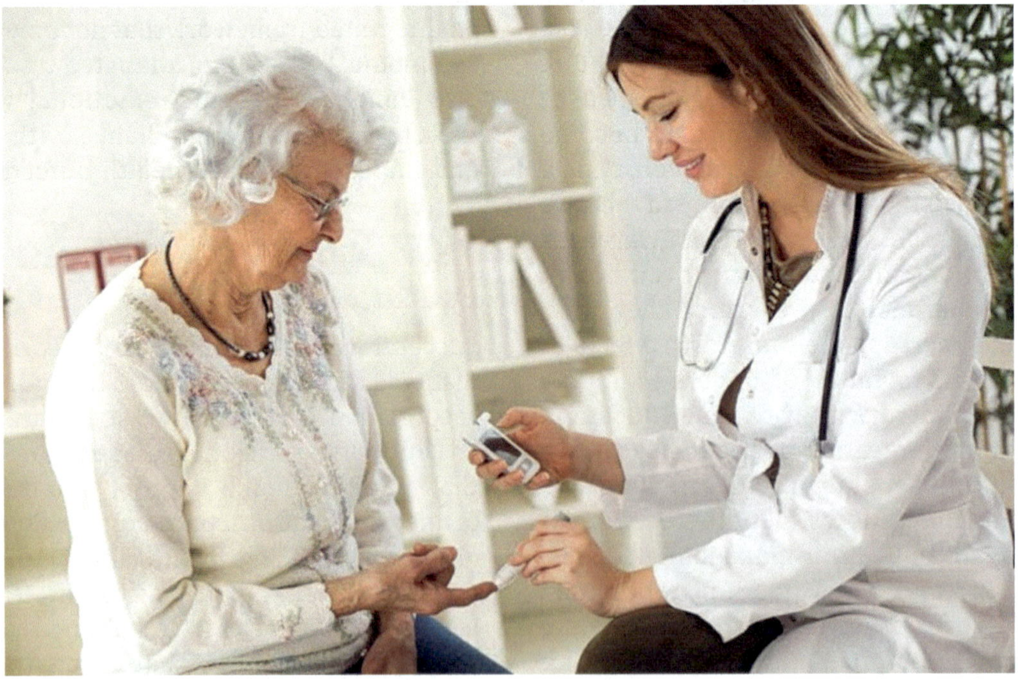

Figure 9.14. Patient education in diabetes management.

Source: https://www.nurseregistry.com/wp-content/uploads/2016/10/diabetic-senior-with-doctor-1200x800.jpg.

9.5.2. Resources for Patients and Families

Management of endocrine disorders, in this case diabetes, involves a comprehensive range of resources focused on patients and families. Resources are educational materials, ease of access to medical professionals, and community support systems. Education in managing diabetes shares information with families about the disease, risk factors, and prevention. One example is family workshops that demonstrate the role of nutrition and exercise in managing blood glucose levels. This proactive activity not only enhances understanding but also promotes collaboration and a positive environment for families to support one another in their diabetes journey, evidencing the educator, counselor, and healthcare provider roles in the efficient management of chronic diseases (Wahyudi et al., 2024). In addition to educational interventions, health professionals also play the crucial role of connecting families with suitable mental health services, particularly given that most comorbid disorders, such as depression, are associated with diabetes (Forman-Hoffman et al., 2016). Primary care settings are an essential site of contact for the identification and treatment of mental illness, wherein practitioners can initiate care and refer the patient for specialty services when appropriate. With the application of collaborative care programs incorporating mental health care, patients with endocrine disorders stand a better chance of improved health status as well as increased quality of life. Aside from this, community resources enable the delivery of ongoing care to families and patients with the complexities of diabetic management. Local diabetes support groups and online forums offer spaces for sharing experiences, discussing coping strategies, and addressing common difficulties. Peer-initiated efforts can also help moderate the isolation that those suffering from chronic diseases tend to experience. Access to such technology as diabetes apps also allows families to track health information and receive medicine and appointment reminders. Overall, use of these varied resources is an important vital in maximizing the efficacy of diabetes management, thereby achieving better health outcomes and patient and family resilience (Wahyudi et al., 2024).

9.5.3. Strategies for Effective Communication

Clear communication is critical in nursing, especially when treating patients with endocrine diseases and diabetes. Nurses must employ various communication strategies to provide patients with concise, accurate, and compassionate information about their disease and treatment. Good communication encourages patients to speak openly about their symptoms and concerns, leading to improved management of their diabetes. When nurses practice active listening and validate patient feelings, they build rapport and trust with the patient, which reinforces the overall therapeutic relationship. This provides a foundation for more participatory care, with patients empowered to become involved in their treatment planning, become educated about the medications they take, and understand the importance of lifestyle modification. These modes of communication not only increase patient adherence but also lead to better health outcomes in the management of chronic diseases, such as diabetes (Halvorsen et al., 2022). The use of educational materials and resources can also make it easier to present information to patients more clearly and memorably. Visual tools, such as diagrams and charts, may be particularly helpful in demonstrating complex concepts related to insulin injections or changes in diet. Also, the utilization of teach-back techniques helps nurses determine patients' comprehension of their health conditions and directions by having them paraphrase the information in their own words. This technique not only supports learning but also determines areas of misunderstanding that require additional clarification. By integrating these pedagogical approaches into regular nursing practice, healthcare providers can ensure that patients with endocrine disorders are properly educated, thereby improving their self-management skills and confidence (Schneider et al., 2021). Lastly, culturally sensitive communication needs to be developed to address the diverse needs of patients with endocrine disorders. Cultural competence in nursing entails the recognition of the distinctive values, beliefs, and practices of various individuals and incorporating this information into care delivery. Cultural differences in health literacy and communication are what can be recognized and dealt with by nurses so they can modify messages for a more effective connection with different communities. This, besides respecting patients' background, makes patients more engaged in health-care interaction. Since the management of diabetes often requires lifestyle changes, culturally sensitive communication can significantly impact patients' readiness to adopt these changes. Thus, the implementation of a culturally sensitive communication approach is paramount in managing endocrine disorders and providing equitable care to all patients (Halvorsen et al., 2022) (Figure 9.15).

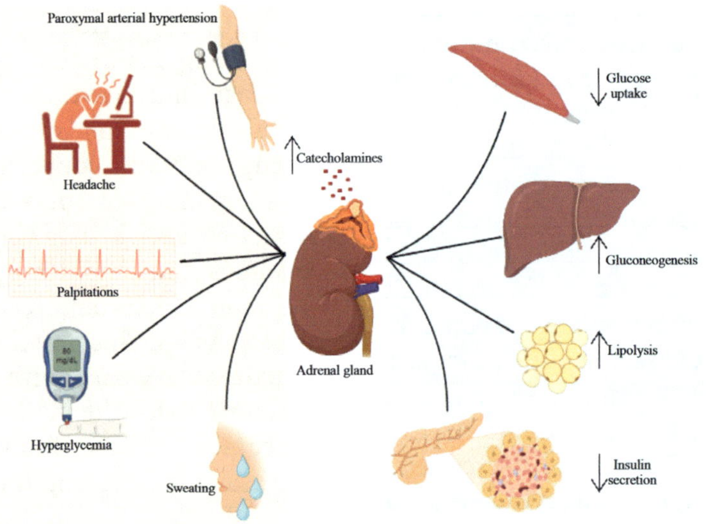

Figure 9.15. Diabetes mellitus secondary to endocrine diseases: an update of diagnostic and treatment.

Source: https://www.mdpi.com/ijms/ijms-24-12676/article_deploy/html/images/ijms-24-12676-g003.png.

Test Your Knowledge

1. Why is individualized education important for promoting patient self-care?
2. How can nurses support patients in managing lifestyle changes related to chronic illness?

9.6. Role of Nurses in Managing Endocrine Disorders

Learning Outcome

1. Describe the collaborative care and interdisciplinary teams of endocrine disorders
2. Define the advocacy for patient needs and rights
3. Identify the continuing education and professional development

Nurses occupy the pivotal role in the management of endocrine diseases, such as diabetes care. Their function extends beyond universal patient education to a profound understanding of the complex mechanisms that control hormonal balance and metabolic health. Due to the increasing prevalence of endocrine diseases, such as diabetes, nurses must be equipped with high-level knowledge to diagnose signs, manage complications, and enable lifestyle modifications. A healthy patient-nurse relationship promotes an interactive atmosphere where nurses can assess individualized needs, administer medications, and provide ongoing support. Moreover, as health care team members, nurses play a significant role in multidisciplinary care practices that enhance overall patient well-being.

By combining medical data with empathetic communication, nurses can achieve closure of the clinical care versus patient adherence gap, ultimately enhancing outcomes for individuals with endocrine diseases. Cultural competency with sensitivity in attending to diverse groups, such as transgender clients who may have special endocrine concerns, is a second critical element of nursing here. The nurses must be informed of the specific needs related to hormone therapy and how it may impact health, as well as relevant mental health issues that may arise during treatment. The nurses can better manage the challenges of care that transgender patients face by adopting a culturally responsive practice. This involves tailoring educational materials to meet the individual needs of patients and establishing a safe environment where patients feel at ease discussing their medical problems. As mandated, there is new vocabulary to learn in the evolving landscape of patient care, with primary emphasis on ongoing education for nursing practitioners.

In achieving successful resolutions to these scenarios, there are opportunities for improved patient satisfaction and wellness, solidifying the nurse's role as caregiver and advocate within the healthcare system (Markwick et al., 2016). Nurses also must be sensitive to the psychosocial implications of endocrine disease, where stress and mental health have a significant impact on physical health outcomes.

The dynamic between stressors and hormonal response necessitates an integral nursing practice that intertwines mental health screening with traditional diabetes care interventions. Nurses are particularly positioned to observe patients' mental status, screen for evidence of stress, and intervene appropriately in order not to exacerbate endocrine disease. Recognizing that stress is a predominant determinant of health and disease throughout the life cycle necessitates the urgency for nurses to integrate stress management skills into their day-to-day practice (Estrine et al., 2006). Such positive thinking not only adheres to the physiological management of diseases like diabetes but also enhances the overall quality of life for patients. Therefore, the broad role of nurses in addressing endocrine disease extends far beyond the clinical environment, encompassing the emotional and psychological aspects of health that are essential to comprehensive diabetes management (Figure 8.16).

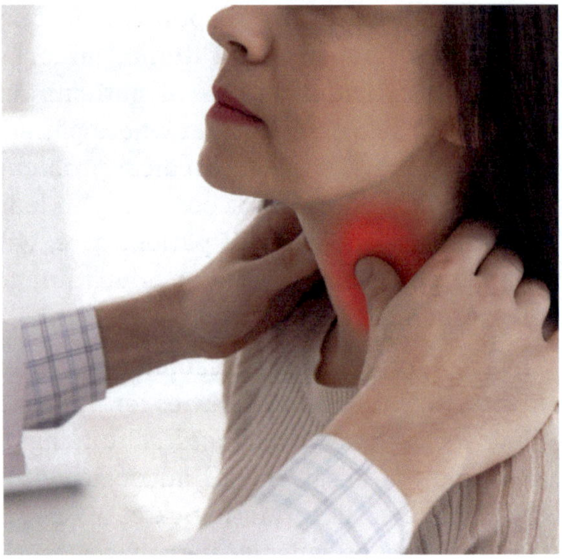

Figure 9.16. Managing endocrine disorders.

Source: https://external-content.duckduckgo.com/iu/?u=https%3A%2F%2Fgreenwich.peakwellness.com%2Fwp-content%2Fuploads%2Fsites%2F3%2F2024%2F05%2FManaging-Endocrine-Disorders.png&f=1&nofb=1&ipt=e5e82fe211abe6c74419a664d0519fe0936a867138bf7af82111aa9b22aecad6.

9.6.1. Collaborative Care and Interdisciplinary Teams

The complex nature of endocrine diseases, and in particular diabetes, necessitates a structured model of patient care to facilitate harmonious collaboration among healthcare professionals. System models of collaborative care highlight the need to integrate multidisciplinary knowledge, enabling health teams to address not only the medical but also the psychological and social aspects of managing chronic diseases. Enhanced communication and shared decision-making between physicians, nurses, dietitians, and mental health professionals promote patient outcomes through a comprehensive consideration of all aspects of a patient's health. Such multidisciplinary interaction enables the development of individualized treatment plans tailored to each patient's values and priorities, ultimately leading to better adherence to recommended lifestyle modifications and medication regimens. The coordination of multidisciplinary teams is crucial in the treatment of patients with metabolic-kidney-cardiovascular syndrome-related diseases, as described by existing research. The complexity of the inter-relationship among metabolic diseases calls for a comprehensive response more than using traditional treatment methodologies. For example, while physicians focus on pharmacologic therapy, nutritionists can create specific diets that lower obesity and diabetes risk factors. In addition, social worker interventions can address the external determinants of health that influence a patient's capacity to maintain lifestyle changes. Evidence for this interprofessional intervention is supported by literature that documents the benefits of coordinated systems of care in improving patient outcomes, particularly in the context of interacting complexity of endocrine conditions and cardiovascular risk factors, despite ongoing challenges in implementing positive changes (Ndumele et al., 2023). Furthermore, the role of continuous education and training among health professionals in interdisciplinary teams cannot be overstated. All specialists involved in the care of patients with endocrine diseases should have current knowledge of evidence-based practices, as this directly influences the management and prevention of complications. Training initiatives may enhance teamwork and communication skills, fostering a culture where information is openly shared and decisions regarding care are informed by a comprehensive understanding of patient health. New strategies, such as telehealth services, also enhance collaboration by removing geographical boundaries, allowing diverse teams to communicate effectively in real-time. Thus, the promotion and establishment of interdisciplinary models in diabetes care are needed not only to address patients' needs within a short time span, but also to ensure long-term health outcomes (Halvorsen et al., 2022).

9.6.2. Advocacy for Patient Needs and Rights

In the context of nursing practice, patient rights and needs advocacy is an integral part that can significantly influence the treatment of endocrine disorders and diabetes. Nurses are valuable bridge players between patients and the healthcare system, enabling individuals to access proper care that best suits their unique health requirements. This advocacy is particularly critical for disadvantaged populations, e.g., those with multicultural backgrounds or specific health complications. For example, the care of the health of transgender patients involves culturally competent care, and these patients may develop unique mental health and substance abuse problems depending on treatment and hormone therapy. Nurses, therefore, must be well-equipped to advocate for such patients, all with their own needs, and reverse any care barriers that can be experienced in a clinical setting (Markwick et al., 2016). Patient empowerment in their own healthcare is also a key feature of patient advocacy among nurses. Patients with endocrine disorders such as diabetes are may have a range of problems that tend to jeopardize their capability for self-care. Education is a key element in this process, as better-educated patients are better equipped to make informed decisions about their treatment and lifestyle adjustments. Nurses should ensure that they provide comprehensive diabetes education, focusing on dietary control, medication adherence, and regular monitoring. This not only manages the condition but also instills a sense of power and responsibility in patients, stimulating them to become active participants in their own health. Thus, successful advocacy through education can lead to improved health outcomes because patients are more willing to take charge of their conditions and advocate for themselves to healthcare providers (Burman et al., 1995). Moreover, addressing systemic barriers in healthcare is crucial in solving advocacy issues relating to patient needs and rights. Most marginalized groups do not have access to quality healthcare services,—which aggravates their situation. Several determinants, including geographic proximity, availability of resources, and socioeconomic status, may influence patient care and access to necessary interventions. Residents in reservations, for instance, do not always have adequate access to skilled home health care services, which can hinder effective disease management for diabetes and other endocrine disorders. Nurses can advocate for policy changes that promote equitable access to healthcare resources such that all patients are given the care they deserve, regardless of their circumstance. By addressing such systemic issues, nursing advocacy seeks not only to address the immediate needs of patients but also to achieve a more equitable healthcare environment in the broader sense (Burman et al., 1995; Markwick et al., 2016) (Figure 9.17).

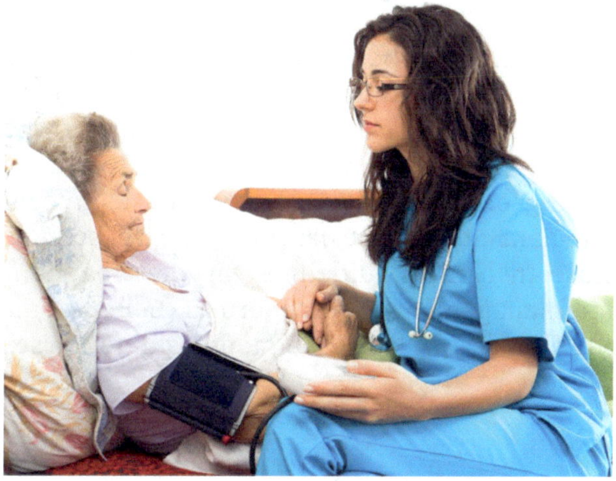

Figure 9.17. Advocacy for patient needs and rights.

Source: https://images.wisegeek.com/nurse-in-blue-scrubs-near-elderly-patient.jpg.

9.6.3. Continuing Education and Professional Development

In the rapidly evolving field of healthcare, particularly in the management of endocrine disorders and diabetes, the importance of continuing education and professional development cannot be overstated. Nurses who engage actively in continuous learning opportunities will deliver quality patient care and aid in improving chronic diseases. Through their knowledge of the latest clinical guidelines, treatment patterns, and interdisciplinary approaches, nursing practitioners can enhance their abilities and confirm they are providing evidence-based practices. For instance, with recent updates to diabetes care guidelines, nurses can obtain essential information on patient education methods and therapies through workshops or conferences. This proactive strategy promotes a culture of continuous improvement, ultimately leading to enhanced patient outcomes in both clinical and home care settings. In addition, integrating evidence-based practices in nursing education translates directly to professional growth. Regular continuing education programs are implemented to bridge the gap between theoretical practice and actual application, particularly in disease management, such as diabetes. To illustrate, the diverse management approaches reflected by leading organizations are designed to inform clinicians about best practices in care, such as those in clinical guidelines for the treatment and management of osteoporosis (LeBoff et al., 2022). Not only do these models guide nurses in assessing and treating patients, but they also highlight the necessity of continuous learning because they must adapt to the emergence of new knowledge and changes in patient populations. Active participation in continuous education not only satisfies regulatory requirements but also maximizes the intensity of practice, ensuring interdisciplinary collaboration between healthcare teams. Mentorship and peer-to-peer learning schemes can also be at the forefront in promoting professional development among nursing personnel who are affected by endocrine disorders. Through the establishment of an environment conducive to the exchange of experiences and expertise, health organizations can foster a culture of knowledge sharing. These measures encourage the application of holistic models of care with multidisciplinary opinion across specialties, as evident in the attempt to manage scarce immune-related adverse events of cancer therapy (Schneider et al., 2021). This coordination is essential for the effective management of not only patients' short-term clinical needs but also their long-term planning, which contributes to achieving long-term health outcomes. Continuing professional development through mentorship and shared learning facilities gradually promotes responsibility, ensures compliance with best practice, and cultivates a workforce able to address the nuances of endocrine illness and diabetes management.

Test Your Knowledge

1. What are the key nursing responsibilities in the care of a patient with diabetes mellitus?
2. How can nurses help monitor and manage complications of thyroid disorders?

SUMMARY

Diabetes and endocrine diseases highlight the absolute necessity of nursing intervention and treatment in patient management. Endocrine disorders, particularly diabetes, necessitate proper control through an early detection and prevention-based multidisciplinary approach. As exemplified by studies of pediatric obesity, primary care providers must be vigilant for at-risk patients as the burden of such disease extends beyond acute medical management to incorporate lifestyle modifications and long-term support. By committing themselves to closing the gaps in diagnosis and treatment, nursing professionals can significantly improve patient outcomes and lay the groundwork for lifelong health management, particularly among young populations (Gelement et al., 2014). Furthermore, it is significant that nursing professionals engage in continuous education on the complexity of endocrine disorders. Increased consciousness of the nuances of diabetic care, and particularly acute problems like symptomatic hypoglycemia, can lead to more effective pre-hospital therapy. Experience indicates that emergency patients often leave without adequate follow-up instructions, which exposes them to repeated attacks (Booley et al., 2015). Nurses are in the best position to bridge this gap by providing comprehensive discharge planning and education, ensuring patients are well-equipped to care for themselves upon discharge from the hospital. This forward-thinking approach is not only crucial to improving care for individual patients but also public health outcomes more broadly. ~~Last but not least,~~ In addition, effective management of endocrine disorders hinges on an interdisciplinary collaboration, and nursing is the cornerstone of such a collaborative process. Building up habits of communication among caregivers, patients, and providers is crucial in offering unbroken care and preventing complications of diabetes. By embracing evidence-based practice to promote the total well-being of patients, nurses can enhance better health outcomes for individuals with endocrine disorders. Adherence to these principles will allow nursing practitioners to spearhead revolutionary changes in healthcare provisioning that ultimately make societies healthier (Glement et al., 2014; Booley et al., 2015).

To address the intricacies of endocrine disorders, particularly in diabetes management, there is a need to understand the complex nature of these complications. Endocrine disorders directly impact metabolic processes and overall well-being, thus necessitating a holistic approach to nursing intervention. For instance, stress has been identified as a significant factor well known to disrupt hormonal levels and glucose metabolism. An understanding of the interaction between endocrine and brain responses is at the heart of nurses' comprehension, who are often in the position of leadership for the treatment of patients. This adherence to values of holistic care intervenes more easily suited to individuals, emphasizing the pivotal role of nursing in endocrine disorder care and optimizing outcomes related to diabetes (Estrine et al., 2006). Additionally, diabetes management encompasses not only pharmacological interventions but also lifestyle modifications. This is of particular interest in populations with hypertension, where improved management can prevent complications. There is evidence that lifestyle changes, including increased exercise and weight loss, can have a significant impact on blood pressure and, consequently, diabetes management. In South Africa, practice guidelines advise delaying drug therapy for hypertension in preference to lifestyle change in the majority of patients. This integrated approach emphasizes patient education on the beneficial impact of a change in lifestyle, reinforcing nurses' dual roles as educators and managers of chronic diseases (Collard et al., 2014). Additionally, facilitating effective communication and collaboration among healthcare teams enhances care for endocrine diseases and diabetes. By fostering an environment in which patient problems and interdisciplinary solutions can be openly discussed, nurses can close the gap between specialties whose staff treat a patient. In addition to attempting to better understand the needs of particular patients in a more coordinated manner, the team-based approach also utilizes the healthcare framework to its maximum potential by addressing every aspect of a patient's problem. Finally, these combined forces, coupled with a greater focus on educating patients about the impact of stress and lifestyle on hormonal well-being, lead to better control of outcomes in endocrine disease and diabetes management in nursing practice.

KEY TERMS FROM THIS CHAPTER

- Addison's disease
- Cushing's syndrome
- Diabetic ketoacidosis (DKA)
- Foot care in diabetes
- Hyperglycemia
- Hyperthyroidism
- Insulin
- Oral hypoglycemic agents
- Thyroid disorders
- Blood glucose monitoring
- Diabetes self-management education (DSME)
- Endocrine function tests
- Hemoglobin A1c (HbA1c)
- Hyperosmolar hyperglycemic state (HHS)
- Hypoglycemia
- Insulin pump therapy
- Pituitary gland disorders
- Type 1 diabetes mellitus

CRITICAL THINKING QUESTIONS

1. **Which hormone is deficient in Type 1 Diabetes Mellitus?**
   a. Glucagon
   b. Insulin
   c. Cortisol
   d. Thyroxine
2. **A classic symptom of hyperthyroidism is:**
   a. Weight gain
   b. Bradycardia
   c. Cold intolerance
   d. Heat intolerance
3. **What is the primary goal of diabetes management?**
   a. Increase insulin resistance
   b. Prevent weight gain
   c. Maintain blood glucose within normal range
   d. Eliminate the need for insulin
4. **Which of the following is a sign of hypoglycemia?**
   a. Flushed skin
   b. Slow pulse
   c. Sweating and confusion
   d. Increased urination
5. **What is the nurse's first action when a diabetic patient is found unconscious?**
   a. Administer insulin
   b. Check for pulse
   c. Start CPR
   d. Administer glucose or glucagon

Short Answer Questions

1. What is the primary function of insulin in the body?
2. What is the difference between Type 1 and Type 2 diabetes?
3. Name one complication of uncontrolled diabetes.
4. What nursing action is essential when managing a patient with hypothyroidism?
5. Explain the nursing assessment and management of a patient experiencing hypoglycemia.
6. Discuss the pathophysiology, clinical features, and nursing care of a patient with hyperthyroidism.
7. Describe the components of a practical diabetes self-care education plan for newly diagnosed patients.
8. Explain the long-term complications of diabetes mellitus and the role of nursing in prevention.

Answers to Critical Thinking Questions

1. (b) 2. (d) 3. (c) 4. (c) 5. (d).

REFERENCES

1. Abdu, A., & Bakrey, H. (2025). Comprehensive Review of Gestational Diabetes: Pathophysiology, pharmacological management and the role of Pharmaceutical care. *Current Drug Safety, 20*. https://doi.org/10.2174/0115748863348681250117111223Agabiti-Rosei, E., Cruickshank, J. K., Dominiczak, A., Erdine, S., et al. (2016). 2016 European Society of Hypertension guidelines for the management of high blood pressure in children and adolescents. https://core.ac.uk/download/46165193.pdf (accessed on 30th June 2025).
2. Amber, K. T., Brooks, L., Ference, T., Hadi, S., et al. (2015). Assessing the prevalence of autoimmune, endocrine, gynecologic, and psychiatric comorbidities in an ethnically diverse cohort of female fibromyalgia patients: Does the time from hysterectomy provide a clue? https://core.ac.uk/download/46954518.pdf (accessed on 30th June 2025).
3. Annagur, A., Beck, B., Cronin, D., Dennett, D., Dowdy, D., et al. (2018). Polycystic ovary syndrome across the life span of women: A wellness-based integrative intervention. https://core.ac.uk/download/213088882.pdf (accessed on 30th June 2025).
4. Booley, R., Mohamed, S., & Welzel, T. (2015). A cross-sectional analysis of the short-term outcomes of patients receiving prehospital treatment for symptomatic hypoglycemia in Cape Town. https://core.ac.uk/download/pdf/82225708.pdf (accessed on 30th June 2025).
5. Bordoni, A., Dupont, D., Gille, D., Kachal, J., et al. (2015). Understanding the gastrointestinal tract of the elderly to develop dietary solutions that prevent malnutrition. https://core.ac.uk/download/286575279.pdf (accessed on 30th June 2025).
6. Browne, N. T., Snethen, J., Greenberg, C. S., Frenn, M., Kilanowski, J. F., Gance-Cleveland, B., Burke, P. J., et al. (2020). When pandemics collide: The impact of COVID-19 on childhood obesity. *Journal of Pediatric Nursing, 56*, 90–98. https://doi.org/10.1016/j.pedn.2020.11.004.
7. Burman, M. E., Indian Health Service, Billings Area Indian Health Service, Public Health Nursing Division, & Jansa, N. (1995). Benchmarking home health care and public health nursing services. https://core.ac.uk/download/151599904.pdf (accessed on 30th June 2025).
8. Cheng, J. (2017). The mechanisms of psychological therapy with people with long-term physical health conditions. https://core.ac.uk/download/96838376.pdf (accessed on 30th June 2025).
9. Collard, J., Gafane, L., Nell, T., Rennie, K., et al. (2014). Physical activity and hypertension in South African adults. https://core.ac.uk/download/29852228.pdf (accessed on 30th June 2025).
10. Copeland, L., James, D., Duinkerken, M., Kelsey, G., et al. (2019). Jefferson Digital Commons quarterly report: October–December 2019. https://core.ac.uk/download/286097805.pdf (accessed on 30th June 2025).
11. Dieleman, J. L., Baral, R., Birger, M., Bui, A. L., Bulchis, A., Chapin, A., Hamavid, H., et al. (2016). US spending on personal health care and public health, 1996–2013. *JAMA, 316*, 2627–2627. https://doi.org/10.1001/jama.2016.16885.
12. Dunger, D. (1998). *Childhood and Adolescent Diabetes.* https://www.semanticscholar.org/paper/84e710c7a6c0f1a2c80c9568debc2035baedadb2 (accessed on 30th June 2025).
13. Estrine, J., & DeLisle, L. (2006). Stress: Putting the brain back into medicine. https://core.ac.uk/download/71356692.pdf (accessed on 30th June 2025).

14. Farseena, K., & Deshpande, S. (2025). A case report on Ayurvedic management of type 2 diabetes mellitus. *The Bioscan.* https://www.semanticscholar.org/paper/f21c3ea5c1aafc644b0235f16bfa4e040c09aa29 (accessed on 30th June 2025).

15. Forman-Hoffman, V., McClure, E., McKeeman, J. L., Wood, C., Middleton, J., Skinner, A., Perrin, E. M., et al. (2016). Screening for major depressive disorder in children and adolescents: A systematic review for the U.S. Preventive Services Task Force. *Annals of Internal Medicine, 164*, 342–349. https://www.semanticscholar.org/paper/a0da04d57415ae7ef5db7e778b4341a0c9443268 (accessed on 30th June 2025).

16. Gelement, J. E. (2014). Pediatric obesity: Taking advantage of well-child visits for early identification. https://core.ac.uk/download/232575619.pdf (accessed on 30th June 2025).

17. Gustafsson, U., Scott, M. J., Hübner, M., Nygren, J., Demartines, N., Francis, N., Rockall, T., et al. (2018). Guidelines for perioperative care in elective colorectal surgery: Enhanced Recovery After Surgery (ERAS®) Society recommendations: 2018. *World Journal of Surgery, 43*, 659–695. https://doi.org/10.1007/s00268-018-4844-y.

18. Halvorsen, S., Mehilli, J., Cassese, S., Hall, T. S., Abdelhamid, M., Barbato, E., De Hert, S., et al. (2022). 2022 ESC guidelines on cardiovascular assessment and management of patients undergoing non-cardiac surgery. *European Heart Journal, 43*, 3826–3924. https://doi.org/10.1093/eurheartj/ehac270.

19. Hasni, Y., Nouira, S., El Fekih, H., Thabet, M., Ssafi, W., Thabet, N., Halloul, I., et al. (2024). Management strategies for mixed GH and prolactin-secreting macroadenomas following surgical failure: A case report. *Journal of Innovations in Medical Research*. https://www.semanticscholar.org/paper/675902c6358b9beb71c1f5b016a6b9a894969b68 (accessed on 30th June 2025).

20. Hogan, P., Nikolov, P., & Dall, T. (2025). Economic costs of diabetes in the U.S. in 2002. https://core.ac.uk/download/pdf/9315084.pdf (accessed on 30th June 2025).

21. Iqbal, S. (2016). A clinical study on the dermatological manifestations of obesity. https://core.ac.uk/download/235662077.pdf (accessed on 30th June 2025).

22. Kapke, D. R. (2015). Childhood type II diabetes: The risks and complications. https://core.ac.uk/download/58826199.pdf (accessed on 30th June 2025).

23. Kiełczewska, A., Kiełczewska, A., & Szcześniak, G. (2025). Obesity-related endocrine disorders. *Journal of Education, Health and Sport*. https://www.semanticscholar.org/paper/3368028645db9b5f07b6d6f4439b7cd57b8f5231 (accessed on 30th June 2025).

24. LeBoff, M. S., Greenspan, S. L., Insogna, K., Lewiecki, E. M., Saag, K. G., Singer, A., & Siris, E. S. (2022). The clinician's guide to prevention and treatment of osteoporosis. *Osteoporosis International, 33*, 2049–2102. https://doi.org/10.1007/s00198-021-05900-y.

25. Marazuela, M., Giustina, A., & Puig-Domingo, M. (2020). Endocrine and metabolic aspects of the COVID-19 pandemic. *Reviews in Endocrine and Metabolic Disorders, 21*, 495–507. https://doi.org/10.1007/s11154-020-09569-2.

26. Markwick, L. (2016). Male, female, other: Transgender and the impact in primary care. https://core.ac.uk/download/48623404.pdf (accessed on 30th June 2025).

27. Miao, X., Fu, Z., Luo, X., Wang, J., Ren, Z., Wang, Y., Mei, G., et al. (2024). Evidence-based management strategies for endocrine complications after pituitary adenoma surgery. *Ibrain.*

https://www.semanticscholar.org/paper/4e7912e29745739886c04126be2144e4c43f2c7e (accessed on 30th June 2025).

28. Ndumele, C. E., Neeland, I. J., Tuttle, K. R., Chow, S. L., Mathew, R. O., Khan, S. S., Coresh, J., et al. (2023). A synopsis of the evidence for the science and clinical management of cardiovascular-kidney-metabolic (CKM) syndrome: A scientific statement from the American Heart Association. *Circulation, 148*, 1636–1664. https://doi.org/10.1161/cir.0000000000001186.

29. Oh, T. (1990). *Intensive Care Manual*. https://www.semanticscholar.org/paper/6dc9376e40514aa091f866707e3f62dff35b498c (accessed on 30th June 2025).

30. Petrakis, D., Margină, D., Tsarouhas, K., Tekos, F., Stan, M., Nikitovic, D., Kouretas, D., et al. (2020). Obesity–A risk factor for increased COVID19 prevalence, severity and lethality (Review). *Molecular Medicine Reports, 22*, 9–19. https://doi.org/10.3892/mmr.2020.11127.

31. Rizwan, A. (2025). Perioperative management of endocrine disorders–practical considerations. *Journal of the Pakistan Medical Association*. https://www.semanticscholar.org/paper/99407d6207cb84d19db2201d1b2b42c7b9117edf (accessed on 30th June 2025).

32. Salimian, M. R., Injinari, N., Azizi, R., Nikkhah, H., & Namiranian, N. (2024). Prevalence and impact of thyroid disorders on glycemic control in patients with type 2 diabetes mellitus: A cross-sectional study. *Iranian Journal of Diabetes and Obesity*. https://www.semanticscholar.org/paper/723fa3efe83c411c659d7ae0db542f83cc581677 (accessed on 30th June 2025).

33. Schneider, B. J., Naidoo, J., Santomasso, B., Lacchetti, C., Adkins, S., Anadkat, M. J., Atkins, M. B., et al. (2021). Management of immune-related adverse events in patients treated with immune checkpoint inhibitor therapy: ASCO guideline update. *Journal of Clinical Oncology, 39*, 4073–4126. https://doi.org/10.1200/jco.21.01440.

34. Shah, A. K., Niroula, P., Yadav, P. K., & Mautsa, R. M. (2024). Management of severe dyselectrolytemia in an elderly patient with normal pressure hydrocephalus. *Journal of Pharma Insights and Research*. https://www.semanticscholar.org/paper/0d30ac2cb2e7cdae79309f8c270eab4f8790361c (accessed on 30th June 2025).

35. Speiser, P., Arlt, W., Auchus, R. J., Baskin, L. S., Conway, G. S., Merke, D. P., Meyer-Bahlburg, H. F. L., et al. (2018). Congenital adrenal hyperplasia due to steroid 21-hydroxylase deficiency: An Endocrine Society* clinical practice guideline. *The Journal of Clinical Endocrinology & Metabolism, 103*, 4043–4088. https://doi.org/10.1210/jc.2018-01865.

36. Upadhyay, R. T., & Upadhyay, A. K. (2025). Integrative approaches to diabetes management: Evaluating the impact of naturopathy, diet, yoga, and herbal therapy compared to conventional treatments. *Journal of Ayurveda and Integrated Medical Sciences*. https://www.semanticscholar.org/paper/e7c47f2436b578817a60ff4a5a532d2df749e50d (accessed on 30th June 2025).

37. Yan, M., Yu, Y., Li, S., Zhang, P., & Yu, J. (2024). Effectiveness of King's theory of goal attainment in blood glucose management for newly diagnosed patients with type 2 diabetes: Randomized controlled trial. *Journal of Medical Internet Research, 26*. https://www.semanticscholar.org/paper/6b211fc34e7cf97c3062e8635a181113787a3eb0 (accessed on 30th June 2025).

38. Yelne, S., Gawai, J., Kasturkar, P., Meshram, P., Uke, T., & Taksande, V. (2025). Mental health nursing care for people with diabetes mellitus: A narrative review. *Multidisciplinary Reviews*. https://www.semanticscholar.org/paper/dab295a95d8cc4763e07fff087eb14cb4f13dcc0 (accessed on 30th June 2025).

RENAL AND URINARY TRACT FUNCTION: ASSESSMENT AND INTERVENTIONS

10

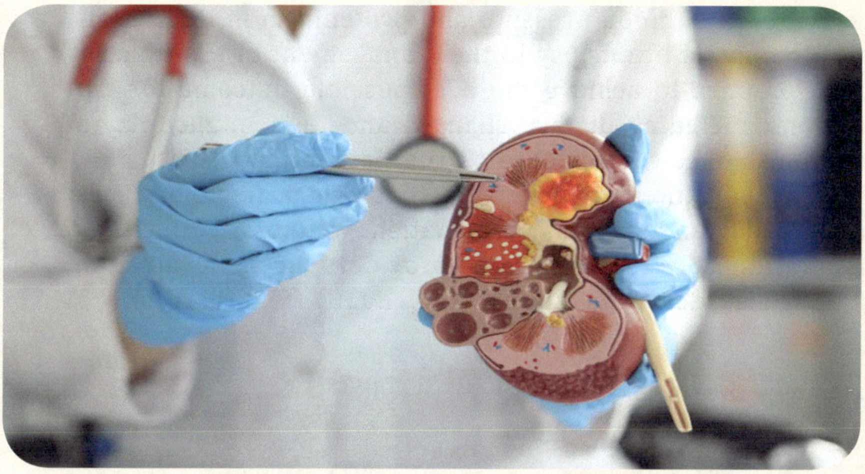

LEARNING OBJECTIVES

After studying this chapter, you will be able to:

1. Understand the anatomy of the renal system
2. Explain the physiology of renal function
3. Discuss the common renal and urinary tract disorders
4. Focus on assessment techniques for renal function
5. Learn about interventions for renal health
6. Evaluate the preventive measures for renal and urinary health

Introduction

The urinary tract and renal system play a crucial role in helping maintain homeostasis in the human body by assisting fluid balance, electrolyte regulation, and the elimination of waste. The kidneys, which contain millions of nephrons, filter blood to discard wastes through urine while preserving vital nutrients and water, thereby maintaining good health. Impaired renal function can lead to severe health conditions, such as chronic kidney disease (CKD) and end-stage renal failure, which mandate proper monitoring and intervention methods. Providers require an in-depth understanding of renal and urinary tract physiology to navigate the complexities of numerous pathologies involving these systems (Gustafsson et al., 2018). This context provides the groundwork for reporting current evaluation techniques and interventions employed to manage issues related to renal and urinary tract function. Renal function testing typically involves both laboratory work and imaging studies, which serve as valuable markers of an individual's kidney health. Laboratory studies that are most often utilized include serum creatinine concentration, estimated glomerular filtration rate (eGFR), and urinalysis, which can reflect kidney dysfunction as well as other related conditions. Additionally, imaging modalities such as ultrasonography or computed tomography scans are used to visualize anatomical derangements or obstructions within the urinary tract. The multimodal approach to evaluation is crucial for the early diagnosis of renal pathologies, enabling prompt interventions that can halt further decline in kidney function. Evidence-based guidelines, such as those of the American Urological Association and the Enhanced Recovery After Surgery Society, form the basis of good patient care, ensuring that interventions are suitably tailored to a patient's individual needs (Assimos et al., 2016). Treatment for renal and urinary tract dysfunction encompasses a wide range of therapeutic approaches, including pharmacological therapies, surgical procedures, and lifestyle modifications. Pharmacologic treatment may involve the use of diuretics to decrease fluid overload or medications that control blood pressure and proteinuria in individuals with CKD. Surgical interventions, such as the use of lithotripsy in the management of urolithiasis, require unwavering adherence to clinical practice to achieve the best possible outcome for the patient. Furthermore, lifestyle modifications, including dietary changes and fluid intake, play a crucial role in maintaining kidney function and may contribute to the prevention of recurrent urinary tract infections and stone formation. An integrative method that brings together these disparate modalities is required to optimize renal function and overall patient wellness, highlighting the necessity of interprofessional collaboration between healthcare providers for the evaluation and management of renal and urinary tract disorders (Gustafsson et al., 2018) (Figure 10.1).

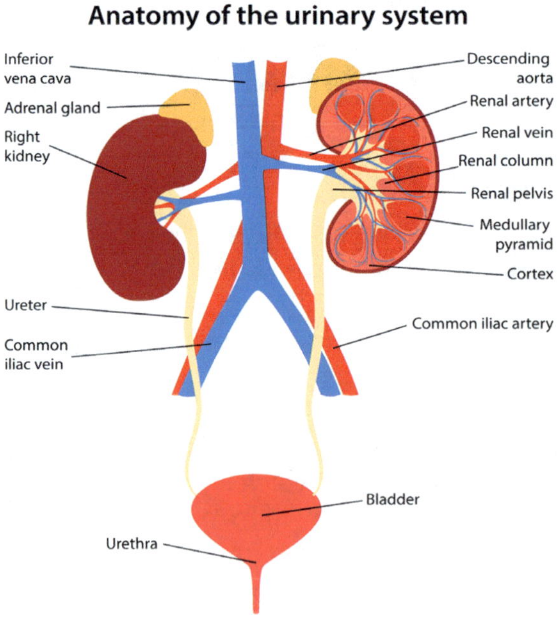

Figure 10.1. Diagram of the urinary system anatomy urinary tract.

Source: https://as1.ftcdn.net/v2/jpg/02/75/63/34/1000_F_275633487_rNMSRoJDTWTetipZmrwOYFn6EvDL37Wl.jpg.

Overview of Renal and Urinary Tract Functions

The renal and urinary tract systems play a very crucial role in maintaining homeostasis in the human body. The kidneys, which are the central organs in the renal system, purify blood to remove waste products, excess material, and toxins, which are expelled as urine. Each kidney contains approximately one million nephrons, which are functional units responsible for filtration, reabsorption, and secretion. The regulated processes of glomerular filtration and tubular reabsorption are necessary to maintain fluid, electrolyte, and acid-base balance. Essentially, such a complex interaction ensures that waste is efficiently removed and valuable substances, such as glucose and certain electrolytes, are conserved, highlighting the kidneys' critical function in maintaining overall metabolic equilibrium. The urinary tract, or the ureters, bladder, and urethra, is responsible for the storage and elimination of urine. The ureters transport urine from the kidneys to the bladder, where it is stored temporarily awaiting expulsion. The bladder wall being muscular permits it to distend with increasing content and relax upon emptying. Micturition involves voluntary and involuntary muscular regulation, emphasizing coordination of nervous and muscular mechanisms. The urinary tract also offers a pathway for the elimination of many hormones and metabolic end products. Preservation of the normal functioning of this system is essential for preventing urinary tract infections and other consequences of dysregulation, making a thorough assessment strategy imperative to practice. Renal and urinary function is multifaceted in its evaluation, encompassing both technology and clinical assessment. Serial laboratory investigations, including serum creatinine and blood urea nitrogen (BUN), provide an initial indication of the kidneys' function and efficacy in waste elimination. Imaging modalities, including ultrasound and CT scans, enable practitioners to visualize anatomical structures, thereby assisting in the location of obstructions or malformations. These tests are essential, as they guide interventions that are not only detection-related but also condition management for conditions such as chronic kidney disease and bladder dysfunction. The worth of evidence-based guidelines, such as those discussed in Cosentino et al. (2019) and Gustafsson et al. (2018), also stems from the need for healthcare practitioners to be current with renal and urinary tract practice, so that patients' outcomes are optimized (Figure 10.2).

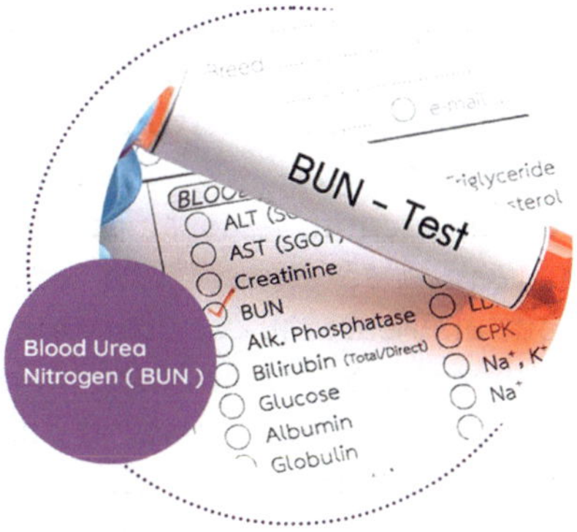

Figure 10.2. Blood urea nitrogen (BUN).

Source: https://mediscanlab.com/wp-content/uploads/2022/03/Blood-Urea-Nitrogen-BUN-770x641.png.

Importance of Assessment in Renal Health

Appropriate assessment of renal function is crucial in detecting kidney failure and its potential complications early. The kidneys are also tasked with homeostasis through the regulation of electrolyte balance, blood pressure, and the excretion of waste products. Regular follow-up of renal function through laboratory tests such as serum creatinine and glomerular filtration rate (GFR) allow clinicians to determine changes in kidney function. Early detection of renal injury can prevent irreversible damage and delay in appropriate intervention, with a resultant effect on better patient outcomes. This is particularly crucial in the context of the increased incidence of chronic kidney disease (CKD) due to diabetes and hypertension, which are prevalent among the population. Hence, periodic assessment is a basis upon ~~which~~ diagnosis, planning for treatment, and educating the patient; supplementing overall management of renal health as well as referring patients to experts at the right time (Chapple et al., 2010). Urinary tract function also requires proper evaluation, as urinary health bears a close relationship with renal function. Assessment of the urinary system can give critical information regarding underlying renal disease or systemic disease and hence allow interventions to be made appropriately in a timely fashion. Several, detecting abnormalities like hydronephrosis or urinary obstruction. Assessment of urinary symptoms can also detect not only acute infection but also chronic conditions amenable to surgical correction. Combining nephrology and urology assessments assists in delineating complex cases, and ultimately, the care of renal and urinary tract illnesses (Cody et al., 2012). Hence, the application of a multi-dimensional modality to renal assessment enhances the validity and efficacy of tailored treatment regimens. Secondly, patient education is crucial in renal health screening, as educated patients can participate more effectively in their own care. Educating patients about the importance of routine screening, symptoms of kidney failure, and lifestyle changes can empower them to become active participants in their own health. For instance, reading about the relationship between diet, fluid intake, and kidney function can motivate individuals to adopt kidney-friendly lifestyles. In addition, patient education on drug adherence, especially in diseases that adversely affect renal function, is crucial in preventing the progression of kidney disease. By developing a patient-participatory health environment where patients understand the importance of frequent monitoring, clinicians can facilitate earlier detection of complications, leading to improved adherence to management regimens and ultimately better renal health outcomes (Chapple et al., 2010).

10.1. Anatomy of the Renal System

Learning Outcome

1. Describe the structure of the kidneys
2. Focus on components of the urinary tract
3. Learn about the relationship between renal anatomy and function

Knowledge of the anatomy of the renal system lies at the heart of understanding its intricate function in the maintenance of fluid balance, electrolyte homeostasis, and waste elimination in the human body. The kidneys are at the hub of the system and are retroperitoneal organs located on either side of the vertebral column at levels T12 to L3. There are two kidneys, approximately the size of a human fist each, that are enclosed by adipose tissue, renal fascia, and a fibrous capsule to protect them against infection and trauma. The renal cortex, in which the nephron, the functional unit of the kidney, is found, is beneath the fibrous capsule, and the renal medulla, in which the renal pyramids, which are responsible for concentrating urine, are found. This organ design supports the effective filtration and treatment of blood, leading to the formation of urine, which is then pumped through the ureters into the bladder to be stored before excretion. Besides its structural components, the vascular supply to the renal system has a significant role to play in its operation. The kidneys receive a substantial amount of blood supply, consisting of approximately 20% of the cardiac output, from the renal arteries. These arteries branch directly from the abdominal aorta and, subsequently, branch into segmental and interlobar arteries within the kidney. The blood then flows into the afferent arterioles that branch off the glomeruli, where there is filtration. The blood then returns to the circulation via the efferent arterioles, which flow into peritubular capillaries and eventually the renal veins. This highly intricate vascular bed not only supports the metabolic demands of renal tissue but also enables the regulation of systemic blood pressure and fluid balance, underscoring the kidneys' pivotal role in homeostasis, as evidenced in clinical standards that outline renal function assessment techniques (Lerner et al., 2021). The urinary system comprises various anatomical parts that work together with the kidneys to facilitate the efficient removal of waste from the body.

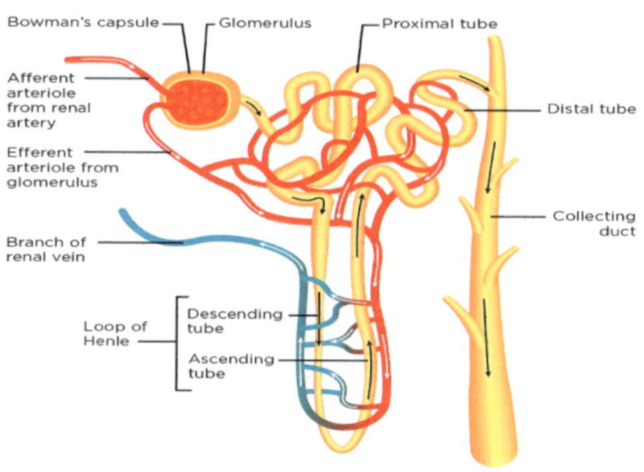

Figure 10.3. The anatomy and physiology of the kidneys.

Source: https://s3-eu-west-1.amazonaws.com/emap-moon-prod/wp-content/uploads/sites/3/2023/01/Fig-3.-Anatomy-of-a-nephron-1024x793.jpg.

Following the production of urine in the kidneys, it moves down through the muscular tubes known as the ureters via peristaltic contractions into the bladder, a temporary storage organ for urine until it is voluntarily excreted. The internal and external sphincter of the urethra plays a vital role in the regulation of urine outflow during voiding. Dysfunction or irregularity of any part of this apparatus may lead to significant clinical issues, for instance, retention of urine or incontinence, which should be evaluated and treated appropriately. Identifying these anatomical features enables health practitioners to develop personalized management plans for conditions affecting renal and urinary tract function, as supported by various evaluation methods outlined in clinical guidelines (Cosentino et al., 2019) (Figure 10.3).

10.1.1. Structure of the Kidneys

The structure of the kidneys is crucial to their function in maintaining fluid and electrolyte balance, excreting waste, and ensuring homeostasis. The kidney is approximately the size of a fist and is located on either side of the spinal column in the upper part of the back. The renal anatomy comprises several distinct regions: the cortex, medulla, and pelvis. The external layer is the cortex, which contains thousands of nephrons, the structural and functional units responsible for purifying the blood. In the medulla, renal pyramids facilitate urine concentration through a precisely organized pattern of tubules and collecting ducts. The renal pelvis is a funnel that directs urine into the ureters. Such structural conformity ensures kidneys efficiently perform their life-supportive roles, which emphasizes the importance of anatomical integrity in renal and urinary tract assessment and treatment. The nephrons, which represent the basic structural and functional units of the kidneys, serve a vital role in the filtration process. Every kidney has an average of one million nephrons, each with a renal corpuscle and a renal tubule. The renal corpuscle, constituted of Bowman's capsule and glomerulus, is the point at which blood filtration begins. The filtrate, which consists of waste products, electrolytes, and water, passes through the renal tubule, further classified as the proximal tubule, loop of Henle, and distal tubule. Each segment has specialized functions: the proximal tubule reabsorbs water and required nutrients, and the loop of Henle produces an osmotic gradient necessary for the concentration of the urine. The distal tubule, along with collecting ducts, regulates urine composition. The complex structure of the nephron is at the heart of kidney function, underscoring its value in diagnostic and intervention planning for urinary tract diseases. An understanding of kidney structure is particularly important in assessing kidney function and detecting potential pathologies. Alteration of kidney architecture, secondary to chronic disease or trauma, can exert a profound influence on urinary tract function. For instance, damage to renal tubules can disrupt sodium and water reabsorption, leading to the sequelae of electrolyte imbalance and fluid overload. Structural alterations in the kidney can also predispose systemic complications, such as hypertension and cardiovascular risk. As global temperatures rise, heat stress also affects the health of the kidneys by causing acute damage or chronic disease, complicating renal function (Butler-Dawson et al., 2019). Knowing the structure of the kidneys helps clinicians develop focused interventions to offer patients proportionate care to maintain renal health despite intra- and extrinsic stressors (Figure 10.4).

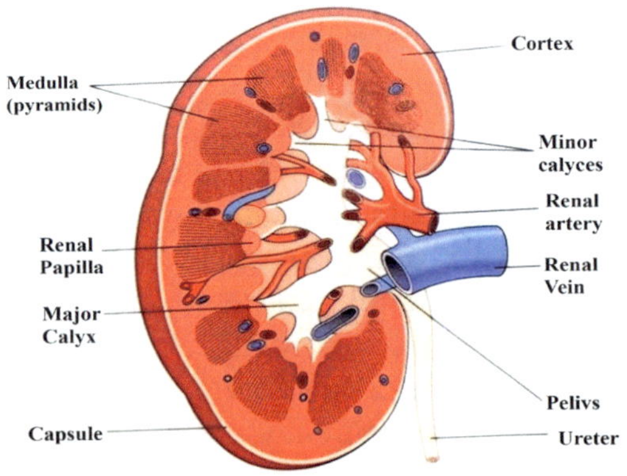

Figure 10.4. Structure of the kidneys.

Source: https://external-content.duckduckgo.com/iu/?u=https%3A%2F%2Fwww.studyread.com%2Fwp-content%2Fuploads%2F2019%2F09%2Fkidney_structure.jpg&f=1&nofb=1&ipt=0363ad53b14719bb1ae89a80c514605944b1d2c2075f2171f2e78c65c5672f6d.

10.1.2. Components of the Urinary Tract

The urinary system is a sophisticated network that is an integral part of the body's capacity to filter, store, and discharge waste products from the blood. It is composed of the kidneys, ureters, bladder, and urethra, each with its own characteristic structures and functions. The kidneys, located in the retroperitoneal space, carry out filtration and excretion; they filter out waste but conserve essential components, thereby preserving fluid and electrolyte balance. The ureters convey urine from each kidney to the urinary bladder, a muscular reservoir for storing urine until a socially convenient time for excretion. In this system, the urethra is the last passage for urine to leave the body, featuring specific mechanisms that control voiding under both voluntary and involuntary control. The functioning of the urinary tract is crucial for maintaining homeostasis. Specifically, the kidneys play a vital role in controlling blood pressure through the renin-angiotensin-aldosterone system and in red blood cell production by releasing erythropoietin in response to low oxygen levels. In addition to these control mechanisms, the urinary tract and kidneys maintain acid-base balance by excreting hydrogen ions and reabsorbing bicarbonate in proportion. Dysfunction in any component of the urinary tract can cause serious health problems, such as urinary tract infections (UTIs), which are particularly common and can lead to renal damage if left untreated. The possible implications of impaired urinary tract function make timely evaluation and proper intervention measures quite crucial. Evidence regarding the impact of urinary tract dysfunction suggests that such disorders do not have an age or gender bias. To add, children with chronic kidney disease (CKD) are most susceptible to urinary tract complications, with research indicating a high rate of lower urinary tract (LUT) dysfunction among this population (Öborn et al., 2014). Diagnosing LUT dysfunction involves an intensive evaluation process that may include bladder diaries, uroflowmetry, and several questionnaires used to assess quality of life and related symptoms. It is essential to recognize and manage these complications to the immediate health of the victims, but also to their long-term quality of life, as evidenced by research showing reduced well-being among those who experience incontinence or recurrent UTIs (Öborn et al., 2014). The incorporation of such assessment tools into practice can enhance care and intervention approaches for individuals struggling with urinary tract dysfunction (Figure 10.5).

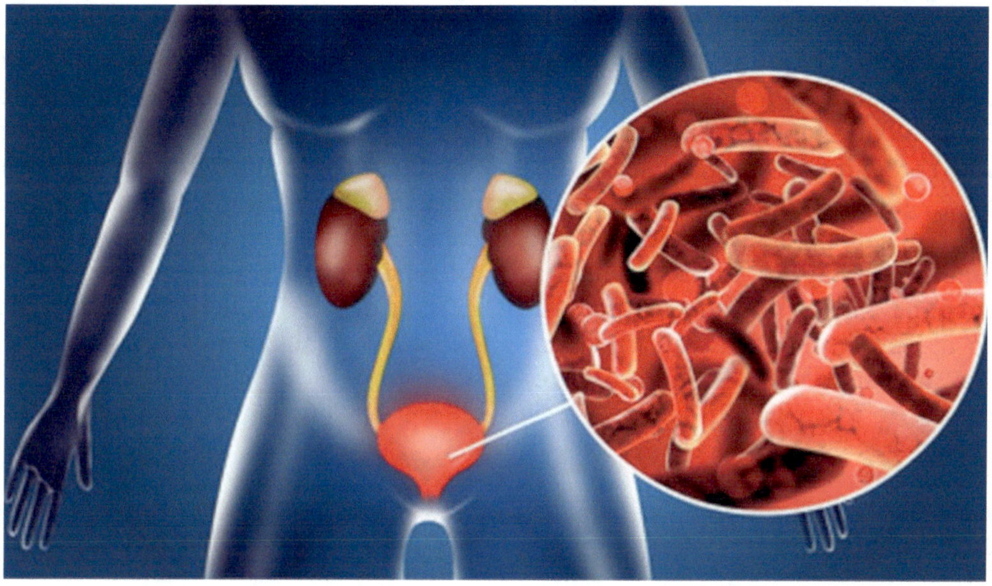

Figure 10.5. Urinary tract infections.

Source: https://urologyclinics.com/wp-content/uploads/2023/06/Image-depicting-how-Urinary-Tract-Infections-look-within-the-body-and-where-theyre-located-1024x613.jpg.

10.1.3. Relationship Between Renal Anatomy and Function

The subtle interrelation between the renal structure and function is one of the most critical keys to homeostasis in humans. The kidneys, with their sophisticated structures such as nephrons, play a crucial role in urine formation and the regulation of various body functions. Each nephron contains a glomerulus and a renal tubule, which together enable blood filtration, reabsorption of essential substances, and secretion of waste products. This renal arrangement allows the kidneys to filter 150-180 liters of blood daily, producing approximately 1-2 liters of urine. Variability in renal anatomy, such as nephron count and integrity, can significantly impact renal function, demonstrating the body's ability to manage electrolytes, modulate blood pressure, and filter toxins. Thus, knowledge of renal anatomy is necessary to assess kidney function and diagnose potential complications resulting from anatomical variations. Additionally, renal anatomy has a direct impact on certain renal functions that are crucial for maintaining urinary tract health. The distribution of specialized roles within renal anatomy enhances overall kidney performance; for instance, the loop of Henle plays a crucial role in urine concentration, while the proximal convoluted tubule is essential for nutrient reabsorption. Furthermore, the glycogen storage diseases (GSDs) provide a prototype of how structural and functional abnormalities can lead to renal complications. In these situations, patients suffer from renal impairment—hyperfiltration or proximal renal tubular acidosis—secondary to a metabolic derangement affecting renal structure. As observed in recent studies, timely and thorough evaluations of the renal anatomy are critical to the explanation of such dysfunctions to facilitate interventions at the right times and improve patient outcomes (Reyes-Apodaca et al., 2025). Evaluating both renal function and structure through an integrative model can enhance diagnostic value and treatment outcomes within a clinical environment. Lastly, the advancement of imaging modalities, such as renal ultrasound, has significantly improved the ability to assess the relationship between renal function and anatomy. The noninvasive technique provides superb information about kidney size, shape, and vascular flow and aids in the thorough assessment of renal health. For instance, ultrasound can reveal anatomical abnormalities that are correlated with biochemical markers of kidney function, such as serum creatinine and glomerular filtration rate. Studies comparing otherwise healthy patients have shown that incidental findings on renal ultrasounds can influence clinical decisions and prompt additional testing (Yakubu et al., 2024). These diagnostic functions highlight the importance of integrating anatomic assessment with functional analysis in renal health evaluation. Ultimately, an understanding of renal anatomy and its functional implications is crucial for the development of interventions aimed at maintaining renal and urinary tract integrity.

Test Your Knowledge

1. What are the main functions of the kidneys in the renal system?
2. How do the ureters, bladder, and urethra work together in urine excretion?

10.2. Physiology of Renal Function

Learning Outcome

1. Explain the filtration processes in the kidneys
2. Define the role of nephron in urine formation
3. Discuss the regulation of electrolytes and fluid balance

The physiology of renal function must maintain homeostasis within the body. The kidneys play a crucial role in regulating fluid balance, electrolyte composition, and waste removal. This intricate process begins with glomerular filtration, where blood filters through the glomeruli, allowing water and solutes to pass through while leaving behind larger molecules, such as proteins. Upon filtration, reabsorption and secretion are performed by the renal tubules, which are processes that fine-tune the urinary composition and maintain the body's internal environment. These functions are better understood through research on the effects of long-term conditions, such as diabetes and hypertension, on renal physiology, which can trigger a sequence of functional impairments unless well controlled in clinics (Davies et al., 2018). Besides, the kidneys not only function in filtration but also play an essential role in maintaining systemic blood pressure through the renin-angiotensin-aldosterone system (RAAS). This system operates in response to changes in blood circulation, sodium concentration, and overall fluid status within the body. When blood pressure is reduced or, in the case of decreased sodium, the kidneys release renin, which leads to the formation of angiotensin II, a potent vasoconstrictor that increases systemic vascular resistance and blood volume. This intricate feedback mechanism illustrates the kidneys' role in cardiovascular health and describes how renal function can affect more universal systemic states. Alterations in this system can significantly impact outcomes in patients with cardiovascular disease and chronic kidney disease, necessitating constant monitoring and targeted interventions to decrease risk factors (Liguori et al., 2018).

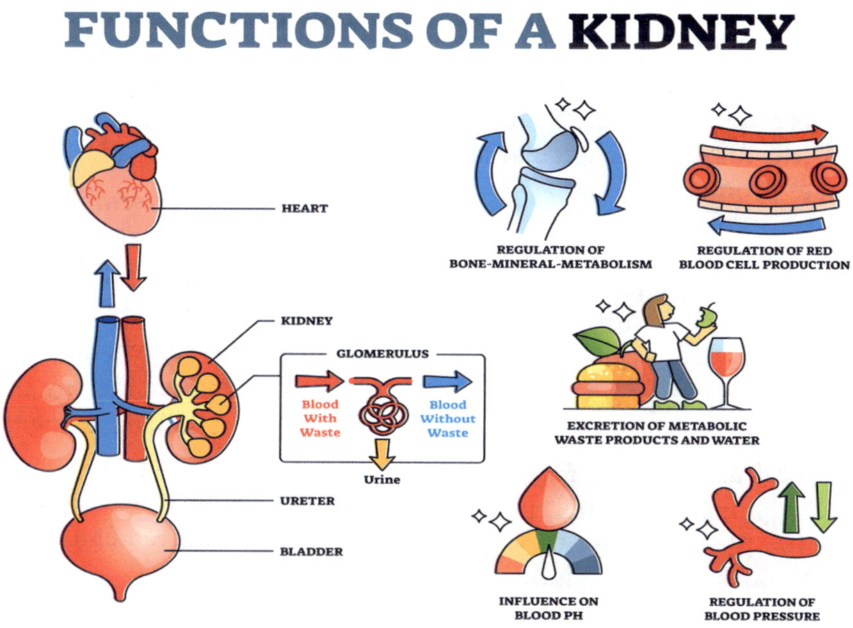

Figure 10.6. Physiology of renal function.

Source: https://i.pinimg.com/originals/b7/68/b6/b768b60de7cf59cb7e7de5d15dcff170.jpg.

In addition to these regulatory functions, the kidneys also play a central role in metabolic processes, including hormone production such as erythropoietin and calcitriol. Erythropoietin stimulates red blood cell production during hypoxia, and calcitriol, the active form of vitamin D, is essential for maintaining calcium homeostasis and promoting bone health. These mechanisms demonstrate the interconnection between renal physiology and overall metabolic requirements, showing that renal insufficiency can lead to complications such as anemia and bone mineral imbalance. The assessment of renal function, therefore, transcends clinical measures such as glomerular filtration rate (GFR) to include a comprehensive image of patient well-being. Understanding these physiological factors plays a crucial role in designing effective management plans and interventions for patients with renal and urinary tract diseases (Davies et al., 2018) (Figure 10.6).

10.2.1. Filtration Processes in the Kidneys

The kidneys play a crucial role in the mechanism of homeostasis through their complex filtration mechanisms. The primary role of the kidneys is to filter blood for the removal of waste products, excess substances, and toxins, ultimately resulting in the formation of urine. The nephrons, located in the renal cortex, are the primary working units of the kidneys, comprising glomeruli and renal tubules. The initial filtration occurs at the glomerulus, where blood pressure forces plasma, solutes, and water through the glomerular membrane. Selective permeability permits required contents such as proteins and blood cells to remain in circulation, but eliminates waste products.

The efficiency of such filtration is regulated by numerous determinants, including renal blood flow, glomerular filtration rate, and systemic blood pressure, and therefore, the kidneys become a target for interventions in the regulation of renal and urinary tract function during clinical assessment. Following initial filtration in the glomerulus, renal tubules subsequently treat the filtrate further through reabsorption and secretion mechanisms. When the filtrate flows through the proximal convoluted tubule, essential nutrients such as glucose, amino acids, and electrolytes are reclaimed from the filtrate and pumped back into the blood. This is important for sustaining the body's basic components as well as maintaining fluid homeostasis. Distal portions of the nephron contribute to controlling the composition of urine by excreting excess ions and drugs, thus perfecting the body's electrolyte and acid-base state. The interplay among filtration, reabsorption, and secretion demonstrates the kidney's ability to modify urinary output in response to the body's shifting physiological needs. Understanding these processes is crucial for clinicians during the assessment of kidney function and for developing appropriate interventions to offset renal impairment. Lastly, an understanding of the filtration activities in the kidneys is crucial for effective assessment and intervention in renal and urinary tract function. Clinical examinations typically utilize parameters such as glomerular filtration rate (GFR) and urine output to assess kidney function. The change in these parameters can represent underlying pathologies, which would necessitate directed therapeutic measures. For instance, with the worsening of GFR due to pathophysiological conditions such as hypertension or diabetes mellitus, adjustments in drug therapy or diet might be required to mitigate the load on renal function. Additionally, medical standards emphasize the importance of individualized treatment for patients in determining intervention measures, particularly within the framework of established clinical evidence and research. Health professionals must be cautious in considering the complex nature of kidney function, ensuring their interventions align with optimal practices documented in the literature, as demonstrated by Cosentino et al. (2019) and Visseren et al. (2021) (Figure 10.7).

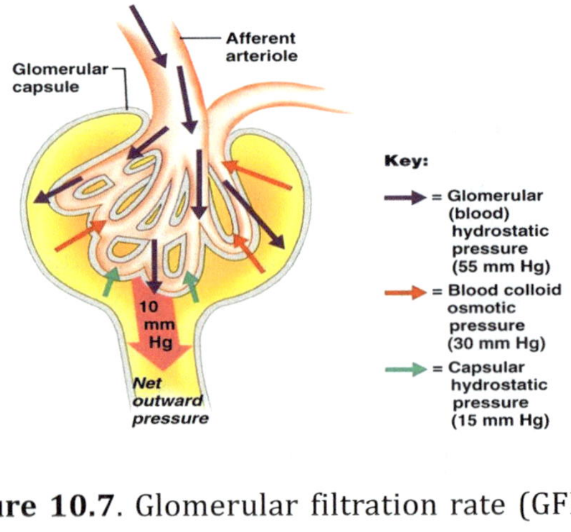

Figure 10.7. Glomerular filtration rate (GFR).

Source: https://image3.slideserve.com/6542370/glomerular-filtration-rate-gfr2-l.jpg.

10.2.2. Role of Nephron in Urine Formation

The functional unit of the kidney, the nephron, plays a crucial role in urine formation through three primary processes: filtration, reabsorption, and secretion. Located in the renal cortex and medulla, each nephron is made up of a glomerulus, proximal tubule, loop of Henle, distal tubule, and collecting duct. The formation of urine begins with glomerular filtration, in which blood plasma is filtered from the glomerular capillaries into Bowman's capsule. This process of filtration lets water, ions, and small molecules pass selectively while retaining large proteins and blood cells. This initial filtration plays an essential role in renal function assessment as it reflects the effectiveness with which the kidneys remove waste products and excess material from the bloodstream.

From an appreciation of nephrons' filter capacity, clinicians can deduce potential renal dysfunction or the presence of conditions such as congenital anomalies. Following filtration, the nephron undergoes reabsorption, a crucial process in which essential substances are recovered from the filtrate and returned to the blood. Approximately 65% of the filtrate volume is reabsorbed within the proximal tubule, which efficiently restores valuable nutrients, including glucose, amino acids, and considerable amounts of sodium and water. Additional reabsorption occurs as the filtrate passes into the loop of Henle, which emphasizes the nephrons' ability to concentrate the urine. The function of the countercurrent multiplier plays a critical role here, as it enables the potential to create more concentrated urine than blood. Through the nephron, hormonal control, underpinned by antidiuretic hormone (ADH) and aldosterone, regulates reabsorption rates to maintain homeostasis. Compromise during this process can lead to clinical problems, such as dehydration or electrolyte disturbances, and highlights the crucial role of nephrons in renal and overall health. Besides reabsorption and filtration, secretion is the third prominent function of the nephrons in the generation of urine. Secretion involves active secretion of waste products, excess ions, and other substances from the blood into the renal tubule.

Potassium, hydrogen ions, and certain metabolic end products, such as urea, are among the substances secreted ~~actively~~ into the tubular fluid. This role is particularly significant for regulating acid-base balance and detoxifying the blood. The capacity of the nephrons to adjust their secretion of single ions based on the body's needs is at the heart of homeostasis, especially in reacting to shifting physiological circumstances. Clinically, awareness of the secretory role of the nephrons can highlight potential dysfunctions that are indicators of more severe renal states, such as chronic kidney disease, which could compromise the kidneys' ability to regulate these processes effectively. Through a thoughtful assessment of nephron function, health professionals can implement suitable interventions to improve renal health and function (Figure 10.8).

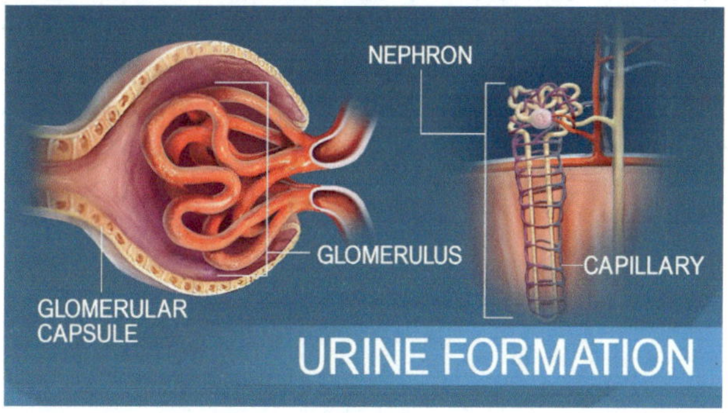

Figure 10.8. Urine formation.

Source: https://www.visiblebody.com/hubfs/1C_Urine_Formation.jpg.

10.2.3. Regulation of Electrolytes and Fluid Balance

Electrolyte balance and fluid control are fundamental renal functions required for homeostasis and efficient physiological functions. The nephron, the functional unit of the kidney, plays a pivotal role in controlling these processes, particularly in the reabsorption and excretion of sodium (Na+) and water. Dysfunctions in the nephrons' ability to control electrolyte levels could lead to significant health problems, including hypertension. Research has shown that excessive salt consumption in the diet is strongly linked to alterations in sodium homeostasis, affecting blood pressure regulation and cardiovascular health. Importantly, the thick ascending limb of the loop of Henle has been identified as a significant site of sodium reabsorption, emphasizing the central role played by this nephron segment in the pathogenesis of salt-sensitive hypertension, particularly when the processes of sodium reabsorption become dysregulated (Dominiczak et al., 2017). Moreover, the consequences of electrolyte imbalance are deeply entangled with renal development determinants. The evidence suggests that maternal diet, particularly increased salt intake during pregnancy, is capable of predisposing later life kidney and cardiovascular disease. For instance, rat model research has shown that maternal exposure to high salt levels can alter fetal kidney development to disrupt sodium handling and cause subsequent life hypertension (da Silva et al., 2013). Such findings highlight the multifaceted interaction between dietary habits, nephron function, and susceptibility to long-term adverse health effects, as well as the necessity for prudent control of salt intake during developmental stages of vulnerability. Therefore, it is essential to understand the mechanisms of regulation of electrolytes and fluid balance to design effective therapeutic measures for the prevention of hypertension and related disorders. In managing electrolyte and fluid balance, physicians need to consider both assessment and intervention plans that target the nephron's reabsorptive capabilities. Routine monitoring of electrolytes, fluids, and kidney function studies is an integral part of patient assessment, particularly for patients at risk of developing electrolyte disturbances. Therapeutic measures may involve diet, drugs, or lifestyle modifications aimed at maximizing the excretion of sodium and ensuring fluid balance. Diuretics, for example, are commonly employed to provide the maximum excretion of sodium and water, particularly in hypertensive patients. In addition, education on the effect of excessive salt intake and promotion of dietary sodium monitoring behavior can empower patients to neutralize the risks of electrolyte disturbances. As our understanding of renal physiology and its relationship to sodium balance expands, it becomes increasingly possible to implement interventions tailored to individuals' differing needs, promoting success in renal and cardiovascular wellness.

Test Your Knowledge

1. How do the kidneys help regulate blood pressure?
2. What role do nephrons play in the filtration of blood?

10.3. Common Renal and Urinary Tract Disorders

Learning Outcome

1. Explain the chronic kidney disease (CKD)
2. Define the urinary tract infections (UTIs)
3. Describe the kidney stones and their implications

Chronic kidney disease, or CKD, is the most prevalent renal function disorder, with a progressive loss of kidney function over months or years. It is most often secondary to concurrent disease such as diabetes and hypertension, which lead to insidious damage to the nephrons, the functional units of the kidney. Early diagnosis and treatment are critical, as CKD may advance to end-stage renal disease requiring dialysis or transplantation for survival. Renal function ~~is most commonly~~ can be estimated by the testing of glomerular filtration rate (GFR), with urinalysis for the detection of proteinuria, hematuria, and other abnormalities to indicate kidney dysfunction. Systemic monitoring and intervention strategies, such as lifestyle modifications and pharmacological treatment, are essential to retard the progression of the disease and prevent complications associated with CKD, including cardiovascular conditions that frequently occur in conjunction with renal insufficiency (Ginsberg et al., 2021). Urinary tract infections (UTIs) are a common disorder associated with renal and urinary tract disease. These infections can occur in any component of the urinary system, including the ureters, kidneys, bladder, and urethra, with the bladder being the most frequently affected. The clinical presentation ranges from dysuria to urgency to systemic signs such as fever and malaise, particularly with pyelonephritis. Urinary tract infection treatment is typically achieved with antibiotics. Still, their–they should be used cautiously ~~of~~ with the increasing concerns about resistance to these drugs. In recurring UTI subjects or patients with intrinsic neurogenic lower urinary tract dysfunction, evaluation of risk factors and symptoms is necessary (Visseren et al., 2021). Treatment can be extended to include behavioral modification, education, and, in severe cases, surgery to prevent recurrence and structural pathology of the urinary tract. Benign prostatic hyperplasia (BPH) is a highly significant condition in renal and urinary health among men, particularly in aging men. BPH leads to enlargement of the prostate gland, which causes urinary symptoms of increased frequency, urgency, and nocturia that may severely compromise quality of life. The pathophysiology of BPH is primarily due to hormonal changes, most notably the action of dihydrotestosterone on prostatic tissue. Diagnosis typically consists of a comprehensive history and physical examination, as well as measures such as the International Prostate Symptom Score (IPSS) to quantify the severity of the symptoms. Therapy can range from watchful waiting for minimal symptoms to pharmacotherapy in the form of alpha-blockers and 5-alpha reductase inhibitors. Surgical approaches are reserved for patients with severe obstruction or bladder retention problems. Individualized treatment plans are necessary to enhance patients' outcomes and alleviate the pain associated with BPH (Ginsberg et al., 2021) (Figure 10.9).

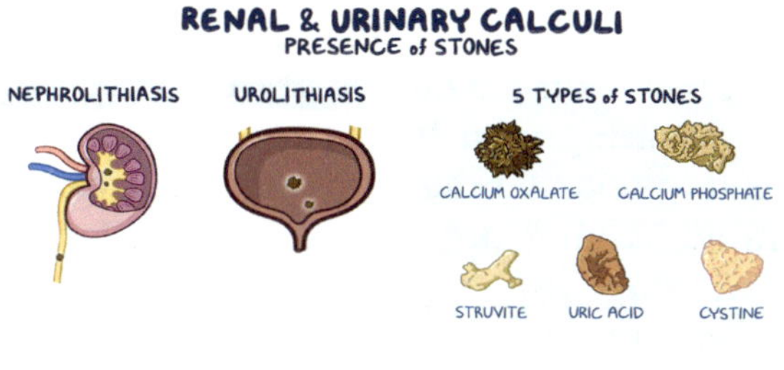

Figure 10.9. Renal and urinary calculi.

Source: https://d16qt3wv6xm098.cloudfront.net/5318zK8gR2moXHwGtiS-NgNcQ-_K5SrV/_.jpg.

10.3.1. Chronic Kidney Disease (CKD)

Chronic kidney disease (CKD) is a significant public health problem, primarily due to its increasing incidence and morbidity. CKD is a persistent loss of renal function over time until it advances to end-stage renal disease (ESRD) if left untreated. CKD is a pathophysiologic process resulting from numerous risk factors, including diabetes, hypertension, and glomerulonephritis, that significantly contribute to renal injury. As kidney function declines, patients are likely to experience a cascade of complications including anemia, mineral bone disease, and cardiovascular disease. These sequelae also highlight the importance of early diagnosis and intervention in CKD and the ability to alter disease course and patient outcomes fundamentally. Understanding the intricate, multifaceted nature of CKD is important to enable healthcare clinicians to develop assessment and intervention optimally approaches to address individual patient needs. Assessment of CKD is a comprehensive evaluation of renal function, typically initiated by the application of routine laboratory tests such as serum creatinine and urine protein. The glomerular filtration rate (GFR) is a critical index of renal dysfunction, helping to guide clinical judgment and therapeutic options. Estimation of renal damage is also performed by following up on relevant biomarkers and imaging studies to establish potential etiologies and complications of the disease. CKD is staged based on the degree of GFR, with stage 1 representing mild impairment and stage 5 indicating anuria requiring renal replacement therapy. Staging not only aids clinicians in establishing the appropriate intervention but also allows for easier communication to patients regarding prognosis and management approach, ultimately contributing to reducing the impact of CKD on the healthcare system. CKD management interventions are designed to retard the progression of the disease and reduce complications. Lifestyle adjustments, including dietary restrictions, physical exercise, and smoking cessation, are the cornerstones of CKD management. Pharmacologic therapies, such as antihypertensives, diuretics, and glycemic agents, also serve a central role in treating co-morbid illnesses frequently linked with CKD, namely diabetes and hypertension. Close observation and early therapy adjustment are necessary to optimize patient outcomes. Furthermore, therapies such as dialysis and renal transplant might be required in patients who progress to ESRD. The best practices of CKD care are based on multidisciplinary care, ensuring that patients receive proper treatment tailored to their personalized needs, and promoting drug compliance and overall quality of life (Assimos et al., 2016; Bischoff et al., 2014) (Figure 10.10).

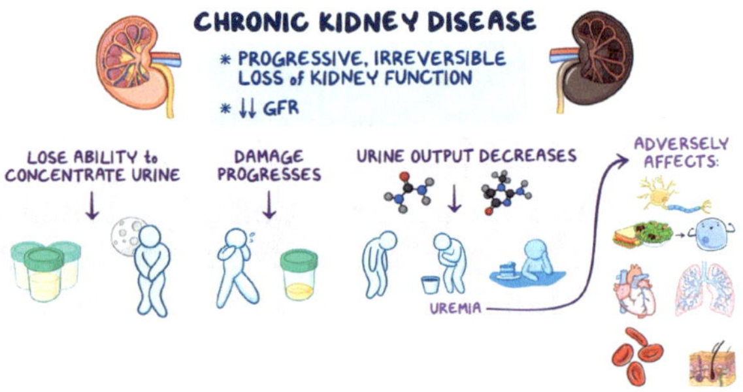

Figure 10.10. Chronic kidney disease (CKD).

Source: https://osmose-it.s3.amazonaws.com/aXSj3_JeTKOrsmgxbZsX33mhRiaWuImy/_.jpg.

10.3.2. Urinary Tract Infections (UTIs)

The prevalence of urinary tract infections (UTIs) is a significant clinical problem, particularly in the pathophysiology of renal and urinary tract function. UTIs are caused by bacterial invasion of the urinary tract, which can lead from mild discomfort to life-threatening complications. UTIs are most frequently seen in women due to anatomic and hormonal differences that put them at risk for infection. Recurrent UTIs may also be caused by etiologies such as inadequate bladder emptying or structural abnormalities that mandate a complete evaluation by physicians. A complete evaluation, including a history and urinalysis, according to guidelines, is crucial for determining the etiology of the UTI and instituting proper interventions that minimize long-term sequelae. Effective management and diagnosis not only treat immediate symptoms but also reduce incidence rates through concentrated prevention strategies (Ginsberg et al., 2021). Understanding the correlation between UTIs and conditions is vital in making an effective treatment plan. In neurogenic lower urinary tract dysfunction (NLUTD) patients, the onset of recurrent UTIs is much more probable. Such a patient is likely to develop bladder dysfunction that prevents significant urine flow, making it easier for bacteria to thrive. Determining the connection between NLUTD and UTIs gives the practitioner insight into probable complications for risk stratification and management protocols. Therapy should thus incorporate not only the use of antibiotics but also those measures that enhance bladder function to prevent recurrence of infections. In individuals with recurrent episodes of UTIs despite adequate management, additional tests such as imaging can be performed to rule out anatomical causes (Visseren et al., 2021). An overall approach that includes assessing urinary function is thus imperative for successful treatment. Preventive strategies are significant in preventing the incidence of UTIs and must be made according to each patient's unique circumstances. Education regarding proper personal hygiene, hydration, and post-coital voiding can significantly reduce the incidence of UTIs, particularly in high-risk groups. In patients with NLUTD, utilization of clean intermittent catheterization techniques will reduce the likelihood of bacteriuria and subsequent infection. Healthcare practitioners must also be mindful of asymptomatic bacteriuria in this population; treatment is not routinely indicated and can lead to adverse antibiotic resistance (Ginsberg et al., 2021). Therefore, the implementation of evidence-based guidelines and patient education is crucial to successful UTI management, ensuring clinical practice aligns with the latest research and guidelines. Such practices not only help resolve acute health complications but also lead to improved urinary tract health in the future (Figure 10.11).

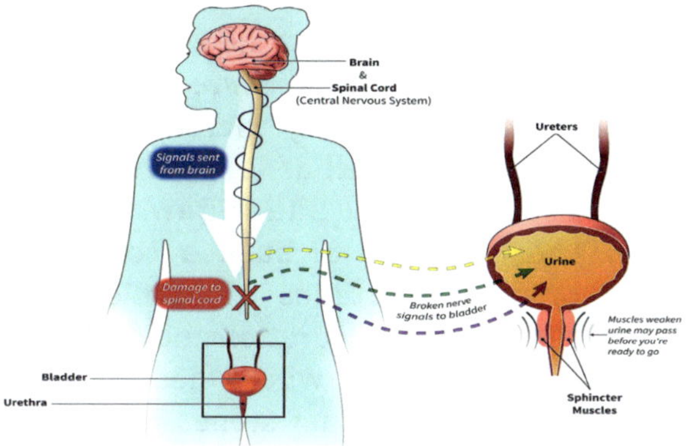

Figure 10.11. Neurogenic lower urinary tract dysfunction (NLUTD).

Source: https://surgery.wustl.edu/app/uploads/2022/04/Neurogenic-Bladder_News-Page-01-1024x677.jpg.

10.3.3. Kidney Stones and Their Implications

Kidney stones, also known as renal calculi, are solid deposits of minerals and salts that form within the kidneys. Their formation is a multifactorial process that typically begins with an imbalance of urine contents. Dehydration, diet, and genetic factors are some of the causes that can significantly raise chances of developing such calculi. The implication of kidney stones extends beyond the immediate physical pain that they cause; they may lead to obstructive uropathy, infection, and chronic kidney disease in the case of neglect. Furthermore, their chronic nature may be associated with significant healthcare costs and a lowered quality of life for patients, making the importance of early diagnosis and effective management practices evident (Anson et al., 2014). The effect of kidney stones is particularly severe in populations that have to deal with extreme environmental conditions. With the rising global temperature, the incidence of heatwaves increases dehydration at a rapid rate, a proven causative factor for kidney stones. Under such environmental stress, the kidneys may lose their ability to maintain fluid and electrolyte balance, thereby further complicating urinary tract health. Research indicates that frequent exposure to heat and inadequate hydration may increase the risk of kidney stones, as well as long-term chronic kidney disease (CKD) (Butler-Dawson et al., 2019). The existence of such a connection highlights the importance of public health campaigns focused on hydration and education, particularly in regions where heat stress is prevalent. Moreover, kidney stones also require treatment as well as preventative strategies, both of which necessitate a multidisciplinary approach. Patients are typically advised to alter their dietary patterns, increase fluid intake, and adopt lifestyle changes that can help reduce the recurrence of stones. These aside, complicated stones or large stones may require more sophisticated medical procedures, such as lithotripsy and surgery. Continuous research and intervention are necessary, particularly because the changing climate presents new challenges. The interaction between kidney stones and environmental factors underscores the need for an interdisciplinary approach, combining urology, nephrology, and public health in developing effective prevention and treatment strategies (Anson et al., 2014).

Test Your Knowledge

1. What are common symptoms of a urinary tract infection (UTI)?
2. How does chronic kidney disease (CKD) affect overall body function?

10.4. Assessment Techniques for Renal Function

Learning Outcome

1. Identify the laboratory tests in assessing renal and urinary tract function
2. Define the imaging studies- ultrasound and CT scans
3. Describe the urinalysis and its significance

Renal function measurement is crucial in the diagnosis and management of renal and urinary tract diseases. Techniques applied in renal function measurement are serum creatinine measurements, urinalysis, and imaging studies. Serum creatinine is a widely used biomarker for assessing kidney function by determining creatinine clearance from the blood. An increase in serum creatinine is ~~typically most frequently~~ a sign of impaired renal function and can be employed to identify abnormalities such as acute kidney injury or chronic kidney disease. Further, urinalysis and urine analysis also provide valuable information regarding the presence of protein, blood, or glucose, which may indicate underlying renal pathology. By integrating these methods, clinicians can generate a better comprehensive picture of a patient's renal disease and establish prompt intervention and treatment. Imaging modalities, including ultrasound and CT scans, serve an ancillary function in renal function testing. These provide visualization of the urinary tract and can identify structural defects, obstructions, or lesions that result in reduced kidney function. For instance, hydronephrosis can be identified through the use of an ultrasound, whereas a CT scan can detect tumors or stones that block the urinary tract. Additionally, Doppler ultrasound can measure renal blood flow, which reflects the state of the vascular system in relation to kidney function. It is essential to understand the interaction of these measurement methods, as imaging procedures often influence clinical decisions, such as whether to operate or order additional diagnostic tests, like renal biopsies. Consequently, a comprehensive approach leads to a more thorough understanding of renal pathology.

Beyond conventional assessments, newer techniques such as antenatal intervention for congenital urinary tract malformations have evolved, reflecting the importance of prophylactic evaluation. For instance, studies on fetal intervention in congenital lower urinary tract obstruction (LUTO) have reported promising results in improving perinatal survival and postnatal renal function. By procedures such as the employment of vesico-amniotic shunts, clinicians can make early intervention to avoid potential in utero renal injury, eventually leading to better outcomes following the birth of the newborn. These advancements point to the progression of renal function testing, where early intervention and detection can significantly alter clinical outcomes. As research in these disciplines continues, combining new methods into routine assessment protocols will lead to the development of improved management techniques in renal and urinary tract wellness, ultimately resulting in enhanced patient care (Cody et al., 2012; Arduino et al., 2020).

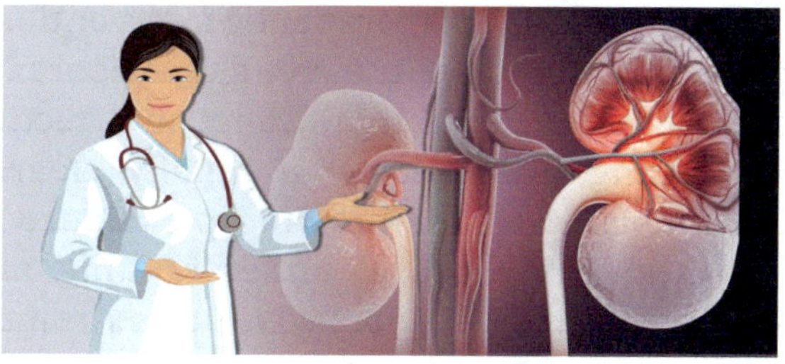

Figure 10.12. Assessment techniques for renal function.

Source: https://study.com/cimages/videopreview/qt7d82ihm0.jpg.

10.4.1. Laboratory Tests (e.g., Blood Urea Nitrogen, Creatinine)

Renal and urinary function is assessed through laboratory testing by the measurement of some biomarkers such as blood urea nitrogen (BUN) and creatinine. BUN is a body marker of the body's nitrogen status and a product of protein breakdown. Elevated BUN is suggestive of compromised renal function, dehydration, or excessive protein intake and thus needs assessment to ascertain the etiology of the dysfunction. Creatinine, a metabolite of muscle metabolism, is utilized as a more accurate measure of renal function. Creatinine remains quite stable and is not much affected by diet and is therefore helpful in diagnosing and treating chronic kidney disease. Both of these tests are included in a full metabolic panel, and both provide crucial information on kidney function and potential dysfunction. Beyond BUN and creatinine, the value of the creatinine clearance test cannot be exaggerated. It is utilized to estimate the glomerular filtration rate (GFR) which measures the kidneys' capacity for filtering. Through 24-hour urine collection and measurement of serum creatinine, clinicians can assess the kidneys' ability to clear creatinine, thereby determining the extent of renal impairment. Profound GFR measurement is important in making the diagnosis of chronic kidney disease and directing optimal therapeutic interventions. Moreover, the result of the creatinine clearance test may be of crucial significance in directing drug dosing, particularly of renally cleared medications. With the growing prevalence of chronic kidney disease, understanding and use of these laboratory tests will be extremely important in optimizing patient outcomes and care in the renal health sector. Laboratory tests, such as BUN and creatinine levels, can be helpful in evaluating renal function. However, it is also essential to understand that demographic factors, including a patient's race and ethnicity, can influence these results. Clinical measurements based on ~~these~~ parameters that do not reflect race or ethnicity can lead to inconsistency in diagnosis and treatment regimens. Healthcare providers should thus report these tests with care, drawing on an educated understanding of the patient's history and context, and employing multilevel approaches to care. Myoken et al. Professionals must remain informed about the significance of laboratory results, particularly as advancements in kidney assessment methods continue to evolve, necessitating balanced and informed patient assessment procedures (Crabb et al., 2019; Vyas et al., 2020).

10.4.2. Imaging Studies (e.g., Ultrasound, CT Scans)

Imaging studies play a crucial role in evaluating renal and urinary tract function, providing detailed information that enables accurate diagnosis and treatment regimens. Ultrasound is commonly employed as the first imaging study due to its non-invasive nature and ability to provide real-time visualization of renal anatomy. It is particularly useful in detecting renal masses, hydronephrosis, and urinary tract obstructions. Furthermore, ultrasound may guide procedural interventions, such as the drainage of obstructed urine collections. Computed tomography (CT) scans provide a comprehensive overview of the urinary tract, enabling the identification of calculi and the characterization of complex lesions. It has emphasized the importance of such imaging modalities in the case of diseases such as nephrolithiasis, in which early detection and precise localization of stones can directly influence the success of treatment (Bove et al., 2013). CT scans, in fact, provide more detail compared to ultrasonography, enabling clinicians to see not only the kidneys but also surrounding tissues, which facilitates differential diagnosis of diseases such as nephrolithiasis. In urolithiasis, CT scanning is a cornerstone for measuring renal stone size, position, and type, which directly influences treatment, ranging from medical expulsive therapy to surgery. Recent refinements of CT technology, including lower doses of radiation exposure and improved three-dimensional reconstruction, have further solidified its role in the routine assessment of renal pathology. Additionally, multi-phase CT imaging can identify changes in renal perfusion and function, offering insight into renal ischemia or injury that may not be well appreciated on other modalities (Bove et al., 2013).

Thus, incorporating practice with CT imaging has the potential to enhance individualized interventions based on patient needs. In addition, the evolution of imaging modalities has led to the emergence of new procedures, such as laser ablation, for treating conditions like ureteroceles, particularly in veterinary medicine.

Laser ablation under cystoscopic and fluoroscopic guidance has been an effective modality for the relief of obstruction by ureteroceles, as evidenced by studies that have revealed significant improvement in urinary dynamics and decreased postoperative complications. The ability to precisely target obstructive sites with minimal tissue injury to the surrounding tissues is a substantial advancement in interventional methods. Imaging follow-up of procedures is crucial to assess the efficacy of the intervention and monitor the recurrence of obstructive lesions. Multi-modality imaging, integrated in this way, significantly enhances diagnostic yields as well as the therapeutic value, providing new options for the more effective treatment of renal and urinary tract diseases (Figure 10.13).

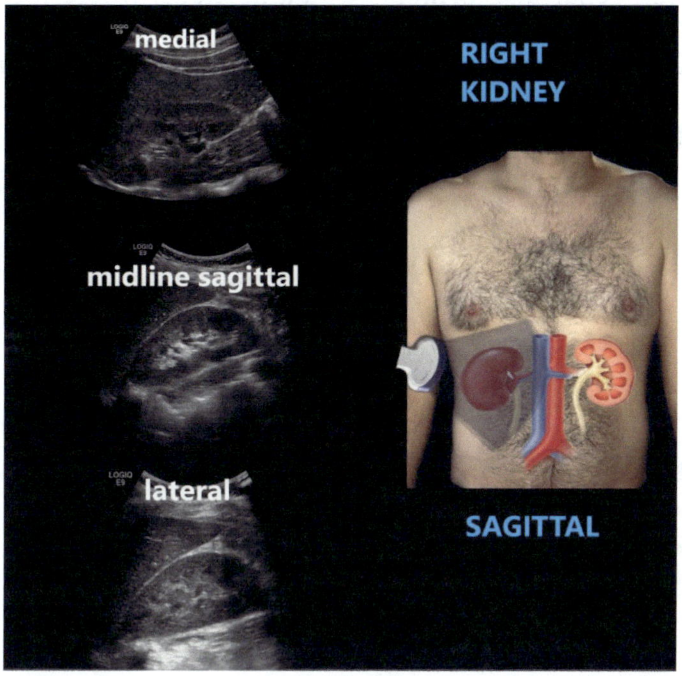

Figure 10.13. Renal ultrasound.

Source: https://sonographictendencies.com/wp-content/uploads/2021/03/1.jpg?w=1024.

10.4.3. Urinalysis and Its Significance

Urinalysis is the most important diagnostic test in renal and urinary tract function testing, providing crucial information regarding the standard and pathological conditions of the urinary system. It is a non-invasive diagnostic test that investigates various components of urine, i.e., its physical, chemical, and microscopic properties. Urinalysis can detect a range of conditions, from benign urinary tract infections to serious renal illnesses. For instance, the presence of chemicals such as protein or glucose may indicate current issues, such as diabetes or nephrotic syndrome, while abnormal electrolyte concentrations may indicate an electrolyte imbalance that can compromise renal function. The function of urinalysis is not merely for diagnosing disease; it is also vital in monitoring conditions and evaluating the response to therapeutic regimens, in conjunction with a holistic approach to renal health. In addition to its diagnostic application, urinalysis is highly significant in guiding clinical interventions. Clinicians often use urinalysis findings to inform appropriate decisions when treating their patients. For example, urine culture is used to detect specific pathogens in urinary tract infections, allowing for the appropriate antibiotic therapy to be directed towards these infections and thereby improving the treatment outcome and minimizing the risk of antibiotic resistance. Urinalysis can be further incorporated into routine screening programs for at-risk groups with renal disease, allowing for early detection and intervention. This progressive process is crucial in improving patient outcomes and potentially reducing the cost burden associated with complex renal diseases. Thus, urinalysis not only serves as a diagnostic tool but also as a preventive care tool, which places it at the forefront of assessing renal and urinary tract function. The evolving status of healthcare further positions the value of urinalysis today. Advances in urinalysis methods and laboratory testing technology have made determinations more rapid and accurate, enabling doctors to take swift action in the clinical setting. As highlighted in current guidelines, urinalysis is now routinely incorporated into the patient's diagnostic workup on a systematic basis. In addition, its application extends beyond the clinical setting to research and public health applications, where it informs epidemiological studies that identify the endemicity of renal conditions in populations. The multi-dimensional significance of urinalysis thus makes it a critical component of renal health assessment and intervention strategies, thereby enhancing the need for ongoing education and training among healthcare workers on its proper use in clinical practice (Campbell et al., 2017; Zeng et al., 2020).

Test Your Knowledge

1. What is the significance of monitoring urine output in assessing renal function?
2. How does a serum creatinine test help evaluate kidney health?

10.5. Interventions for Renal Health

Learning Outcome

1. Describe the pharmacological treatments for renal health
2. Define the dietary modifications and lifestyle changes
3. Discuss the dialysis and transplantation options

Effective intervention in renal health involves a multifaceted approach, combining diet modification, lifestyle changes, and medication. Nutrition plays a critical role in renal maintenance, particularly in the case of patients with CKD. Low-sodium, phosphorus, and potassium diets significantly lighten the load on the kidneys, hence preserving their filtering capacity. Moreover, the ingestion of good-quality proteins such as lean meat and plant products leads to a lowering of urea production and waste build-up management. Regular physical exercise also improves vascular health, thereby improving overall renal perfusion. All these interventions not only promote kidney health but also help mitigate the risks of the comorbid conditions of hypertension and diabetes that prevail in the renal population. Interprofessional collaboration between patients and healthcare professionals plays a central role in designing customized intervention programs that yield optimal outcomes. In renal medicine, emerging diagnostic technologies continue to transform the management of kidney disease. An example of this is the urinary proteome-based classifier, CKD273, which enables early prediction and detection of CKD progression. Using capillary electrophoresis in combination with mass spectrometry, this sophisticated diagnostic tool utilizes specific urinary peptides to identify individuals at risk. The extensive validation of CKD273 by large-scale studies, involving populations of over 1,000 patients, underscores its importance in clinical practice. Enabling prompt interventions, clinicians can begin preventative actions earlier, which ultimately benefits the patient. Regulatory backing by the likes of the US Food and Drug Administration for CKD273 supports greater backing for emerging biomarkers for use in the evaluation of renal function.

This diagnostic improvement marks a shifting landscape, with anticipatory evaluation driving effective care and therapeutic treatment of chronic kidney diseases (Mischak et al., 2017). Drug therapy remains the cornerstone of renal health management, to optimally utilize the kidneys' function and halt the progression of disease. Medication treatment using drugs such as angiotensin-converting enzyme (ACE) inhibitors or angiotensin receptor blockers (ARBs) can significantly reduce the incidence of hypertension as well as albuminuria among participants with existing kidney disease. In addition, there is new evidence suggesting that sodium-glucose cotransporter 2 (SGLT2) inhibitors have not only therapeutic benefits in the treatment of diabetes but also offer renal protective benefits. The medications have been shown to slow the rate of renal function decline, indicating their therapeutic potential. Education of the patient regarding medication adherence and potential side effects is crucial for achieving the maximum benefit from these drug therapies. Finally, an integrated approach, incorporating concomitant lifestyle modifications, state-of-the-art diagnostics, and targeted pharmacotherapy, is essential for enhancing renal health and ensuring long-term kidney function (Ohk et al., 2012) (Figure 10.14).

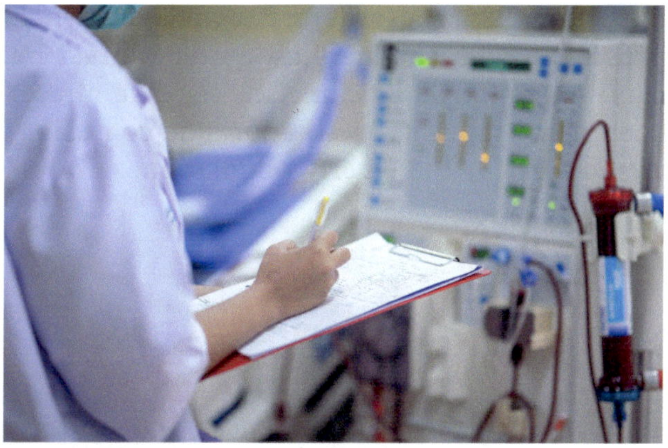

Figure 10.14. Effective nursing interventions for managing acute renal failure.

Source: https://simplenursing.com/wp-content/uploads/2018/06/iStock-1124361636-scaled.jpg.

10.5.1. Pharmacological Treatments

Pharmacological therapy is a crucial element in the management of renal and urinary tract illnesses, particularly in the case of NLUTD patients. Effective pharmacotherapy relies on a thorough consideration of both the urological symptoms and the underlying neurological disease state. Clinicians should consider patient-specific factors, such as cognitive status, mobility, and social support, when personalizing pharmacologic therapies, thereby achieving maximal therapeutic outcomes and enhancing the quality of life for NLUTD patients. This approach encourages collaborative decision-making between clinicians and patients, ensuring the optimal alignment of treatment plans with patients' needs and preferences, thereby maximizing compliance with prescribed treatments. Furthermore, pharmacological management can include anticholinergic therapy for overactive bladder or autonomic dysreflexia medication, and this suggests the necessity for individualized treatment programs in the diverse patient group (Ginsberg et al., 2021). Healthcare providers must consider the potential side effects and complications of pharmacologic therapies for urinary tract disorders. For instance, when prescribing anticholinergics, patients must be closely monitored by clinicians for side effects such as dry mouth, constipation, and confusion, particularly in the elderly population.

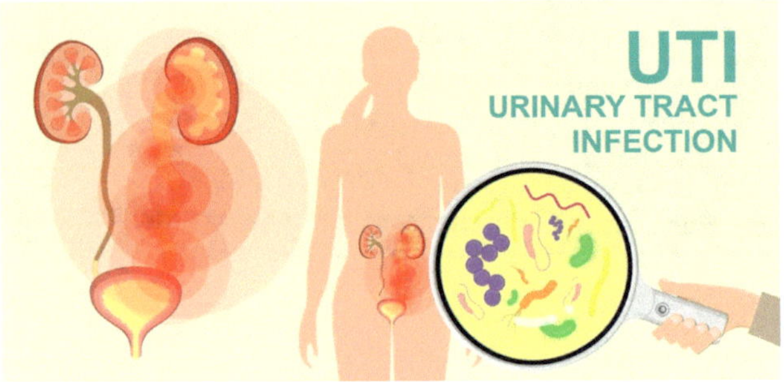

Figure 10.15. Managing urinary tract infections (UTIs).

Source: https://nursesrevisionuganda.com/wp-content/uploads/2023/01/ezgif.com-gif-maker-5-1-1024x503.jpg.

Additionally, long-term administration of the drugs can lead to an increased risk of urinary retention, for which constant monitoring of the patient's bladder function is essential. Follow-ups and continuous monitoring of patient symptoms are necessary to detect any early alteration that would warrant modification of the pharmacotherapy regimen. Lastly, maintaining open communication with patients will achieve better control and even avert complications caused by medication abuse or misadaption (Visseren et al., 2021). Upon treating urinary tract infections (UTIs), medical practitioners ought to be judicious in handling pharmacological regimens, especially for groups prone to high recurrence, such as those presenting with NLUTD. It is essential to avoid the temptation of using antibiotics where they are not needed, especially among asymptomatic cases of bacteriuria, since this can cause antibiotic resistance—a fact alarming to contemporary medicine. Treatment should be withheld for certain UTIs based on clinical presentation and supportive laboratory data. Clinicians must ensure the use of culture-specific antibiotics to optimize effective treatment while practicing responsible antibiotic stewardship. An interdisciplinary approach involving urologists, primary care providers, and pharmacists is necessary to enhance patient education about UTI symptoms and signs, thereby improving patient compliance and treatment outcomes in such patients (Ginsberg et al., 2021) (Figure 10.15).

10.5.2. Dietary Modifications and Lifestyle Changes

Renal and urinary tract function maintenance also relies on dietary adjustments and lifestyle modifications. Proper dietary planning, specifically tailored to address the requirements of kidney function, can alleviate renal anatomy stress and improve overall function. The reduction of sodium intake is typically part of dietary modifications used to offset the resultant hypertension, a common comorbidity in patients with renal dysfunction. Additionally, protein consumption may need to be adjusted; low protein intake can reduce stress on the kidneys while providing necessary nutrients. By employing these dietary forms, medical practitioners can establish an environment conducive to renal health, which will ultimately aid in the healing of chronic diseases that afflict the urinary tract. Thus, it becomes highly essential to unravel the intricate interaction of diet and renal function for optimal therapy to benefit patient outcomes in renal medicine (Visseren et al., 2021). Along with dietary alterations, lifestyle modifications become a significant component in maintaining urinary tract and renal well-being. Regular exercise plays a vital role in regulating weight, promoting cardiovascular health, and enhancing insulin sensitivity, which in turn relates to kidney function. Regular exercise may be pivotal in the prevention of kidney disease and also in modulating the disease once it is established. Furthermore, relaxation and mindfulness exercises for stress management can also enhance physical health; chronic stress causes elevated blood pressure and blood glucose levels, which can both adversely impact renal function. In combination, these lifestyle interventions, when implemented in the daily routines of patients, can lead to remarkable improvement in renal function and strengthen resistance to urinary tract infection complications (Mach et al., 2019). Moreover, education and counseling by medical experts are integral factors in guiding individuals through diet and lifestyle modifications. Comprehensive educational programs can provide patients with the correct information to make informed decisions about their health. Since dietetic modifications, as recommended by medical practitioners, can significantly influence kidney function, healthcare workers must emphasize the importance of adherence and regular monitoring of eating patterns. Besides, long-term support promotes a team-based model of care that helps patients ~~to~~ sustain lifestyle changes towards optimizing renal health. Healthcare professionals should also pay attention to the specific needs of individual patients, tailoring interventions to accommodate their individual tastes and food cultural intake habits. Effective communication of dietary guidance can facilitate patients and lead to improved self-management and kidney outcomes (Visseren et al., 2021).

10.5.3. Dialysis and Transplantation Options

The management of end-stage renal disease (ESRD) is predominantly dialysis and kidney transplantation, the two therapies with significant impact on patient outcomes. Dialysis serves as a life-saving bridge for patients who cannot maintain sufficient kidney function, based on mechanisms such as hemodialysis and peritoneal dialysis to remove waste products and fluid overload from the blood. Hemodialysis, which is ~~most often~~ performed in special dialysis clinics or even at home, employs an artificial kidney to cleanse the blood, while peritoneal dialysis uses the patient's abdominal membrane to remove waste. Both procedures can prolong life as well as enhance the quality of life, yet they have challenges, including dietary limitations, fluid balance, and complications like infection or vascular access complications. Recognition of the strengths of both modalities allows health practitioners to tailor treatment to individual patient requirements, increasing overall care outcomes in renal procedures. Transplantation is regarded as the optimal treatment of choice for ESRD, providing patients with the guarantee of greater longevity and improved quality of life. Transplantation is the surgical introduction of a viable donor kidney into the recipient's body, allowing for enhanced renal function compared to dialysis. Whether the donor is living or dead holds many implications for the health of patients, with a living donor transplant typically yielding better results due to earlier function and lower rejection rates. However, the supply of organs and the possibility of matching donors can represent a significant hurdle. As shown in current guidelines, the use of multidisciplinary support teams is essential for pre-transplant assessment and post-operative management optimization, covering aspects such as immunosuppression and complications related to graft function. The choice of transplantation as a treatment option, therefore, needs to be decided cautiously as part of the overall scope of renal and urinary tract interventions (Steffel et al., 2018). Technological advances and improved medical techniques are continually redefining the field of dialysis and transplant. Developments, such as improvement in immunosuppressive therapy protocols and sophisticated operative methods, have optimistically enhanced transplant success. Furthermore, research into the application of bioengineered organs and xenotransplantation offers promising frontiers for future therapy. Simultaneously, dialysis patient management is also being developed, with actions centered on individualizing treatment modalities and improving patient adherence to treatment. With the renal care field evolving further, there is a necessity to integrate evidence-based interventions—such as those highlighted by the KDIGO guidelines for chronic kidney disease—into clinical settings in order to further improve patient outcomes and address care complexity issues (N/A, 2017). By integrating technological advances and patient-centered care approaches, stakeholders can optimize renal well-being interventions to manage ESRD more effectively, both through dialysis and transplant (Figure 10.16).

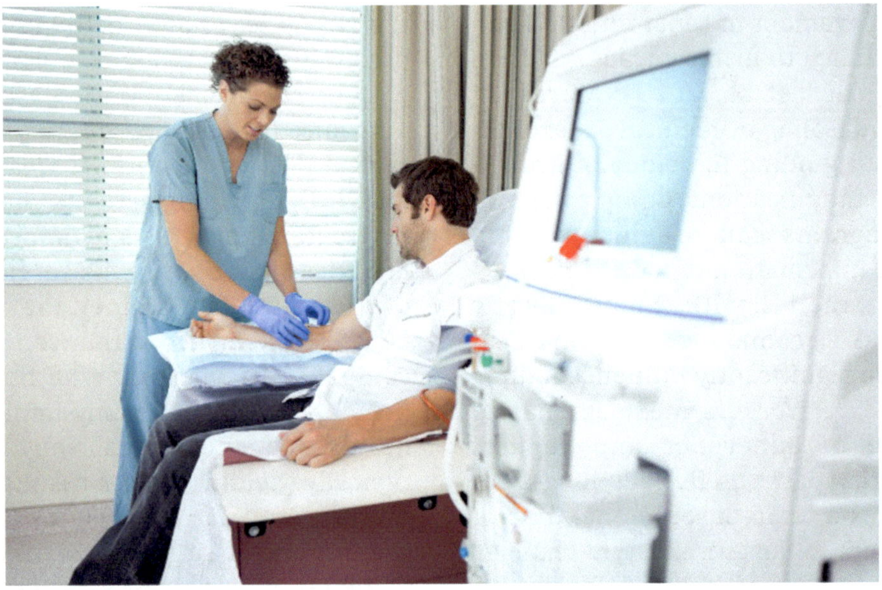

Figure 10.16. Dialysis and transplantation options.

Source: https://nhsbtdbe.blob.core.windows.net/umbraco-assets-corp/20882/dialysis.jpeg.

Test Your Knowledge

1. How can fluid management help in preventing complications in patients with kidney disorders?
2. What dietary modifications are commonly recommended for patients with chronic kidney disease?

10.6. Preventive Measures for Renal and Urinary Health

Learning Outcome

1. Describe the importance of hydration
2. Define the regular health screenings
3. Identify the education on risk factors and symptoms of renal and urinary tract disorders

The importance of preventive measures to renal and urinary health cannot be stressed enough, since preventive intervention is the cornerstone of prevention of urinary tract infection (UTI) and other renal problems. Hydration is key; adequate fluid intake helps keep the urine diluted, allowing it to effectively flush out the causative bacteria.

One should aim to drink at least eight glasses of water daily, depending on the level of activity and weather conditions. Good personal hygiene is also vital in preventing UTI occurrence, particularly in women due to their greater susceptibility to anatomical factors. Frequent urination as much as possible, particularly after sexual intercourse, is also a highly effective preventive measure that can help reduce UTI incidence. These affirmative measures not only benefit the urinary health but also the overall functioning of the renal system, anticipating the interconnectivity of preventive care in a broader field of renal and urinary tract health. Dietary modifications also play a pivotal role in enhancing renal and urinary health. Consuming a healthy diet rich in fruits, vegetables, and whole grains can help enhance nephron function and maintain renal integrity. Some foods, such as those rich in antioxidants found in berries and cruciferous vegetables, can help combat oxidative stress, which has been linked to negatively affecting kidney function. Additionally, reducing sodium consumption to lower blood pressure can decrease the risk of chronic kidney disease, a growing public health concern. Attention should be given to the number of processed foods with high content of preservatives since these have the potential of elevating renal workload. Education on these dietary interventions is essential because they allow people to make intelligent choices that ensure long-term kidney health and have a multiplier effect on public health outcomes related to renal diseases and urinary dysfunction.

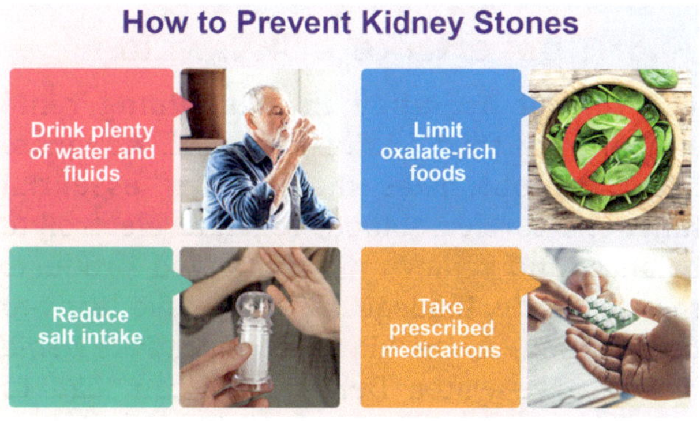

Figure 10.17. Understand the difference between kidney stones.

Source: https://external-content.duckduckgo.com/iu/?u=https%3A%2F%2Fwww.elitecarehc.com%2Fwp-content%2Fuploads%2F2023%2F05%2FEliteCare-SubBlog-4-02-03-2022.jpg&f=1&nofb=1&ipt=5d34864e4dc31146d738df41760beeb3b940ab2ba762eb704b01c11dc68849c1.

Regular medical screening and clinical evaluation are also critical in the early identification of renal and urinary tract disorders. Regular blood pressure monitoring, as well as proteinuria or urinary blood tests, may reveal concealed conditions that are likely to cause major complications, such as hypertension or diabetic nephropathy (Agabiti-Rosei et al., 2016). Preventive health programs should also educate the population regarding renal condition symptoms so that appropriate medical consultation is obtained as early as possible. Furthermore, the application of models of mutual care, as used with the successful management of other diseases, could facilitate greater family participation in kidney disease management through improved support and communication (Sebern et al., 1996). Through these multistage preventive measures, fluid consumption, dietary elements, and early medical visits—individuals can actually reduce the risk of kidney and urinary system diseases and, therefore, improve quality of life and health status (Figure 10.17).

10.6.1. Importance of Hydration

The role of hydration in maintaining renal and urinary tract health is crucial. Adequate hydration optimizes the kidneys' essential functions to clear blood, regulate electrolyte balance, and remove metabolic end products through urine. Inadequate fluid intake leads to dehydration, as the kidneys concentrate urine to conserve water. Dehydration can lead to kidney complications like acute kidney injury and exacerbation of chronic kidney disease. Furthermore, dehydrated patients are more likely to experience urinary tract infection (UTI) from concentrated urine, that will support infection risk. Therefore, an optimal hydration state is paramount not only for the well-being of the kidneys but also for the integrity of the entire urinary system. Clinically, hydration status needs to be assessed when renal function is considered, particularly in patients who are going to undergo an intervention and can compromise their renal well-being. For instance, contrast medium administration during imaging exams has been associated with renal toxicity, especially for individuals with pre-existing renal dysfunction (Orlacchio et al., 2022). Pre-procedure hydration has been identified as the best preventive measure against preventable complications such as post-contrast AKI. The guidelines emphasize that intravenous hydration can substantially minimize renal risk and therefore enhance patient safety during diagnostic assessment or interventional therapy. Thus, clinicians need to prioritize hydration assessment and intervention as a regular part of patient management for patients with compromised renal function. Additionally, the importance of hydration extends beyond acute renal protection to encompass broader health-related aspects. Hydration maintains hemodynamics at optimal levels and prevents overloading of renal tissue, which ultimately leads to functional deterioration. Studies have confirmed that sufficient fluid intake helps prevent comorbidities that can compromise renal function, including diabetes mellitus and hypertension (Mach et al., 2019). Health practitioners are thus required to educate patients about the long-term benefits of consistent hydration patterns. Through knowledge of hydration's key role in renal and urinary tract well-being, clinicians can empower patients to take a more active role in their health, adopting a proactive approach to the care of the kidneys through management of hydration.

10.6.2. Regular Health Screenings

Regular health checks play a central role in the early detection and treatment of urinary and renal illnesses. Through regular checks, medical care providers can identify abnormalities that would otherwise go undetected until they develop into symptomatic or advanced conditions. For instance, congenital urinary tract lesions typically occur due to pregnancy issues, an indication of the importance of pregnancy ultrasounds undertaken in early pregnancy, which enable timely intervention (Berendt et al., 2019). Such preventive measures not only facilitate immediate treatment methods but also enhance long-term health benefits by allowing for planned postnatal care, hence enhancing the prognosis among affected infants. This highlights the need to integrate intensive screening protocols into healthcare interventions in order to monitor kidney function as well as urinary tract health effectively. Apart from congenital diseases, regular health screenings are also a crucial tool for detecting acquired conditions, such as urinary tract infections (UTIs) and chronic kidney disease (CKD). The insidious nature of CKD leads to the generation of minimal early symptoms, and regular laboratory testing becomes the key to detecting diminished renal function. With known risk factors, such as diabetes or hypertension, routine screening allows patients and healthcare providers to collaborate on early interventions to prevent acute kidney injury and disease progression. Furthermore, engaging patients in tailored disease control through frequent measurements fosters a sense of responsibility and adherence to treatment regimens, ultimately leading to improved patient outcomes.

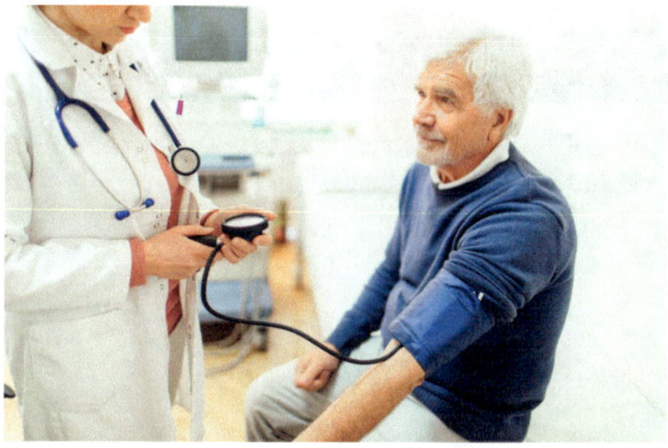

Figure 10.18. The importance of regular check-ups for your health.

Source: https://external-content.duckduckgo.com/iu/?u=https%3A%2F%2Fwww.nurseregistry.com%2Fwp-content%2Fuploads%2F2017%2F01%2FiStock-500457696-1024x683%402x.jpg&f=1&nofb=1&ipt=4a493526e93c646a6f2b4044c3721f69c30f28c438a6ba1e244a52d72f037763.

Moreover, the "shared care" term emphasizes the importance of reciprocal relationships between patients, families, and health professionals in achieving proper health screening management. Reciprocal engagement has a direct effect on preventive practice and health outcomes. For example, patients whose relatives are honest with each other about symptoms and treatment response are likely to adhere more closely to preventive care interventions, thereby reducing renal complications, as indicated by results of recent research (Sebern et al., 1996). Thus, establishing a culture that fosters engagement in collaborative care not only enhances the effectiveness of regular health screenings but also ensures that patients are assisted from the beginning of their treatment phase, which is crucial for managing community health (Figure 10.18).

10.6.3. Education on Risk Factors and Symptoms

Educational interventions addressing risk factors and symptoms of kidney and urinary tract diseases are imperative to effective prevention and control. Effective understanding of these factors can enable patients, as well as medical practitioners, to make educated decisions regarding healthcare intervention. Common risk factors include refractory hypertension, diabetes mellitus, and susceptibility due to genetics, all of which need to be actively screened and counseled to the patient. Through the education of patients comprehensively regarding these risks, medical professionals can educate them about early interventions that can make a great difference in relieving the course of kidney ailments. This setting up of information is the building block for patients to assume healthier life habits and regular screening, instilling personal responsibility and potentially relieving the healthcare burden. Kidney and urinary tract disorders will typically present with slowly developing symptoms, making it hard to detect and treat early. Patient education about; is paramount for early medical attention. Detection of minimal changes in urinary patterns or pain will encourage individuals to seek assessment before the development of early disorders into advanced complications. Sustained discussion within the clinical setting about these symptoms not only heightens awareness but also promotes an alertness culture among the patients. This positive approach is part of larger public health goals for early diagnosis and intervention, ultimately benefiting patient outcomes. By emphasizing symptom awareness, healthcare workers can initiate timely assessments and appropriate interventions, hence treating kidney health as a whole. Moreover, interagency collaboration between public health agencies and healthcare workers is important in delivering beneficial education about renal and urinary tract disease risk factors and symptoms. The collaborative effort can lead to tailored educational initiatives that are sensitive to various patient populations, thereby making information accessible and relevant to specific cultural contexts. Technology programs, such as internet websites and mobile apps, can be utilized to enhance outreach and engagement. Notably, health professionals should also incorporate proven clinical guidelines into such education, taking into account the most current findings and recommendations. As noted by renowned medical experts, health workers are expected to be updated and disseminate the latest clinical practice guidelines, thus empowering patients with the information required to take control of their renal status and battle for their well-being (Cosentino et al., 2019; Visseren et al., 2021).

Test Your Knowledge

1. How does staying well-hydrated help in preventing urinary tract infections?
2. Why is controlling blood pressure important for maintaining kidney health?

SUMMARY

Assessment of renal and urinary tract function is essential in modern clinical practice, especially with regard to increasing cases of renal disease and its complications. Proper evaluation measures, such as serum creatinine and new biomarkers, such as urinary NGAL (uNGAL), enhance early diagnosis of acute kidney injury (AKI) in patients. The findings of more recent research indicate that uNGAL and the accompanying urinary creatinine ratio well exceed standard serum creatinine approximations in canine AKI diagnosis, and therefore, it suggests the necessity for further research and validation of such markers in human patients. Recognizing these signs earlier can lead to timely interventions, reducing the likelihood of complications due to renal impairment and thereby improving patient outcomes and maintaining effective management programs in clinical settings (Cowgill et al., 2016). Additionally, the interactive relationship between gastrointestinal health and renal function has further highlighted the complexity of patient care in patients undergoing treatments such as hemodialysis. The potential for improved intestinal permeability in individuals on dialysis would contribute to the severity of their renal disease, suggesting that a comprehensive approach to their treatment is essential. Established evidence highlights the importance of conducting robust research on the effects of hemodialysis on the body's overall systems, including the gastrointestinal system, which is particularly sensitive to fluctuations in blood volume during procedures. It is required to understand these interactions to develop integrated treatment protocols that not only improve renal function but also consider the general physiological consequences of interventions performed in dialysis (Bischoff et al., 2019). In conclusion, the importance of quantifying renal and urinary tract function extends beyond the precision of diagnosis; it truly shapes the clinical management and therapeutic decisions surrounding patient treatment. Incorporating new biomarkers will progressively improve diagnostic pathways to ensure interventions are timely and responsive to each patient's needs. With an appreciation of the intricate interplay between renal and other body systems, it is hoped that healthcare providers will be prompted to employ a multidisciplinary approach, promoting teamwork among specialties to optimize patient outcomes. Further emphasis on education and investigation in this field will eventually improve our capability to manage the complexities of renal disease in a successful way and improve the overall quality of patient care.

The urinary and renal systems play a critical role in regulating homeostasis, maintaining water balance, balancing electrolytes, and excreting waste. The system's important organs, including the kidneys, ureters, bladder, and urethra, all work together to purify the blood, reabsorb essential materials, and excrete toxins through urine. Renal function testing typically encompasses a combination of history-taking, physical examination, laboratory tests, and imaging tests. These assessments not only allow for the detection of acute and chronic kidney disease but also allow health care providers to monitor the evolution of renal pathology. By understanding the intricate pathways and mechanisms of renal function, clinicians can tailor interventions to individual patient needs, promote health, and enhance patient outcomes. Interventions to optimize renal and urinary tract function encompass both non-pharmacological and pharmacological methods. Non-pharmacologic interventions consist of lifestyle modifications such as diet changes, exercise, and fluid management that directly influence the health of the kidneys. A low-sodium diet with high fruit and vegetable intake, for instance, can manage blood pressure, one of the key risk factors of chronic kidney disease. Diuretics for enabling the loss of fluid or medication for managing underlying conditions like diabetes and hypertension can constitute the pharmacological intervention. In addition, understanding the risk factors for renal impairment, such as age, heredity, and comorbidities, is crucial during the process of undertaking early prevention. The multi-factorial process aims to ensure that individuals at risk of renal dysfunction are properly identified and managed to reduce the likelihood of further complications. Additionally, evidence-based guidelines are crucial in informing interventions for renal and urinary tract dysfunction. Current recommendations emphasize the need for routine screenings and assessments to identify renal impairment among groups deemed to be at risk. For instance, repeated assessments of kidney function markers, such as serum creatinine and urine albumin, detect early manifestations and allow for intervention, resulting in the provision of suitable care in a timely manner. Furthermore, a multidisciplinary team approach facilitates comprehensive patient care based on both physical and psychosocial determinants of health. By adopting an evidence-based, holistic strategy tailored to respective patient profiles, healthcare professionals can improve renal and urinary tract conditions. Adherence to the current guidelines and continuous professional learning are key factors in supporting optimal renal health outcomes, ultimately enhancing the patients' quality of life (Cosentino et al., 2019; Crabb et al., 2019).

KEY TERMS FROM THIS CHAPTER

- Acute kidney injury (AKI)
- Blood urea nitrogen (BUN)
- Cystoscopy
- Fluid and electrolyte balance
- Glomerular filtration rate (GFR)
- Kidney transplantation
- Peritoneal dialysis
- Serum creatinine
- Urinary incontinence
- Urinary tract infection (UTI)
- Bladder training
- Chronic kidney disease (CKD)
- Diuretic therapy
- Foley catheterization
- Hemodialysis
- Nephrostomy
- Renal biopsy
- Urinalysis
- Urinary retention
- Urine specific gravity

CRITICAL THINKING QUESTIONS

1. Which laboratory test is most commonly used to assess kidney function?

a. Hemoglobin level

b. Serum creatinine

c. Blood glucose

d. Prothrombin time

2. A key symptom of a urinary tract infection (UTI) is:

a. Increased appetite

b. Flank pain and dysuria

c. Dry skin

d. Shortness of breath

3. Which of the following is a nursing intervention to prevent catheter-associated urinary tract infection (CAUTI)?

a. Irrigate the catheter every shift

b. Clamp the catheter to retain urine

c. Maintain a closed drainage system and ensure perineal hygiene

d. Use antibiotics prophylactically

4. Which fluid and electrolyte imbalance is commonly seen in acute kidney injury (AKI)?

a. Hypernatremia

b. Hypokalemia

c. Hyperkalemia

d. Hypocalcemia

5. What is the nurse's priority during the assessment of a patient with suspected urinary retention?

a. Measure blood glucose

b. Monitor for edema in the legs

c. Palpate the bladder and assess voiding patterns

d. Check bowel sounds

Short Answer Questions

1. What is the normal function of the kidneys?
2. Name two signs of urinary tract infection (UTI).
3. Which lab tests are commonly used to assess renal function?
4. What is urinary retention, and how can it be assessed?
5. Explain the nursing assessment and care of a patient with acute kidney injury (AKI).
6. Discuss the causes, symptoms, and nursing interventions for chronic kidney disease (CKD).
7. Describe the nursing management of a patient with urinary incontinence.
8. Discuss the nursing responsibilities in caring for a patient undergoing hemodialysis.

Answers to Critical Thinking Questions

1. (b) 2. (b) 3. (c) 4. (c) 5. (c).

REFERENCES

1. Lurbe, E., Agabiti-Rosei, E., Cruickshank, J. K., Dominiczak, A., Erdine, S., Hirth, A., Invitti, C., Litwin, M., Mancia, G., Pall, D., Rascher, W., Redon, J., Schaefer, F., Seeman, T., Sinha, M., Stabouli, S., Webb, N. J., Wühl, E., & Zanchetti, A. (2016). 2016 European Society of Hypertension guidelines for the management of high blood pressure in children and adolescents. *Journal of Hypertension, 34*(10), 1887–1920. https://doi.org/10.1097/hjh.0000000000001039Anson, K., Burr, J., Kilonzo, M., Lam, T., et al. (2014). Use of drug therapy in the management of symptomatic ureteric stones in hospitalized adults (SUSPEND), a multicenter, placebo-controlled, randomized trial of a calcium-channel blocker (nifedipine) and an α-blocker (tamsulosin): Study protocol for a randomized controlled trial. https://core.ac.uk/download/20664049.pdf (accessed on 30th June 2025).
2. Arduino, B., Berghella, V., D'Alessandro, P., Escolino, M., et al. (2020). Antenatal intervention for congenital fetal lower urinary tract obstruction (LUTO): A systematic review and meta-analysis. https://core.ac.uk/download/195735545.pdf (accessed on 30th June 2025).
3. Assimos, D. G., Krambeck, A. E., Miller, N. L., Monga, M., Murad, M. H., Nelson, C. P., Pace, K. T., et al. (2016). Surgical management of stones: American Urological Association/Endourological Society Guideline, Part I. *The Journal of Urology, 196*, 1153–1160. https://doi.org/10.1016/j.juro.2016.05.090.
4. Ather, M. H., Ettinger, S., Hoffman, S., Martin, R. A., McLoughlin, M. A., Ross, L. A., Scott, R. C., et al. (2019). Endoscopic laser-ablation for the treatment of orthotopic and ectopic ureteroceles in dogs: 13 cases (2008–2017). https://core.ac.uk/download/213444929.pdf (accessed on 30th June 2025).
5. Berendt, A. M., & Wójtowicz-Marzec, M. (2019). Prenatal diagnosis of urinary tract defects. https://core.ac.uk/download/587242948.pdf (accessed on 30th June 2025).
6. Bischoff, S. C., Barbara, G., Buurman, W. A., Ockhuizen, T., Schulzke, J. D., Sérino, M., Tilg, H., et al. (2014). Intestinal permeability–A new target for disease prevention and therapy. *BMC Gastroenterology, 14*. https://doi.org/10.1186/s12876-014-0189-7.
7. Bischoff, S. C., Bjarnason, I., Bornet, F., Camilleri, M., Carrero, J. J., Dasgupta, P., et al. (2019). Acute hemodynamic changes during hemodialysis do not exacerbate gut hyperpermeability. https://core.ac.uk/download/287581728.pdf (accessed on 30th June 2025).
8. Bove, P., Finazzi Agrò, E., Kim, F. J., Miano, R., Micali, S., Rosa, M., & Usai, P. (2013). Recent findings and new technologies in nephrolithiasis: A review of the recent literature. https://core.ac.uk/download/pdf/54580708.pdf (accessed on 30th June 2025).
9. Butler-Dawson, J., Diaz, H. F., Garcia, G., Hernando, A., et al. (2019). Climate change and the kidney. https://core.ac.uk/download/322973173.pdf (accessed on 30th June 2025).
10. Campbell, S. C., Uzzo, R. G., Allaf, M. E., Bass, E. B., Cadeddu, J. A., Chang, A., Clark, P. E., et al. (2017). Renal mass and localized renal cancer: AUA guideline. *The Journal of Urology, 198*, 520–529. https://doi.org/10.1016/j.juro.2017.04.100.
11. Chapple, C., Guideline Development Group, Hill, J., Jones, C., et al. (2010). Management of lower urinary tract symptoms in men: Summary of NICE guidance. https://core.ac.uk/download/370446.pdf (accessed on 30th June 2025).
12. Cody, J. D., Dublin, N., McClinton, S., Nabi, G., et al. (2012). Urinary diversion and bladder

reconstruction/replacement using intestinal segments for intractable incontinence or following cystectomy. https://core.ac.uk/download/20454622.pdf (accessed on 30th June 2025).

13. Cosentino, F., Grant, P. J., Aboyans, V., Bailey, C. J., Ceriello, A., Delgado, V., Federici, M., et al. (2019). 2019 ESC Guidelines on diabetes, pre-diabetes, and cardiovascular diseases developed in collaboration with the EASD. *European Heart Journal, 41*, 255–323. https://doi.org/10.1093/eurheartj/ehz486.

14. Cowgill, L. D., Kanakubo, K., Kowalkowski, K. L., LeRoy, B. E., et al. (2016). Urinary neutrophil gelatinase-associated lipocalin as a marker for identification of acute kidney injury and recovery in dogs with gentamicin-induced nephrotoxicity. https://core.ac.uk/download/323068609.pdf (accessed on 30th June 2025).

15. Crabb, D. W., Im, G. Y., Szabó, G., Mellinger, J. L., & Lucey, M. R. (2019). Diagnosis and treatment of alcohol-associated liver diseases: 2019 practice guidance from the American Association for the Study of Liver Diseases. *Hepatology, 71*, 306–333. https://doi.org/10.1002/hep.30866.

16. da Silva, A. A., Guyton, A. C., Patterson, A. J., Sparrow, A. J., Egan, B. M., Mao, C., Gray, C., et al. (2013). Excess maternal salt intake produces sex-specific hypertension in offspring: Putative roles for kidney and gastrointestinal sodium handling. https://core.ac.uk/download/33573800.pdf (accessed on 30th June 2025).

17. Davies, M. J., D'Alessio, D. A., Fradkin, J., Kernan, W. N., Mathieu, C., Mingrone, G., Rossing, P., et al. (2018). Management of hyperglycemia in type 2 diabetes, 2018. A consensus report by the American Diabetes Association (ADA) and the European Association for the Study of Diabetes (EASD). *Diabetes Care, 41*, 2669–2701. https://doi.org/10.2337/dci18-0033.

18. Dominiczak, A., Ferreri, N. R., & Graham, L. A. (2017). The role of renal transporters and novel regulatory interactions in the TAL that control blood pressure. https://core.ac.uk/download/82893296.pdf (accessed on 30th June 2025).

19. Erdbrügger, U., Blijdorp, C. J., Bijnsdorp, I. V., Borràs, F. E., Burger, D., Bussolati, B., Byrd, J. B., et al. (2021). Urinary extracellular vesicles: A position paper by the Urine Task Force of the International Society for Extracellular Vesicles. *Journal of Extracellular Vesicles, 10*. https://doi.org/10.1002/jev2.12093.

20. Ginsberg, D. A., Boone, T. B., Cameron, A. P., Gousse, A. E., Kaufman, M. R., Keays, E., Kennelly, M., et al. (2021). The AUA/SUFU guideline on adult neurogenic lower urinary tract dysfunction: Diagnosis and evaluation. *The Journal of Urology, 206*, 1097–1105. https://doi.org/10.1097/ju.0000000000002235.

21. Gustafsson, U., Scott, M. J., Hübner, M., Nygren, J., Demartines, N., Francis, N., Rockall, T., et al. (2018). Guidelines for perioperative care in elective colorectal surgery: Enhanced Recovery After Surgery (ERAS®) Society recommendations: 2018. *World Journal of Surgery, 43*, 659–695. https://doi.org/10.1007/s00268-018-4844-y.

22. Janjua, H. S., Lam, S. K., Gupta, V., & Krishna, S. (2019). Congenital anomalies of the kidneys, collecting system, bladder, and urethra. *Pediatrics in Review, 40*, 619–626. https://doi.org/10.1542/pir.2018-0242.

23. Lerner, L. B., McVary, K. T., Barry, M. J., Bixler, B. R., Dahm, P., Das, A. K., Gandhi, M. C., et al. (2021). Management of lower urinary tract symptoms attributed to benign prostatic hyperplasia: AUA guideline Part II—Surgical evaluation and treatment. *The Journal of Urology, 206*, 818–826. https://doi.org/10.1097/ju.0000000000002184.

24. Liguori, I., Russo, G., Curcio, F., Bulli, G., Aran, L., Della-Morte, D., Gargiulo, G., et al. (2018). Oxidative stress, aging, and diseases. *Clinical Interventions in Aging, 13*, 757–772. https://doi.org/10.2147/cia.s158513.

25. Mach, F., Baigent, C., Catapano, A. L., Koskinas, K. C., Casula, M., Badimón, L., Chapman, M. J., et al. (2019). 2019 ESC/EAS guidelines for the management of dyslipidemias: Lipid modification to reduce cardiovascular risk. *European Heart Journal, 41*, 111–188. https://doi.org/10.1093/eurheartj/ehz455.

26. Mischak, H., & Pontillo, C. (2017). Urinary peptide-based classifier CKD273: Towards clinical application in chronic kidney disease. https://core.ac.uk/download/84148675.pdf (accessed on 30th June 2025).

27. N'Dow, J. M. O., & Wilt, T. (2008). Benign prostatic hyperplasia: Part 1–diagnosis. https://core.ac.uk/download/4193266.pdf (accessed on 30th June 2025).

28. Öborn, H. (2014). Lower urinary tract dysfunction in children with chronic kidney disease: Before and after renal transplantation. https://core.ac.uk/download/70341161.pdf (accessed on 30th June 2025).

29. Ohk, B. (2012). Mental and emotional health. https://core.ac.uk/download/46604325.pdf (accessed on 30th June 2025).

30. Orlacchio, A., Guastoni, C., Beretta, G., Cosmai, L., Galluzzo, M., Gori, S., Grassedonio, E., et al. (2022). SIRM-SIN-AIOM: Appropriateness criteria for evaluation and prevention of renal damage in the patient undergoing contrast medium examinations—Consensus statements from Italian College of Radiology (SIRM), Italian College of Nephrology (SIN) and Italian Association of Medical Oncology (AIOM). *La Radiologic Medica, 127*, 534–542. https://doi.org/10.1007/s11547-022-01483-8.

31. Reyes-Apodaca, M., Consuelo-Sánchez, A., Vázquez-Frias, R., Rodríguez-Espino, B. A., & Medeiros, M. (2025). Integral kidney function assessment in pediatric patients with glycogen storage diseases. *Frontiers in Pediatrics, 13*. https://www.semanticscholar.org/paper/a819ed259ba260b20d8ba2b4df553555dd52bb48 (accessed on 30th June 2025).

32. Sebern, M. (1996). Explication of the construct of shared care and the prevention of pressure ulcers in home health care. https://core.ac.uk/download/213077275.pdf (accessed on 30th June 2025).

33. Steffel, J., Verhamme, P., Potpara, T., Albaladejo, P., Antz, M., Desteghe, L., Hæusler, K. G., et al. (2018). The 2018 European Heart Rhythm Association practical guide on the use of non-vitamin K antagonist oral anticoagulants in patients with atrial fibrillation. *European Heart Journal, 39*, 1330–1393. https://doi.org/10.1093/eurheartj/ehy136.

34. Visseren, F. L. J., Mach, F., Smulders, Y. M., Carballo, D., Koskinas, K. C., Bäck, M., Bénétos, A., et al. (2021). 2021 ESC Guidelines on cardiovascular disease prevention in clinical practice. *European Heart Journal, 42*, 3227–3337. https://doi.org/10.1093/eurheartj/ehab484.

35. Vyas, D. A., Eisenstein, L. G., & Jones, D. S. (2020). Hidden in plain sight–Reconsidering the use of race correction in clinical algorithms. *New England Journal of Medicine, 383*, 874–882. https://doi.org/10.1056/nejmms2004740.

36. Yakubu, A., Umar, A., Muhammad, B. J., Akwaeze, C. G., Sidi, M., Ali, A., Abba, M., et al. (2024). The role of renal ultrasound and its correlation with biomarkers in the medical screening of apparently healthy individuals in a Nigerian university. *African Scientific Reports*. https://www.semanticscholar.org/paper/b165a50f15c4bfbbdb0583a72be51baeb2c05086 (accessed on 30th June 2025).

37. Zeng, Y., Xu, X. L., He, X., Tang, S., Li, Y., Huang, Y. Q., Harypursat, V., et al. (2020). Comparative effectiveness and safety of ribavirin plus interferon-alpha, lopinavir/ritonavir plus interferon-alpha, and ribavirin plus lopinavir/ritonavir plus interferon-alpha in patients with mild to moderate novel coronavirus disease 2019: Study protocol. *Chinese Medical Journal, 133*, 1132–1134. https://doi.org/10.1097/cm9.0000000000000790.

REPRODUCTIVE HEALTH: GENDER-INCLUSIVE ASSESSMENT AND CARE

11

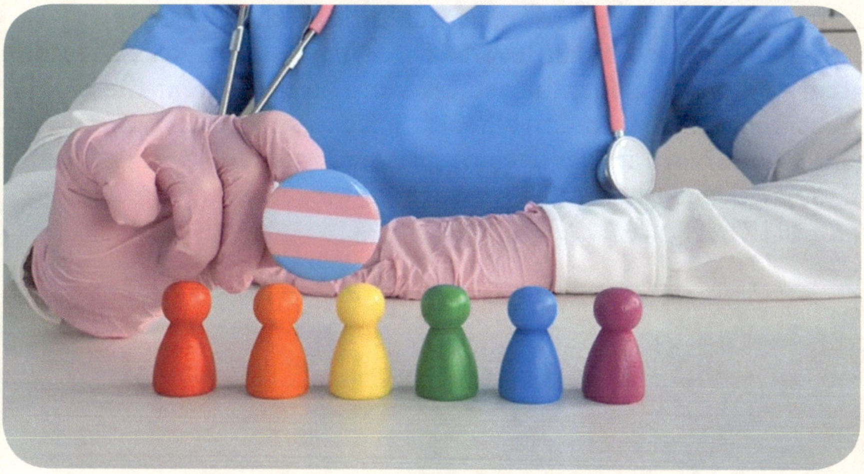

LEARNING OBJECTIVES

After studying this chapter, you will be able to:

1. Understand the historical context of reproductive health
2. Explain the current state of reproductive health services
3. Discuss the gender-inclusive assessment practices
4. Focus on reproductive health education
5. Learn about policy and advocacy for gender-inclusive care
6. Evaluate the case studies of successful gender-inclusive programs

Introduction

Reproductive health is ~~presently realized to be~~ recognized as an intrinsic part of the broader vision of gender equality as well as social justice. With evolving societies, the priority to cater to reproductive health demands through the lens of gender sensitivity has become greater. This is not just because it caters specifically to the challenges faced by different genders, but also because it aims to offer inclusive care encompassing physical, emotional, and psychological needs. Reproductive health is a significant driver of overall health outcomes and plays a central role in empowering individuals to make informed choices about their bodies and futures. By establishing a culture in which gender-sensitive assessments are the norm, healthcare systems can better serve marginalized communities and provide equitable access to essential health services. The World Bank's Gender Equality as Smart Economics action plan is the type of initiative to incorporate gender issues into development strategies. This project focuses on the imperative of having overarching strategy for improving reproductive health care, particularly in places where gender disparities are most glaring. The plan outlines specific actions focused on advancing gender equality and places a high value on crafting interventions tailored to the diverse needs of individuals. Through gender-responsive measures, these policies aim to establish a more gender-balanced healthcare environment, thereby enabling all individuals from all sectors to access basic reproductive healthcare. The association between gender equality and reproductive health highlights the need to implement targeted measures in health screenings that align with the overall objectives of sustainable development. Achieving gender-equitable reproductive health care not only addresses short-term health demands but also contributes to achieving broader social goals established in the 2030 Agenda for Sustainable Development. The agenda addresses a range of global challenges, including health-related and gender equality issues, with a vision to eradicate poverty and reduce inequalities worldwide. By linking reproductive health initiatives directly to the Sustainable Development Goals (SDGs), stakeholders can leverage existing systems to make a compelling case for equitable and integrated care. As member states work to implement these goals, the need for gender-inclusive assessments in reproductive health becomes more and more urgent. These accomplishments can make a difference in the lives of girls and women, leading to a healthier and more just world for all, as evidenced by initiatives such as those documented in the N/A (2010) and Austin-Evelyn et al. (2017) (Figure 11.1).

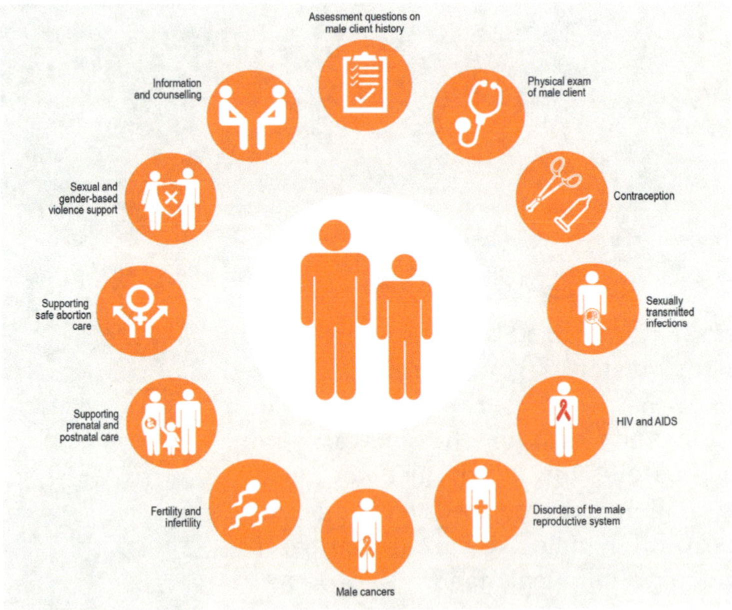

Figure 11.1. Reproductive health.

Source: https://1.bp.blogspot.com/-kNWLjto6_n8/WxISRyrESpI/AAAAAAAAAeg/XfAjujmlVVQcraj1C5_i1v_-udHSH0ozACLcBGAs/s1600/Reproductive%2Bhealth.PNG.

Definition of Reproductive Health

Reproductive health encompasses a broad area of physical, mental, and social well-being related to the reproductive system across all life stages. The definition above is more than just being free from disease or dysfunction; it is said that people should reach a level of wellness that enables them to participate fully in reproductive decisions without discrimination. Gender sensitivity is essential in such a scenario, since reproductive health affects individuals differently in relation to their gender identity. Unabridged awareness also demands an understanding of the reproductive rights that are increasingly viewed as universal human rights, facilitating the exercise of informed choices in relation to reproduction, including family planning and access to necessary healthcare services. Education on reproductive health is also basic but often in fault and not sensitive. For instance, most of the New York State public school districts have been found to implement incomplete and biased sex education programs, which do not equip students with adequate information on their reproductive health options (Yager et al., 2012). Not only do these educational failures take away from personal autonomy but also reinforce societal misconceptions about reproductive health. A gender-sensitive approach addresses such inequalities by advocating inclusive, evidence-based sexual and reproductive health education that addresses the diverse needs of all learners and thereby empowers them to make informed choices about their reproductive lives. Apart from educational concerns, reproductive rights must be recognized within a socio-cultural framework that acknowledges their complexity among diverse populations. Such rights are also closely associated with broader human rights, specifically the right of individuals to control their childbearing, i.e., spacing and number of children (Bhat et al., 2011). Making things worse are social attitudes and institutional barriers that exclude specific groups, such as disabled individuals or those with a different background, from the reproductive health discussion. Therefore, a gender-sensitive evaluation of reproductive health must consider these inequalities and demand policies and practices that enhance and protect reproductive rights for everyone, with equal access to reproductive health care and education.

Importance of Gender Inclusivity in Reproductive Health

The demand for gender inclusiveness in reproductive health cannot be overemphasized, as it addresses and recognizes the diverse needs of both persons in the gender spectrum. Reproductive health systems have commonly emphasized ciswomen at the cost of non-binary individuals, transmen, and others whose reproductive health needs differ considerably. By bringing in a more comprehensive paradigm, health professionals enable fuller understanding of sexual and reproductive health issues outside of conventional parameters. Improved not only by quality care, but also by patient-physician relationships, this expandability produces the potential for more sophisticated health intervention that addresses individuals' lived experiences and selves. Besides, gender inclusivity is key to dismantling systemic obstacles faced by marginalized communities in gaining access to reproductive health services. Evidence proves that inclusive practices work best in dispelling harmful stigma and discrimination against individuals identifying outside the traditional gender binary. Healthcare systems that actively advocate for gender inclusivity become a societal system that supports patients in pursuing care without fear of prejudice or misinterpretation. Such efforts are essential in the development of health policies that recognize and address the unique needs of these groups, thereby enhancing public health as a whole, as well as promoting social justice in accessing healthcare. In addition, incorporating gender sensitivity into reproductive health ensures improved overall health and well-being, which enhances community contribution and empowerment. By recognizing and validating different identities, health systems are able to enable individuals to become actively involved in their reproductive health. This involvement leads to better educated choices and guarantees of understanding the complexities of reproductive health issues. Additionally, inclusive learning within health facilities equips providers with the necessary information and skills to deliver culturally competent care, thereby promoting patients' health literacy. Hence, the integration of inclusive practices within reproductive health not only helps satisfy the demand for short-term health but also the long-term transformation and acceptability at the societal level and ultimately the overall healthier communities (Figure 11.2).

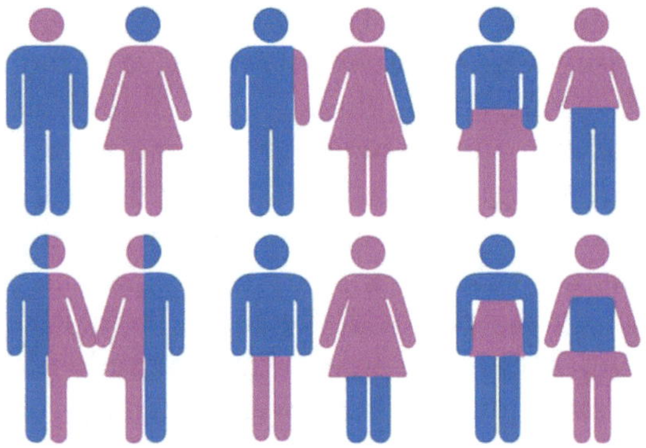

Figure 11.2. Gender inclusivity in reproductive health.

Source: https://miro.medium.com/v2/resize:fit:552/1*yFRDVAJXl-SDKIxLpK9WOA.jpeg.

11.1. Historical Context of Reproductive Health

Learning Outcome

1. Describe the evolution of reproductive health policies
2. Focus on gender disparities in historical healthcare practices
3. Learn how to impact of social movements on reproductive rights

It requires an understanding of the history of reproductive health to grasp the evolution of gender-inclusive evaluation and treatment fully. There was cultural, societal, and political determinism of reproductive health, which dictated access and outcomes, specifically in the past. For many decades, reproductive health services were typically siloed and with primary focus on female care without any regard for transgender and nonbinary communities. Women's health movements during the late 20th century began to challenge these inequalities, urging the provision of holistic reproductive health services that recognized the unique physiological and sociocultural needs of both sexes. This change was a critical turning point towards inclusivity for reproductive health, resulting in a far more sophisticated understanding of healthcare requirements in diverse groups, which continue to be pertinent currently. The emergence of critical works in the second half of the 20th century, particularly along the axis of gender, race, and sexual orientation, provided further depth to the reproductive health discussion. One of the areas of concern for the campaigners was that structural impediments needed to be addressed and removed so that marginalized groups could have equal access to reproductive health. Research indicated that institutionalized stigma and discrimination had a significant impact on LGBTQ+ individuals' reproductive health. These discoveries fueled the development of policies to promote inclusivity, including the official inclusion of sexual and gender minorities as priority groups in reproductive health policies. As a result, healthcare systems began to move towards the inclusion of culturally relevant and gender-sensitive tests that respect multiple identities and deliver maximum care to all patients. Despite these developments, there is still much to be done to achieve true equity in reproductive health. The legacy stigma associated with certain specific identities remains an obstacle to access, underscoring the need for sustained reform and advocacy. Outdated codes of law and discriminatory practices persist in much of the globe, excluding universal provision of inclusive care to persons of all gender identities. Inequitable access to education and health services also perpetuates cycles of inequality, particularly among marginalized groups. Breaking these disparities requires collective action from healthcare providers, policymakers, and communities in order to advocate for systemic changes that enhance inclusive practice. By understanding the history of reproductive health, stakeholders will be able to comprehend the complexities involved and work together towards dismantling obstacles, ultimately striving for equal, gender-neutral care for all individuals (Figure 11.3).

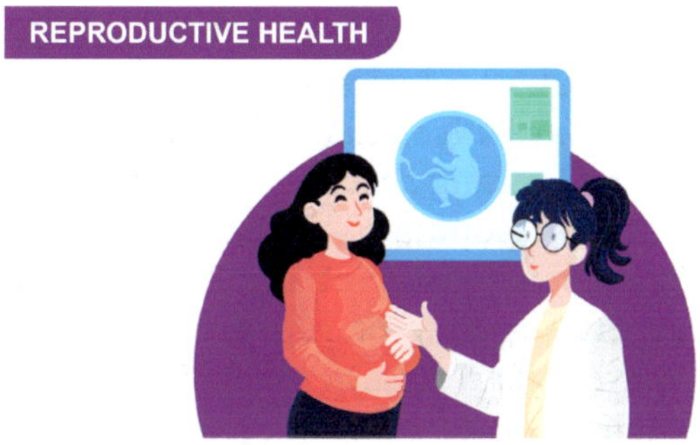

Figure 11.3. Context of reproductive health.

Source: https://cdn1.byjus.com/wp-content/uploads/2017/08/Reproductive-Health.png.

11.1.1. Evolution of Reproductive Health Policies

The evolution of reproductive health policy can be traced in distinct milestones, which have shaped societal and state orientations towards health and gender. Initially, reproductive health was articulated mainly in terms of population control rather than comprehensive care. Over time, women's rights activism and social awareness of gender equality stimulated the shift towards the notion of reproductive health as a universal human right. This shift, which was driven by social movements and scholarly inquiry, underscores the need for policies that not only provide access to reproductive healthcare but also address and eradicate inequalities rooted in these systems. Such a change reflects the ideals of social justice as prescribed in current paradigms, with an emphasis on incorporating multiple gender perspectives when formulating health policies, an occurrence driven by shifting societal values regarding reproductive rights. The implications of these shifting policies are extensive, particularly in terms of their impact on service access and overall well-being. Reproductive health policies that prioritize inclusiveness understand the intersectionality of geographic location, gender, and socio-economic status. As is argued in current academic research, the nexus between sustainable development and gender equality is utmost; ensuring women's equal access to reproductive health not only advances their status in society but also serves other development ambitions. Such realization has created platforms that advocate for complete care, embracing the totality of reproductive health needs, from family planning to maternal care. As a result, reproductive health policy now increasingly addresses the multifaceted challenges faced by women, catering to the evolving priorities and cultural contexts of societies worldwide. In summary, the evolution of reproductive health policy reveals a significant paradigm shift towards an inclusive and gender-equitable approach to healthcare. This reflects an expanded conception of reproductive health as both an aspect of individual rights and collective welfare. In addition, as reaffirmed in the dispute over sustainable development, policies must aim to serve access to resources, favoring reproductive health advances fairly. Initiatives and programs aligned with social justice principles act not only to advance the health indicators of individuals but also of society, advancing gender equality and sustainability as building blocks towards a health-focused future. Hence, knowledge of reproductive health policies from a gender perspective is not only an intellectual exercise but also a necessity for promoting equitable health systems (Figure 11.4).

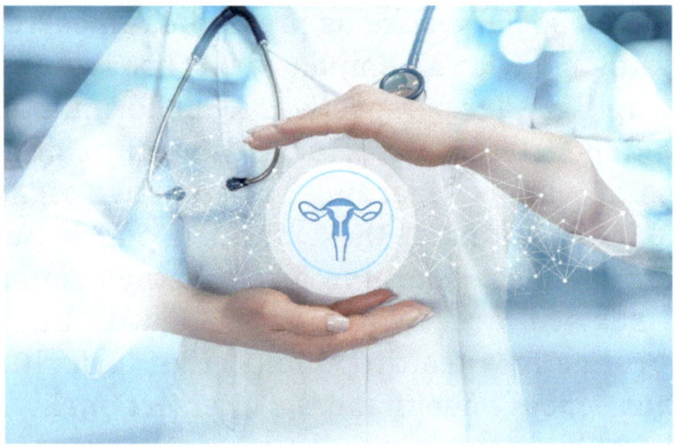

Figure 11.4. Promote reproductive health and wellness.

Source: https://parentinghealthybabies.com/app/phb-data/uploads/2022/06/reproductive-health-scaled.jpeg.

11.1.2. Gender Disparities in Historical Healthcare Practices

The historical context of health practices reveals such stark gender disparities that have determined the reproductive health experience of women. Over centuries, women's health issues have been relegated secondary to men's, and access to related healthcare services has been denied. This institutional neglect is particularly evident in medical practices where male viewpoints have extensively controlled standards of treatment. Particularly, past documents identify instances where women would be disregarded or misdiagnosed by male doctors when they presented with symptoms that male physicians did not fully grasp, leading to an immense lack of confidence within the healthcare system. These disparities have far-reaching impacts beyond personal health results, influencing the perception of society regarding women's health demands as well. Thus, general consideration of past practices is necessary when creating gender-sensitive healthcare models that accurately capture the complexity of reproductive health. Moreover, gender's role in medicine has become encumbered by sociopolitical factors that have silenced women's voices in the medical community. Underrepresentation within medical practice and research has resulted in a lack of data regarding female-specific health issues, giving rise to myths and stereotypes. For instance, studies have historically focused on male groups, resulting in a dearth of holistic insight regarding reproductive health complications disproportionately affecting women. Such studies, which shed light on such disparities, and particularly where interventions like HIV/AIDS are involved, suggest a dire need for gender-sensitive approaches in health policy designed to address women's special challenges. Wherever it occurs, as is generally the case in sub-Saharan Africa, the ramifications of this neglect are dire, exacerbating health inequalities and limiting access to treatment for already vulnerable populations, such as women and their children (Miller et al., 2010). This emphasizes the urgency of representation in policy formation and health research. Given these imbalances, it is clear that a paradigm shift in healthcare practices is essential for resolving the inequities experienced by women. Traditional healthcare systems tended to focus on male health priorities, unintentionally creating a narrative that marginalized women's experiences and reproductive health priorities. Attempts to address this imbalance should begin with the acknowledgment of past injustices and an understanding of how these gender-based disparities have persisted in influencing modern healthcare. Ensuring that there is a gender-sensitive assessment included in reproductive health care is significant because it promotes awareness and respect for women's unique health needs. This approach not only enhances the provision of healthcare but also empowers women by giving them a voice and ensuring they are heard in decision-making. It is therefore important to create cooperative relationships between researchers, healthcare providers, and policymakers to create a conducive healthcare setting for both men and women (Locke et al., 2001) (Figure 11.5).

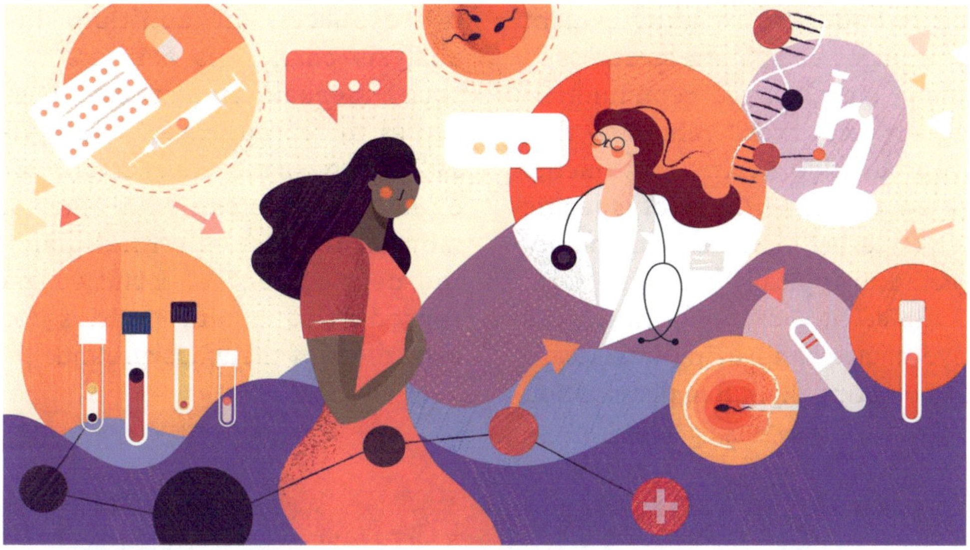

Figure 11.5. Gender disparities.

Source: https://cosmosmagazine.com/wp-content/uploads/2022/03/IWD-data-gap-header-alternative-1200.jpg.

11.1.3. Impact of Social Movements on Reproductive Rights

Social movements have played a significant role in shaping reproductive rights across various historical contexts and geographical spaces. Through collective action, activism, and mobilization, social movements have sought to transcend power dynamics that seek to oppress people's agency over their reproductive lives. For instance, the feminist movement of the 1960s and 1970s pushed open discourse about issues like access to birth control and rights to abortion on the grounds of gender equality in reproductive health.

This campaign institutionalized reproductive rights as core aspects of general human rights, which prompted subsequent movements to address inequalities and stigmas surrounding reproductive healthcare. When activists confront the challenges facing marginalized communities, the intersectional nature of these movements highlights how race, class, and gender are interconnected and influence access to and experience of reproductive health. Interestingly, the rise of ultraconservative efforts opposing reproductive rights has also contributed to a renewed wave of activism from gender equality champions. These mobilizations position themselves as defenders of traditional values and stage campaigns against "gender ideology" as a response to issues of alleged threat posed by feminist and progressive forces. This is strongly politicized in nature and is closely tied to the broader political landscape, particularly the rise of right-wing populism in the early 2010s, as opposition movements capitalize on the public anxieties about social transformations caused by neoliberal policies. Reproductive rights are typically framed here as a battlefield of war within larger contests of ideological war, enlisting a multivalent corps of activists to resist these retrograde narratives. The intersectional necessity of a feminist mass movement to counter these ultraconservative efforts underscores the imperative for understanding the influence of economic, social, and cultural processes on access to reproductive health (Graff et al., 2021). Additionally, the impact of social movements on reproductive rights is evident through policy changes and enhanced access to healthcare among marginalized communities. By advocating for healthcare remedies that incorporate reproductive health, movements have highlighted the timeliness of specific approaches in addressing individual community issues. Such activism typically takes the form of campaigns aimed at increasing awareness of reproductive choice, improving healthcare facilities, and promoting equitable distribution of resources. In addition, intersectional analysis challenges activists to tackle root social inequalities that lead to disparities in access to reproductive health (AT-Maia et al., 2021). Thus, the engagement of community organizations, along with other social justice movements, fosters critical dialogue towards the development of inclusive and equitable reproductive health policies for everyone, regardless of their background.

Test Your Knowledge

1. Why is regular screening essential for maintaining reproductive health?
2. How do hormones regulate the male and female reproductive systems?

11.2. Current State of Reproductive Health Services

Learning Outcome

1. Explain the of reproductive health services
2. Define the barriers to access for marginalized genders
3. Discuss the role of technology in improving service delivery of reproductive health

The current situation of reproductive health care is dominated by vast inequalities that reveal greater social disparities and access limitations between demographic groups. Globally, many women and clients requiring reproductive health interventions face barriers such as restricted access to family planning, prenatal care, and abortion. The World Health Organization has noted a growing need for integrated reproductive health services addressing both physical health outcomes and emotional well-being. Efforts to improve these services must also take into account ~~of~~ the socio-economic determinants of access, which vary by geographic region and cultural context. By embracing a gender-sensitive approach to reproductive health, policymakers can help overcome these disparities so that everyone has the right to make informed choices regarding their reproductive health without societal or institutional obstacles. Apart from access barriers, the character of reproductive health education plays a critical role in defining individuals' perceptions of their reproductive rights. Evidence is that sex education programs in most places, even some regions of the United States, remain archaic, biased, and not holistic enough. The programs omit crucial aspects of sexual health, such as consent and safer sex practices, that can expose individuals to risk for not being able to make well-informed choices about their reproductive lives. Specifically, outcomes in Birds, Bees and Bias: How Absent Sex Ed Standards Fail New York's Students illustrate the necessity of a national re-evaluation of sex education standards. Such a learning shortcoming not only perpetuates stigma around reproductive health but also maintains cycles of misinformation that preclude informed decision-making. Thus, an integrated strategy focusing on proper, complete education is essential in empowering individuals to assert their reproductive health rights. Furthermore, reproductive health services that enhance gender equity also have significant possibilities for raising investments. According to a study by the UN Foundation and BNY Mellon, economic benefits from the closure of the global gender gap, and in more significant areas, such as health, are staggering. The report predicts a potential market impact of nearly $300 billion by 2025 through investments in telecommunications, family planning, childcare, water, and energy. These sectors not only provide investors with financial yields but also have key roles in enhancing women's health and agency globally. By funding investments that foster gender equality, the stakeholders will be able to encourage innovation in reproductive health services that are inclusive, accessible, and innovative, ultimately resulting in a better future for all (Figure 11.6).

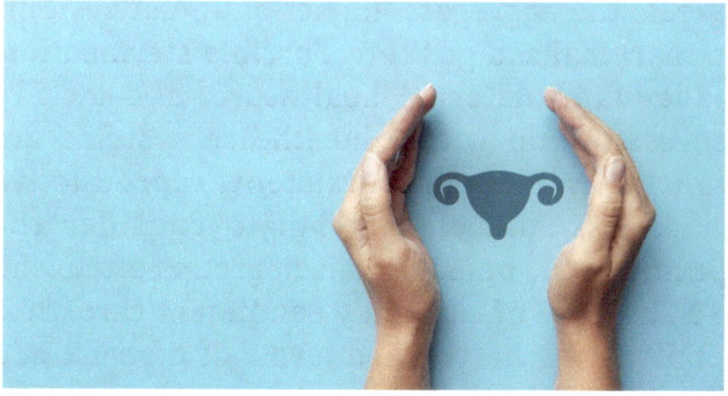

Figure 11.6. Good care of your reproductive system.

Source: https://www.toplinemd.com/ideal-women-health-care/wp-content/uploads/sites/258/2022/12/How-To-Take-Good-Care-Of-Your-Reproductive-System.jpg.

11.2.1. Availability of Services Across Different Demographics

The provided presence of reproductive health services across different populations suggests the dramatic inequities that compromise the aims of equitable care. Ethnic origin, socioeconomic status, and geographic location have a strong influence on access to essential reproductive health care services like contraception, prenatal care, and abortion. Rural areas tend to face insurmountable barriers in the shape of limited healthcare facilities, diminished healthcare providers, and a lack of specialized care, posing the risk to exacerbate poor reproductive health outcomes. The impact is further exacerbated in at-risk populations, where institutionalized race-based, gender identity-based, and socioeconomic-based disparities further exacerbate barriers to necessary care. Knowledge of these differences is essential for designing interventions that are specifically tailored to diverse populations. Access-enhancing strategies must confront resource reallocation and policy adjustments to ensure the optimum availability of services for every demographic group. Cultural practices and beliefs significantly influence the utilization of reproductive health services among diverse demographic groups. Women in traditional communities, or other religious or ethnic communities, may be stigmatized or discriminated against in receiving reproductive health care. Such a cultural environment not only influences the desirability to use services but also the type of care regarded as acceptable or appropriate. For instance, gender minority patients often face additional barriers, including a lack of providers who are competent to offer gender-affirming care, and this discourages them from seeking adequate reproductive health care. Moreover, many healthcare providers ~~usually get~~ are not educated to differentiate between sex and gender, which leads to inadequate recognition and understanding of the distinct health concerns of gender minorities. Solving these issues requires extensive training for healthcare providers to develop a more equitable environment that embraces and values the richer cultural narratives shaping patients' experiences and decisions in reproductive healthcare. The implementation of national policies aimed at enhancing the provision of reproductive health services is crucial for reducing disparities and promoting equity. Recent recommendations by organizations such as the National Academies of Sciences, Engineering, and Medicine emphasize the importance of collecting disaggregated data on sex, gender identity, and demographic factors to comprehend the barriers faced by different groups. Resources such as the SAGER guidelines have developed guidelines for inclusive data collection that can inform health practice and policy. By embracing such programs, health systems can design specialized programs that respond to the varying needs of populations, particularly those who are marginalized and face uneven access to healthcare. Not only do such programs enable correct delivery of healthcare, but they also enable improved policymaking based on the dynamics of the terrain of reproductive health, eventually establishing an environment which fosters increased health benefits for all segments of society, irrespective of demographic context (Figure 11.7).

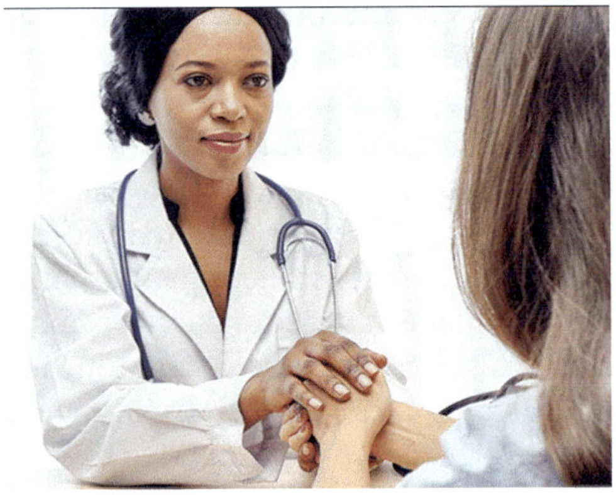

Figure 11.7. Allegheny reproductive health center.

Source: https://alleghenyreproductive.com/wp-content/uploads/2020/07/abortion-services-m.png.

11.2.2. Barriers to Access for Marginalized Genders

Understanding the barriers to access experienced by marginalized genders in reproductive health is vital to planning inclusive care approaches. Marginalized genders generally experience systemic inequities combined with socio-economic disadvantages, discriminatory mechanisms, and weak health infrastructure. Structural racism, violence against gender, and economic marginalization exist in configurations that restrict access to critical reproductive health care and lead to adverse health outcomes and deep-rooted disparities. For instance, individuals in marginalized populations may find it difficult to access family planning and contraception services by virtue of geographic, economic, or sociocultural obstacles, making their reproductive autonomy even more challenging. A thorough examination of such obstacles reveals not only the immediate health effects but also the long-term societal effects on individuals and groups of people who suffer within an unjust health system. Further, the historical context of reproductive justice reveals the aggregate impact of unjust systems on marginalized genders. Forcible sterilization, inadequate maternal healthcare, and lack of representation within healthcare systems are stark examples of persistent reproductive injustices. Policies that fail to consider the specific needs of marginalized groups often lead to a shortage of culturally competent care, thus perpetuating heightened levels of distrust and alienation from healthcare systems. The broader paradigm of reproductive justice seeks to rectify these historical injustices and offers insight into how current policies concerned with health may be revised to provide equitable access to care. By placing medicine within the context of reproductive justice values, physicians can begin to dismantle structural barriers and champion engaged, participatory involvement by the very individuals most affected by these inequalities. Finally, integrating reproductive justice-oriented education curricula into medical school education is key to educating healthcare providers on how to address the unique challenges marginalized genders face. By providing medical students with an understanding of the ethical and social determinants of health inequity, future professionals will be better positioned to advocate for complete care and enact policies that value inclusion. Emergent curricula that incorporate experiential education on the lives of marginalized genders can foster empathy and cultivate critical consciousness regarding the systems that impact reproductive health. These lines of study not only prepare medical professionals to overcome these barriers, but challenge them to reform these models of care. It is proactive in pursuing the goal of equitable reproductive healthcare where marginalized groups are not only seen as patients but also as participants in the health conversation (Ojo et al., 2022).

11.2.3. Role of Technology in Improving Service Delivery

The integration of technology in reproductive health has revolutionized delivery services, making them more efficient and accessible to diverse populations. Mobile health applications have contributed significantly to the delivery of reproductive health education and care, particularly to marginalized populations. Through smartphones and other devices, health workers can disseminate significant information about sexual and reproductive rights, family planning, and available health facilities. This increased access not only enables individuals to make their own health decisions but also provides a more egalitarian space in which women and men can access vital resources without stigma. Technology, therefore, serves to bridge the gap, bringing underserved populations to essential reproductive health care that they would otherwise miss due to geographic or social limitations. Furthermore, the technology-enhanced collection and management of data have significantly enhanced the quality of reproductive health care. Electronic health records (EHRs) enable the better tracking of patient histories and treatment outcomes, allowing medical professionals to tailor their services to the unique needs of each individual. For gender-responsive care and assessment, application of the technologies can enable crucial understanding of the usually singular issues faced by various groups, in particular women. Examination of trends and patterns in reproductive health data enables policymakers to create evidence-informed interventions that address inequities in service delivery. Such an evidence-based approach is consistent with the realities presented in Bank (2013), which indicates the central role of information in designing policies that enhance opportunities for women in core sectors, such as reproductive health. The role of technology is also best demonstrated in telehealth services, which have expanded access to reproductive health care for individuals residing in remote or underserved locations. Telehealth systems enable patients to communicate with medical experts via video conferencing, thereby reducing the need for physical mobility and associated costs. This is particularly helpful in areas where reproductive health services are scarce, enabling timely consultations, follow-ups, and health education. Moreover, telehealth can be most beneficial in solving gender-related health issues by enabling access to reproductive health care for women subtly and at convenience. These developments in service delivery underscore the need for incorporating technology into public health agendas, as emphasized in N/A (2014), to address the significance of specific policies that can effectively cope with emerging challenges in development within the context of reproductive health.

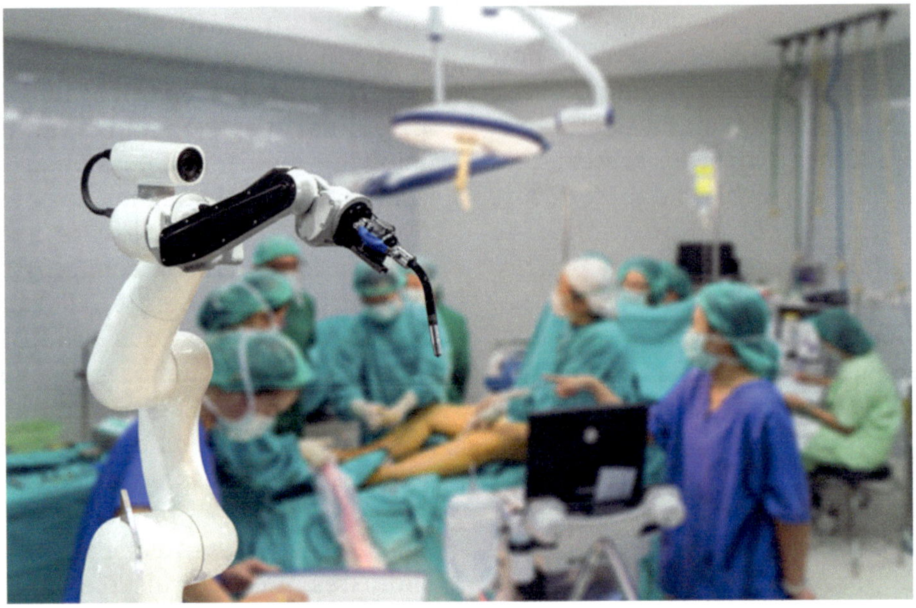

Figure 11.8. Role of technology in improving service delivery.

Source: https://www.roboticstomorrow.com/images/upload/images/Depositphotos_207824992_xl-2015.jpg.

Test Your Knowledge

1. What are some key barriers to accessing reproductive health services in underserved communities?

How have recent policy changes influenced the availability of family planning and maternal care?

11.3. Gender-Inclusive Assessment Practices

Learning Outcome

1. Explain the importance of understanding diverse gender identities
2. Define the training of healthcare providers in gender sensitivit
3. Describe the tools and methods for inclusive assessments in reproductive health

The implementation of gender-inclusive assessment strategies is most crucial within reproductive health, as it attempts to address disparities and biases that typically define traditional models of healthcare. By recognizing and addressing the varied experiences and needs of individuals along the gender spectrum, healthcare providers are able to construct a more inclusive environment. This approach not only enhances the quality of care provided but also enhances the ability of patients to be actively involved in their healthcare. For instance, the integration of gender identity and expression in the process of assessment allows practitioners to understand better the that the patients can pose, thereby improving communication and treatment interventions. Such interventions are crucial in enabling a holistic understanding of reproductive health outside the of gender, hence towards improved healthcare outcomes in all individuals irrespective of gender identity. Furthermore, collaboration in decision-making in reproductive health care has been proven to contribute significantly to the outcomes of care. Findings indicate that within settings where both partners engage actively in reproductive health care discussions, the agreement regarding access to health facilities directly affects the choice of ~~delivery~~ birth location. In Tanzania, for example, Danworth et al, (2009) found that when couples are consistent with healthcare beliefs, then there are more likely chances that women would embrace facility-based deliveries as opposed to the use of traditional birth attendants only. This emphasizes the acute necessity for healthcare professionals to engage both partners in evaluations and decision-making. From a gender-sensitive point of view, practitioners can enhance the agency of all stakeholders so that women's voices are not only heard but prioritized when it comes to making decisions regarding reproductive health, thereby influencing favorable health-related outcomes (Danforth et al., 2009). Lastly, adolescent-focused health service design and delivery play a crucial role in promoting gender-sensitive practice in reproductive health. Designing services to meet the unique needs of adolescents aged between 14-25 years is essential in effective healthcare delivery. Evidence suggests that varied models of care delivery, ranging from school-linked to community-based, have been proven to enhance the reach of care to adolescents significantly. By incorporating adolescent feedback on their healthcare needs, practitioners can create strategies that engage this age group and foster an attitude of ownership and responsibility for their reproductive health. A gender-sensitive service design approach thus not only addresses the short-term healthcare issues but also teaches adolescents to take responsibility for their reproductive health in the long run (Ryan et al., 2015) (Figure 11.9).

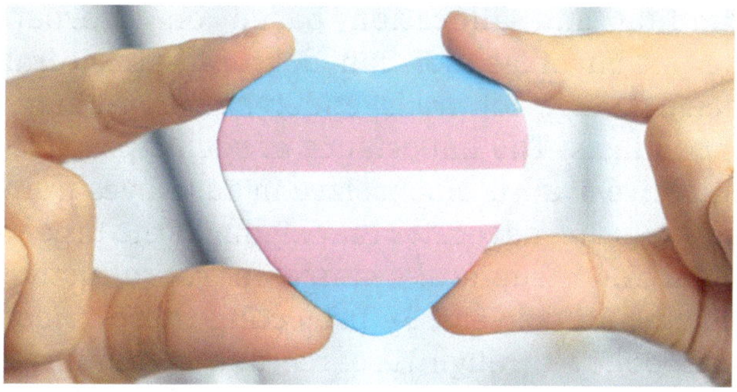

Figure 11.9. Gender-inclusive assessment practices.

Source: https://www.nursinginpractice.com/wp-content/uploads/2023/06/how-can-we-be-more-inclusive-to-transgender-patients-539x282.jpg.

11.3.1. Importance of Understanding Diverse Gender Identities

The recognition and comprehension of various gender identities are pivotal in ensuring equal and effective reproductive health care. While the traditional binary understanding of gender is no longer adequate, healthcare professionals are required to expand their knowledge to include a variety of identities beyond male and female. ~~By~~ With practitioners being open, patients can comfortably approach care, which ultimately results in better health outcomes in the long term. When examining structural causes of discrimination, it is discovered that subordinated groups usually have barriers to the provision of reproductive health services. Eliminating these barriers would involve prioritizing diverse gender identities in healthcare policies and practices, allowing for a holistic approach to reproductive health that considers the distinctive needs of all stakeholders involved. Furthermore, the effects of multiple gender identities extend to policy development and public health interventions. An awareness of how various identities intersect with social determinants of health allows for tailored interventions that are more responsive to inequalities. For instance, funding and allocation based on a broad definition of gender can decrease structural disadvantage for transgender and non-binary individuals. The importance of such a practice, inclusive of all, is emphasized in narratives from activists and advocates that highlight the urgent need for structural change in reproductive healthcare delivery. By projecting these voices into policy through research and community-level mobilization, reproductive health policies become a reflection of the circumstances that all communities face, ensuring justice and equity within healthcare settings, as highlighted in initiatives that target systemic change (Villarosa et al., 2014).

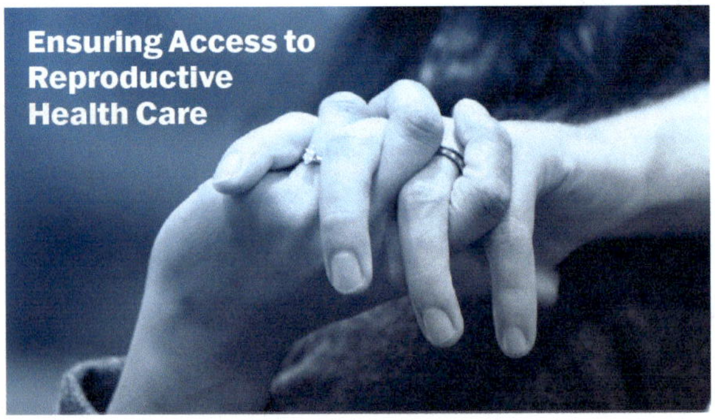

Figure 11.10. Ensuring access to reproductive health care.

Source: https://health.mil/-/media/Images/MHS/Hero-Images/Repro_Spotlight.ashx.

Also, placing diverse gender identities on the reproductive health agenda restores the significance of intersectionality in health. Intersectionality understands that individuals do not exist in isolation from identity and that intersections of variables such as race, socioeconomic status, and sexual orientation intersect with gender identity to impact health outcomes. Therefore, a comprehensive understanding of these complex intersections is necessary to deliver gender-inclusive care. Services that facilitate access to reproductive services, for example, must understand and respond to the unique barriers faced by individuals at the intersection of multiple marginalized identities. Evidence-based results indicate that identifying and intervening at these intersections leads to improved health literacy and outcomes, ultimately enabling people to advocate for their reproductive health and rights. Detailed evaluations that appreciate diverse gender identities are, therefore, central in facilitating health equity, aided by demands for reproductive health research structures to be inclusive (Locke et al., 2001) (Figure 11.10).

11.3.2. Training Healthcare Providers in Gender Sensitivity

Educating healthcare professionals in gender sensitivity is a fundamental component of enhancing reproductive health services, particularly in communities where cultural gender roles tend to impact the delivery and access to healthcare. Through the inclusion of gender sensitivity in medical training curriculum programs, healthcare professionals will be better equipped to identify and address the unique social, cultural, and psychological factors that affect patient experiences more effectively. For instance, understanding the influence of gender norms on health-seeking behavior informs more effective communication and intervention. In addition to amplifying clinical competency, this type of training provides a context where patients can hear and appreciate their voices. This holistic approach can significantly enhance patient outcomes, as it provides an opportunity for discussion about the values and desires that patients bring to their care. In addition, there are gender-sensitive training interventions that may be applied to deconstruct stereotypes present in health settings. These stereotypes usually limit the involvement of both women and men in discussions regarding family planning. For example, the CHARM intervention focuses on engaging men in family planning discussions, demonstrating that gender-focused training can lead to more equitable health practices. When health workers are trained to acknowledge the shared responsibility for reproductive health, they can constructively promote gender equality among couples, thereby eliminating barriers to access and enhancing the effectiveness of contraceptive use. By incorporating an integrated approach with both genders, the healthcare system would benefit, ultimately resulting in more effective and holistic reproductive health services. In addition to improving patient care, gender sensitivity training of healthcare workers has broader policy and practice implications for healthcare policy.

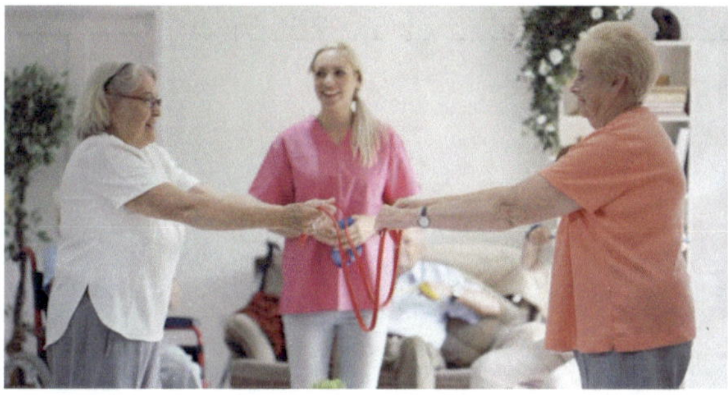

Figure 11.11. LGBTQ sensitivity training for nurses.

Source: https://terranova.org/wp-content/uploads/2020/11/UnderstandingDifferences_LGBTQ_5_womenexercising.png.

Knowledge of the intricacy of gender dynamics can inform the formulation of health programs targeted to reach the needs of groups of diverse populations, such as marginalized groups. Research indicates that women, particularly minority women, are likely to receive poor health care services that do not cater to their unique circumstances, as reflected in the research findings regarding California-based incarcerated women (N/A, 2006). By adding gender sensitivity training into the curriculum of medical education, professionals are better placed to advocate for policy change aimed at addressing areas of care deficiencies. This aligns with ongoing efforts to provide reproductive health care that is accessible and equitable to all parts of society, thereby contributing to healthier populations and reductions in healthcare disparities in access and outcomes (Figure 11.11).

11.3.3. Tools and Methods for Inclusive Assessments

Practical tools and strategies for inclusive reproductive health screenings must target the quality collection of data that addresses the various needs of various gender identities. This includes the integration of gender-sensitive surveys and focus group discussions that respond to the realities and perceptions of each member of the community, particularly vulnerable groups. Building an inclusive environment in these assessments enables a more precise identification of obstacles faced by individuals seeking reproductive health services. Additionally, the combination of quantitative measures with qualitative data can enable a more comprehensive analysis of access and satisfaction levels among different groups of people, thereby enhancing the overall level of service quality provided. Through such strategies, health service providers can identify specific service gaps and tailor interventions to provide equal access to healthcare for both men and women, thereby improving reproductive health outcomes in communities. Beyond data collection techniques, the use of gender action plans (GAP) is a key tool in designing frameworks to ensure gender equity in reproductive health programs. As shown in the Urban Primary Health Care Project, the GAP specifically identifies aims and strategies for increasing access to healthcare among women and girls, as well as for addressing gender matters more broadly. Elements of such a plan may include outreach programs targeted at specific groups, education among community members regarding reproductive health rights, and gender-sensitive training of healthcare personnel. By tracking progress systematically against the determined indicators, these action plans not only hold health systems accountable but also empower communities to demand improved services. Such frameworks need to be incorporated into reproductive health programs to create sustainable changes that effectively meet the needs of both genders, particularly in settings where inequalities are stark (Bank, 2015). Finally, innovative interventions on male involvement in family planning are excellent examples of inclusive assessments and care. The Counseling Husbands to Achieve Reproductive Health and Marital Equity (CHARM) intervention emphasizes the participation of men in the reproductive health discourse while promoting gender equity. This program promotes education and support for husbands and wives through encouraging joint decision-making around family planning and the use of contraceptives. The result of this intervention, utilizing randomized controlled study designs and multi-session programming, provides evidence of increased contraceptive use and marital equity when gender dynamics are addressed inclusively. Such programs not only improve the reproductive health environment but also facilitate realignments in cultural norms that encourage male involvement in reproductive health decision-making, thereby promoting a more holistic approach to assessment and treatment (Balaiah et al., 2016).

Test Your Knowledge

1. Why is it important to use inclusive language during reproductive health assessments?
2. How can healthcare providers create a safe environment for patients of all gender identities?

11.4. Reproductive Health Education

Learning Outcome

1. Identify the need for comprehensive sex education
2. Define the tailoring of educational materials for diverse audiences
3. Describe the role of community outreach in education

Reproductive health education is crucial in ensuring that an individual is well-informed about their reproductive choices and the health implications associated with them. Given the existing increase in knowledge about gender diversity, reproductive health education must incorporate a gender-responsive framework. Such a focus values the unique reproductive wants of various gender identities, including those of the LGBTQ+ individuals, who have historically been marginalized in matters of health. By understanding the special healthcare needs of these groups, education programs can introduce an inclusive dialogue that equips individuals to use appropriate reproductive healthcare. In addition to empowering individuals, these programs also enhance the effectiveness of healthcare systems in promoting reproductive well-being across diverse communities, as reflected in shifting demographic trends in reproductive needs (N/A, 2023). Incorporating comprehensive and adequate reproductive health education into curriculum can assist in closing gaps in care, particularly among LGBTQ populations. Evidence indicates that such groups are prone to having disparate health outcomes and experiencing higher rates of complications in the reproductive outcomes since they lack access to appropriate health services. Lesbian and bisexual women, for example, experience lower pregnancy success rates than their heterosexual counterparts (Croll et al., 2022). Moreover, transgender and non-binary people face particular challenges during pregnancy, hormone treatment, and mental illness. Educators and medical practitioners need to prioritize training courses that address these disparities, educating future healthcare professionals with the facts and compassion necessary for inclusive care. By developing an understanding of these complexities, reproductive health education can be a transformative agent in achieving equitable health results. Lastly, empowering patients through gender-responsive reproductive health education will not only enhance their healthcare experience but also increase their engagement with healthcare systems. Quality education should aim at informed consent, reproductive rights to make a choice, and the place of mental health in reproduction. As evidence illustrates that LGBTQ+ individuals often experience higher perinatal stress and mental health problems, a safe and understanding health environment is required (Croll et al., 2022). Healthcare workers must provide spaces for individuals to report their concerns and needs without fear of discrimination or prejudice. By making reproductive health education inclusive, we can help to dismantle the barriers that block access to essential reproductive health care and ultimately improve overall health outcomes for all, not just based on sexual orientation or gender identity (Figure 11.12).

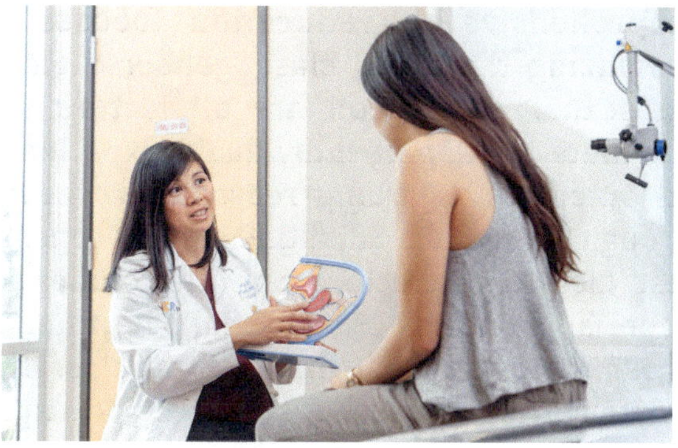

Figure 11.12. Sexual and reproductive health care services.

Source: https://health.universityofcalifornia.edu/sites/default/files/2024-08/women-student-health.jpg.

11.4.1. Need for Comprehensive Sex Education

Comprehensive sex education (CSE) is a key pillar in the encouragement of reproductive health and gender-sensitive assessment and care. Merging sex education in the context of reproductive health enables individuals to be armed with all the information regarding their bodies, sexual health, and rights. Adequate CSE not only teaches individuals about the biological aspects of reproduction but also about the emotional, social, and ethical issues involved in sexuality. This system of education provides an atmosphere of autonomy and prudent decision-making, thereby reducing the occurrence of unintended pregnancies and sexually transmitted infections (STIs) in teenagers and young adults. Furthermore, good sex education can be an effective tool for dismantling toxic stigmas of sexuality and giving an empowered voice to marginalized communities through diversity and representation in curriculum design, hence ensuring increased reproductive justice (N/A, 2023). The implementation of CSE in the classroom is also important in tackling the inequality faced by historically excluded communities. Intersectional comprehensive sex education focuses on recognizing that race, class, gender identity, and sexual orientation are all factors that contribute to shaping individuals' experiences and outcomes regarding reproductive health. Through curriculum adjustments that consider these factors, instructors can offer students a deeper appreciation of the social determinants responsible for producing inequalities. This analytical framework aligns with the principles of reproductive justice, which aim to ensure equal access to reproductive health services for all individuals, particularly those in vulnerable circumstances (Ojo et al., 2022). In this regard, proper sex education is not just an educational requirement but also an ethical imperative to ensure that all individuals have the knowledge and means at their disposal to make decisions regarding their reproductive health.

The need for CSE transcends the typical school environment, necessitating modification of societal attitudes towards sexual health. Public health initiatives and community programs are vital for disseminating CSE to a diverse array of people, thereby solidifying the perception that sexual health is integral to overall well-being. Moreover, as disinformation is found on numerous media platforms, successful outreach can counteract such propaganda with correct and affirming reproductive health data, fostering healthier relationships and improved health. Significantly, in-depth sex education addresses the specific issues of LGBTQ+ communities, creating an environment of respect and acceptance that encourages frank communication regarding sexual health. All these combined unlock the way for a healthier society, where comprehensive sex education is recognized as an inalienable right, not an indulgence, ultimately leading to improved reproductive health outcomes (Ojo et al., 2022) (Figure 11.13).

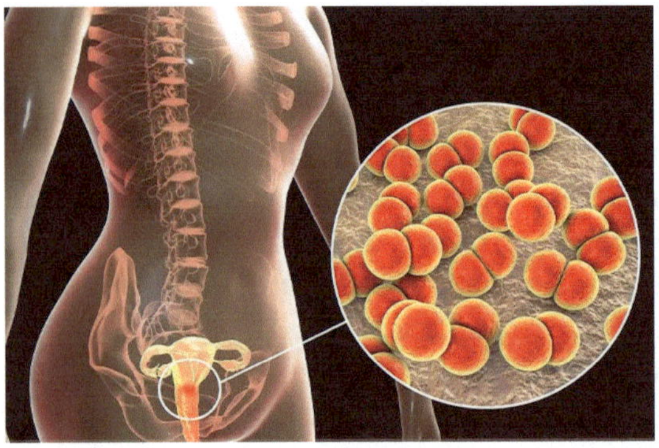

Figure 11.13. Sexually transmitted diseases (STDs).

Source: https://images.medicinenet.com/images/Article/main_image/female-gonorrhea-ovaries-medical-concept-illustration-rendering.jpg?output-quality=75.

11.4.2. Tailoring Educational Materials for Diverse Audiences

In reproductive health education, tailoring materials to suit various audiences is essential to prevent exclusivity and achieve effectiveness. This tailoring considers the reality that individuals have varying backgrounds, each with its own set of cultural, social, and educational contexts that shape their understanding of reproductive health. For example, educational materials need to address the specific needs of the oppressed women of color or LGBTQ+ by providing culturally relevant information and perspective. Tailoring it not only enhances knowledge but also confidence and engagement, ultimately leading to better health. By employing a range of formats—ranging from interactive workshops to paper-based materials and electronic media—teachers can reach diverse populations and foster understanding across demographic lines, thereby creating a more inclusive foundation for reproductive health education. Additionally, the use of multiple educational approaches can significantly enhance the impact of disseminating reproductive health information. Employing case studies enables the use of teaching methods in field contexts. As explained in Abrash et al. (2011), effective communication within the arena of social problem documentaries relies on design to address specific audiences, explaining how specifically designed learning materials can engage them effectively. Through these specialized approaches, instructors can craft messages that directly address their audiences, trigger responses specific to unique beliefs across cultures, avoid linguistic conflicts, and appeal to various levels of existing knowledge. This not only facilitates active engagement but also allows for group discussion, where students can interact and share experiences in a safe environment.

This critical thinking is essential because it enables the realization of people's ability to make own choices over their reproductive health, which encourages informed decisions. In addition, the intersection of reproductive health education and social environments, such as poverty and resource availability, underscores the importance of an integrated approach to curriculum adaptation. The presentation of reproductive health within the framework of socioeconomic disparities highlights the need for teachers to integrate contextual data that addresses actual issues encountered by different communities. As cited in N/A (2003), the cycle of poverty across generations has the potential to widen health disparities, and thus, there is a necessity for resources that not only educate but also advocate for change at the system level. With the inclusion of advocacy components, teachers can spark a movement towards enhancing reproductive health care accessible to all, regardless of their socioeconomic status. Ultimately, a well-rounded and inclusive education system fosters a greater level of awareness about reproductive health, enabling communities and individuals to make informed health choices and advocate for broader social change.

11.4.3. Role of Community Outreach in Education

Community outreach is a key component of the educational landscape, particularly in reproductive health, where decision-making must be grounded in accurate knowledge. Outreach is what fills the gaps that separate health systems from local societies, and is especially needed in low and middle-income countries (LMICs) where access to health care is most often blocked by socio-economic barriers. By facilitating direct interaction between communities—through workshops, educational sessions, and collaboration with local leaders—reproductive health education can be tailored to the specific cultural and contextual needs of different populations. Such initiatives empower people, particularly women and vulnerable groups, to access care and claim their health rights, thereby easing trust building between providers and communities. As discussed in the section on fair health systems, establishing such trust is crucial for any long-term improvement in health outcomes (Kruk et al., 2018). Outreach in the community is also a key factor in surmounting the challenges different populations experience for reproductive health education. Groups who are marginalized, including women and adolescents who are in insecure environments, are likely to experience disproportionately poor health outcomes because they have limited available information and resources. Effective outreach programs increase access to educational materials and also encourage gender-sensitive care practices that are responsive to the needs of diverse populations. Engaging community health workers educated in indigenous traditions and vernaculars supports better communication as well as the reinforcement of key health information. Furthermore, such programs can maximize the participation of communities, leading to greater advocacy for reproductive health care services and policies aligned with the interests of all individuals, particularly the marginalized by conventional health systems (N/A, 2018). Lastly, the sustainability of outreach programs in communities depends on establishing long-term partnerships with educational institutions, governments, and non-profit organizations. Collaborative practice ensures the sharing of resources and assured constant interaction with the served populations, leading to healthier education systems. Medical schools can become invaluable by integrating outreach into education, so the future generation of health professionals prioritizes community needs and participation in their work. This extension of the education strategy, along with strengthening the knowledge base for reproductive health, fosters a culture of shared learning and responsibility in both healthcare systems and communities. Institutionalizing these connections advances the agenda of gender-sensitive care, ultimately resulting in more equitable, resilient, and responsive health systems that meet the health and education needs of everyone (Kruk et al., 2018) (Figure 11.14).

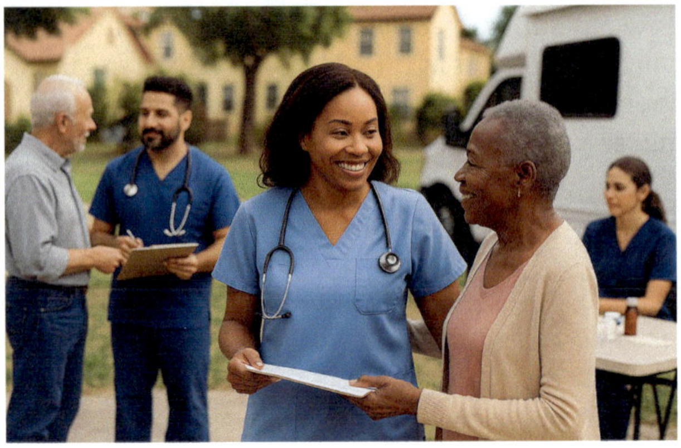

Figure 11.14. Role of community outreach in education.

Source: https://ceufast.com/imgs/community-outreach-blog.jpg.

Test Your Knowledge

1. How does comprehensive reproductive health education benefit adolescents?
2. Why is it important to include consent and healthy relationships in reproductive health curricula?

11.5. Policy and Advocacy for Gender-Inclusive Care

Learning Outcome

1. Describe the current reproductive health policies
2. Define the advocacy efforts for inclusive legislation
3. Discuss the role of non-profit organizations in policy change

Policy development advancing gender-inclusive care is necessary to reverse the disparities in reproductive health outcomes. Systemic barriers have been sustained through the historical marginalization of LGBTQ+ communities, and these sustain health inequities. Ongoing advocacy efforts aim to address these inequities by implementing practices that acknowledge and affirm diverse gender identities. Legislative measures, such as the Equality Act, aim to enhance antidiscrimination protection in healthcare settings, ensuring that gender-diverse individuals are treated fairly and receive necessary services. Those efforts must include comprehensive training for healthcare professionals to decrease prejudices and enhance their knowledge of gender diversity, thereby developing a culturally competent healthcare system. The merging of policy with advocacy work is a strong tool for fighting against the stigmatization of LGBTQ+ identities and subsequently advancing the quality of reproductive health care for everybody, regardless of their gender identity (N/A, 2023). The inclusion of gender-inclusive care in health policy frameworks also entails insight into the intersectionality of identities. LGBTQ+ populations also experience intersectional discrimination based on gender, race, and socioeconomic status that needs targeted interventions in their care. Intersectional thinking is integrated into policies to effectively dismantle structural barriers as well as promote holistic health outcomes. Data collection, including disaggregation of health statistics by gender identity and sexual orientation, is needed to recognize the targeted health issues faced by these populations. By ensuring that research informs policy directly, healthcare systems can create more just solutions that consider the specific needs of marginalized groups. Through this, good policy and advocacy can lead to drastic changes within healthcare environments, promoting inclusive practices that ultimately result in enhanced reproductive health outcomes for all, particularly for those who are gender-diverse (Soled et al., 2022). Finally, ongoing education and public advocacy campaigns are essential to sustain the development of gender-inclusive care policy. With shifts in societal attitudes toward the LGBTQ+ population, health care professionals and policy-makers must continually be educated about new concerns and practices in gender inclusivity. Training health professionals can help facilitate better sexual and gender minority understanding through respectful practice of care and communication that takes into consideration the profound disparities these populations have. Community engagement programs can also facilitate LGBTQ+ individuals in asserting their own health needs, giving them a voice in policy creation. As the face of reproductive health keeps evolving, sustained advocacy and policy reforms are needed to create an inclusive health care system that supports the rights and needs of all individuals and forges a favorable environment where equitable health care becomes the norm (Soled et al., 2022; N/A, 2023) (Figure 11.15).

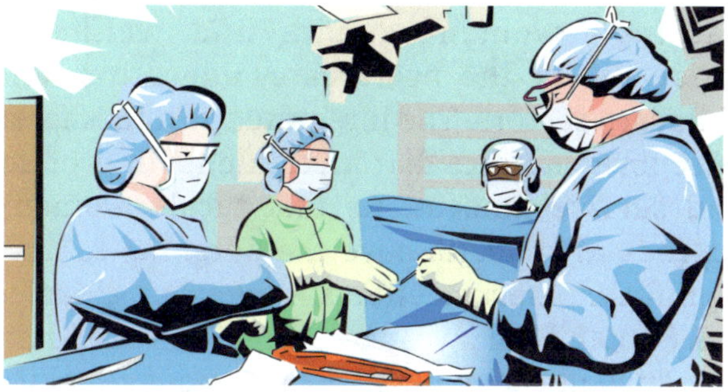

Figure 11.15. Perioperative care of the transgender and gender-diverse patient.

Source: https://aornjournal.onlinelibrary.wiley.com/cms/asset/18472c0a-205e-46eb-9df3-fee541c9d74f/aorn14242-gra-0007-m.jpg.

11.5.1. Overview of Current Reproductive Health Policies

The contemporary landscape in reproductive health policies is complex and often shaped by diverse socio-political realities. Most countries are embarking on significant reforms to improve access to reproductive health services, especially for marginalized groups. Policymakers are increasingly appreciating the imperative of having gender-sensitive analyses that can determine obstacles women and gender minorities may encounter in accessing reproductive services. This transition to inclusion is not only set to foster equal health outcomes but also to confront those ingrained system inequalities that have been present in healthcare systems for years. In addition, the rise of initiatives that champion reproductive health demonstrates a greater commitment to sustainable development, particularly with respect to United Nations Sustainable Development Goal 5, which aims to attain gender equality and empower all women and girls, thereby prompting governments to assess policies from a gender perspective. Investment in reproductive health is also gaining increased scrutiny as a key driver towards attaining gender equality. Reports say that there is significant scope for investors to match their portfolios to gender-sensitive investments, backing women's health and wellbeing, especially in the healthcare, education, and childcare sectors. The integrated results shared in reports indicate that investments in product and service innovations that tackle women's reproductive health have the potential to have significant market effects, valued at close to U.S. $300 billion a year by 2025. Such economic statistics not only highlight the money-making potential of gender-lens investing but also point to the social imperative of investing in healthcare systems that benefit women directly, such as those that enhance access to family planning and related services. Thus, reproductive health policy is more and more linked to economic opportunities that promote gender equality and women's empowerment, with a consequent favorable climate for long-term investment. The gender and development approach, over the past several decades, has provided the foundation for improvements in reproductive health policy globally in major institutions such as the World Bank. The Banks Gender Equality as Smart Economics program highlights that mainstreaming gender in economic development plans is not only a moral obligation but an economic imperative. Drawing from experience with previous applications of gender action plans, policies are being streamlined to meet the specific reproductive health needs of varying populations. The political commitment to the forceful implementation of gender policies in these development frameworks emphasizes the significant role played by global finance and organizational aid in determining reproductive health outcomes. As institutions promote advancement through focused funding and policy measures, they also help break down institutional barriers that prevent access to reproductive health services, ultimately resulting in healthier, more equitable communities.

11.5.2. Advocacy Efforts for Inclusive Legislation

Advocacy campaigns for equal reproductive health legislation play a critical role in helping to promote equal access to related healthcare services among all people in society, regardless of their gender identity or socio-economic status. Advocacy campaigns are crucial in shaping public policy, legislative change, and awareness regarding gender disparities in health outcomes. By means of inclusive policy advocacy, organizations aim to eradicate structural barriers that often marginalize groups of individuals, above all, women and non-binary individuals. Campaigns and community outreach programs advocate for the recognition of diverse reproductive health needs and ensuring that these needs are addressed in health policies. This priority aligns with the regulations outlined in guidelines such as the UN Development Assistance Framework, which prioritizes human rights and gender equality in policy-making efforts to enhance health impact among marginalized groups (N/A, 2014). The call for inclusive lawmaking with a gender focus extends beyond reproductive healthcare, encompassing broader socioeconomic determinants that influence accessibility and equity. Various lobbying groups focus on the connection between equitable growth and economic empowerment, the latter of which is seen as a key factor in promoting women's health. A case in point is the G20 commitment to remove barriers preventing women's participation in the economy, an action that builds upon the interdependence of inclusive growth and improved health (N/A). As women gain access to education, secure jobs, and healthcare, they are in a much better position to become masters of their own reproductive health. Advocacy in this context aims to integrate gender-sensitive policies into economic policy, thereby promoting reproductive health rights, economic well-being, and social well-being. In connecting public health objectives with economic empowerment, advocates aim to create an integrated system that addresses the intersectionality of health and gender. Additionally, sustained advocacy for enabling laws entails the coordination of efforts among multiple stakeholders, such as the government, civil society organizations, and community leaders. Multi-sector collaboration ensures an interdisciplinary understanding of the various determinants that influence reproductive health outcomes, enabling more impactful policy interventions. From the realization that emerges from advocacy, legislation can be crafted that reflects the realities faced by excluded populations. In addition, effective monitoring and evaluation systems are required in such advocacy to enable stakeholders to establish the effect of the policies implemented and correct them accordingly. Therefore, fostering a culture of inclusion in the legislative process is the most important step toward achieving equal reproductive health outcomes for all, demonstrating that promoting public health is not merely a legal exercise but a moral imperative (N/A, 2014) (Figure 11.16).

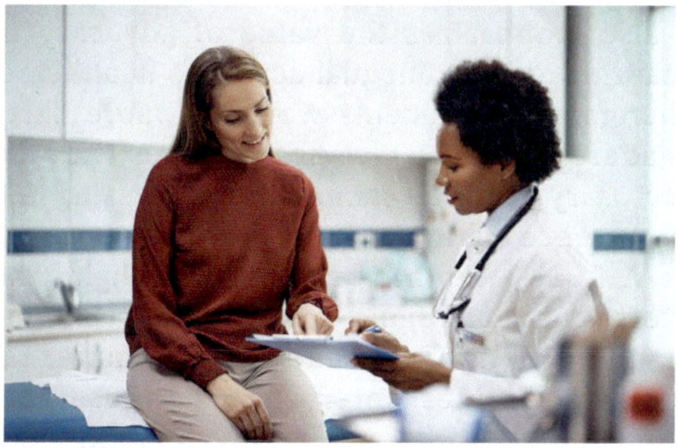

Figure 11.16. New research shows higher risk of reproductive disorders for women.

Source: https://celiac.org/wp-content/uploads/2024/04/Womens-Health-iStock-1461330630-768x512.jpg.

11.5.3. Role of Non-Profit Organizations in Policy Change

Non-profit organizations play a crucial role in initiating policy reform campaigns to promote reproductive health and gender-sensitive care. Through grassroots mobilization, the organizations make sure that marginalized communities are heard in policy forums and included in policy debates. By applying evidence-based research and sharing information, they create awareness about the need for diverse, gender-inclusive reproductive healthcare. For instance, women's health centers commonly collaborate with schools of learning to gather evidence supporting the positive impacts of access to complete reproductive care. Their findings highlight not just individual health improvements but also enhanced society-wide health benefits, thus providing a robust argument for policymakers to enact legislative measures necessary primarily to eliminate barriers to healthcare delivery. In the context of non-profit activism, the pragmatic use of partnerships enhances policy activities. By engaging in collaboration with various constituencies, such as government agencies, healthcare providers, and community-based organizations, nonprofits are in a position to create multifaceted strategies to address the complex realities of reproductive health issues. Through coalition building, they tap on collective resources and expertise, making themselves heard in policy circles. Policies closely aligned with the United Nations' Sustainable Development Goals (SDGs) underscore the interconnectedness of gender equity and sustainable health outcomes as a compelling policy argument. As seen by evidence, women's equal access to reproductive health resources not only ensures their own well-being but allows for the health of society to be sustained, which requires a broad policy lens (Herklotz et al., 2012). Moreover, non-state actors can engage in lobbying activities specifically targeting legislative organs to push for reproductive health reforms. Through mobilization of public opinion and via social media platforms, the mentioned non-state organizations can influence policymakers to accept gender-sensitive appraisal and treatment on their agendas. United Nations member states' adoption of the 2030 Agenda for Sustainable Development is proof of an international movement towards solving differences, including those regarding women's reproductive rights. In this respect, non-profits play a crucial role as intermediaries that translate global agendas into local actions that resonate within communities. Through their consistent advocacy, they shape policies that not only safeguard reproductive health rights but also aid in the realization of global goals towards poverty reduction and equality promotion (Austin-Evelyn et al., 2017).

Test Your Knowledge

1. How can healthcare policies promote equitable access to care for gender-diverse individuals?
2. Why is advocacy important in advancing gender-inclusive practices in reproductive health?

11.6. Case Studies of Successful Gender-Inclusive Programs

Learning Outcome

1. Describe the examining reproductive health across various countries
2. Define the analysis of program outcomes in gender-inclusive reproductive health
3. Identify the lessons learned and best practices of gender-inclusive reproductive health care

In seeking out successful gender-responsive programs, it is essential to identify diverse initiatives that prioritize reproductive health as a fundamental human right. A model case can be cited in curricula practice that places reproductive justice (RJ) at the forefront and strives to address systemic inequalities and historical injustices experienced by vulnerable populations. For instance, a case-based, interactive curriculum aimed at medical students has shown significant impacts on enhancing trainees' sensitivity to reproductive injustices and improving their understanding of complex socio-political health determinants of outcomes. Not only does this new model of instruction promote greater awareness of the unique vulnerabilities of various groups, but it also emphasizes the value of advocacy in guarding against unequal access to healthcare. Therefore, the students would be more likely to address reproductive health issues with the necessary cultural competence, stressing the importance of RJ in future clinical practice (N/A, 2023). Another case study highlights the effectiveness of gender-sensitive interventions in identifying and addressing maternal health disparities. Interventions whose goal is to improve access to family planning and equitable prenatal care have been instrumental in lessening maternal morbidity and mortality for historically disenfranchised women. These interventions involve the use of community health workers who are from the targeted population, thereby creating trust and enhancing patient-provider interaction. Applications of culturally responsive models of care offer the possibility of tailored educational materials that address the unique concerns and interests of different populations. The model highlights the convergence of social, economic, and environmental factors on reproductive health, aligning with the call for inclusive processes in planning and implementing programs (N/A, 2023). Additionally, successful gender-inclusive programs have been found to have a tangible impact in fueling the participation of underrepresented genders in reproductive health research.

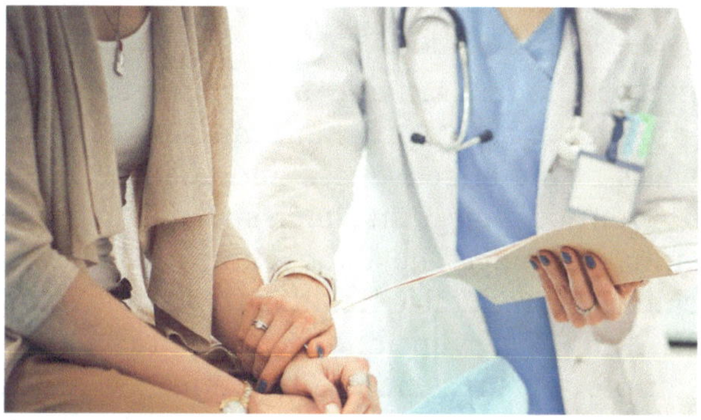

Figure 11.17. Reproductive health & justice.

Source: https://lwvfl.org/wp-content/uploads/2021/03/01-LWVFL-Reproductive-Health.jpg.

By intentionally planning frameworks with an appreciation of gender diversity, researchers are in a position to bridge gaps in information focused on the particular reproductive health concerns of diverse gender groups. Such an approach fosters cooperation among researchers, community stakeholders, and policy proponents in ways that ensure diverse perspectives are integrated into health research agendas. The emphasis on participatory research enhances the validity of outcomes and engages communities in the development of health interventions that are grounded in their realities. As these methods continue to advance, there is a need to maintain the momentum in promoting inclusive practices that will ultimately result in improved reproductive health outcomes for all, regardless of gender identity (Ojo et al., 2022) (Figure 11.17).

11.6.1. Examples From Various Countries

When reproductive health is examined across various countries, striking disparities in access and care are found, reflecting varying cultural traditions and political policies. Sweden, for instance, offers augmented reproductive health services characterized by open-ended policies focused on accessibility and education. Such models ensure the delivery of timely and non-discriminatory services to people irrespective of their gender identity, essentially providing not only physical health needs but emotional well-being as well. On the other hand, those countries with restrictive reproductive health policies tend to reinforce health disparities. For example, various parts of the United States still have ongoing debates concerning reproductive rights that disproportionately impact marginalized constituents by and significant owing to political dynamics and cultural stigmas. This dichotomy mirrors the important role that governmental systems play in dictating reproductive health access and underscores the need for gender-sensitive assessments that embrace all under health systems, as seen in N/A (2023). Reproductive health services globally have a trend of embracing inclusion that is far different from work being done in most regions. Others, such as Canada, have gender-sensitive frameworks that attempt to counter the odds that confront LGBTQ+ communities. The incorporation of sexual orientation and gender identity (SOGI) data collection into health policy indicates increased awareness of the particular challenges of these communities. Such a measure allows more targeted data, which in turn can be used to inform more targeted services. On the other hand, Poland depicts a striking example where new legislation threatens not only reproductive rights but also the overall health and dignity of gender and sexual minorities. The conflicting examples are indicative that, despite advancements, there remain considerable setbacks in attaining fair reproductive health care, as contended in Soled et al. (2022). The work of reproductive health and gender sensitivity is made even more complex by sociocultural determinants that vary internationally. In nations such as India, where gender and reproduction are deeply influenced by cultural values, negotiating healthcare systems becomes particularly difficult for gender-diverse populations.

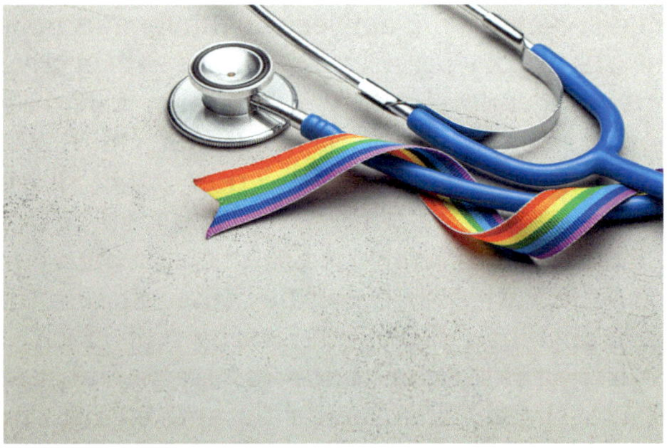

Figure 11.18. LGBTQ-inclusive health care.

Source: https://external-content.duckduckgo.com/iu/?u=https%3A%2F%2Fbcbstwelltuned.com%2Fwp-content%2Fuploads%2F2022%2F06%2FGettyImages-1177401202-scaled-e1654711176708.jpg&f=1&nofb=1&ipt=4a672b8e31df75759d7fd3fd26ab0c2ee874f0f001a598cdef1597e234fd45d2.

Strengthening the comprehension of gender-inclusive health care is essential to changing entrenched societal norms and advancing integrative care. Conversely, countries like New Zealand have adopted models that actively incorporate the views of marginalized groups into policymaking for health, thereby developing environments in which reproductive healthcare is tailored to meet diverse needs. These practices are themselves models with which other countries are striving to comply in a quest to eradicate health disparities and extend all members, regardless of gender identity, necessary reproductive health care. Achieving these goals requires ongoing collaboration and advocacy in creating a more balanced global health framework, with a focus on the importance of gender-sensitive assessments in reproductive services, as presented in Soled et al. (2022) (Figure 11.18).

11.6.2. Analysis of Program Outcomes

Outcome measurement of gender-sensitive reproductive health programs measure essential results of the effectiveness and adaptability of interventions targeting men's engagement in family planning. The Counseling Husbands to Achieve Reproductive Health and Marital Equity (CHARM) intervention is the paradigmatic example of this model through its multi-session delivery and targeting of both the male attendants and their spouses. A review of the program across a demographically heterogeneous rural population within Maharashtra, India, yields significant findings. The intervention design, which involved gender equity counseling, successfully addressed long-standing cultural norms of family planning decision-making. The data obtained through surveys and pregnancy testing identified not only changes in the use of contraception but also changes in marriage relationships as they relate to reproductive responsibilities. These factors are crucial in informing evidence-based interventions that will be integrated into the fabric of society and meet the needs of the rural population, thereby contributing to increased program success. Moreover, compliance with the intervention protocol in the process assessment also supports the program's implementation and effects on participants' involvement. The fact that there was a positive response to CHARM sessions, as indicated by husbands, wives, and village health providers (VHPs), bears witness to the importance of direct involvement and open communication in enhancing reproductive health. In-depth interviews conducted at the 18-month mark enabled an in-depth exploration of the participant's experience, highlighting successes and pitfalls. Qualitative feedback to this quantitative data suggests the worth of an extended evaluation strategy in determining program effectiveness. Through understanding how well the constituents align with the program's themes, subsequent iterations can be fashioned to address the needs of communities more effectively, and in so doing, further the replication of gender-inclusive reproductive health efforts. The relevance of such integrated program assessments also extends beyond immediate reproductive health implications and may encompass wider gender equity strategies. As seen in the World Bank Group's Gender Equality as Smart Economics (GAP) strategic frameworks, analysis of results from gender-targeted programs can provide lessons that are invaluable and help inform future policy decisions. The evidence built up from analyzing programs like CHARM can assist in reconstructing the functioning models for integrating gender considerations into health policy. This convergence can then be used to enhance the efficiency of reproductive health programs globally, promoting synergistic benefits in gender and development. Thus, a sound analysis not only highlights the direct benefits of such programs but also advances the debate on the necessity of integrating gender perspectives into public health programs, ensuring that everyone is engaged and empowered.

11.6.3. Lessons Learned and Best Practices

In the pursuit of gender-sensitive reproductive health care, several key lessons have been learned that underscore the importance of inclusive stakeholder engagement. Interacting with various voices, especially marginalized groups, creates a better awareness of the special challenges they experience in terms of reproductive health. Such stakeholders' feedback helps in pinpointing loopholes within the available services, and ensure that policies remain responsive to the needs of both genders. For instance, Generations Ahead's intervention in addressing social justice challenges surrounding genetic technologies gave positive lessons from stakeholders that revealed the significance of participatory discussion in developing effective health policies (N/A, 2012). By focusing on stakeholder engagement, reproductive health programs can create environments that not only address specific health issues for individuals but also promote greater social equity, leading to more effective and sustainable health interventions. Yet another important lesson that is learned relates to the mainstreaming of gender perspectives into health policy and programming. The lessons from the World Bank Group's Gender Equality as Smart Economics action plan serve to highlight this well (N/A, 2010). By integrating gender analysis into Bank instruments and frameworks, institutions can pre-emptively identify and address gender-specific health inequalities. It not only makes reproductive health services more efficient but also shifts the focus of health programs from mere service delivery to establishing an equitable health environment. Some of the best practices in this regard include the adoption of gender-responsive budgeting, the introduction of key performance indicators with a focus on gender equity, and regular impact monitoring that takes into consideration the different experiences of all genders. In achieving this, health systems are able to effectively leverage the power of gender-sensitive policies to improve overall health outcomes. Lastly, the need for constant review and re-adjustment of reproductive health programs is a lesson that cannot be overlooked. The dynamism of gender issues and health trends necessitates the adaptive implementation of policies and the delivery of services. Reproductive health programs must have mechanisms for periodic review so that changes are made in good time based on emerging needs and users' feedback. The culture of constant improvement ensures best practices based on established effectiveness in practice, ultimately enhancing the quality and accessibility of services provided. In addition, open reporting of evaluation findings and lessons gained can help build the broader knowledge base so that other organizations can implement evidence of practical approaches. By establishing a culture of learning and adaptation, reproductive health programs can remain sensitive and effective amid the continually changing context of gender-sensitive care.

Test Your Knowledge

1. What key strategies contributed to the success of a gender-inclusive healthcare program you have studied?
2. How did community involvement enhance the effectiveness of a gender-inclusive initiative?

SUMMARY

The examination of reproductive health from a gender-sensitive viewpoint emphasizes the need to emphasize the undeniable link between gender equality and health results. The United Nations' 2030 Agenda for Sustainable Development emphasizes that the world's biggest challenges have interconnected solutions, recognizing the transformative potential of this agenda in the lives of girls and women everywhere (Austin-Evelyn et al., 2017). By advocating for gender-sensitive care practices and evaluations, health systems can address the distinct needs of diverse populations, ultimately improving reproductive health outcomes in the long run. This suggests that advocating for gender equity is not merely a moral imperative; it is also necessary to improve health statistics and ensure equitable access to care for both genders. Besides, the empirical evidence gathered from interventions to promote men's involvement in family planning illustrates the necessity of integrating male participation in reproductive health services. As discovered by the study from rural India, programs focusing on gender equity counseling are linked to more informed decision-making, which leads to improved use of contraceptive methods and low rates of unintended pregnancies (Balaiah et al., 2016). These findings only further reinforce the imperative importance of reaching out to the social dynamics of reproductive health because male involvement has the potential to revolutionize the complexion of family planning. By engaging men in discussions about reproductive health, we can establish an enabling environment that promotes shared decision-making and ultimately leads to healthier families and communities. Overall, enhancing reproductive health through gender-sensitive diagnosis and treatment demands a holistic approach that tackles systemic barriers alongside encouraging collaboration between genders. An understanding of gender roles, particularly in multicultural environments, plays a crucial role in developing effective health policies and programs. As we strive to achieve comprehensive reproductive health solutions, the spirit of inclusivity must be upheld to hear and heed every voice in the discussion about reproductive health. The inclusive method possesses the transformative ability not only to align with the Sustainable Development Goals but also to craft a future where everyone has equal access to reproductive healthcare, regardless of gender.

The reproductive health discourse has increasingly acknowledged the need for gender-sensitive assessment and treatment. The fundamental point is that infrastructure directly impacts exposure to reproductive health care, particularly for women. The traditional masculine-dominated models ignore some of the demands and decisions of women, which presents a barrier blocking their empowerment and well-being. Weak infrastructure could exacerbate safety concerns and limit women's agency, thus necessitating that policymakers integrate gender concerns into health systems. (OECD, 2021) Such an observation suggests that providing more voice to women's views on healthcare infrastructure would be key to creating a space that increases reproductive health equity. Moreover, education is an area that needs to be discussed, especially concerning the LGBTQIA+ population. Health disparities impacting this group are staggering, and there are significant gaps in sexual orientation and gender identity education in medical education in pediatric clinical settings. More recent initiatives, such as resident and faculty workshops, aim to equip healthcare providers with the proper training to address disparities. Through a train-the-trainer model, these programs address both clinical skills and the necessity of educating the future healthcare provider. (Paul et al., 2021) Such educational interventions are instrumental in advancing culturally competent care and developing a safe healthcare environment that respects diverse identities across reproductive health services. Finally, the recognition of sexual orientation- and gender identity-based health disparities requires a complete overhaul of medical school curricula. The integration of gender-inclusive practices into medical education can have a direct impact on patient outcomes. As medical professionals become more skilled at addressing reproductive health concerns in LGBTQIA+ environments, they are also better positioned as patient advocates. Workshops that are structured to reach clinical practitioners and educators, focusing on practice and knowledge gaps, are critical to closing these gaps. Such lasting development in these learning settings will enable tomorrow's healthcare professionals to react to reproductive health in a well-informed manner that focuses on inclusivity and respect for all identities, ultimately striving for health equity in outcomes for all (Paul et al., 2021)

KEY TERMS FROM THIS CHAPTER

- Consent and confidentiality
- Culturally competent care
- Gender dysphoria
- Hormone replacement therapy (HRT)
- LGBTQIA+ health
- Pap smear
- Prostate examination
- Sexual health education
- STI screening
- Contraceptive counseling
- Fertility assessment
- Gender identity
- Inclusive language
- Menstrual health
- Prenatal care
- Reproductive rights
- Sexual orientation
- Transgender health

CRITICAL THINKING QUESTIONS

1. **What is a key principle of gender-inclusive reproductive health care?**
   a. Avoid discussing gender identity to prevent discomfort
   b. Use only binary gender language in documentation
   c. Provide respectful, affirming care regardless of gender identity
   d. Refer all nonbinary patients to mental health services
2. **Which of the following best reflects inclusive language in reproductive health documentation?**
   a. "Women's health visit"
   b. "Male reproductive exam"
   c. "Annual reproductive health screening"
   d. "Gynecology visit for female patient"
3. **Why is it important to ask about a patient's chosen name and pronouns?**
   a. It helps verify insurance information
   b. It improves cultural humility and promotes patient dignity
   c. It is required by law in all clinics
   d. It avoids having to use medical terminology
4. **Which of the following should a nurse prioritize during a reproductive health assessment with a transgender patient?**
   a. Assuming their reproductive organs match their gender identity
   b. Asking only questions listed in the standard form
   c. Explaining why each question is being asked and ensuring comfort
   d. Referring them to another provider
5. **What is one barrier that gender-diverse individuals often face in accessing reproductive health care?**
   a. Free health services
   b. Long clinic hours
   c. Stigma and lack of provider training
   d. Easy access to care

Short Answer Questions

1. What does gender-inclusive care mean in reproductive health settings?
2. Why is it important to ask for a patient's pronouns during assessment?
3. List two barriers gender-diverse individuals may face in reproductive healthcare.
4. How can inclusive language be used in documenting reproductive health visits?
5. What is one way nurses can make clinical environments more welcoming for LGBTQ+ patients?
6. Discuss the importance of gender-affirming communication in reproductive health care and its impact on patient outcomes.
7. Describe the steps a nurse should take when conducting a reproductive health assessment with a nonbinary patient.

Answers to Critical Thinking Questions

1. (c) 2. (c) 3. (b) 4. (c) 5. (c).

REFERENCES

1. Abrash, B., & Clark, J. (2011). *Social Justice Documentary: Designing for Impact.* https://core.ac.uk/download/71357451.pdf (accessed on 30th June 2025).
2. Amorim-Maia, A. T., Anguelovski, I., Chu, E., & Connolly, J. (2021). Intersectional climate justice: A conceptual pathway for bridging adaptation planning, transformative action, and social equity. *Urban Climate, 41*, 101053. https://doi.org/10.1016/j.uclim.2021.101053Asian Development Bank. (2013). *Gender Equality in The Labor Market in the Philippines.* https://core.ac.uk/download/19523858.pdf (accessed on 30th June 2025).
3. Asian Development Bank. (2015). *Gender Equality Results Case Study–Bangladesh: Second Urban Primary Health Care Project.* https://core.ac.uk/download/33606861.pdf (accessed on 30th June 2025).
4. Austin-Evelyn, K., & Wood, S. Y. (2017). *Power Lessons: Women's Advocacy and the 2030 Agenda.* https://core.ac.uk/download/80511059.pdf (accessed on 30th June 2025).
5. Averbach, S., Battala, M., Begum, S., Bharadwaj, P., et al. (2019). A gender synchronized family planning intervention for married couples in rural India: Study protocol for the CHARM2 cluster randomized controlled trial evaluation. https://core.ac.uk/download/323064081.pdf (accessed on 30th June 2025).
6. Bhat, U. S., Hegde, V. N., Kosgi, S., Pai, K., et al. (2011). Women reproductive rights in India: Prospective future. https://core.ac.uk/download/pdf/332897.pdf (accessed on 30th June 2025).
7. Croll, J., Sanapo, L., & Bourjeily, G. (2022). LGBTQ+ individuals and pregnancy outcomes: A commentary. *BJOG: An International Journal of Obstetrics & Gynecology, 129*, 1625–1629. https://doi.org/10.1111/1471-0528.17131 (accessed on 30th June 2025).
8. Danforth, E. J., Galea, S., Kruk, M. E., Mbaruku, G., et al. (2009). Household decision-making about delivery in health facilities: Evidence from Tanzania. https://core.ac.uk/download/pdf/11306866.pdf (accessed on 30th June 2025).
9. Davis, H., Assaf, G., McCorkell, L., Wei, H., Low, R., Re'em, Y., Redfield, S., et al. (2021). Characterizing long COVID in an international cohort: 7 months of symptoms and their impact. *EClinicalMedicine, 38*, 101019–101019. https://doi.org/10.1016/j.eclinm.2021.101019 (accessed on 30th June 2025).
10. Donta, B., Battala, M., Dasgupta, A., Ghule, M., et al. (2016). CHARM, a gender equity and family planning intervention for men and couples in rural India: Protocol for the cluster randomized controlled trial evaluation. https://core.ac.uk/download/323065021.pdf (accessed on 30th June 2025).
11. Graff, A., & Korolczuk, E. (2021). *Anti-Gender Politics in The Populist Moment.* https://doi.org/10.4324/9781003133520 (accessed on 30th June 2025).
12. Herklotz, A., Nayar, A., Agarwal, B., Archer, C., Tirado, C., Elson, D., Maceachern, D., et al. (2012). *Powerful Synergies: Gender Equality, Economic Development and Environmental Sustainability.* https://core.ac.uk/download/75779706.pdf (accessed on 30th June 2025).
13. Janus, K. K. (2013). Finding common feminist ground: The role of the next generation in shaping feminist legal theory. https://core.ac.uk/download/62560161.pdf (accessed on 30th June 2025).

14. Kruk, M. E., Gage, A., Arsenault, C., Jordan, K., Leslie, H. H., Roder-DeWan, S., Adeyi, O., et al. (2018). High-quality health systems in the Sustainable Development Goals era: Time for a revolution. *The Lancet Global Health, 6*, e1196–e1252. https://doi.org/10.1016/s2214-109x(18)30386-3 (accessed on 30th June 2025).

15. Locke, C., & Zhang, H. X. (2001). Rights, social policy and reproductive wellbeing: The Vietnam situation. https://core.ac.uk/download/2779862.pdf (accessed on 30th June 2025).

16. Miller, C. (2010). *Children Affected by AIDS: A Review of The Literature on Orphaned and Vulnerable Children.* https://open.bu.edu/bitstream/2144/1304/1/hhdp_10_lit_review.pdf (accessed on 30th June 2025).

17. OECD. (2021). *Women in Infrastructure.* Public governance policy papers. https://doi.org/10.1787/9eab66a8-en (accessed on 30th June 2025).

18. Ojo, A., Singer, M. R., Morales, B. M., Merz, A. A., Molina, R. L., Pelletier, A., del Carmen, A., et al. (2022). Reproductive justice: A case-based, interactive curriculum. *MedEdPORTAL.* https://doi.org/10.15766/mep_2374-8265.11275 (accessed on 30th June 2025).

19. Paul, C. R., Wolfe, A. D., Catallozzi, M., Jirasevijinda, T., Kutscher, E., & Lurie, B. (2021). Teaching sexual orientation and gender identity in pediatric clinical settings: A training workshop for faculty and residents. *MedEdPORTAL.* https://doi.org/10.15766/mep_2374-8265.11137 (accessed on 30th June 2025).

20. Ryan, G. (2015). *Review of the Evidence for Adolescent and Young Person Specific, Community-Based Health Services for NHS Managers.* https://core.ac.uk/download/84342214.pdf (accessed on 30th June 2025).

21. Schier, H., Gunther, C., Landry, M. J., Ohlhorst, S. D., & Linsenmeyer, W. (2022). Sex and gender data collection in nutrition research: Considerations through an inclusion, diversity, equity, and access lens. *Journal of the Academy of Nutrition and Dietetics, 123*, 247–252. https://doi.org/10.1016/j.jand.2022.09.014 (accessed on 30th June 2025).

22. Soled, K. R. S., Clark, K. D., Altman, M. R., Bosse, J. D., Thompson, R., Squires, A., & Sherman, A. D. F. (2022). Changing language, changes lives: Learning the lexicon of LGBTQ+ health equity. *Research in Nursing & Health, 45*, 621–632. https://doi.org/10.1002/nur.22274 (accessed on 30th June 2025).

23. Subramaniam, B. (2015). *Colonial Legacies, Postcolonial Biologizes: Gender and the Promises of Biotechnology.* https://core.ac.uk/download/323083653.pdf (accessed on 30th June 2025).

24. Villarosa, L., & Potapchuk, M. (2014). *Moving Forward on Racial Justice Philanthropy.* https://core.ac.uk/download/75778734.pdf (accessed on 30th June 2025).

25. Win, E. (2015). *Health and Reproductive Rights Portfolio: A Look Back at The Last 14 Years of Thematic Grantmaking and Recommendations for Moving Forward.* https://core.ac.uk/download/75784731.pdf (accessed on 30th June 2025).

26. Yager, A., Lok, E., Miller, J., Noel, K., Goodman, M., & Santamaria-Schwartz, R. (2012). *Birds, Bees and Bias: How Absent Sex Ed Standards Fail New York's students.* https://core.ac.uk/download/71361426.pdf (accessed on 30th June 2025).

INTEGUMENTARY AND SENSORY FUNCTION: DISORDERS AND INJURY MANAGEMENT FOR NURSING

12

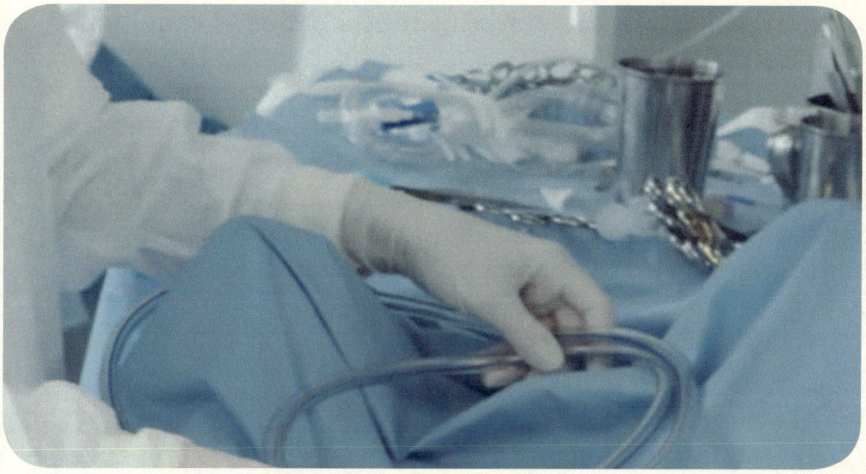

LEARNING OBJECTIVES

After studying this chapter, you will be able to:

1. Understand the anatomy of the integumentary system
2. Explain the common integumentary disorders
3. Discuss the sensory functions of the skin
4. Focus on assessment of integumentary disorders
5. Learn about nursing interventions for integumentary disorders
6. Evaluate the management of sensory function disorders

Introduction

The integumentary system, comprising the skin, hair, nails, and associated glands, serves as a vital barrier to protect the human body from the external world while also being a critical component of sensory perception. The body's largest organ, the skin, regulates body temperature and moisture while also serving as a component of the body's immune defense and maintaining general homeostasis. Nurse practitioners must be well-versed in this complex system to effectively assess and treat a wide range of disorders and injuries. An overview of the system highlights its application in clinical assessment, where symptom identification will optimize patient benefit. Understanding integumentary function provides a foundation for evaluating skin integrity and the effects of injury, which is essential for nurses seeking to ensure quality care in various healthcare settings. Evaluation and management of integumentary disorders must be guided by clinical judgment and culturally appropriate care, with an emphasis on the role of theory integration in practice in nursing education. As discussed in the resource "Introduction to Health Assessment for the Nursing Professional," such education plays a central role in acquiring the skills required to prioritize care based on clinical findings and patient needs (Accettola et al., 2023). In addition to the skills in technology, this education system encourages professional competence through the use of interactive education and formative assessments that enhance learner critical thinking. This not only prepares the learners for nursing practice but also equips them with the tools to advocate for patient safety and equitable outcomes by using evidence-based care. Reiterating the importance of cultural competence, nursing education supports efficient communication and tailored care plans that consider patients' unique experiences based on different backgrounds. When exploring sensory functions, special attention is to be given to the interconnectedness of the integumentary system and sensory perception. Receptors in the skin provide the sensations of touch, pain, heat, and pressure that are significant in the assessment of a patient's condition. Thus, integumentary system trauma can lead to sensory processing dysfunction, and recovery and management become more complex. Nursing diagnostics terminology enhances the ability to identify and manage these interconnected factors effectively, both in clinical practice and in nursing education (Vecchiato et al., 2014). Because nursing professionals are exposed to a variety of integumentary and sensory disorders, their ability to apply clinical knowledge to practice is eminently crucial in delivering holistic, individualized care. Having an understanding that is readily available for these systems in turn enhances nursing practice and prepares students for upcoming practice-related challenges (Figure 12.1).

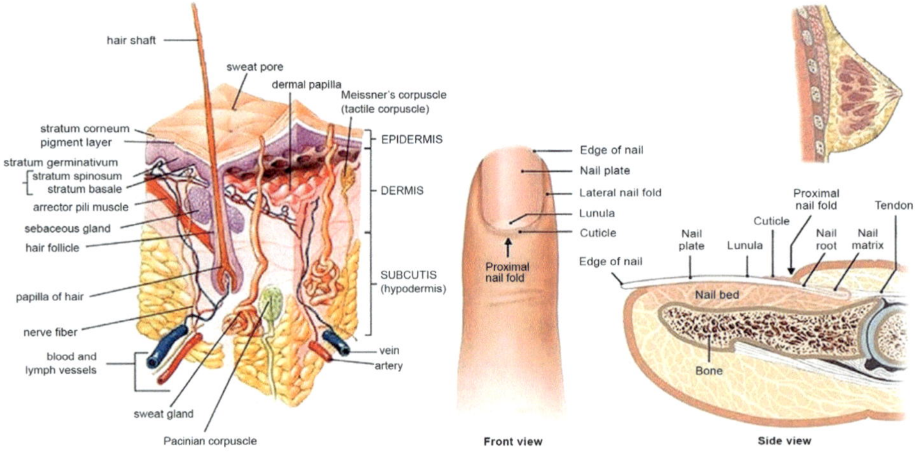

Figure 12.1. Integumentary system.

Source: https://microbenotes.com/wp-content/uploads/2020/06/Integumentary-System.jpg.

Definition of the Integumentary System

The integumentary system is a barrier that encompasses skin, hair, nails, and associated glands, and has important functions in protection, thermoregulation, and sensation. As the body's initial line of defense, the skin protects internal tissues from damage and disease, in addition to preventing dehydration. This is all accomplished through several layers, primarily the epidermis, dermis, and hypodermis, each with distinct functions required to maintain homeostasis. In addition, the integumentary system is also responsible for the sense of perception by facilitating the body to feel changes in the environment through specialized receptors. The intricate system not only regulates body temperature through sweat and blood flow but also synthesizes Vitamin D, which highlights its importance in holistic healthcare as well as nursing interventions towards the preservation of patient health. Knowledge of the integumentary system is essential in nursing for practical assessment and management of integumentary disorders. Nurses should be knowledgeable of the anatomy and physiology of the integumentary system to assess clinical deterioration in patients. For example, the identification of abnormal skin lesions, color, or texture can reveal precious information regarding a patient's general health status. Proper comprehension of the system also enables the early detection of pressure ulcers, skin infections, and other dermatological conditions. A comprehensive and culturally appropriate model of health evaluation, as discussed in texts like "Introduction to Health Assessment for the Nursing Professional," allows nursing students to construct more acute clinical judgment and care prioritization through quality skin examinations (Accettola et al., 2023). Furthermore, the function of the complex integumentary systems extends beyond mere protection to involve complex interactions with the other body systems. The interdependence is exemplified in the immune response function of the skin, which assists in detecting and reacting to the causative agents of infection. Additionally, the integumentary system has a close relationship with the nervous system, providing sensory information to facilitate the response of the body to stimulation. Such integration highlights the significance of a ~~successful~~ adequate understanding of the integumentary system within nursing practice, particularly when handling disorders and injury. Through an understanding of the complete functions of this system, nursing practitioners can use targeted intervention and education practices ~~in order~~ to successfully manage integumentary-related complications, ultimately improving patient outcomes (Ntusi et al., 2019).

Importance of Sensory Functions

Sensory function has a significant role in maintaining physical health, overall well-being, and quality of life. One of the most important parts of the sensory system is the integumentary system, which consists of skin, hair, and nails. The skin is rich in receptors that detect pressure, temperature, and pain, and plays a vital role in protecting the body against injury. The integration of these sensory inputs enables individuals to respond appropriately to their environment and influence behaviors designed to preserve safety and survival. As healthcare practitioners come to realize the value of these functions, how sensory impairment influences patient care assumes even greater importance, particularly in the management of injuries, thereby directly connecting to nursing's ultimate objectives in patient advocacy and care delivery (Banta-Wright et al., 2000). Also, the onset of disease in the integumentary and sensory systems can lead to severe challenges in patient care and management. Sensory impairment, particularly in children and critically ill patients, poses severe issues with their susceptibility to injury and the presence of any potential underlying conditions that might be present as a skin complication. Conditions such as pressure ulcers demonstrate the negative impacts of impaired sensory function, as failure to feel pressure or pain can lead to tissue loss and life-threatening complications. The increased prevalence rates of pressure ulcers in intensive care units underscore the need to establish preventive measures, such as implementing integrated care bundles. Nurses play a crucial role in this preventive treatment, as evidenced by studies that show a significant reduction in the prevalence of ulcers when best practices are applied (Schindler et al., 2010). Effective nursing administration depends on a keen awareness of the importance of sensory activities, particularly in relation to the integumentary system. Specialization enables nurses to utilize interventions that mitigate the adverse effects associated with sensory loss, thereby enhancing patient outcomes. For instance, training in skin examination and sensitivity to routinely repositioning patients can avert the development of pressure ulcers. The use of regular surveillance, good nutrition, and tailored skin care protocols through multidisciplinary practice can reinforce the protective mechanisms of the body's integumentary system. Lastly, the enforcement of sensory functions in practice and nursing education leads to more effective holistic care strategies that not only treat dominant disorders but also successfully prevent injuries (Banta-Wright et al., 2000; Schindler et al., 2010) (Figure 12.2).

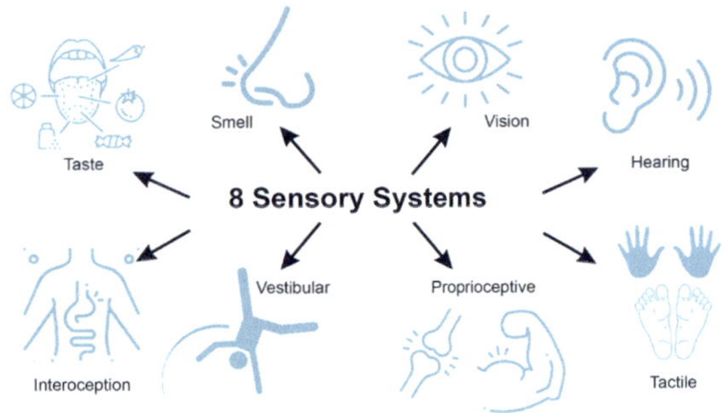

Figure 12.2. Sensory-systems occupational-therapy.

Source: https://developlearngrow.com/wp-content/uploads/2023/05/8-Sensory-Systems-Occupational-Therapy.png.

Overview of Disorders and Injury Management in Nursing

An effective approach to the management of integumentary disorders and injuries is based on the appreciation of patient assessments Nursing professionals must deliver evaluations that are not only comprehensive of the physical indicators of an illness but also of the patient as an individual. This multi-faceted assessment is crucial in determining the advent of signs of complications, i.e., pressure ulcers, which can have a significant impact on patient's recovery pattern. Development of clinical judgment is of prime importance, as highlighted in an open educational resource for nursing students, where strategies are included to elicit effective responses to patient signs and symptoms. With the advancement of decision-making skills, nurses can maximize interventions to ensure patient safety and improve health outcomes, ultimately leading to better management of disorders and injuries in diverse clinical settings (Accettola et al., 2023). Among various possible injuries and disorders affecting the integumentary system, pressure ulcers are a point of serious concern, particularly in critical care units and long-term care. Localized areas of tissue damage, pressure ulcers develop because of sustained external pressure that leads to impaired blood flow, traditionally affecting those patients with mobility constraints. The incorporation of evidence-based practices, such as turning protocols and nutrition care, is essential in the reduction of risk. Research indicates that the application of an effectively integrated pressure ulcer prevention bundle can significantly reduce occurrence rates, supporting that large-scale nursing practice and education are essential in the effective addressing of such complex health issues (Schindler et al., 2010). For the management of pressure ulcers and other disorders, sustained education and engagement with health teams by all nursing practitioners are necessary. The challenge brought about by the critical care setting, where patients are more acutely involved and receive full attention, renders prevention difficult. Time and resource constraints as barriers can hamper nurses' application of the best practices, and therefore, support by organizations in clinical settings becomes essential. Understanding these dynamics enables nursing professionals to advocate for necessary changes, such as improved staffing levels or the implementation of preventive measures. Through involvement in quality improvement activities and interprofessional collaboration, nurses can spearhead innovations in injury care, thereby ensuring that holistic care is consistently delivered and patients' outcomes are optimized in various healthcare environments (Accettola et al., 2023).

12.1. Anatomy of the Integumentary System

Learning Outcome

1. Describe the structure of the skin
2. Focus on accessory structures (hair, nails, glands)
3. Learn about role of the integumentary system in homeostasis

The skin, hair, nails, and associated glands make up the body's first line of defense against harmful agents from the environment. Structurally, the skin is composed of three layers that are responsible for the entire protective and sensing functions of the system: the epidermis, dermis, and hypodermis. The outer layer, the epidermis, provides a barrier against infectious agents and regulates moisture loss, while the dermis contains connective tissue, blood vessels, and nerve endings to facilitate sensation and regulate body temperature.

The hypodermis also supports the skin and the underlying tissues, storing fat for energy maintenance and insulation. Knowledge of the complexity of these layers is essential to nursing practice, especially when evaluating for injuries or disorders that reduce the skin's protective and integrity function. Beyond its physical barriers, the integumentary system is also important in sensory perception. This sensory role is facilitated by numerous receptors present within the skin that detect stimuli such as temperature, pressure, and pain. For nurses, detection of alteration in these sensations is important for the diagnosis of disorders underlying. For instance, diabetic neuropathic patients may lose their protective sensation, leading to unnoticed injuries and consequent complications.

Nursing education must therefore emphasize the anatomy related to the integumentary system and the clinical presentation of sensory dysfunction. Such knowledge enables nurses to effectively prioritize care and apply preventive interventions tailored to patients' specific needs, particularly in populations at risk of integumentary disorders. Integumentary system disorder management, such as pressure injury, requires an interlinked approach underpinned by knowledge of the anatomy of the skin and physiological processes. Evidence-based practice is crucial for treating and preventing such injuries, particularly in high-risk populations, such as those in intensive care (Pomerleau et al., 2021).

This includes the assessment of risk factors using standardized scales and the implementation of educational programs to improve nursing competence and knowledge regarding integumentary assessment (Accettola et al., 2023). Institutional efforts to improve compliance with best practices in wound care can significantly reduce the incidence of hospital-acquired pressure injuries. By integrating systematic evaluation and evidence-based measures to prevent injury into nursing practice, patient safety can be enhanced and outcomes maximized in patients vulnerable to compromised skin integrity (Figure 12.3).

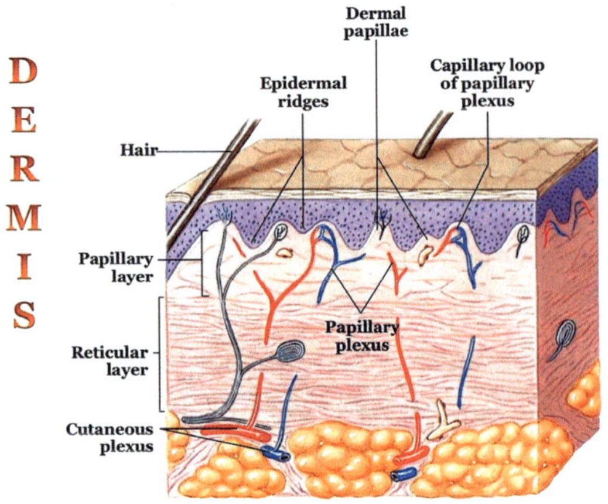

Figure 12.3. The integumentary system.

Source: https://image.slidesharecdn.com/theintegumentarysystem-130515100247-phpapp02/95/the-integumentary-system-21-1024.jpg?cb=1368612221.

12.1.1. Structure of the Skin

The skin, the largest organ of the body, plays a significant role in covering internal structures while being engaged in sensory perception and thermoregulation. It has a layered structure divided into three principal layers: epidermis, dermis, and hypodermis. The epidermis represents the external layer, composed predominantly of keratinocytes that are regularly cycled through the process of differentiation and regeneration. This stratified structure allows the skin not only to protect itself against mechanical trauma but also to generate a potent defense against chemicals and infectious agents. The value of the intact epidermis is best appreciated in the clinic when disturbances in this barrier function lead to increased susceptibility to infection and other cutaneous diseases. Thus, nursing professionals must understand the epidermal anatomy for formulating appropriate prevention and intervention strategies with respect to skin integrity and health. Beneath the epidermis lies the dermis, a dense layer of connective tissue that contains principal structures, including blood vessels, nerve endings, and appendages such as hair follicles and sweat glands. The dermis is further divided into two layers: the papillary dermis, which supports the epidermis and enhances nutrient exchange, and the reticular dermis, which imparts mechanical strength and elasticity to the skin. The presence of sensory receptors in the dermis underscores its crucial role in the body's sensory capabilities, enabling the perception of touch, temperature, and pain. In clinical practice, particularly in wound care and pressure ulcer prevention, understanding the anatomy of the dermal layer becomes essential. Effective injury treatment depends on the complete understanding of how the components are integrated to support the functionality and stability of the skin during healing procedures, especially among vulnerable groups, such as critically ill patients (Schindler et al., 2010). Finally, the hypodermis or subcutaneous tissue forms the foundation of the skin structure as a whole, performing the functions of insulation, cushioning, and energy storage site. The loose connective tissue and adipose cells in the layer enable the skin to attach to deeper structures while helping maintain body heat through thermoregulation. Understanding the hypodermic layer is essential to nursing practitioners, particularly in the assessment and management of injuries. For instance, alterations in the integrity of the hypodermis, such as pressure ulcers, might play a significant role in the patient's outcome. Determining the layers of the skin and their interacting functions might enhance clinical judgment and decision-making as a nurse. By stimulating complete knowledge about the structure of the skin, practitioners can enhance their response to the barriers in the integrity of the skin and take care of disorders or injuries due to this complex organ (Accettola et al., 2023) (Figure 12.4).

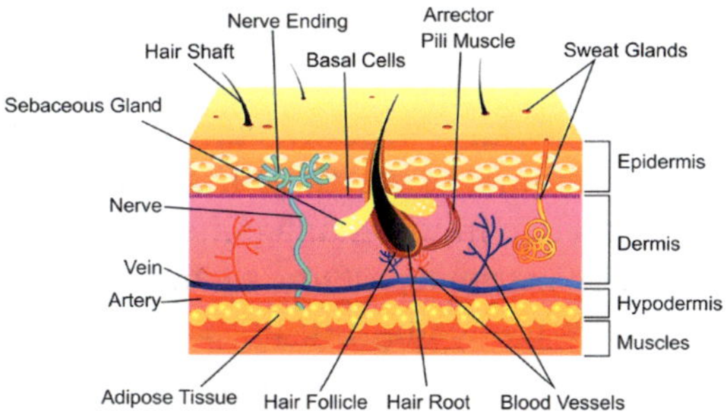

Figure 12.4. Structure of the skin.

Source: https://thumbs.dreamstime.com/z/human-skin-structure-vector-illustration-isolated-background-human-skin-structure-vector-illustration-isolated-white-background-128739887.jpg.

12.1.2. Accessory Structures (Hair, Nails, Glands)

The integumentary system also includes specific accessory structures, like hair, nails, and glands, which play essential roles in maintaining overall skin function and well-being. Hair is formed by follicles embedded within the dermis and plays varied functions, such as protection against UV light, temperature regulation, and contribution to sensory perception. Hair growth depends on many factors, including hormones and nutrient levels. Nursing professionals must understand the structure and function of hair and recognize disorders such as alopecia, which have significant psychological effects on patients. Treatment of hair disorders incorporates a balanced rendering of physiological reactions engaged and social meanings of baldness in diverse populations in accordance with the practice of culturally-sensitive care outlined in nursing educational models, and this is centered on individualized assessment practices identified in Accettola et al., (2023). Nails are another part of the integumentary system, serving both protective and functional roles for the fingers. The nail structure, composed mainly of keratin, provides protection from environmental trauma while also facilitating fine motor activity. Nail color changes may signal an underlying disease or nutritional deficiency. For example, clubbing of the nail with respiratory or cardiovascular disease requires immediate medical assessment. Nurses must be capable of assessing nail health as part of a broader skin examination, thereby enhancing their clinical judgment and ability to identify early clinical deterioration. Additionally, the inclusion of anatomical knowledge, guided by the learning outcomes of nursing education models, ensures that nursing practitioners possess a solid foundation in assessing such accessory structures effectively, ultimately improving patient outcomes, as noted in Akinsanya et al. (2018). Sebaceous and sweat glands in the skin are further evidence of the functionality and complexity of the accessory structures of the integumentary system. Sebaceous glands secrete sebum, which is essential for maintaining skin hydration and its barrier function. Conversely, sweat glands play a crucial role in thermoregulation and the excretion of metabolic waste. Dysregulation of the sweat and sebaceous glands can lead to various skin disorders, including acne and hyperhidrosis. Nursing care needs an awareness of the endocrine and exocrine activity of sweat and sebaceous glands and how they affect skin integrity and patient comfort. Effective condition assessment and management for glandular function require a thorough understanding of pathological processes, as well as effective treatment. Such knowledge not only supports optimal practice in nursing but also allows for patients to be educated about skin health and measures of hygiene to assist with overall patient education and patient health literacy among diverse populations, in alignment with educational goals outlined in Accettola et al., (2023).

12.1.3. Role of the Integumentary System in Homeostasis

The integumentary system, comprising skin, hair, nails, and various glands, helps maintain homeostasis within the human body. Such a complex system is the body's first line of defense against foreign pathogens and physical injury, safeguarding against dehydration and the invasion of infectious agents. The outermost layer of skin is the epidermis, which offers a barrier, while the one beneath it, the dermis, contains elements such as sweat glands and blood vessels. These structures function together to regulate body temperature and permit sensation, both of which are vital elements of homeostasis. For instance, thermoregulation is enhanced through the dilation and vasoconstriction of dermal blood vessels, allowing central body temperature to be maintained under varying external conditions, thereby demonstrating the integumentary system's significance in adaptive physiologic functions. Aside from its defensive functions, the integumentary system plays a crucial role in sensory perception, enabling the body to respond meaningfully to its environment. The skin is rich in a vast network of sensory receptors that are sensitive to touch, temperature, and pain. They play an essential role in feedback mechanisms that convey information to the central nervous system about the state of the environment. The ability to detect alterations in temperature or pressure makes it possible to respond appropriately either through protective action or through adjustment of conduct in various circumstances. Such a sensory process not only guarantees personal safety but also enables the performance of actions crucial to survival, such as evading hazardous situations or seeking refuge from excessive heat or cold, thereby preserving the integrity of homeostasis. Furthermore, disturbances of the integumentary system can significantly impact total homeostasis, thus underscoring the value of effective injury management in nursing practice. For instance, wounds can impair skin barrier integrity, leading to infection and fluid loss, both of which can disrupt homeostatic balance. Additionally, eczema or psoriasis can alter skin integrity and sensation, further aggravating challenges of temperature control and infection prevention. As future healthcare providers, nursing students must understand the integumentary system's role in maintaining homeostasis and learn how to assess and effectively treat skin disorders. Educational resources that reinforce knowledge of clinical judgment and culturally-sensitive health screens are critical in equipping nursing students with the information that will facilitate equalized health outcomes for all patients, warranting the interdependence of integumentary health and systemic homeostasis (Dunphy et al., 2013; Accettola et al., 2023) (Figure 12.5).

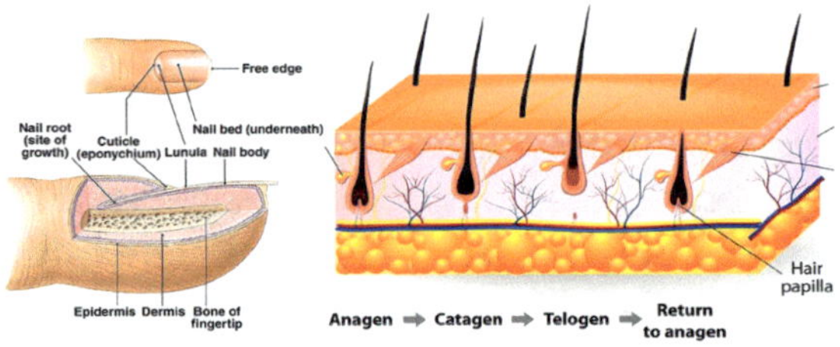

Figure 12.5. Label the parts of the integumentary system.

Source: https://i.ytimg.com/vi/7nR2FEWYIl0/maxresdefault.jpg.

Test Your Knowledge

1. What are the three main layers of the skin and their basic functions?
2. How do hair and nails form as part of the integumentary system?

12.2. Common Integumentary Disorders

Learning Outcome

1. Explain the dermatitis and eczema
2. Define psoriasis
3. Discuss the Skin infections (bacterial, viral, fungal)

The integumentary system, which includes the skin, hair, nails, and accessory glands, is the body's first defense against the external environment. Acute and chronic integumentary conditions, such as eczema, psoriasis, and acne, can have a significant impact on patients' quality of life and require sensitive nursing evaluation and management. Eczema, characterized by an inflammatory reaction of the skin, presents as red, itchy patches, often triggered by allergens or irritants.

Nurses are also key in identifying triggers and instructing patients in proper skin care measures to manage flare-ups. Meanwhile, psoriasis is a chronic autoimmune condition characterized by thick, scaly plaques on the skin, which pharmacologic and non-pharmacologic therapy. With an integrative health assessment, particularly one that is culturally competent, nurses can best facilitate healthy skin and enhance positive health outcomes for multicultural populations (Accettola et al., 2023). Complications of integumentary disorders can also potentially cause significant physical and psychological repercussions for patients. Acne, for instance, even though regarded as a benign condition, has profound effects on the patient's self-esteem and psychological well-being, particularly during adolescence. In this regard, nursing care would entail not only the treatment of the skin but also counseling and support to cope with the emotional distress involved with the condition. The integration of interactive clinical judgment activities in nursing education enhances nurses' ability to recognize the multifaceted nature of integumentary disorders. This type of learning platform enables nursing students to acquire skills necessary for recognizing clinical deterioration cues, potentially leading to a broader application in patient care practice (Ntusi et al., 2019). The management of these integumentary disorders requires in-depth understanding of causative factors, presentation, and treatment.

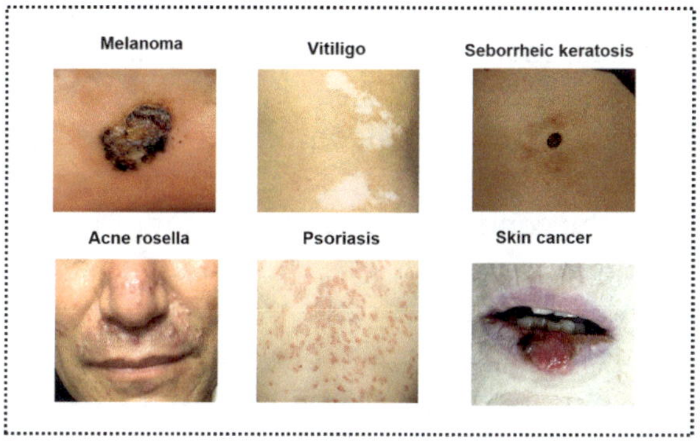

Figure 12.6. Chart of six common types of skin disease.

Source: https://www.mdpi.com/2075-4418/13/23/3506.

For example, the selection of appropriate topical interventions for the treatment of eczema and psoriasis will be determined by whether the assessment of the disorder reveals if it is chronic in nature or the severity of the symptoms. Nurses must be capable of assessing the effectiveness of such intervention and the consequences of long-term use, for example, skin thinning or infection. Since these disorders repetitively recur, teaching the patient is essential in empowering individuals to understand and actively participate in their care. By fostering awareness of their condition and improving compliance with treatment, nurses play a crucial role in maintaining successful patient outcomes. Lastly, the integration of multidisciplinary teams in diagnosis and care enables an even more holistic approach to integumentary disorders, which are often encountered, and is crucial in maintaining long-term health as well as convalescence (Accettola et al., 2023) (Figure 12.6).

12.2.1. Dermatitis and Eczema

Eczema and dermatitis are a spectrum of inflammatory diseases of the skin that are characterized by redness, inflammation, and itchiness of the integumentary system. The conditions can be caused by a range of etiologies, including hereditary predisposition, environmental influences, or immune system dysfunction. Of the encompassing broad term eczema, atopic dermatitis is the most prevalent type of the condition, especially among children, and commonly leads to significant discomfort and impairment of ordinary functioning. The nursing implications are profound, as effective management requires understanding not just the clinical presentations but also the psychological effects on patients. Nurses play a significant role in educating patients about their disease, teaching them good skin care, and reminding them of the importance of compliance to treatment regimens to attain maximal healing and comfort (Chukwu et al., 2018). Treatment of eczema and dermatitis involves individualized treatment plans that typically incorporate both non-pharmacological and pharmacological interventions. Topical corticosteroids are ~~also~~ widely used to reduce inflammation and promote skin healing, with newer modalities, such as biologic therapies, transforming the treatment landscape for severe cases. Furthermore, implementing skincare regimens with moisturizers and barrier creams can significantly enhance the skin's ability to retain moisture and withstand irritation. Nurses must carefully screen each patient for potential triggers, whether allergens or irritants, and then collaborate to develop a comprehensive care plan. By fostering a positive nurse-patient relationship, health professionals can empower patients with the information and skills necessary for effective self-management, ultimately leading to an improved health-related quality of life (Areosa et al., 2017). Besides, the psychosocial aspects of eczema and dermatitis must be managed in patient care. ~~The~~ Many of these patients with these types of skin diseases are embarrassed, socially stigmatized, and anxious, all contributing to increasing the severity of their diseases. Health care providers must be empathetic when caring for such patients, with insight into these psychological conditions. Educational interventions can promote improved understanding and acceptance in the patient's family and community, providing a supportive environment. Furthermore, ongoing research into the roles of dermatology nurses highlights their key role in facilitating treatment compliance, patient education about their condition, and access to available healthcare resources. Empowering nurses to work in such varied positions can significantly improve patient outcomes and keep the care patient-centered and effective (Chukwu et al., 2018) (Figure 12.7).

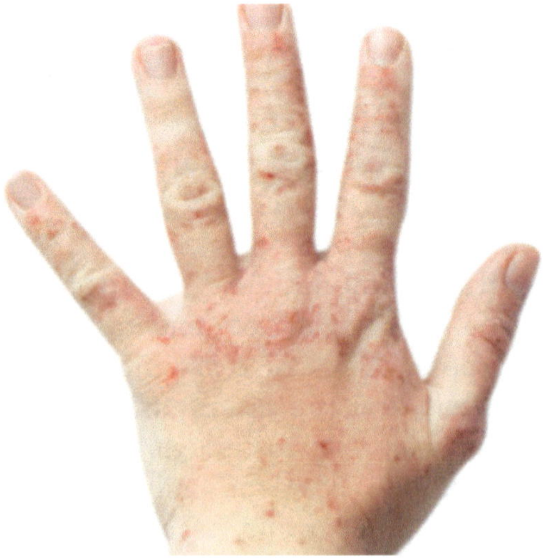

Figure 12.7. Dermatitis: skin surgery clinic.

Source: https://skinsurgeryclinic.co.uk/wp-content/uploads/2020/02/dermatitis-eczema-condition-3-scaled.jpg.

12.2.2. Psoriasis

Psoriasis is a chronic dermatosis of inflammatory nature caused by the increased proliferation of skin cells, leading to the development of scaly plaques on extensor surfaces, the scalp, and the lower back. Although its precise etiology is multifactorial in nature, it is a fact that psoriasis is a result of an interaction between an environmental precipitant and a genetic predisposition, such as infections, stress, and certain medications. The condition is also associated with systemic comorbidities, including an increased risk of cardiovascular disease, obesity, and metabolic syndrome, and this calls for an integrated focus on patient care. Nurses play a vital role in identifying such correlations and can provide monitoring techniques to address not only the cutaneous manifestations of psoriasis but also related health risks.

This integrated perspective enhances the quality of care provided to patients, highlighting the interrelatedness of skin health and overall well-being. Psoriasis treatment is advanced and multidisciplinary, demonstrating a need for interactions among dermatologists, primary care doctors, and nurses. Treatment plans can include topical therapies, phototherapy, and systemic medications based on the extent and severity of the disease.

Nursing intervention is crucial in educating the patients concerning therapy, highlighting the importance of adherence and coping with potential side effects. Proper patient education can also enable the patient to play an active role in controlling their disease, resulting in improved treatment outcomes. The nurses must also assess the psychosocial impact of psoriasis since the visibility of the condition renders them stigmatized and depressed. By facilitating empathetic communication and connecting patients with resources, nursing practitioners make a crucial contribution to the overall care of patients affected by psoriasis. Moreover, dermatology nurses are ideally positioned to optimize patient recovery and education, enabling patients with knowledge and with the skills necessary to care for their disease efficiently. As outlined in recent literature, nurse interventions have been shown to promote patient adherence through education, enhancing patient awareness of skin disease and treatment. Specifically, education provided by dermatology nurses informs patients of the importance of lifestyle modifications, such as reducing stress and maintaining a healthy weight, which play a significant role in exacerbating psoriasis. Building trust relationships between nurses and patients also reinforces motivation, which encourages adherence to the treatment regimen. Nurses, in return, are not only caregivers but also advocates for patient education and empowerment, ensuring integrated care that results in improved outcomes for the management of psoriasis (Chukwu et al., 2018; Accettola et al., 2023) (Figure 12.8).

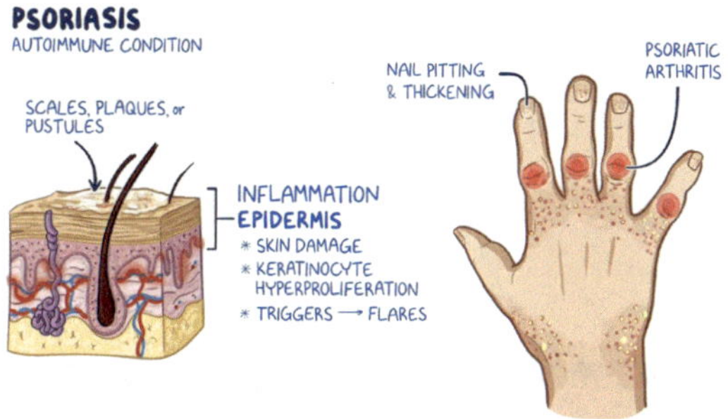

Figure 12.8. Psoriasis.

Source: https://d16qt3wv6xm098.cloudfront.net/Wswl_jD3SRCE-p2kQV9i3V1cTVerGhXF/_.jpg

12.2.3. Skin Infections (Bacterial, Viral, Fungal)

Infections of the skin caused by bacterial, viral, and fungal pathogens are a significant issue in clinical practice nursing due to their varied presentations and potential complications. Bacterial infections such as cellulitis and impetigo result from direct invasion of the skin and may lead to systemic symptoms if left untreated. Understanding the pathophysiology of such infections, as discussed in texts such as Introduction to Health Assessment for the Nursing Professional, is essential for nursing students and professionals to properly allocate care. Nurses must possess the knowledge to recognize clinical signs of deterioration, facilitate early intervention, and educate patients on measures to prevent infection and maintain hygiene, thereby reducing the risk of complications associated with bacterial skin infections (Accettola et al., 2023). Viral skin infections, such as herpes simplex and varicella-zoster virus, require a systematic approach to managing them, as well as implementing isolation interventions if necessary. Presentation of such infections is usually vesicular lesions necessitating various therapy approaches. Nursing management involves relieving symptoms and providing patient education in prevention, especially considering the infectious potential of certain viruses. Further, knowledge from the series of pathophysiology course notes emphasizes the importance of understanding the immune system reaction to such an infection, which can be applied in nursing practice and patient education (Sargsyan et al., 2020). By acquiring comprehensive knowledge about the clinical presentation and transmission patterns of viral infections, nurses can maximize patient health and safety. Fungal skin dermatological infections, such as tinea pedis and candidiasis, are another serious issue in integumentary health. These infections are generally opportunistic in nature, often occurring in immunocompromised patients or on compromised skin. Good practice in nursing entails recognizing signs, adhering to standard treatment procedures, and educating patients on prevention. Knowledge grounded in pathophysiological principles and clinical models, such as those outlined in health education documents, empowers nurses to promote healthier lifestyles and effectively contain outbreaks (Sargsyan et al., 2020). In addition, with the growing prevalence of antifungal resistance, nurses must be ~~sensitive to shifting trends~~ understand the changes in treatment patterns to optimize patient outcomes in the management of fungal skin infections and thereby actualize their role as agents of vast patient care.

Test Your Knowledge

1. What are typical symptoms of eczema that nurses should assess for?
2. How does psoriasis differ from a fungal skin infection?

12.3. Sensory Functions of the Skin

Learning Outcome

1. Explain the mechanoreceptors and touch perception
2. Define the thermoreceptors and temperature regulation
3. Describe the nociceptors and pain sensation

Skin is also a significant interface between the body and the outside world, and it is a highly specialized sensory organ. It consists of many varied receptors that allow detection of a variety of stimuli, including touch, temperature, pain, and pressure. Mechanoreceptors, for example, respond to tactile stimuli and allow for the detection of light touch via specialized structures such as Merkel cells and Meissner's corpuscles. While thermoreceptors are crucial for sensing temperature changes, which is necessary for regulating homeostasis and preventing potentially dangerous circumstances, such as excessive heat or cold. This intricate system of sensory receptors not only enhances environmental perception but also profoundly affects behavioral responses, thereby solidifying the skin's role in overall well-being and safety. It is essential for nursing professionals to understand these sensory functions, as they must be able to recognize how skin disorders can impact sensory perception (Accettola et al., 2023). Damage or disorder to the skin can have a profound impact on its sensory functions, resulting in impaired perception of environmental conditions. For instance, disorders like neuropathy can diminish the ability to sense pain, which can lead to injuries going unnoticed. The implication is particularly strong in diabetic or other chronic populations, in which sensory input is crucial for avoiding injury. In these situations, sensory assessment by nurses is of vital importance for monitoring changes in skin integrity and ensuring patient safety. Furthermore, recognizing the connection between compromised sensory function and increased risk of skin breakdown reinforces the benefit of early intervention. Sound management strategies, like thorough skin examination and patient education, are essential in averting complications with skin diseases and injury. Active management ultimately results in better patient outcomes in the clinical setting (Ntusi et al., 2019). Moreover, the interaction between sensory function and the integumentary system has implications for pain management and rehabilitation in nursing practice. In addition to being an organ of sensation, the skin also plays a role in emotional responses to stimulation and influences pain perception through processes involving both physiological and psychological factors.

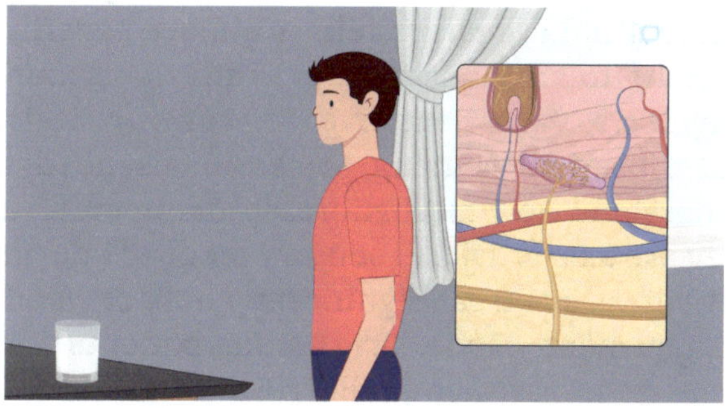

Figure 12.9. Sensory functions of the skin.

Source: https://www.jove.com/files/media/science-education/science-education-thumbs/13887.jpg.

For instance, both burns and pressure ulcers can lead to long-term syndromes of pain that must be treated by employing numerous different paths. Nurses should understand the complexity of such sensory functions to adequately fulfill the needs of patients in pain resulting from skin-damaging conditions. Therapeutic management may entail drug therapy, physical therapy, or other modalities such as mindfulness and cognitive-behavioral approaches, the goals of which include reduction of sensory deficits and healing. By facilitating an understanding of the skin's sensory role, nursing personnel can effectively encourage and implement care plans that meet the diverse needs of their patients (Accettola et al., 2023) (Figure 12.9).

12.3.1. Mechanoreceptors and Touch Perception

Mechanoreceptors are sensory nerve endings embedded in the skin and other tissues that are tasked with detecting touch. Mechanoreceptors transduce mechanical stimuli, such as pressure, vibration, and texture, into electrical signals that the nervous system interprets. Various mechanoreceptors, including Merkel cells, Meissner's corpuscles, Pacinian corpuscles, and Ruffini endings, respond to multiple aspects of tactile stimuli. Merkel cells are more sensitive to light touch and texture, while Meissner's corpuscles are sensitive to varying touch and vibration. Nursing professionals need to understand how mechanoreceptors operate, as they are also crucial in sensory feedback during patient care and can significantly impact wound management, particularly among patients with sensory impairments (Barroso et al., 2019). In the management of injury, the role of mechanoreceptors becomes increasingly critical. When skin is broken, whether due to a chronic wound or acute trauma, mechanoreceptive pathways can become compromised in terms of integrity, this not only affects patients' perception of touch but also their perception of potentially damaging stimuli, leaving them vulnerable to further injury. For instance, neonates are most susceptible to skin damage by virtue of having thin skin and increased sensitivity, as indicated in recent research examining the multifactorial causes of neonatal injury, with evidence of poor prevention efforts (August et al., 2022). An understanding of such risks empowers nurses with the knowledge to implement the most effective care interventions, ensuring the protection and rehabilitation of sensory function. Moreover, advances in wound care technology confront the issue raised by compromised mechanoreceptive function. Advances such as bioengineered skin substitutes and growth factor therapies can facilitate healing and restore both structural and sensory integrity to injured skin. These methods, if implemented within nursing practice, have the ability to decrease the long-term consequences of skin injury significantly, commensurate with improved patient outcomes. Understanding the relationship between mechanoreceptors, the perception of touch, and the healing process provides nurses with valuable information for patient care, ultimately guiding therapeutic treatments that enhance recovery and the well-being of individuals suffering from wounds and skin conditions (Barroso et al., 2019).

12.3.2. Thermoreceptors and Temperature Regulation

Thermoreceptors play a critical role in regulating body temperature as integral components of the integumentary and sensory systems. Thermoreceptors are specialized sensory receptors located in the skin and other tissues that respond to temperature changes and send this information to the central nervous system. There are two main types of thermoreceptors: warm receptors, which are stimulated by increasing temperatures, and cold receptors, which are stimulated by decreasing temperatures. This intricate detection system enables the body to maintain homeostasis by regulating physiological functions, including blood circulation and sweating. It is essential for nursing professionals to learn about thermoregulation, particularly in assessing patients at risk of temperature-related conditions. Misidentification of maladaptive responses can have serious clinical consequences, such as hypothermia or heat exhaustion, and hence requires an integrated approach to patient monitoring and management across various healthcare environments. The path of response from the activation of thermoreceptors to the physiological reactions generated by the body is highly complex and involves several mechanisms. Upon detecting a deviation from the set point of approximately 98.6°F (37°C), signals are transmitted through afferent pathways to the hypothalamus, resulting in various thermoregulatory responses. Rising body temperature, for instance, may result in vasodilation and excessive sweating, facilitating heat dissipation. Conversely, a drop in body temperature triggers reactions such as shivering and vasoconstriction to conserve heat. : The interaction of these responses highlights the importance of thermoregulators in clinical practice, with interventions potentially being required to restore the body to its normal balance. Application of evidence-based interventions, including environmental components' monitoring and managing individual variance in thermoregulation, is an important essential in ensuring the optimization of patients' outcomes as well as avoiding injury or disorders caused by temperature. Moreover, recent evidence supports the application of impaired thermoreceptor function to clinical conditions; therefore, adopting preventive practices is essential when treating patients. For instance, in diabetic neuropathy, thermoreceptor sensitivity can be altered, impairing the body's ability to regulate temperature. Nursing professionals should be vigilant for signs of thermoregulation disorder, especially in high-risk populations such as the elderly or patients with chronic diseases. Patient education on extreme temperatures and taking ~~up~~ precautions against environmental hazards is part of the management. Individualized care plans that incorporate features of thermoregulation will enable nurses to provide anticipatory and therapeutic care, ultimately contributing to improved health outcomes. By bridging the gap between practice and theoretical training in the clinical environment, nurses can improve their capacity for identifying and treating disorders of thermoregulation more effectively, as highlighted by current nursing education frameworks that aim to promote whole-person assessment of health (Vecchiato et al., 2014; Accettola et al., 2023) (Figure 12.10).

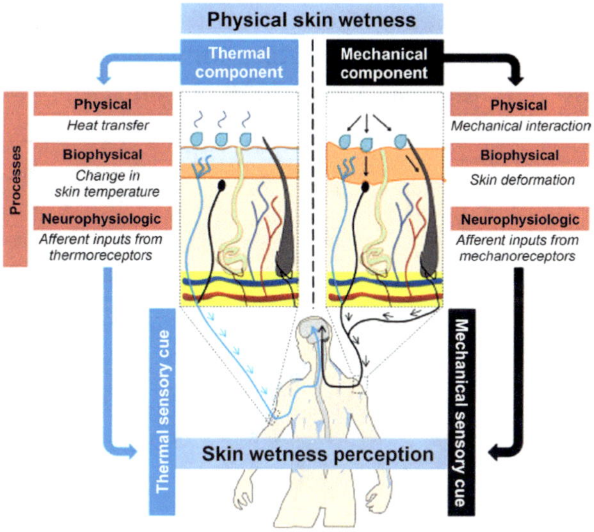

Figure 12.10. Thermoreceptor.

Source: https://ars.els-cdn.com/content/image/1-s2.0-B9780444639127000059-f05-02-9780444639127.jpg.

12.3.3. Nociceptors and Pain Sensation

Understanding nociceptors and their role in the perception of pain is central to nursing practice, particularly integumentary and sensory function. Nociceptors are specialized sensory receptors that detect noxious stimuli, which can lead to tissue injury, thereby playing a key role in the pain process. Nociceptors are predominantly located in the skin, muscles, joints, and some internal organs and serve as the body's front line of protection against potential injury. Following stimulation by painful stimuli—ranging from mechanical trauma to thermal extremes—nociceptors convey information to the central nervous system, initiating both reflex action and the perception of pain. The dual role underscores the importance of nociceptors in the recognition and regulation of pain, which nurses, charged with the examination and treatment of patients' pain, must be aware. By altering the perception of pain, nociceptors play a crucial role in the body's protective mechanisms. The perception of pain varies significantly due to individual differences, including genetic factors, life experiences, and emotional states, all of which influence pain processing and perception. Pain is either acute or chronic, and chronic pain occasionally becomes a disabling disorder requiring worldwide management measures. Nurses must be capable of assessing such differences in patients' pain experiences and determining the need for individualized care plans addressing physiological and psychosocial dimensions of pain.

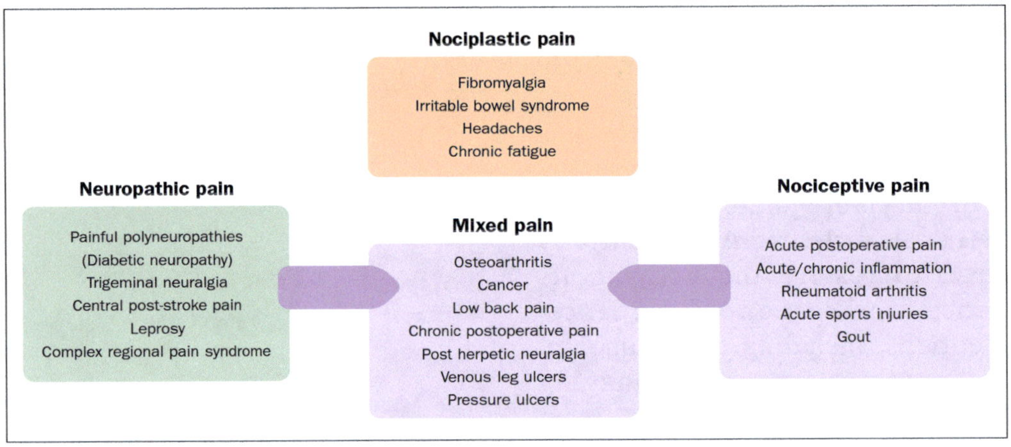

Figure 12.11. Nociceptors and pain sensation.

Source: https://www.britishjournalofnursing.com/media/cm5ewyf0/bjon202332258_f02.jpg.

The inclusion of culturally sensitive approaches within health assessment is necessary, as evident in Accettola et al., (2023), to ensure the optimal effectiveness of pain management plans and foster patient-centered care in nursing practice. Furthermore, advances in controlling pain are also spurred by greater knowledge about nociceptors and their pathways. Pain treatment requires not only pharmacological management but also a change of life, psychological therapy, and alternative methods. Such a multifaceted approach addresses the overall objectives of health promotion and the prevention of disability related to pain in nursing practice. Resources like pain management literature become invaluable for nurses, whose feedback translates into worthwhile strategies tailored to every patient's personalized requirements, as emphasized in N/A (2021). By considering both the biological and behavioral aspects of pain, nurses are able to significantly improve patient outcomes, delivering an integrative style of care crucial to treating integumentary and sensory system disorders (Figure 12.11).

Test Your Knowledge

1. How do sensory receptors in the skin help detect environmental changes?
2. What role does the skin play in the perception of pain and temperature?

12.4. Assessment of Integumentary Disorders

Learning Outcome

1. Identify the visual inspection techniques in nursing
2. Define the palpation and physical examination within the nursing profession
3. Describe the diagnostic tests (biopsies, cultures)

A detailed analysis of integumentary disorders is crucial for nurses because it directly impacts patient care and outcomes. The integumentary system comprises skin, hair, nails, and accessory glands, which can exhibit numerous disorders that reflect systemic issues that must be addressed promptly. In clinical practice, assessment begins with a thorough history and physical examination to detect changes in skin color, temperature, turgor, and texture, which can be signs of underlying pathologies. Such step-by-step assessments not only facilitate the diagnosis of common dermatoses, such as dermatitis and infections, but also increase knowledge regarding chronic diseases, including psoriasis and eczema. With the use of clinical judgment and culturally sensitive health assessment techniques, nurses can identify the subtle signs of decline, thereby promoting patient safety and facilitating effective interventions (Accettola et al., 2023). Classification and identification of pressure ulcers are an essential area of focus in integumentary disorder assessment, particularly among at-risk populations. Pressure ulcers, also known as bedsores, occur when the skin is subjected to constant pressure, which limits blood flow and, in severe cases, leads to tissue necrosis. Risk factors need to be evaluated, including immobility, poor nutrition, and moisture, which are leading causes of ulcers. It occurs particularly in critically ill patients, who are more likely to develop pressure ulcers due to the severity of their illness and vigorous treatment protocols. Evidence shows that incorporating prevention measures, such as the S.K.I.N. care package—encompassing support surfaces, frequent repositioning, incontinence care, and nutrition advice—can effectively lower incidence rates. Familiarity with these techniques makes nursing professionals well placed to manage possible integumentary disorders in their practice (Schindler et al., 2010). The contribution of education in the assessment and management of integumentary disorders cannot be overemphasized. Nursing education models must prioritize comprehensive training in skin exams and sensitivity to the diverse range of disorders that may arise among various populations.

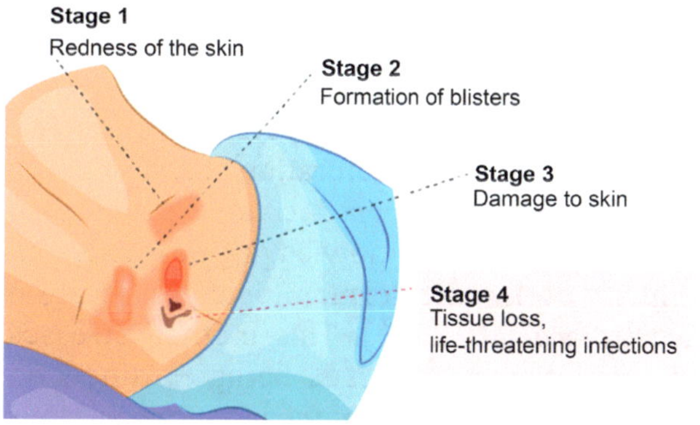

Figure 12.12. Stage 4 bedsore – nursing home neglect & pressure ulcers.

Source: https://www.nursinghomeabusecenter.com/wp-content/uploads/2021/04/stage-4-bedsore-illustration.png.

This would include knowledge of cultural differences that affect skin conditions, such as variations in pigmentation and common dermatological responses. By incorporating a holistic system of health assessment, nursing programs can better equip students to address the unique needs of a diverse patient population. Moreover, the combination of theoretical knowledge and practical skills enhances clinical judgment, enabling future nurses to identify and treat skin disorders effectively. Such a holistic approach not only enables enhanced nursing practice but also improves patient experiences and outcomes in the context of integumentary health (Accettola et al., 2023) (Figure 12.12).

12.4.1. Visual Inspection Techniques

Effective visual assessment techniques are essential in nursing as they form the foundation of observing and monitoring integumentary and sensory function. Nurses employ these techniques to identify abnormal states of the skin, hair, and nails, which are valuable markers for underlying disease processes. When performing an assessment, clinicians must use a systematic approach, such as noting skin color, texture, and temperature. These visual cues typically provide instant information regarding potential dermatologic conditions or systemic disease, which can direct timely interventions. Furthermore, cultural competence cannot be overstated; the varied coloration of skin renders it essential to have an inclusive process of visual assessment, acknowledging how race and ethnicity do impact dermatologic presentation (Accettola et al., 2023). This method stresses the importance of nurses being –trained on visual examination techniques to increase their clinical judgment and enhance patient safety. The use of advanced visual inspection devices has revolutionized the practice of examining skin diseases. High-definition imaging and dermatoscopic equipment enable nurses to conduct more rigorous examinations, facilitating the diagnosis of skin lesions and conditions, such as melanoma or psoriasis. Such technologies not only enhance visual accuracy but also support decision-making processes by providing clear, recorded evidence upon which to make further analysis. Nurses trained with this kind of training can identify key warning signals that may indicate more rigorous diagnostic investigation or specialist referral (Jefferson et al., 2016). This enhances the quality of patient care while allowing nurses to manage health proactively. Therefore, an emphasis on continuing education and the infusion of technology into practice is necessary to enhance the effectiveness of visual inspection techniques. Visual inspection techniques are not merely observation; they involve critical thinking and the integration of information received visually during patient evaluation. The nurse must consider certain factors, including the patient's medical history and current conditions, to assess potential hazards effectively.—Documenting findings not only gives a point of reference for future evaluation but also is a crucial instrument for the tracking of change over time, and therefore facilitating early intervention where required. By recognizing the relationship between the sensory function and integumentary health, nurses can more clearly identify the broader consequences of their visual examination. Therefore, establishing a solid foundation in visual inspection skills is crucial for achieving enhanced patient outcomes in nursing through the provision of practitioners who are sufficiently skilled to manage both immediate and long-term care needs efficiently (Accettura et al., 2023).

12.4.2. Palpation and Physical Examination

Palpation is a fundamental element of physical examination within nursing practice and is highly significant in assessing integumentary and sensory function. During palpation, healthcare professionals use their fingers to assess the skin and underlying tissue for temperature, tenderness, and texture, thereby enabling them to detect any anomalies. This technique is particularly relevant to recognizing signs and symptoms of inflammation or infection, as well as assessing circulatory status and tissue integrity. For instance, palpation can ~~pick up~~ detect changes in skin temperature associated with dermatitis or cellulitis, both of which are common in patients with impaired integumentary function. To conduct a practical, thorough assessment, nurses should be proficient in recognizing various tactile cues and be guided by this knowledge to implement clinical judgment and decision-making skills, which result in improved patient outcomes as required in nursing practice education materials (Accettola et al., 2023). A physical exam, with palpation as one of its key components, plays a substantial role in the treatment of integumentary system disorders and injuries. A comprehensive assessment involves not only palpation but also visual inspection and a patient's history as a guide for nursing action. Together, these methods enable nursing clinicians to identify and categorize skin conditions, ranging from benign to more complex diseases, such as pressure ulcers or infections. For example, when observing a patient with a new knee arthroplasty, a nurse can inspect the surgical area and surrounding tissue for signs of redness or diminished circulation. Through tactile examination, they assess temperature, swelling, and the degree of pain, which are key considerations for evaluating post-operative care needs and the efficacy of rehabilitation strategies, as described in surgical recovery case studies (Holm et al., 2015). Furthermore, coordination of palpation and physical assessment skills is crucial for facilitating effective nursing interventions related to sensory function and responsiveness to injury. Nurses should remain attentive to the identification of unusual findings, as early observation of slight changes can be crucial in treatment. For instance, cold or abnormally textured skin may indicate circulatory issues or impending necrosis that require prompt intervention. Secondly, these assessments inform patient teaching and engagement in the recovery process, teaching patients how to monitor their own skin integrity within the home setting. Overall, the ability in palpation and physical assessment not only informs nurses' power in clinical settings but also strengthens patient safety by detecting probable complications early (Accettola et al., 2023) (Figure 12.13).

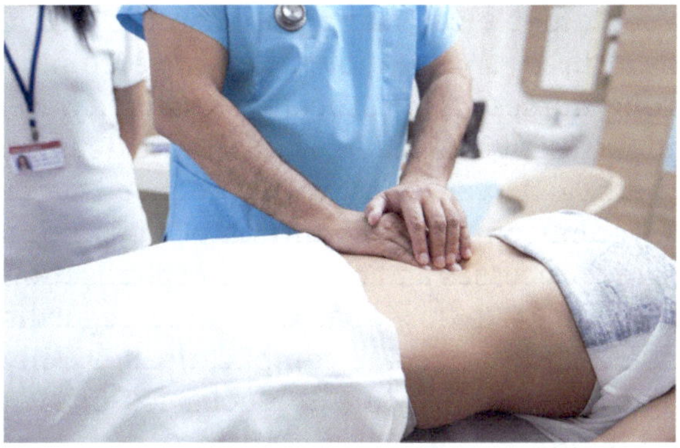

Figure 12.13. The role of palpation in medicine.

Source: https://www.verywellhealth.com/thmb/IlUQdgpwPAX-QKpYNlY3zWFOsWY=/1500x0/filters:no_upscale():max_bytes(150000):strip_icc()/GettyImages-533539909-80bd5f8ad7af46929a8d199384efef09.jpg.

12.4.3. Diagnostic Tests (Biopsies, Cultures)

Diagnostic procedures such as biopsies and cultures are paramount in the management and assessment of integumentary diseases. With these diagnostic procedures, clinicians can make a solid diagnosis and thus select the appropriate therapeutic management. Biopsies, where tissues are removed for histological examination, are particularly crucial in evaluating skin lesions or cancers suspected thereof. The pathological test provides information regarding the cellular changes that are the basis for, hence ~~enabling~~ conditions like skin cancer, dermatitis, and autoimmune disorders to be diagnosed. Coupled with clinical tests, these tests enable nurses and clinicians to provide personalized treatment plans, ultimately leading to improved patient outcomes and quality of life. Cultures, yet another fundamental diagnostic tool, are crucial for determining infectious agents in the integumentary system. By culturing samples obtained from wounds, skin lesions, or other suitable sites, clinicians can identify the causative pathogens and thereby guide antibiotic selection and treatment. For instance, diabetic foot ulcer management relies heavily on cultures, a condition now more common among nurses with associated morbidity. New evidence suggests that early, accurate detection of pathogens can significantly reduce the risk of systemic infections, ultimately promoting healing processes and reducing hospitalizations. As highlighted in global discourse regarding diabetic foot syndrome complications, efficient diagnostic examination is crucial for effective management and intervention measures, particularly in exposed populations (N/A, 2021). Additionally, integrating diagnostic tests into nursing practice optimizes the overall patient care structure. Nurses are often the first point of assessment, and therefore, their role in ordering and interpreting such tests becomes pivotal. Familiarity with indications, procedures, and potential outcomes of biopsies and cultures equips nurses with the knowledge necessary to represent their patients effectively. In addition, ongoing education about advancements of diagnostic techniques is required to remain up to date with evolving clinical practice. Although healthcare systems continue to grapple with the rising prevalence of sensory and skin diseases, the utilization of stringent diagnostic methods will be a crucial tool in achieving timely and effective treatment of these diseases (Department of Education et al., 2020).

Test Your Knowledge

1. What key features should be documented when assessing a skin lesion?
2. Why is it essential to assess for changes in skin color and texture?

12.5. Nursing Interventions for Integumentary Disorders

Learning Outcome

1. Describe the wound care and management
2. Define the patient education on skin care
3. Discuss the pharmacological treatments (topical and systemic)

Nursing interventions for integumentary disorders encompass a broad range of interventions aimed at promoting the healing and maintenance of skin integrity. One of the fundamental principles of such interventions is regular skin assessment to identify any potential issues early. Nurses must be able to identify early pressure ulcers, which are regions of affected tissue localized to an area as a result of prolonged pressure on the skin, particularly in patients who are immobile or critically ill. Efficient assessment skills enable nurses to plan care allowbased on clinical experience, facilitating timely intervention and ultimately enhancing patient safety and health outcomes, as outlined in the open educational resource for health assessment in nursing practice (Accettola et al., 2023). Systematic evaluation of skin conditions enables nurses to create individualized care plans that meet specific needs and result in enhanced recovery pathways. In addition, the application of evidence-based practice has an essential part in managing integumentary disorders, especially in preventing pressure ulcers. The most well-known intervention is the use of the

S.K.I.N. care bundle, such as support surfaces, repositioning at regular intervals, managing incontinence, and nutrition consultation. For example, turning a patient every two hours can significantly decrease the incidence of pressure ulcers, as supported by research indicating a substantial reduction in major incidents after implementing these standards (Schindler et al., 2010). Further, nutrition is addressed to ensure adequate input for skin healing and overall well-being. These comprehensive, structured interventions emphasize the importance of team and multidisciplinary approaches in patient care, providing an environment conducive to healing while minimizing complications associated with skin integrity.

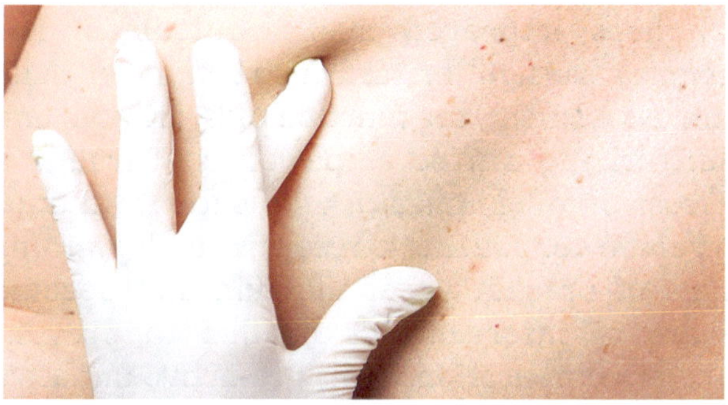

Figure 12.14. Comprehensive skin assessment.

Source: https://www.medline.com/wp-content/uploads/2019/11/STK_SkinAssessment_RGB_840x473.jpg.

A patient education component is also a valuable component of nursing interventions in integumentary disorders. Empowering patients and families regarding skin care, the importance of skin hygiene, and the earliest indications of skin breakdown can increase compliance with preventive interventions. Nurses play a vital role in educating patients on performing skin assessments in their own environment and the importance of making environmental adjustments, such as maintaining a clean, well-hydrated skin surface. Addressing the psychosocial problems, such as the emotional impact of visible skin disease, will also facilitate treatment adherence. By providing an educative and supportive environment, nurses not only foster the physical health of patients but also their emotional and psychological well-being. Such an integrative approach is crucial in the effective management of integumentary diseases and the improvement of quality of life (Figure 12.14).

12.5.1. Wound Care and Management

Effective wound management and care are of utmost importance in nursing, particularly in patients with compromised integumentary and sensory functions. Wound care is not merely a matter of cleaning and dressing the wound; it requires an in-depth approach to understanding the cause or etiology of compromised skin integrity, which can range from ischemic disorders to inflammatory reactions. For example, pressure ulcers, also known as bedsores, occur when soft tissue is subjected to a continuous force of pressure, especially in immobile patients, such as those bedridden in critical care units. Intravascular and inflammatory etiologies can progress further, necessitating that nursing professionals have focused interventions in place. Recognition of at-risk patients early on and the adoption of an active approach to wound care can significantly decrease complications and enhance rates of recovery. Recent data confirm the effectiveness of bundles of interventions designed to prevent pressure ulcer development in high-risk populations. In a trial of infants in a pediatric intensive care unit, an intensive pressure ulcer prevention bundle called S.K.I.N. comprised support surface selection, frequent repositioning, incontinence management, and nutritional guidance. The implementation of this model resulted in a significant decrease in pressure ulcer incidence, reducing the rate from 18.8% to 6.8%. Such evidence-based practices underscore the necessity of continuous assessment and targeted intervention measures tailored to the diverse needs of different patient populations. Thus, being nurses, awareness of these structured approaches facilitates an overall care environment that aims at maintaining skin health and overall patient well-being. It is also necessary to highlight the deterrents that face healthcare professionals in order to adopt pressure ulcer prevention measures. Rival competing demands on nurses' time were the single most significant barrier to effective implementation of the S.K.I.N. bundle in the study as mentioned earlier.

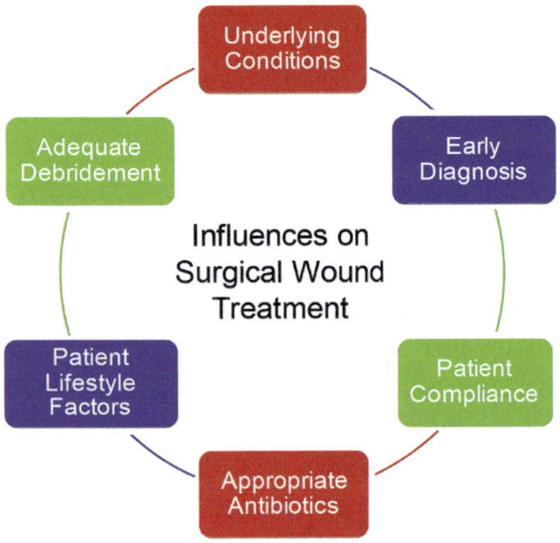

Figure 12.15. Influences on surgical wound treatment in the wound care center.

Source: https://www.researchgate.net/profile/Gregory-Bohn-3/publication/310439210/figure/fig5/AS:593795636805637@1518583320745/nfluences-on-Surgical-Wound-Treatment-in-the-Wound-Care-Center.png.

This highlights an important aspect of wound care management: the need for systemic transformation within healthcare settings to provide nurses with an acceptable level of support. By making equipment and supplies available, health care administrators can allow nurses to have wound care in their control without the stress of the lack of resources. With changing nursing practices, building cooperative environments and promoting health awareness among the public will be crucial to proper wound management, thereby improving patient care delivery in all available clinical settings (Figure 12.15).

12.5.2. Patient Education on Skin Care

The importance of patient skin care education cannot be overemphasized, especially in nursing and the management of injuries. Nurses play a crucial role in educating patients on proper skin care techniques, particularly those at risk of pressure injuries due to their underlying conditions. Education of patients and caregivers produces an educated support system that enhances improved health outcomes. For instance, straightforward instruction on daily skin assessment, the function of hydration, and moisturizing can be empowering. Through a discussion of skin health with patients, nurses can empower patients to recognize early warning signs of breakdown of the skin and become aware of interventions needed to prevent further complications. This pro-active initiative not only supports patient independence but also enhances overall adherence to prescribed treatment regimens and preventive measures. Furthermore, education programs targeting individuals must address the unique needs of diverse patient populations, such as intensive care patients who are particularly vulnerable to hospital-acquired pressure injuries. As can be seen through quality improvement initiatives, integrating evidence-based educational suites into practice has significantly improved nurses' knowledge and practice areas regarding skin care and wound prevention strategies. Applying standardized assessment instruments and documentation practices among health professionals has been crucial to enable consistent skin examinations. For instance, the significant increase in compliance with visual documentation of risky anatomy, from 17% to 65%, is a testament to the success of collaborative educational interventions (Pomerleau et al., 2021). Organized interventions ensure accountability among nurses, leading to enhanced patient safety and improved quality of care during clinical practice. Lastly, the establishment of interdisciplinary collaboration in patient education has the potential to significantly contribute to skin care management in any healthcare setting. Nurses should actively involve other healthcare professionals, such as physical therapists and dietitians, in educating patients about the various aspects of skin integrity. This interdisciplinary approach leverages the available diversity of expertise to provide comprehensive care that addresses all possible risk factors for skin breakdown, including nutritional status and mobility restrictions. As seen from recent research, joint participation by an interdisciplinary team ensures a robust education platform in which skin care is fully integrated into the overall patient health management framework (Laslo et al., 2020). Collaborative joint participation enables the healthcare team to reinforce the necessity of proper skin care processes collectively, and hence the incidence of pressure injuries is reduced, while patient outcomes are enhanced in all types of clinical settings (Figure12.16).

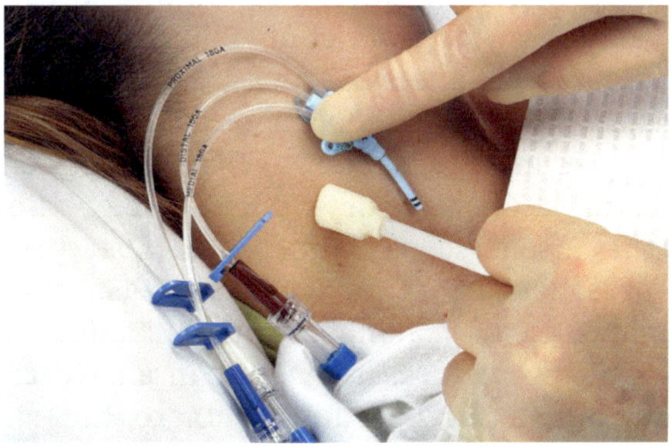

Figure 12.16. Advanced skin care.

Source: https://s7d9.scene7.com/is/image/mmmspinco/1655_app03:XS--mobile?ts=1730385532709&cropN=0,.0,.8,1&dpr=on,2.625.

12.5.3. Pharmacological Treatments (Topical and Systemic)

Treatment of integumentary disorders is most often pharmacological, topical, and systemic, aimed at alleviating symptoms and promoting healing. Topical treatment is often the first line, particularly for those that are localized to the skin. Corticosteroids, anti-inflammatory medications, and antimicrobial ointments are prescribed for conditions such as eczema, psoriasis, and bacterial infections. The advantage of local drug therapy is its localized action at the disease site, which reduces systemic side effects and enhances therapeutic effectiveness. Additionally, preparations such as creams, ointments, and gels possess the added advantage of restoring skin hydration and barrier function, which are essential for integumentary healing and maintenance. Thus, pharmacodynamic knowledge and the appropriate use of these agents become critical for nursing professionals interested in optimizing patient outcomes in skin health care. Conversely, systemic pharmacologic treatment becomes necessary in cases where local use would be insufficient or when the disease process is more extensive. Oral medication, such as systemic corticosteroids, antibiotics, and newer biologic drugs, plays a crucial role in managing episodic or severe cutaneous diseases that cause chronic pain and a decreased quality of life. Such chronic illnesses would best be treated with a multidisciplinary approach that integrates pharmacological treatment with lifestyle modifications and other therapeutic regimens (Goodman et al., 2022). Nurses play a critical role in monitoring patients' responses to systemic therapy, minimizing side effects, and enhancing patient education to promote medication adherence and identify potential interactions. With ongoing pharmacological advancements, it is essential that nurses stay up to date on new therapies that can improve patient outcomes. Besides, the pharmacologic interventions' knowledge are tied with pain management principles, particularly in individuals with chronic wounds and skin injuries. Pain is a critical patient-related issue that, on occasion, remains uncontrolled among this population (Goodman et al., 2022). Pharmacological interventions, such as analgesics and local anesthetics, are necessary to control pain caused by wounds, thereby facilitating improved healing outcomes. Systemic analgesics play a special role in patients who are experiencing significant distress that is producing interference with activities of daily living. Additionally, the ability to establish effective pain relief has a significant impact on the psychological well-being of patients, leading to enhanced compliance with care routines and improved clinical outcomes. Hence, nursing education must incorporate an extensive understanding of both pharmacological options and their application for fostering whole-patient care in the realm of integumentary and sensory health.

Test Your Knowledge

1. What nursing interventions are essential for preventing pressure ulcers in immobile patients?
2. How can nurses manage itching and discomfort in patients with dermatitis?

12.6. Management of Sensory Function Disorders

Learning Outcome

1. Describe the assessment of sensory deficits
2. Define the rehabilitation strategies for sensory loss
3. Identify the role of assistive devices in sensory management

Optimal intervention for sensory function disorders is crucial to enhance patient outcomes, particularly in nursing practice. Nurses are at the forefront of detecting signs and symptoms of sensory dysfunction that result from numerous underlying conditions. Their clinical judgment and observational skills in assessing sensory capacity are most important for successful intervention. An inclusive model that also considers issues of race and ethnicity, gender, and disability can significantly improve patient care. Such a model, besides being consonant with the fundamental principles of culturally competent care, also enables nursing students to learn necessary critical thinking skills needed during the clinical decision-making process. By employing health assessment strategies that focus on sensory function, nurses can respond to and prevent complications in sensory disorders, as well as effectively advocate for patient-specific care, thereby fulfilling the goal of achieving equitable health outcomes among diverse populations (Accettola et al., 2023). Moreover, the specific challenges involved in managing sensory disorders render targeted intervention strategies indispensable. For instance, patients with impaired sensory function, e.g., those in the intensive care unit, are most prone to pressure ulcers as well as to associated complications. Prolonged immobilization and invasive procedures typical of intensive care units add a further dimension to the risk. Implementing structured prevention bundles, such as regularly turning and lifting the patient, can significantly mitigate these risks. Research has established that the implementation of comprehensive prevention measures leads to substantial reductions in pressure ulcer incidence, underscoring the need for nurses to prioritize these evidence-based methods in their practice protocols. Understanding the barriers to implementing these measures—such as other demands on nursing time—also shapes staff training and resource allocation to maximize patient safety and quality of care (Schindler et al., 2010). Overall, management of sensory function disorder is best served by an interdisciplinary practice that combines patient interaction knowledge with evidence-based practices. Continuous training and education of the nurses are a necessary part of establishing an environment where sensory function disorders are being managed competently and confidently. This continuous professional development not only empowers the nurses but also equips them with the necessary tools to adapt to ever-evolving patient needs. The inclusion of critical thinking and clinical judgment in nursing education enhances the preparedness of future nurses. It enables them to effectively address the complexities of sensory function disorders. Lastly, emphasis on management strategies for these disorders is essential as it impacts patient safety, care quality, and health outcomes in diverse populations (Accettola et al., 2023).

12.6.1. Assessment of Sensory Deficits

Effective measurement of sensory loss is crucial for clinical nursing practice, particularly in the context of various conditions that affect sensory function. Nurses must apply a holistic framework in determining patients' sensory function, including vision, hearing, touch, taste, and proprioception. Evaluation typically encompasses extensive patient history, physical assessment, and specific tests focused on measuring sensory perception. For instance, patients with a cerebrovascular accident (CVA) may present with sensory losses complicating rehabilitation. In these cases, employing standardized measures and patient-tailored interventions such as those used in Neurodevelopmental Treatment (NDT) may promote functional recovery and improve patient outcomes while allowing nurses to monitor and address sensory impairments adequately during treatment (Takatsuki et al., 2014). Furthermore, sensory deficit management incorporates the understanding of its impact on the patient's functioning and quality of life. Sensory impairments can cause problems related to communication, mobility, and self-care, resulting in increased reliance on caregivers. Psychosocial factors must therefore be included in nursing assessment because patients who adjust to sensory deficits could feel frustrated, lonely, or depressed. Interdisciplinary treatment can provide a more holistic approach, as coordination with occupational therapists, speech therapists, and mental health professionals can affirm interventions aimed at improving sensory function and overall health. The emphasis on comprehensive assessment highlights the need for flexibility in nursing practice to address the unique challenges posed by sensory deficits in diverse patient populations. A second critical area of sensory deficit assessment relates to preventive interventions, particularly among high-risk populations such as critically ill patients or vulnerable patients at risk of developing pressure ulcers. For example, infants in pediatric intensive care units are at higher risk for sensory deficits as well as prolonged episodes of immobility and invasive therapy exposure. Use of systematic prevention bundles, for example, the S.K.I.N. care bundle, demonstrates the need to use a systemic approach in assessing and managing sensory impairment associated with hospital stay for an extended period (Schindler et al., 2010). By utilizing systematic sensory assessment and incorporating prevention strategies, complications such as pressure ulcers can be reduced, thereby enhancing patient care and overall outcomes. These preventative measures form the broader aim of perpetuating sensory integration as a cornerstone of effective nursing practice (Figure 12.17).

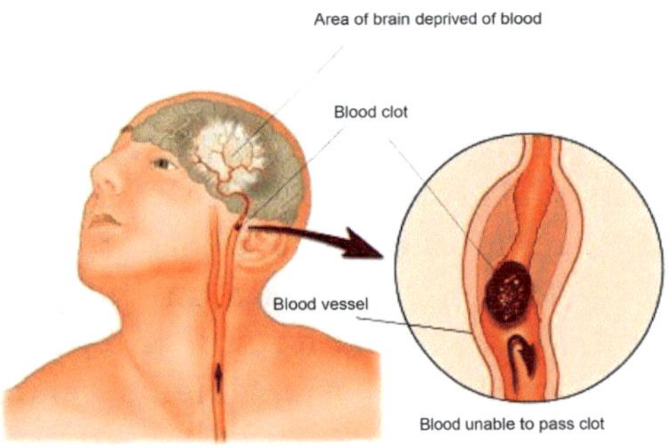

Figure 12.17. Cerebrovascular-accident.

Source: https://www.rnpedia.com/wp-content/uploads/2015/01/Cerebrovascular-Accident.jpeg.

12.6.2. Rehabilitation Strategies for Sensory Loss

Rehabilitation therapy for sensory loss is of paramount importance in enhancing the quality of life for patients with this complication. These therapies employ a comprehensive approach to compensate for the multidimensional aspects of sensory impairment. One of the initial steps in rehabilitation is typically a thorough study to determine the level of sensory loss and its impact on daily activities. Techniques such as sensory re-education, designed to retrain the brain's response to sensory messages, can contribute to this function. Assistive technology could be introduced to enable adaptation to sensory loss and enhance communication and interaction with the environment. By focusing on individualized interventions that address the specific needs of each patient, rehabilitation can significantly improve an individual's overall functional ability, as well as their mental state, and, in doing so, foster a sense of independence and self-esteem among those affected (Ntusi et al., 2019). Multidisciplinary teams cannot be overemphasized in sensory loss rehabilitation. Interdisciplinary collaboration among occupational, physical, and speech therapists is essential for providing comprehensive care that is tailored to the diverse needs of patients. Occupational therapy, for example, can provide training in daily living skills, while speech therapy can assist in overcoming communication difficulties brought about by sensory loss. The teams can also offer an early stimulated environment that enhances patient empowerment and participation throughout the rehabilitation process. Effective communication among the team members ensures that all aspects of a patient's loss of sensation are addressed step by step, leading to better results. It is essential to have a pledge to ongoing evaluation and revision of rehabilitation plans, as this is where adaptive interventions are incorporated that respond to the patient's dynamic needs and improvements over time (Jefferson et al., 2016). Developments in technology have revolutionized rehabilitation practices for sensory loss, introducing new innovations to complement traditional approaches. For instance, virtual reality (VR) is increasingly used to create immersive surroundings to stimulate sensory functions in a controlled setting. Technology allows people to undergo simulated activities that enable sensory integration and re-education in an effective manner. Wearable devices that provide feedback through the senses can also help people develop a greater awareness of their environment. As such, the increasing availability of technology has enormous potential for integrating it into rehabilitation interventions, thereby personalizing care for various populations. It is imperative that healthcare professionals are adequately trained in such technology to achieve their full potential. Through advances in technology, the rehabilitation of sensory loss can become more effective, positively affecting one's recovery process and quality of life (Ntusi et al., 2019).

12.6.3. Role of Assistive Devices in Sensory Management

The integration of assistive equipment is a crucial area of sensory management, exceptionally if executed by nursing practices that address integumentary and sensory disorders and injuries. The equipment ranges from simple aids, such as magnifying glasses for the visually impaired, to highly advanced technology, including electronic mobility aids for individuals with profound motor impairments. Through enhancing the perception of the senses and facilitating interaction with the environment, such devices empower patients and facilitate increased autonomy. Assistive devices can also potentially serve as a key part of rehabilitation, such as in the case of using neurodevelopmental treatment (NDT) methods for patients who involve CVAs, where sensory input and functional movement interaction are a focus (Ntusi et al., 2019). Thus, the incorporation of assistive aids into care activities not only assists with sensory management but also plays a key role within the rehabilitation process, promoting overall well-being. For nursing practice, the selection and utilization of assistive devices should be comprehensive and tailored to individual patient requirements. Assessing the sensory impairments and functional needs of patients who have undergone conditions such as CVAs is essential in deciding the appropriate assistive devices to be utilized. For instance, as explained through rehabilitation case reports, assistive technology can significantly restore mobility and balance, resulting in tangible improvements in a patient's independence and quality of life. The tremendous advancements in assistive technology provide healthcare professionals with diverse devices and options to enhance patient outcomes; however, this requires ongoing evaluation of efficacy in different patient populations to ensure that the selected devices are suitable for therapy (Ntusi et al., 2019). This is why extensive training for nursing staff on such devices is inevitable. Additionally, beyond sensory augmentation, assistive devices have the ability to influence participation and engagement in daily life.

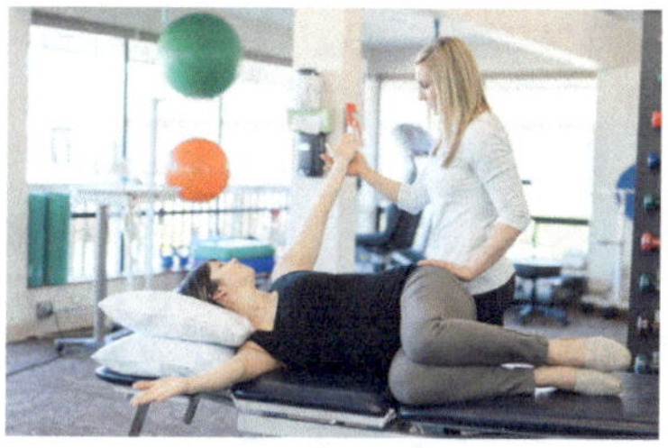

Figure 12.18. Neurodevelopmental treatment (NDT).

Source: https://storage.googleapis.com/physiotherapy-clinic/img/neurodevelopmental-t.jpg.

Particularly in terms of sensory management, assistive devices may augment communication for individuals with hearing loss or cognitive impairments, allowing them to better socially interact and maintain a perception of normalcy. Achievement of functional mobility and sensory awareness through the use of assistive devices enhances the rehabilitative framework in general, where patient-centered interventions emphasize differentiated care policies. The activity can be a very significant factor in patients' mental health, as they are directly engaged in rehabilitation and interact with their environment in greater confidence (Takatsuki et al., 2014). Therefore, understanding the various benefits of assistive devices used in managing the senses provides nursing professionals with information to facilitate whole-person patient care in continuity of healthcare (Figure 12.18).

Test Your Knowledge

1. How can nurses support patients with impaired tactile sensation to prevent injury?
2. What interventions are helpful for patients experiencing chronic itching or neuropathic pain?

SUMMARY

An analysis of the integumentary and sensory functions in nursing reveals that extensive knowledge of these systems is a prerequisite for effective patient care. The integumentary system is not only a protective covering but also plays a role in thermoregulation, sensation, and immunity. Nurses must assess and treat disorders of these functions—such as skin infections, wounds, and dermatological disorders—while considering the complexity involved in their treatment. Psychological and physical health also have a dynamic interrelationship, as skin conditions can carry psychological weight, affecting a patient's overall well-being, and highlighting the importance of holistic treatment in nursing practice. Moreover, developments in dermatological management and treatment provide nurses with the competency to offer evidence-based practice that enhances patient outcomes. The integration of relational caring complexity, based on theories like Ray's and Turkel's, enhances nurses' ability to consider patients' unique backgrounds and experiences when addressing their needs. As nursing develops, an emphasis on evidence-based practice and inter-professional collaboration is increasingly crucial in the effective management of integumentary disorder. Inter-professional collaboration ensures consideration of a patient's overall health, resulting in holistic recovery and facilitating an active role for nursing as a health facilitator and healing agent. Last but not least, the intersection of sensory function and integumentary health reveals an additional layer of complexity in treatment and management protocol. Sensory loss, alongside dermatological conditions, presents complex issues that require specialized interventions on the part of nursing personnel. Understanding the association between sensory input and skin integrity enables nurses to implement measures that improve patients quality of life, especially in vulnerable populations. Ongoing research and education will increasingly enhance nurses' skills in managing these interactions. Therefore, the careful incorporation of information about integumentary and sensory functions is essential in the education of nurses for responding to the evolving demands of the modern healthcare scene, as well as for obtaining optimal outcomes for their patients (Miller et al., 2016; Alcocer-Leon et al., 2020).

Care of integumentary disorders is an integral part of nursing practice, especially in wards like pediatric intensive care units (PICUs) where skin injury is more probable. One of the significant issues is the development of pressure ulcers, which can occur due to prolonged pressure on soft tissue, particularly in critically ill neonates. Studies have shown that the incidence of pressure ulcers among this high-risk population is relatively high, ranging from 10.2% to 27%. When evidence-based prevention strategies are employed, including the S.K.I.N. bundle that addresses support surfaces, frequent repositioning, appropriate incontinence care, and nutritional supplementation, there is a considerable decrease in the incidence of ulcers, from 18.8% to 6.8%. This underscores the necessity of meticulous risk assessment and preventive measures in preventing such complications in vulnerable patients (Schindler et al., 2010). Competence and proficiency in managing integumentary conditions are not only a matter of understanding the underlying pathophysiology but also of acquiring the proper communication skills necessary for patient care. Perhaps the most significant area in nursing education is the acquisition of professional language skills, which are essential for effective communication with international health communities and access to professional literature. This prerequisite becomes more critical now due to the globalized nature of healthcare and the increasing need for nurses to critically analyze and interpret multiple sources of information in order to make informed decisions. The curriculum should therefore consist of significant practice in professional vocabulary, critical thinking, and academic writing. Emphasizing these strengths will better prepare nursing students to address the evolving healthcare practice environment, thus fortifying their skill set for future challenges in this critical profession (Літвінчук et al., 2022). Furthermore, effective management of patients with integumentary disorder conditions involves an interdisciplinary approach that includes physical and psychosocial dimensions of care. Reassessing patients who are at risk for skin breakdown regularly, as well as being aware of their psychosocial needs, is essential to improving overall health. Pain, anxiety, and loneliness can genuinely make a difference in a patient's stay and recovery. Nurses must be alert in assessing not only the physical state of the skin but also the psychological support that a patient will require, particularly in an environment like the PICU, where distress is more likely to occur. Thus, establishing a therapeutic environment that emphasizes empathy, education, and reliable support can enhance patient outcomes and satisfaction. This integrated approach not only reduces the risk of physical complications but also addresses the emotional and psychological aspects of care, demonstrating the holistic approach of nursing in managing integumentary and sensory function (Schindler et al., 2010).

KEY TERMS FROM THIS CHAPTER

- Braden scale
- Burns
- Cataracts
- Cellulitis
- Debridement
- Decubitus ulcer
- Dermatitis
- Eczema
- Glaucoma
- Hearing loss
- Pressure ulcers
- Protective sensation
- Psoriasis
- Sensory perception
- Skin grafting
- Skin integrity
- Tinnitus
- Vision impairment

CRITICAL THINKING QUESTIONS

1. **Which of the following is a common nursing concern for patients with pressure ulcers?**
   a. Fluid overload
   b. Impaired skin integrity
   c. Hyperglycemia
   d. Visual disturbances
2. **A patient with a severe burn injury is at most significant risk for which of the following complications in the first 24 hours?**
   a. Infection
   b. Hypertension
   c. Fluid volume deficit
   d. Constipation
3. **Which skin disorder is characterized by redness, scaling, and itching, often linked to allergies or irritants?**
   a. Psoriasis
   b. Eczema (atopic dermatitis)
   c. Cellulitis
   d. Acne vulgaris
4. **What is a priority nursing action when caring for a patient with decreased visual acuity?**
   a. Keep the room dark and quiet
   b. Place frequently used items within reach and maintain a safe environment
   c. Speak louder to ensure understanding
   d. Administer oxygen therapy
5. **What is the most appropriate intervention for preventing skin breakdown in an immobile patient?**
   a. Encourage fluid restriction
   b. Provide a high-fat diet
   c. Reposition the patient every 2 hours
   d. Administer sedatives to prevent movement

Short Answer Questions

1. What is the primary function of the integumentary system?
2. Name two common causes of pressure ulcers.
3. What are typical signs of a localized skin infection?
4. What does the Braden scale assess?
5. Describe the nursing assessment and management of a patient with second-degree burns.
6. Explain how nurses can support patients with visual impairments to maintain safety and independence.
7. Discuss the pathophysiology, clinical features, and treatment of eczema (atopic dermatitis).
8. Outline a comprehensive nursing care plan for a patient at high risk of developing pressure ulcers.
9. Describe the assessment and care of a patient presenting with acute hearing loss or sensory impairment.

Answers to Critical Thinking Questions

1. (b) 2. (c) 3. (b) 4. (b) 5. (c).

REFERENCES

1. Accettola, E., Bogdan, A., Callahan, S., Chawda, R., et al. (2023). Introduction to health assessment for the nursing professional: Part II. https://core.ac.uk/download/622362029.pdf (accessed on 30th June 2025).
2. Akinsanya, J., Biggs, J., BiNE, General Medical Council, McHanwell, S., Meskell, M., Moxham, J. B., et al. (2018). The Anatomical Society's core anatomy syllabus for undergraduate nursing. https://core.ac.uk/download/520510991.pdf (accessed on 30th June 2025).
3. Jiménez-Zarazúa, O., Vélez-Ramírez, L. N., Alcocer-León, M., Hernández-Domínguez, D. A., Tadeo-González, J. E., Martínez-Rivera, M. A., López-González, M. D. A., Tafoya-Rojas, S. X. L., & Mondragón, J. D. (2020). Paraneoplastic Cerebellar Degeneration Secondary to BRAF Mutant Melanoma Metastasis from an Occult Primary Cancer. *Case Reports in Oncology*, *13*(2), 633–642. https://doi.org/10.1159/000507729Arantón Areosa, L., López De los Reyes, R., Rumbo Prieto, J. M., Vives Rodríguez, J., et al. (2017). Practical guide for moisture associated skin damages. https://core.ac.uk/download/288090144.pdf (accessed on 30th June 2025).
4. August, D. L. (2022). Neonatal skin injuries from mechanical forces: A multicenter, mixed methods study. https://core.ac.uk/download/542341107.pdf (accessed on 30th June 2025).
5. Banta-Wright, S., & Campbell, J. (2000). Neonatal skin disorders: A review of selected dermatologic abnormalities. http://digitalcommons.georgefox.edu/cgi/viewcontent.cgi?article=1004&context=sn_fac (accessed on 30th June 2025).
6. Barroso, A. F. N. (2019). Technological advances in cutaneous wound repair. https://core.ac.uk/download/322655383.pdf (accessed on 30th June 2025).
7. Chukwu, R., & Mankila, J. (2018). Dermatology nurses' job description: Literature review. https://core.ac.uk/download/161432240.pdf (accessed on 30th June 2025).
8. Department of Medical Education. (2020). 2020 Academic Achievement Day. https://core.ac.uk/download/322527423.pdf (accessed on 30th June 2025).
9. Dunphy, J. L., Ireland, M. F., Logan, P., McClean, R., et al. (2013). Six years of teaching human bioscience, pathophysiology and pharmacology: A journey of reflective practice. https://core.ac.uk/download/229408185.pdf (accessed on 30th June 2025).
10. Goodman, L., Jaimangal, R., & Sibbald, G. (2022). Skin and wound care for health care professionals. https://core.ac.uk/download/622361052.pdf (accessed on 30th June 2025).
11. Holm, S. (2015). The use of physical therapy evaluation and treatment to manage a patient following a total knee arthroplasty: A case study. https://core.ac.uk/download/235074390.pdf (accessed on 30th June 2025).
12. Jefferson, N. (2016). A case report: Paraplegia secondary to a failed lumbar fusion. https://core.ac.uk/download/235074354.pdf (accessed on 30th June 2025).
13. Laslo, M. A. (2020). Pressure injury documentation and reporting: A quality gap. https://core.ac.uk/download/346021284.pdf (accessed on 30th June 2025).
14. Miller, T. A. (2016). Essential nursing care for the sole. https://core.ac.uk/download/217655827.pdf (accessed on 30th June 2025).
15. Ntusi, N. A. B. (2019). Guest editorial: Health and rehabilitation sciences in a clinical context. https://core.ac.uk/download/478315380.pdf (accessed on 30th June 2025).

16. Pomerleau, T. A. (2021). Strategies to prevent hospital acquired pressure injuries in the intensive care unit. https://core.ac.uk/download/490617094.pdf (accessed on 30th June 2025).
17. Sargsyan, A. (2020). Essential notes on pathophysiology for advanced practice nurses. https://core.ac.uk/download/323021466.pdf (accessed on 30th June 2025).
18. Schindler, C. A. (2010). More than S.K.I.N. deep: Decreasing pressure ulcer development in the pediatric intensive care unit. https://core.ac.uk/download/67759746.pdf (accessed on 30th June 2025).
19. Takatsuki, J. (2014). PT management of a patient with a CVA focusing on functional training with neurodevelopmental treatment-based interventions in the inpatient acute rehabilitation setting: A case report. https://core.ac.uk/download/146517561.pdf (accessed on 30th June 2025).
20. Vecchiato, S. (2014). Un lexique satellite: Les diagnostics informers. https://core.ac.uk/download/576777577.pdf (accessed on 30th June 2025).

INDEX

C

D

I

J

R

S